NUTRITIONAL INFLUENCES ON ILLNESS

Also by Melvyn R. Werbach

THIRD LINE MEDICINE: MODERN TREATMENT FOR PERSISTENT SYMPTOMS

The Keats Health Reference Library

BRAIN ALLERGIES	• William H. Philpott, M.D. and Dwight K. Kalita, Ph.D.
COMMON QUESTIONS ON SCHIZOPHRENIA AND THEIR ANSWERS	• Abram Hoffer, M.D., Ph.D.
DIET AND DISEASE	• E. Cheraskin, M.D., D.M.D., W. M. Ringsdorf, Jr., D.M.D., J. W. Clark, D.D.S.
GUIDE TO MEDICINAL PLANTS	• Paul Schauenberg and Ferdinand Paris
THE HEALING NUTRIENTS WITHIN	• Eric R. Braverman, M.D. with Carl C. Pfeiffer, M.D., Ph.D.
MEDICAL APPLICATIONS OF CLINICAL NUTRITION	• Edited by Jeffrey Bland, Ph.D.
THE NUTRITION DESK REFERENCE (Second Edition, Revised)	• Robert H. Garrison, Jr., M.A., R.Ph. and Elizabeth Somer, M.A., R.D.
NUTRITION IN NURSING	• Betty Kamen, Ph.D. and E. Lynn Fraley, R.N., Dr. P.H.
NUTRITION AND PHYSICAL DEGENERATION	• Weston A. Price, D.D.S.
NUTRITIONAL INFLUENCES ON ILLNESS	• Melvyn A. Werbach, M.D.
ORTHOMOLECULAR MEDICINE FOR PHYSICIANS	• Abram Hoffer, M.D., Ph.D.
A PHYSICIAN'S HANDBOOK ON ORTHOMOLECULAR MEDICINE	• Edited by Roger J. Williams, Ph.D. and Dwight K. Kalita, Ph.D.
THE SACCHARINE DISEASE	• T. L. Cleave, M.D.
VICTORY OVER DIABETES	• William H. Philpott, M.D. and Dwight K. Kalita, Ph.D.
WELLNESS MEDICINE	• Robert A. Anderson, M.D.
YOUR FAMILY TREE CONNECTION	• Chris M. Reading, M.D. and Ross S. Meillon

NUTRITIONAL INFLUENCES ON ILLNESS

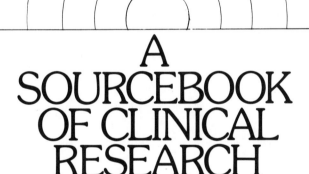

A SOURCEBOOK OF CLINICAL RESEARCH

MELVYN R. WERBACH, M.D.

Keats Publishing, Inc., New Canaan, Connecticut

To my wife, Gail,
and my sons, Kevin and Adam,
for their love and support
which made this book possible.

Although the author has exhaustively researched all sources to ensure the accuracy and completeness of the information contained in this book, we assume no responsibility for errors, inaccuracies, omissions or any inconsistency herein.

The treatment of illness must be supervised by a physician or other licensed health professional. The information presented in this book is intended for education only and does not contain treatment recommendations for the public.

NUTRITIONAL INFLUENCES ON ILLNESS

Copyright © 1987, 1988 by Melvyn R. Werbach, M.D.
All Rights Reserved. No part of this book may be reproduced in any form without the written consent of the publisher.

Published by arrangement with Third Line Press, Inc. Paperback edition published September 1990.

Werbach, Melvyn R.
    Nutritional influences on illness.

    Reprint. Originally published: Tarzana, Calif.:
Third Line Press, c1987.
    Includes index.
    1. Diet therapy—Handbooks, manuals, etc.
2.Nutrition—Handbooks, manuals, etc. 3. Nutritionally induced diseases—Handbooks, manuals,
etc. I. Title. [DNLM: 1. Diet Therapy—abstracts.
2. Disease—etiology—abstracts. 3. Nutrition—
abstracts. ZWB 400 W484n 1987a]
RM217.2.W47 1989   615.8′54   89-2378
ISBN 0-87983-500-1

Printed in the United States of America

Keats Publishing, Inc.
27 Pine Street (P. O. Box 876)
New Canaan, Connecticut 06840

NUTRITIONAL INFLUENCES ON ILLNESS:
A SOURCEBOOK OF CLINICAL RESEARCH

Table of Contents

PART II: APPENDICES

INTRODUCTION

As nutritional science has developed, so have the clinical applications. Clinical nutrition was initially limited to treating general malnutrition and specific nutritional deficiency states. In the past two decades, the field has gradually broadened to include the treatment of subclinical deficiencies and dependencies, as well as the provision of nutrients in massive doses as pharmacologic agents. Unfortunately, early work in this area drew strong criticism due to the premature advocacy of certain treatments despite the lack of adequate scientific validation.

Scientific justification for an expanded definition of clinical nutrition has been considerably strengthened since then. Laboratory tests can provide evidence of inadequate nutriture despite the lack of clincial findings of classical nutritional deficiency syndromes. Even in the absence of laboratory validation of nutritional deficiencies, numerous studies utilizing rigorous scientific designs have demonstrated impressive benefits from nutritional supplementation. It is now well established, for example, that nutritional factors are of major importance in the pathogenesis of both atherosclerosis and cancer, the two leading causes of death in Western countries, and studies validating their importance in the pathogenesis of many other diseases continue to be published.

It is hoped that the material presented in this book will enable all health care professionals to better utilize nutritional science in their practices by summarizing the available data. The bulk of the text consists of a series of chapters covering the major illnesses for which a reasonable amount of nutritional literature exists. Basic dietary factors are discussed first, then vitamins, minerals, other nutrients, "medicinal" foodstuffs, and finally other related factors, with special attention to the influence of food sensitivities on illness.

Each chapter presents a series of statements concerning relevant nutrients, with each statement being followed by selected abstracts from the literature which either substantiate or refute it. (These statements are *not* therapeutic recommendations!) Whenever possible, randomized, double-blind controlled studies are presented; because such studies are often lacking, however, observational (epidemiologic) studies, uncontrolled studies, and animal experiments are included which suggest the relevance of particular nutrients without providing strong scientific validation for treatment with those nutrients. *Each clinician must decide how strong the scientific evidence must be before utilizing a particular nutrient.* In order to assist you in reaching a decision, abstracts from published review articles have been included to provide the advice of acknowledged experts.

Abstracts are presented in the order of their year of publication, with the latest papers listed first. As it is not possible to include all studies, preference has been given to the best, the most relevant, and the most recent.

Several appendices are included. Their suggested use is as follows:

Common Nutritional Deficiencies: Provides an "index of suspicion" since, the more common a deficiency, the more likely it is that it contributes to the patient's symptomatology.

Dangers of Nutritional Supplementation: Should be consulted routinely before initiating nutritional supplementation for information concerning possible adverse effects, especially when the dosages suggested are in the pharmacologic range.

Guidelines to Nutritional Supplementation: Provides suggested guidelines both for adult daily dietary levels of major nutrients and for nutritional therapy to treat specific illnesses.

Laboratory Methods for Nuritional Evaluation: A guide to choosing the best available laboratory method for appraising nutriture for each major nutrient. Methods are listed in rough order of preference.

Nutrient Bioavailability and Interactions: Should be consulted routinely when evaluating specific nutrients in order to identify factors which may be affecting their current levels or which could be utilized to modify such levels.

Syndromes Due to Abnormal Tissue Nutrient Levels: Provides a brief summary of the various signs and symptoms of nutrient deficiencies and toxicities as well as heavy metal toxicities. Should be consulted to discover whether the patient's presentation is consistent with that of a suspected deficiency or toxicity.

A useful sequence for reaching a decision regarding the role of nutrients both as causative factors and as potential therapeutic agents is as follows:

1. Include the patient's dietary history and current eating patterns when taking a medical history.
2. Examine the patient for signs of nutritional deficiencies as part of the medical examination.
3. Review the specific chapters relating to the patient's complaints and/or diagnosis.
4. Review the relevant appendices.
5. If indicated, perform selective evaluative laboratory testing.

All patients deserve appropriate trials of well-validated nutritional interventions. How early in the course of treatment these trials should be undertaken depends upon how they compare to the other therapeutic options in regard to:

1. the evidence that nutritional factors play a causative or a curative role in the illness;
2. their demonstrated safety and efficacy;
3. their cost; and
4. patient preference.

In addition, patients who have failed to respond to well-validated treatments should be considered for appropriate trials of poorly-validated but reasonably safe nutritional interventions.

NOTE: The treatment of such patients is discussed in: Werbach, MR. *Third Line Medicine: Modern Treatment for Persistent Symptoms*. London & New York. Arkana Paperbacks, 1986.

While clinical nutrition provides a complex, highly-sophisticated approach to understanding and treating illness, it is also a young and still primitive field with an often disappointingly inadequate scientific literature. It is hoped that the reader will come away from this book with a deeper appreciation of the state of this rapidly evolving field as it exists today—and will be better able, not only to utilize nutrition in practice, but to answer the many questions concerning nutrition being asked of health professionals by an increasingly sophisticated public.

PART ONE

ILLNESSES AND THE EFFECTS OF NUTRIENTS, TOXICS AND ENVIRONMENTAL SENSITIVITIES

ACNE ROSACEA

NUTRIENTS:

<u>Vitamin B complex</u>:

Supplementation may be beneficial (*Tulipan L. Acne rosacea: A vitamin B complex deficiency. <u>Arch. Derm. Syph.</u> 56:589, 1947; Gross P. Non-pellagrous eruptions due to deficiency of the vitamin B-complex. <u>Arch Dermatol. & Syph.</u> 43:504, 1941*).

- <u>Pyridoxine</u>:

Ref: *Stillians AW. Pyridoxine in treatment of acne vulgaris and rosacea. <u>J. Invest. Dermatol.</u> 7:150, 1946*

- <u>Riboflavin</u>:

Experimental Study: 32/36 pts. with rosacea keratitis had prompt healing following small doses (1-4.5 mg daily orally or by injection) of riboflavin. 9 of these pts. also had cutaneous rosacea and 5 of them improved. It was found that these pts. either had inadequate dietary riboflavin or were hypochlorhydric (*Johnson L, Eckardt R. Rosacea keratitis and conditions with vascularization of the cornea treated with riboflavin. <u>Arch. Ophthalmol.</u> 23:899, 1940*).

OTHER FACTORS:

Rule out <u>hydrochloric acid deficiency</u>.

Note: While gastric anacidity had been reported in the past to be a relatively common condition which was associated with acne rosacea and a number of other illnesses, the presence of achlorhydria is no longer accepted unless a potent parietal-cell stimulant (such as histamine) is employed in gastric analysis. More recent studies suggest that histamine-fast anacidity is uncommon before the fifth decade of life and, although it probably does not occur in a normal stomach, its presence is not necessarily associated with symptoms (Rappaport EM. Achlorhydria: Associated symptoms and response to hydrochloric acid. <u>New Engl. J. Med.</u> 252(19):802-5, 1955).

Experimental Study: 32 pts. with rosacea keratitis (some of whom also had cutaneous rosacea) who responded to riboflavin supplementation were found to either be hypochlorhydric or to have inadequate dietary riboflavin (*Johnson L, Eckardt R. Rosacea keratitis and conditions with vascularization of the cornea treated with riboflavin. <u>Arch. Ophthalmol.</u> 23:899, 1940*).

See Also:

Edwards RL. The significance of achlorhydria and hypochlorhydria in dermatosis. <u>Balyeat Hay Fever and Asthma Clinic Proc.</u> 19(1):28-30, 1949

A plug for acid therapy. <u>Am. J. Digest. Dis.</u> 16(11):418, 1949

Brown WH et al. Fractional gastric analysis in diseases of the skin: Further observation in 316 cases, with special reference to rosacea. Brit. J. Dermatol. Syph. 47:181, 1935

Ryle JA, Barber HW. Gastric analysis in acne rosacea. Lancet 2:1195-6, 1920

Supplementation (along with vitamin B complex) may be beneficial.

Experimental and Observational Study: Of 30 pts. with subacute or chronic conditions which had resisted all forms of local treatment, 12 (40%) had no HCl and only 4 (13%) had normal HCl levels. The severity of the condition seemed to correlate with the extent of the the HCl deficiency and also seemed to be associated with signs of vitamin B complex deficiency. Improvement of the HCl deficient pts. followed treatment with supplemental HCl and vitamin B complex (*Allison JR. The relation of hydrochloric acid and vitamin B complex deficiency in certain skin diseases. Southern Med. J. 38:235-241, 1945*).

Pancreatic enzymes:

Serum lipase concentrations may be deficient.

Observational Study: Pancreatic function was studied in 21 pts. and 21 controls by means of the cerulein infusion test. Compared to controls, pts. had significantly lower lipase concentration and output (with the decrease ranging from 18.5-66% of normal) despite normal flow rate and normal bicarbonate and chymotrypsin concentration and output, suggesting that deficient lipase secretion could be responsible, at least partly, for the clinical manifestations of rosacea (*Barba A et al. Pancreatic exocrine function in rosacea. Dermatologica 165:601-6, 1982*).

Supplementation may be beneficial.

Clinical Observation: When pts. complain of digestive symptoms, the administration of pancreatic extracts may ameliorate both the dyspepsia and the skin lesions (*Barba A - ibid*).

ACNE VULGARIS

BASIC DIET:

General:

The Western diet is associated with an increased incidence of acne (*Rosenberg EW, Kirk BS. Acne diet reconsidered. Arch. Dermatol. 117:193-95, 1981*).

Observational Study: Far less acne was found among the black population in Zambia eating traditional diets than among young blacks in the U.S. (*Rosenberg EW, Kirk BS. Acne diet reconsidered. Arch. Dermatol. 117:193-95, 1981; Ratnam AV, Jayaraju K. Skin diseases in Zambia. Brit. J. Dermatol. 101:449-53, 1979*).

Observational Study: After World War II, Eskimos who changed to Western diets developed a number of new diseases including acne (*Bendiner E. Disastrous trade-off: Eskimo health for white civilization. Hosp. Pract. 9:156-89, 1974*).

Observational Study: Far less acne was found among the black population in Kenya eating traditional diets than among young blacks in the U.S. (*Rosenberg EW, Kirk BS. Acne diet reconsidered. Arch. Dermatol. 117:193-95, 1981; Verhagen ARHB. Skin diseases, in Vogel LC et al, Eds. Health and Diseases in Kenya. Nairobi, Kenya, East African Literature Bureau, 1974, pp. 499-507*).

Low _fat_ diet.

Dietary fat may be associated with excess sebum production (*Frank SB. Acne Vulgaris. Springfield, Illinois, Charles C. Thomas Publisher, 1971, pp. 66-72*).

High _fiber_ diet.

Experimental Study: Pts. showed rapid clearing following supplementation with 1 oz daily of an all-bran cereal, perhaps due to correction of the effects of constipation (*Kaufman WF. The diet and acne. Letter to the Editor. Arch. Dermatology 119(4):276, 1983*).

- -

NUTRIENTS:

Folic Acid:

Supplementation may be beneficial.

Experimental Study: 8 pts. with acne vulgaris were given oral synthetic folic acid 5-10 mg daily. 6 were "much improved" and 1 was "improved" (*Callaghan TJ. The effect of folic acid on seborrheic dermatitis. Cutis 3:583-88, 1967*).

Pyridoxine:

Supplementation may be beneficial, especially for <u>premenstrual acne flares.</u>

Experimental Study: 106 young women pts. received vitamin B$_6$ 50 mg daily for 1 wk. prior to and during menses. 72% improved (*Snider BL, Dieteman DF. Pyridoxine therapy for premenstrual acne flare. Letter to the Editor. Arch. Dermatol. 110:130-31, 1974*).

See Also:

Stillians AW. Pyridoxine in treatment of acne vulgaris and rosacea. J. Invest. Dermatol. 7:150, 1946

Joliffe N et al. Effects of pyridoxine (vit. B$_6$) on persistent adolescent acne. J. Invest. Dermatol. 5:143, 1942

Vitamin A:

WARNING: Because of the potential toxicity of high doses, close medical supervision is necessary

Supplementation may be beneficial.

Experimental Study: 123 cases were treated. Doses below 300,000 I.U. daily were ineffective. After 5 months of treatment there were no serious cases of toxicity. Only 1 pt. had a transient elevation of liver function tests and 1 or 2 patients had transient headaches (*Kligman AM et al. Oral vitamin A in acne vulgaris. Int. J. Dermatol. 20:278, 1981*).

- with Vitamin E:

Vitamin E affects the biologic utilization of vitamin A, and vitamin A absorption is markedly impaired in vitamin E-deficient animals (*Ames SR. Factors affecting absorption, transport and storage of vitamin A. Am. J. Clin. Nutr. 22:934, 1969*).

Supplementation may be beneficial.

Experimental Study: Over 100 pts. had conditions which were successfully controlled with ave. daily doses of 100,000 IU of vitamin A and 800 IU of vitamin E. Most responded within weeks and maintenance of control was obtained with lower doses (*Ayres S Jr., Mihan R. Acne vulgaris and lipid peroxidation: New concepts in pathogenesis and treatment. Int. J. Dermatol. 17:305, 1978*).

- -

Selenium:

- with Vitamin E:

RBC glutathione peroxidase levels may be deficient. If so, levels may normalize with supplementation.

Observational Study: 47 male acne pts. had significantly decreased erythrocyte glutathione peroxidase levels compared to controls, while the levels of 47 female pts. not on oral contraceptives did not differ from those of controls (*Michaelsson G, Edqvist L. Erythrocyte glutathione peroxidase activity in acne vulgaris and the effect of selenium and vitamin E treatment. Acta. Derm. Venereol. (Stockh.) 64(1):9-14, 1984*).

Pts. with low RBC glutathione peroxidase levels and pustular acne respond best to supplementation.

Experimental Study: 29 pts. with severe acne received selenium (Na$_2$ SeO$_3$) 200 mcg and vitamin E (tocopheryl succinate) 10 mg twice daily for 6-12 wks. with "good" results, especially in those with pustular acne and low glutathione peroxidase activity, and improvement was usually paralleled by a slow rise in glutathione peroxidase activity (*Michaelsson - ibid*).

<u>Zinc</u>: 90 - 135 mg. daily with meals (results in 1 - 3 months)

May be deficient.

Observational Study: Compared to controls, both male and female pts. had 28.3% less zinc in their serum, 24.1% less zinc in hair and 26.7% less zinc in nails. RBC zinc levels and alkaline phosphatase activity were not depressed (*Pohit J et al. Zinc status of acne vulgaris patients. J. Applied Nutr. 37(1):18-25, 1985*).

Observational Study: Boys with severe acne had lower serum zinc levels than controls, while both boys and girls with severe acne had lower levels of retinol-binding protein than controls (*Michaelsson G. Diet and acne. Nutrition Reviews 39(2):104-6, 1981*).

See Also:

Amer M et al. Serum zinc in acne vulgaris. *Int. J. Dermatol.* 21:481, 1982

Supplementation may be beneficial.

Review Article: "The use of oral zinc ... has gotten mixed reviews" (*Dobson RL, Nelson. What's new: A review of advances in therapy. J. Am. Acad. Dermatol. 5:323-27, 1981*).

Experimental Placebo-controlled Study: 50 mg. elemental zinc 3 times daily resulted in significant improvement after 6 - 12 weeks with 75% of pts. "content with results" (*Michaelsson G et al. Serum zinc and retinol-binding protein in acne. Brit. J. Dermatol. 96:283, 1977*).

Experimental Double-blind Study: Effervescent zinc sulphate (135 mg. daily) was as effective as tetracycline (750 mg. daily)(70% improvement over 12 wks.) with fewer side effects from chronic use (*Michaelsson G et al. A double blind study of the effect of zinc and oxytetracycline in acne vulgaris. Brit. J. Dermatology 97:561, 1977*).

Experimental Placebo-controlled Study: 48 pts. received 90 mg. zinc daily while others received placebo. After 12 wks. 75% of the zinc-treated pts. were "content with the therapeutic results" (*Hillstrom L. Brit. J. Dermatol. December 1977*).

Experimental Placebo-controlled Study: Zinc sulphate 135 mg. daily was more effective (85% improvement after 12 wks.) than 300,000 I.U. of vitamin A or placebo (*Michaelsson G et al. Effects of oral zinc and vitamin A in acne. Archives Dermatol. 113:31-36, 1977*).

See Also:

Verma KC et al. Oral zinc sulfate therapy in acne vulgaris: a double blind trial. *Acta Dermatovener* 60:337, 1980

Weimar V et al. Zinc sulphate in acne vulgaris. *Arch. Dermatol.* 114:1776-8, 1978

- -

<u>Omega-6 Fatty Acids</u>:

Supplementation along with a low-fat diet may be beneficial.

Experimental Study: Corn oil supplementation appeared to improve the clinical course in acne pts. on low-fat diets (*Hubler WR. Unsaturated fatty acids in acne. Arch. Derm. 79:644, 1959*).

- -

High chromium yeast: 1 tsp. 2 times daily (400 mcg chromium)

Skin glucose tolerance (but <u>not</u> oral glucose tolerance) is significantly impaired in acne vulgaris (*Abdel KM et al. Glucose tolerance in blood and skin of patients with acne vulgaris. Ind. J. Derm. 22:139-49, 1977*).

Supplementation with high chromium yeast improves glucose tolerance and enhances insulin sensitivity (*Offenbach E Pistunyer F. Beneficial effect of chromium-rich yeast on glucose tolerance and blood lipids in elderly patients. Diabetes 29:919-25, 1980*).

The benefits of high-chromium yeast may be due to the effect of insulin on essential fatty acid metabolism, since insulin induces delta-6-desaturase synthesis which is required for conversion of linoleic acid to prostaglandins (*McCarty M. High chromium yeast for acne? Med. Hypotheses 14:307-10, 1984*).

Supplementation may be beneficial.

Experimental Study: 10 pts. rapidly improved following supplementation with high-chromium yeast ("Chromax") 2 tsp daily providing 400 mcg chromium (*Rubin D - reported in McCarty M. High chromium yeast for acne? Med. Hypotheses 14:307-10, 1984*).

- -

OTHER FACTORS:

Rule out <u>food sensitivities</u>.

General:

Negative Experimental Study: 120 pts. underwent intracutaneous allergen testing with 23 of the most important food antigens. Test results on 83/120 (69.2%) were negative. 9 pts. (7.4%) showed an immediate reaction on 4 or more extracts. Almonds showed the most positive reactions (11.6%),then malt (10%), cheese, mustard, red pepper (8.3% each), and wheat flour (7.5%). Pts. were placed on an elimination diet based on the results of skin testing, placed on an "acne diet," or told to follow no diet. After 3 mo. 45 pts. were evaluated and no statistical difference was found between the 3 groups. Although diet is generally not very significant, it can be possibly useful in some cases (*Wuthrich B, Much T. [Acne vulgaris: Results of food allergen tests and a controlled elimination diet.] Dermatologica 157(5):294-95, 1978 (in German)*

Review Article: "There is no well-documented study proving that foods aggravate acne. There are, however, statements of belief that this is so" (*Rasmussen JE. Diet and acne. Int. J. Dermatol. 16:488-92, 1977*).

Negative Experimental Study: Over a 6 yr. period, each new pt. was questioned about prohibited foods and his actual experience linking diet to exacerbations of the acne. 8-10% of pts. claimed chocolate as a cause and 3-4% blamed nuts, cola or milk. Most of the pts. reporting associations believed that their acne worsened substantially within 36hrs. after eating the prohibited food, worsened in proportion to the amt. of food eaten, and the acne flare lasted 3-5 day afterwards. Gps. of 4-8 subjects, all sensitive to the same food ate large amts. of that food daily for 1 week and changes in the appearance of their acne were objectively recorded. Absolutely no major flares of acne were produced by the foods. While 1/3 of subjects developed new lesions during the 10 days of the tests, these were within the expected variation for control patients, and almost half of the pts. showed slight improvement (*Anderson PC. Foods as a cause of acne. Am. Fam. Physician 3(3):102-03, 1971*).

Chocolate:

Review Article: Although there are specific contraindications to the ingestion of chocolate by selected individuals, these do not apply to the general population with high frequency (*Fries JH. Chocolate: A review of published reports of allergic and other deleterious effects, real or presumed. Ann. Allergy 41(4):195-207, 1978*).

Experimental Double-blind Study: Of 500 allergy pts., 16.2% believed that chocolate caused allergic symptoms, but only 10 manifested very specific allergic symptoms within a predictable time after eating chocolate. 8 of these ten were fed both placebos and defatted chocolate in capsule form. In 3/8, the reported clinical symptoms were reproduced after ingestion of the cocoa capsules, but not after the placebos. Only 1 of these 3 had a positive skin test to chocolate (*Maslansky L, Wein G. Effect of chocolate on acne vulgaris. Letter to the Editor. JAMA 211(11):1856, 1970*).

Negative Experimental Double-blind Study: 65 adolescents were feed either unusually large amts. of chocolate or a placebo bar of candy. Evaluation was made in measurement of quantity, composition and comedogenic potency of sebum. Results suggested that "ingestion of high amounts of chocolate did not materially affect the course of acne vulgaris or the output or composition of sebum" (*Fulton JE et al. Effect of chocolate on acne vulgaris. JAMA 210:2071, 1969*).

> *Note: This study has been criticized because the placebo candy bar did not differ sufficiently from chocolate in its fat and sugar content, and the adverse effects of chocolate may be due, in fact, to its high content of molecular carbons, enhanced by the content of sugar and xanthines, which are said to cause diminished fluidiy of sebum (Acne, soap, and chocolate. Editorial. Med. J. Aust. 1:584, 1975; Mackie BS, Mackie LE. Chocolate and acne. Aust. J. Derm. 15:103, 1974).*

Negative Experimental Study: 8 pts. who were certain that chocolate aggravated their acneiform eruptions were fed chocolate without effect (*Grant JD, Anderson PC. Chocolate as a cause of acne: A dissenting view. Mo. Med. 62:459, 1965*).

Milk:

Has been said to aggravate acne due either to its progesterone content or to its animal fat content.

Negative Observational Study: Sex hormones known to produce acne were not detectable in bovine milk when analyzed by methods capable of detecting concentrations less than 10 mcg of testosterone and androsterone and 15 mcg of estradiol glucuronides/liter, suggesting that milk ingestion could not be the cause of acne based on its conjugated hormone content (*Brewington CR et al. Evidence for the absence of the conjugates of acne-causing hormones in cow's milk. Proc. Exp. Biol. Med. 139(3):745-48, 1972*).

Refined Carbohydrates:

Observational Study: In a study of over 1000 physicians, dentists and their wives, five parameters of refined carbohydrate consumption were found to be significantly related (p less than 0.01 to less than 0.001) to the incidence of skin signs and symptoms of dermatoses. Those subjects reporting one or more symptoms and signs consumed a significantly greater quantity of refined carbohydrate compared to those reporting none as measured by each parameter: total calories, calories from refined carbohydrate, percentage of calories from refined carbohydrate, gms. of refined carbohydrate, and tsps. of sugar (*Ringsdorf WM Jr, Cheraskin E. Diet and dermatosis. South. Med. J. 69(6):732 & 734, 1976*).

Negative Controlled Experimental Study: Pts. who were placed on a diet which was restricted in sugar showed no differences from controls (*Cornbleet T, Gigli I. Should we limit sugar in acne? Arch. Dermatol. 83:968, 1961*).

Negative Experimental Study: Acne pts. were treated with IV carbohydrates and improvement was noted (*Crawford GM, Swartz JH. Acne and the carbohydrates. <u>Arch. Dermatol. Syphilol.</u> 33:1035-41, 1936*).

See Also:

> Bett DGG et al. Sugar consumption in acne vulgaris and seborrhoeic dermatitis. <u>Br. Med. J.</u> 3:153-55, 1967

> Mullins JF, Naylor D. Glucose and the acne diathesis: An hypothesis and review of the literature. <u>Tex. Rep. Biol. Med.</u> 20:161-75, 1962

- -

COMBINED NUTRITIONAL REGIME:

Experimental Study: 98 pts. with acne of varying severity were treated. 31/98 had had acne for at least 10 years, and many of them had been unsuccessfully treated with oral antibiotics. On the following regime, 90/98 (92%) had a good to excellent response, 2 (2%) had a poor response and 42 (43%) had 90-100% clearing of their condition in 2 months or less:

1. Avoid <u>inorganic iron</u> (inactivates vitamin E).
2. Avoid <u>female hormones</u> (antagonistic to vitamin E).
3. Avoid extra <u>iodine</u> (can aggravate acne).
4. Avoid commencial soft drinks with brominated vegetable oils (can aggregate acne).
5. Avoid over 1 glass <u>milk</u> daily (hormones can aggravate acne).
6. Avoid <u>vitamin B$_{12}$</u> (can produce or aggravate acne).
7. <u>Vitamin A</u> (water-soluble) 50,000 IU twice daily before meals.
8. <u>Vitamin E</u> (d,alpha-tocopheryl acetate or succinate) 400 IU twice daily before meals.
9. <u>Pyridoxine</u> 50 mg once or twice daily for premenstrual and menstrual acne.
10. <u>Benzoyl peroxide</u> 5% gel applied at night after washing gently with nonmedicated soap.
11. Well balanced diet, low in <u>fat</u> and <u>sugars</u>.

(*Ayres S, Mihan R. Acne vulgaris: Therapy directed at pathophysiologic defects. <u>Cutis</u> 28:41-2, 1981*)

ALCOHOLISM

See Also: "HYPOGLYCEMIA" (FUNCTIONAL)

OVERVIEW:

There are many nutritional deficiencies which may be caused by excessive alcohol ingestion and the deficient nutrient intake often associated with alcoholism. By boosting the nutritional intake, not only may it be possible to reduce the toxic effects associated with alcoholism, but there is preliminary evidence that alcohol craving and the symptoms of alcohol withdrawal may also be ameliorated.

1. Reducing alcohol toxicity.

   Since many of the toxic effects of alcoholism are due, not to alcohol, but to the associated nutritional deficiencies, adding these nutrients to the diets of alcoholics can be protective. These include vitamin A, vitamin B complex, vitamin C, vitamin E, magnesium, selenium, and zinc. In addition, certain accessory nutrients such as D,L-carnitine, catechin, gamma-linolenic acid, glutathione and pantethine may protect the liver from damage due to alcohol.

2. Reducing the craving for alcohol.

   Research is this area is limited, but there are several intriguing preliminary studies which suggest that alcohol craving is associated with poor nutrition. Normals placed on a diet particularly high in raw foods began to spontaneously avoid alcohol (and tobacco), while chronic alcoholics placed on a nutrititious diet along with a multivitamin supplement did far better at follow-up in abstaining from alcohol than did controls. Studies with rats have had similar results. In one study, a "junk food" diet, especially when supplemented with coffee, led to increased alcohol consumption while, in another study, alcohol was preferred by the animals only when they were made B vitamin-deficient.

   Supplementation with certain specific nutrients may reduce craving although, once again, confirmatory studies are needed. Nicotinic acid and pantethine have been said to be beneficial due to their ability to reduce acetaldehyde. L-glutamine has been shown to diminish alcohol craving in rats and may do the same for some alcoholics.

   There is evidence that alcohol can induce reactive hypoglycemia, while hypoglycemia may stimulate alcohol consumption. Food sensitivites have also been accused of causing alcohol craving, but scientific evidence is lacking.

3. Reducing the severity of alcohol withdrawal syndromes.

Although more studies are needed, it is possible that insuring adequate magnesium status prior to withdrawal may be beneficial, and animal studies suggest that the supplementation with the nutritional precursors of prostaglandin E_1 may lessen or prevent withdrawal syndromes.

KEY: C = may affect craving for alcohol
      T = may affect alcohol toxicity
      W = may affect symptoms of alcohol withdrawal

- -

BASIC DIET:

Well-balanced, nutritionally adequate diet.
(C)

Animal Experimental Study (C): One gp. of rats which was fed a typical teenage "junk food" diet continuously increased its alcohol consumption during the study, while another gp. which received a well-balanced control diet maintained a low level of alcohol intake. When supplemented with either caffeine or coffee, both gps. significantly increased their alcohol intake. Results suggest that "metabolic controls to drinking exist which are sensitive to dietary factors" (*Register et al. J. Am. Diet. Assoc. 61:159-62, 1972*).

Increase consumption of raw foods.
(C)

Experimental Study (C): 32 hypertensives ingested an average of 62% of their calories as uncooked food for a mean of 6.7 months. 80% of those who smoked or drank alcohol abstained spontaneously (*Douglass J et al. Effects of a raw food diet on hypertension and obesity. South. Med. J. 78(7):841, 1985*).

- -

NUTRIENTS:

General Review Article: Most specific nutritional deficiencies in alcoholics have their roots in ethanol toxicity. "Alcoholic gastritis causes anorexia, retching and vomiting. The small-intestinal disease leads to diarrhea with electrolyte loss and to difficulties in absorption of specific nutrients, including thiamine, folate, vitamin B_{12}, glucose, and amino acids. Pancreatic disease leads to steatorrhea with malabsorption of essential fatty acids, fat-soluble vitamins, and calcium. Alcoholic liver disease among other things leads to failure of protein synthesis, amino acid imbalance, reduced zinc storage, enhanced metabolism of and failure to store vitamin A, and failure to store vitamin B_6" (*Sherlock S. Nutrition and the alcoholic. Lancet 1:436-8, 1984*).

See Also:

Majumdar SK et al. Vitamin utilization status in chronic alcoholics. Int. J. Vitam. Nutr. Res. 51(1):54-58, 1981

Thomson AD, Majumdar SK. The influence of ethanol on intestinal absorption and utilization of nutrients. Clin. Gastroenterol. 10(2):263-93, 1981

Vitamin A:
(T)

May be deficient.

Observational Study: Plasma levels in 3/25 pts (aged 28-70) were deficient. It is noted that falling plasma levels indicate exhaustion of its hepatic storage and is therefore suggested that supplementation be given along with other polyvitamins during detoxification for ethanol withdrawal to prevent hypovitaminosis A (*Majumdar SK et al. Vitamin A utilization status in chronic alcoholic patients. Int. J. Vitam. Nutr. Res. 53(3):273-79, 1983*).

Review Article: Frequently markedly deficient in the liver (even at early stages of liver involvement) despite normal serum levels; however, its hepatotoxicity is enhanced by chronic alcohol consumption (*Lieber CS. Alcohol-nutrition interaction: 1983. Contemporary Nutrition December 1983*).

See Also:

> *Leo MA, Lieber CS.   Interaction of ethanol with vitamin A.   Alcoholism: Clin. Exp. 7:15, 1983*

Vitamin A plus zinc deficiencies are said to cause such alcoholic disorders as night blindness, cirrhosis, impaired immune function, etc. (*Scholmerich J et al.   Zinc and vitamin A deficiency in liver cirrhosis.   Hepato-Gastroenterol. 30:1333-8, 1982*).

Supplementation when deficient may improve taste and olfactory sensitivity.

> **Experimental and Observational Study (T):** 11/37 pts. who demonstrated diminished taste and olfactory detection compared to controls were deficient in both zinc and vitamin A. All 37 received oral doses of vitamin A 10,000 mg daily. After 4 wks. of treatment, both those with and without zinc deficiency demonstrated a higher degree of taste and olfactory sensitivity (*Garrett-Laster M et al.   Impairment of taste and olfaction in patients with cirrhosis: The role of vitamin A.   Human Nutr.: Clin. Nutr. 38C:203-214, 1984*).

<u>Vitamin B Complex</u>:   100 mg. daily
(*C,T*)

Often deficient in alcoholics (esp.thiamine, pyridoxine and vitamin B_{12} and folate) due both to inadequate intake and impairment in absorption (*Baines M.   Detection and incidence of B and C vitamin deficiency in alcohol-related illness.   Ann. Clin. Biochem. 15:307-12, 1978*).

Deficiency may increase the craving for alcohol.

> **Animal Experimental Study (C):** Rats made deficient in B vitamins were more likely to choose alcohol than water - but supplementation reversed their tastes (*Norton VP.   Interrelationships of nutrition and voluntary alcohol consumption in experimental animals.   Brit. J. Addiction 72(3):205-12, 1977*).

See Also:

> *Pekkanen L.   Effects of thiamine deprivation and antagonism on voluntary ethanol intake in rats.   J. Nutr. 110:937, 1980*

- <u>Folic Acid</u>:

May be deficient.

> **Observational Study:** Although urine volumes did not increase significantly while alcoholic subjects were drinking, urinary folate levels were 20-24% higher than during abstinence in 4/5 patients (*Russell RM et al.   Am. J. Clin. Nutr. 38:64-70, 1983*).

> **Observational Study:** Serum folate was decreased in all 41 pts. with alcoholic liver disease except those with alcoholic hepatitis, while RBC folate was normal for all patients (*Majumdar SK et al.   Blood vitamin status (B_1, B_2, B_6, folic acid and B_{12}) in patients with alcoholic liver disease.   Int. J. Vitamin. Res. 52(3):266-71, 1982*).

See Also:

> *Thornton WE, Pray BJ.   Lowered serum folate and alcohol withdrawal syndromes.   Psychosomatics December 1977, p. 32*

Halstead CH et al.   Intestinal malabsorption in folate-deficient alcoholics. Gastroenterol. 64:526, 1973

- Nicotinic Acid: minimum 500 mg daily
(C,T)

Supplementation may be beneficial.

Theoretical Discussion (C): There is evidence that the degradation of ethanol to acetaldehyde is accelerated in chronic alcoholics while the second step in the degradation of acetaldehyde is slowed down; thus acetaldehyde is elevated. Acetaldehyde has been shown to condense with dopamine in the brain to form tetrahydro-papoveroline, a morphine-like substance, which has been postulated to cause alcohol addiction. Nicotinic acid oxidizes alcohol to reduce acetaldehyde levels and also saturates NAD brain receptors to abolish a possible deficiency of NAD which would cause irritability and restlessness (*Cleary JP. The NAD deficiency diseases. J. Orthomol. Med. 1(3):149-57, 1986*).

Experimental Study (C): 12 alcoholics received nicotinic acid 500 mg daily. Results suggested that supplementation was an effective means of treatment (*Cleary JP. Etiology and biological treatment of alcohol addiction. J. Neuro. Ortho. Med. Surg. 6:75-77, 1985*).

Experimental Study (C,T): 507 alcoholics were treated with nicotinic acid 3 gms or more daily for 5 years. Results suggested that 30% of alcoholics, and 50-60% of "organic" alcoholics, benefit from supplementation both by symptom reduction and reduced recidivism (*Smith RF. Status report concerning the use of megadose nicotinic acid in alcoholics. J. Orthomol. Psychiat. 7(1), 1978; Smith RF. A five-year trial of massive nicotinic acid therapy of alcoholics in Michigan. J. Orthomol. Psychiat. 3:327-31, 1974*).

Experimental Study (T): Nicotinic acid supplementation reduced mortality from 90% to 14% in a large series of pts. who were admitted with severe impairment of consciousness or delirium, and cogwheel rigidity of the limbs with uncontrollable grasping and sucking reflexes, half of whom showed evidence of niacin deficiency (*Jolliffe N et al. Nicotinic acid deficiency encephalopathy. JAMA 114:307-12, 1940*).

- Pyridoxine:
(T)

A functional deficiency is common due to impaired conversion to pyridoxal-5-phosphate (the active form) and enhanced degradation (*Lumeng L. The role of acetaldehyde in mediating the deleterious effect of ethanol on pyridoxal-5-phosphate metabolism. J. Clin. Invest. 62:286-93, 1978*).

Observational Study: All 41 pts. with alcoholic liver disease were deficient in pyridoxal-5-phosphate (*Majumdar SK et al. Blood vitamin status (B₁, B₂, B₆, folic acid and B₁₂) in patients with alcoholic liver disease. Int. J. Vitamin. Res. 52(3):266-71, 1982*).

Observational Study: 11/12 chronic alcoholics were deficient in RBC pyridoxal-5-phosphate (*Majumdar SK et al. Vitamin utilization status in chronic alcoholics. Int. J. Vitam. Nutr. Res. 51(1):54-58, 1981*).

- Riboflavin:

May be deficient.

Observational Study: Out of 41 pts. with alcoholic liver disease, blood riboflavin was deficient only in pts. with histologically normal livers (*Majumdar SK et al. Blood vitamin status (B₁, B₂,*

B6, folic acid and B12) in patients with alcoholic liver disease. Int. J. Vitamin. Res. 52(3):266-71, 1982).

Observational Study: 6/12 chronic alcoholics were deficient in riboflavin as measured by glutathione reductase activity (*Majumdar SK et al. Vitamin utilization status in chronic alcoholics. Int. J. Vitam. Nutr. Res. 51(1):54-58, 1981*).

- Thiamine:
(T)

Thiamine deficiency is known to be responsible for such neurological complications as polyneuropathy and Wernicke's Syndrome.

Observational Study: As judged by serum transketolase activity, 30% of fairly well-nourished pts. with alcoholic liver disease were deficient (*Hoyumpa AM Jr. Alcohol and thiamine metabolism. Alcoholism: Clin. Exp. Res. 7:11-14, 1983*).

Observational Study: All 41 pts. with alcoholic liver disease were deficient in blood thiamine (*Majumdar SK et al. Blood vitamin status (B1, B2, B6, folic acid and B12) in patients with alcoholic liver disease. Int. J. Vitamin. Res. 52(3):266-71, 1982*).

Observational Study: 7/12 chronic alcoholics were deficient in thiamine as measured by RBC transketolase activity (*Majumdar SK et al. Vitamin utilization status in chronic alcoholics. Int. J. Vitam. Nutr. Res. 51(1):54-58, 1981*).

- Vitamin B12:

May be deficient despite normal or elevated serum levels.

Observational Study: Compared to normals, liver content of cobalamin in 27 alcoholics was low while serum cobalamin and RBC cobalamin analogues were high, confirming earlier work which suggested that, in alcoholism and liver disease, cobalamin depletion in tissues may be masked by normal to high serum cobalamin and analogue levels. The failure of damaged liver to take up from the serum cobalamin and analogues, compounded by the release of these compounds and their binders from damaged liver into the serum, can account for these findings (*Kanazawa S, Herbert V. Total corrinoid, cobalamin (viamin B12), and cobalamin analogue levels may be normal in serum despite cobalamin in liver depletion in patients with alcoholism. Lab. Invest. 53(1):108-10, 1985*).

Observational Study: Blood levels were normal in a gp. of 41 pts. with alcoholic liver disease except for those with cirrhosis where it was raised (*Majumdar SK et al. Blood vitamin status (B1, B2, B6, folic acid and B12) in patients with alcoholic liver disease. Int. J. Vitamin. Res. 52(3):266-71, 1982*).

Observational Study: Alcoholism was the most common disease correlate of vitamin B12 elevations in female general hospital patients. 61% of them had a serum B12 concentration greater or equal to 1000 ng/l compared to 17% of non-alcoholics. B12 elevations paralleled high SGOT, GGT and MCV values. In contrast, males far less often exhibited B12 elevations (*Goldman PA et al. A sex difference in the serum vitamin B12 levels of hospitalized alcoholics. Curr. Alcohol. 5:237-49, 1979*).

Vitamin C:
(T)

Usually deficient in alcoholics.

Observational Study: Deficient in 91% of patients with alcohol-related diseases (*Baines M. Detection and incidence of B and C vitamin deficiency in alcohol-related illness. Ann. Clin. Biochem. 15:307-12, 1978*).

Supplementation may reduce the effects of ethanol toxicity.

Experimental Study (T): Supplementation reduced the effects of ethanol toxicity (when combined with zinc sulphate) (*Yunice AA, Lindeman RD. Effect of ascorbic acid and zinc sulphate on ethanol toxicity and metabolism. Proc. Soc. Exp. Biol. Med. 154:146-50, 1977*).

Animal Experimental Study (T): Supplementation reduced the effects of ethanol toxicity (*Yunice AA et al. Ethanol-ascorbate interrelationship in acute and chronic alcoholism in the guinea pig. Proc. Soc. Exp. Biol. Med. 177:262-71, 1984*).

See Also:

Sprince H et al. Protective effect of ascorbic acid and sulfur compounds against acetaldehyde toxicity: Implications in alcoholism and smoking. Agents Actions 5:164, 1975

When taken before or during alcohol ingestion, supplementation may prevent fatty infiltration of the liver (*DiLuzio NR. A mechanism of the acute ethanol-induced fatty liver and the modification of liver injury by antioxidants. Lab. Invest. 15:50-61, 1966*).

Vitamin E:
(T)

May protect against the cardio-toxic effects of alcohol.

Animal Experimental Study (T): Mice pretreated with vitamin E by injection prior to injection of a large dose of alcohol exhibited much less evidence of myocardial cell damage than control mice (*Retzki J et al. J. Toxicol.-Clin. Toxicol. 20:319-31, 1983*).

When taken before or during alcohol ingestion, may prevent fatty infiltration of the liver (*DiLuzio - see above*).

See Also:

Hirayama C et al. Effect of alpha-tocopherol and tocopheronolactone on ethanol induced fatty liver and triglyceridemia. Experientia 26:1306, 1970)

- -

Calcium:

A number of studies have recorded low serum calcium levels in chronic alcoholics, and hypomagnesemia is associated with hypocalcemia which can be reversed by magnesium administration (*Thomson AD. Alcohol and nutrition. Clinics in Endocrinol. & Metabol. 7(2), 405-28, 1978*).

See Also:

O'Brien CC. Experimental evidence in the treatment of alcoholism by intensive calcium therapy. J. Am. Osteopathic Assoc. 51:393, 1952

Magnesium:
(T,W)

Intracellular depletion is common due to renal hyperexcretion and can cause cardiomyopathy (*Burch GE, Giles TD. The importance of magnesium deficiency in cardiovascular disease. Am. Heart J. 94:649-57, 1977*).

See Also:

> *Bohmer T, Mathiesen B. Magnesium deficiency in chronic alcoholic patients uncovered by an intravenous loading test. Scand. J. Clin. Lab. Invest. 42:633, 1982*

Along with alkalosis, deficiency may induce symptoms of delerium tremens (*Victor M. The role of hypomagnesemia and respiratory alkalosis in the genesis of alcohol-withdrawal symptoms. Ann. N.Y. Acad. Sci. 215:235-248, 1973*), although, in one study, magnesium supplementation did not reverse its course (*Brooks BR, Adams RD. Cerebral spinal fluid acid-base and lactate changes after seizures in unanaesthetised man due to alcohol withdrawal seizures. Neurology 25:943-48, 1975*).

Selenium:
(T)

Essential for the activity of glutathione peroxidase which protects against alcohol-induced liver damage.

Often deficient in alcoholics with severe liver disease.

> **Observational Study (T):** Serum selenium was evaluated in relation to hepatic structure in 46 alcoholics and was found to be lower in those with normal liver, fatty liver, alcoholic hepatitis and cirrhosis than in 25 healthy controls. Its level was related to the severity of the liver disease and was lowest in those with decompensated alcoholic cirrhosis (*Korpela H et al. Am. J. Clin. Nutr. 42:147-151, 1985*).

> **Observational Study (T):** Whole blood, plasma and RBC selenium levels were measured in 30 symptom-free alcoholics, 16 alcoholics with severe liver disease and 27 healthy controls. Compared to the controls, both gps. of alcoholics had reduced levels of selenium with the lowest average levels in the gp. with liver disease (*Dworkin B, Rosenthal W. Letter to the Editor. Lancet 1:1015, 1984*).

Zinc:
(T)

Chronic alcohol consumption is associated with zinc deficiency (*McClain CJ, Su L-C. Zinc deficiency in the alcoholic: A review. Alcoholism: Clin. Exp. 7:5, 1983; Wu CT et al. Serum zinc, copper, and ceruloplasmin levels in male alcoholics. Biol Psychiat. 19:1333-8, 1982*).

Zinc deficiency impairs ethanol metabolism, thus increasing the risk of liver damage.

> **Animal Experimental Study (T):** Gps. of young male rats were given zinc adequate or zinc deficient diets in combination with ethanol or isocaloric diets. The addition of alcohol to the diet with or without adequate zinc caused an impairment in body weight gain as did inadequate zinc alone. Both serum and liver zinc levels were depressed in the zinc-deficient gp. (ZD) and the zinc-deficient gp. which received alcohol (ZDE). The gp. which received a zinc-adequate diet and alcohol (CE) also had depressed zinc levels. The activity of acetaldehyde dehydrogenase (ALDH) (needed to oxidize acetaldehyde to acetate) was decreased in the ZD group. Ethanol elimination was impaired in the

ZD and ZDE gps. as compared to controls.   The CE gp. had an increased level of alcohol dehydrogenase activity (needed to oxidize ethanol to acetaldehyde) and ethanol elimination. The activity of ALDH was not affected by zinc deficiency but was increased by ethanol feeding (*Das et al. J. Lab. Clin. Med. 104:610-17, 1984*).

Zinc supplementation (along with ascorbic acid) may be beneficial in preventing alcohol toxicity.

Animal Experimental Study (rats) (T): *Yunice AA, Lindeman RD. Effect of ascorbic acid and zinc sulphate on ethanol toxicity and metabolism. Proc. Soc. Exp. Biol. Med. 154:146-50, 1977*

- -

Amino Acids: (mixed freeform)
(T)

Supplementation may be beneficial in alcoholic hepatitis.

Experimental Controlled Study: 17/35 pts. with alcoholic hepatitis randomly received amino acids 70-85 gm IV daily. All 35 had similar clinical and biochemical features and received a 3000 kcal 100 gm protein diet. After 28 days, ascites and encephalopathy tended to improve more in the study group. Serum bilirubin and albumin improved only in the study group. 4 pts. died in the control gp., but none in the study gp. (*Nasrallah SM, Galambos JT. Aminoacid therapy of alcoholic hepatitis. Lancet 2:1276-7, 1980*).

Carnitine:
(T)

May inhibit alcohol-induced fatty liver, perhaps by facilitating the oxidation of the increased fatty acid load produced by alcohol ingestion.

Animal Experimental Study (T): Rats fed ethanol as 36% of total calories developed typical hepatic steatosis (accumulation of total lipids, triglycerides, cholesterols, phospholipids and free fatty acids). Supplementation of the ethanol diet with 1% D,L carnitine, 0.05% L-lysine and 0.2% L-methionine (carnitine precursors) significantly lowered ethanol-induced increases of various lipid fractions except for free fatty acids. The lipid-lowering effect of carnitine was superior to that of its precursors and their effect together was no greater than that of carnitine alone. The results suggest that a deficiency of functional carnitine may exist in chronic alcoholics (*Sachan DS et al. Ameliorating effects of carnitine and its precursors on alcohol-induced fatty liver. Am. J. Clin. Nutr. 39:738-44, 1984*).

Catechin:
(T)

A naturally occurring flavonoid.

May help prevent ethanol-induced liver damage (*World M et al. (+)-cyanidanol-3 for alcoholic liver disease: Results of a six month clinical trial. Alcohol Alcohol 19:23-9, 1984*).

Evening Primrose Oil: 1/2 - 1 gram three times daily
(T,W)

Supplementation may be beneficial.

Theoretical Discussion: Alcohol blocks the conversion of linoleic acid to gamma-linolenic acid and enhances the conversion of dihommogamma-linolenic acid to prostaglandin E_1; the result is a deficiency in GLA which can be replaced by primrose oil. Supplementation with EPO may theoretically prevent the development of alcohol addiction by preventing the development of tolerance due to DGLA depletion (*Horrobin DF. A biochemical basis for alcoholism and alcohol-induced damage including the fetal alcohol syndrome and cirrhosis: Interference with essential fatty acid and prostaglandin metabolism. Med. Hypotheses 6:929-42, 1980*).

See Also:

> *Glen AL et al. Essential fatty acids in the treatment of the alcohol dependence syndrome, in Birch GG, Lindley MG, Eds. Alcoholic Beverages. London, Elsevier, 1985, pp. 203-21*

> *Karpe F et al. Ethanol dependence in rats on diets high and low in essential fatty acids (EFA) (abstract). Acta Pharmacol. Toxicol. Suppl. 114:143-45, 1985*

> *Segarnick DJ et al. Prostanoid modulation (mediation?) of certain behavioral effects of ethanol. Pharmacol. Biochem. Behav. 23:71-75, 1985*

> *Horrobin DF. Prostaglandins (PGs) and essential fatty acids (EFAs): A new approach to the understanding and treatment of alcoholism. Psychiatry in Practice. August 3, 1984, pp. 19-21*

May reduce the symptoms of alcohol withdrawal.

Animal Experimental Study (W): Mice were exposed to ethanol by inhalation for 4 days prior to withdrawal, the effects of which were lessened by evening primrose oil (*Segarnick DJ et al. Biochemical and behavioral interactions between prostaglandin E_1 and alcohol, in Horrobin DF, Editor. Clinical Uses of Essential Fatty Acids. Eden Press, 1982, pp. 199-204*).

Animal Experimental Study (W): Injections of PGE_1 prevented the alcohol withdrawal syndrome (*Rotrosen J et al. Ethanol and prostaglandin E_1: Biochemical and behavioral interactions. Life Sci. 26:1867-76, 1980*).

May prevent liver damage due to high alcohol intake.

Animal Experimental Study (T): *Ryle PR et al. Effects of gamma-linolenic acid and antioxidant administration on alcoholic fatty liver in the rat (abstract). Proc. Nut. Soc. 44(1):11A, 1985*

Animal Experimental Study (T): *Wilson DE et al. Prostaglandin E_1 prevents alcohol-induced fatty liver. Clin.Res. 21:829, 1973*

See Also: *Horrobin, 1980 (listed above)*

May prevent alcohol-related CNS impairment.

Experimental Double-blind Study (T): 21 pts. received either EPO or placebo for 3 weeks. Compared to controls, the amount of diazepam needed to ease withdrawal symptoms in treated pts. was significantly reduced and cognitive function on 1 of the psychomotor tests improved significantly. 34 pts. were then randomly chosen for a 6-month trial. Again there was some recovery in cognitive function although there were no significant differences in test results (*Glen E et al. Possible pharmacological approaches to the prevention and treatment of alcohol-related CNS impairment: Results of a double blind trial of essential fatty acids, in Edwards G, Littleton J, Eds. Pharmacological Treatments for Alcoholism. London, Croom Heim, 1984, pp. 331-50*).

L-Glutamine: 2 grams (1/2 tsp.) daily in divided doses.
(C)   (Powder may also be licked off teaspoon when craving alcohol.)

May affect the craving for alcohol.

Experimental Single-blind Crossover Study (C): 9/10 subjects as well as their friends and relatives stated that glutamine diminished the desire to drink, decreased anxiety and improved sleep. 2 or 3 subjects continued to do well after placebo substitution, but no subjects responded to placebo unless they had first responded to glutamine (*Rogers LL, Pelton RB. Quart. J. of Studies on Alcohol 18(4):581-7, 1957*).

Animal Experimental Study (C): Administering glutamine to experimental rats materially diminished their physiological urge to drink alcohol (*Rogers LL, Pelton RB, Williams RJ. Voluntary alcohol consumption by rats following administration of glutamine. J. Biological Chem. 220(1):321-3, 1956*).

Glutathione: 300 mg. daily
(T)

May protect the liver from alcohol-induced damage (*Sies H, Wendel A. Functions of Glutathione. New York, Springer-Verlag, 1978*).

Pantethine: 300 mg 2-3 times daily
(C,T)

A metabolic intermediate which is the stable disulfide form of pantetheine, a derivative of pantethenic acid and a precursor of Coenzyme A.

Acetaldehyde, the primary metabolite of alcohol, may promote alcohol addiction by combining with monamine metabolites to form addicting morphine-like alkaloids (*Myer RD. Tetrahydroisoquinolines in the brain: The basis of an animal model of addiction. Alcohol Clin. Exp. Res. 2:145, 1978; Cohen G, Collins MA. Alkaloids from catecholamines in adrenal tissue: Possible role in alcoholism. Science 167:1749-51, 1970; Davis We, Walsh MJ. Alcohol, amines, and alkaloids: a possible biochemical basis for alcohol addiction. Science 167:1005-7, 1970*).

Acetaldehyde has also been implicated in the pathogenesis of alcoholic liver disease and alcoholic cardiomyopathy and may play a role in the development of atherosclerosis as related to ethanol ingestion (*Watanabe A et al. Lowering of blood acetaldehyde but not ethanol concentrations by pantethine following alcohol ingestion: Different effects in flushing and non-flushing subjects. Alcohol Clin. Exp. Res. 9:272, 1985; Sprince H et al. Protection against acetaldehyde toxicity in the rat by L-cysteine, thiamin and L-2-methylthiazolidine-4-carboxylic acid. Agents Actions 4(2):125-30, 1974*).

Supplementation with pantethine may theoretically reduce the adverse effects of acetaldehyde by increasing the activity of aldehyde dehydrogenase, the enzyme which metabolizes it.

Experimental Study (T): Administration of pantethine prior to alcohol ingestion reduced acetaldehyde levels in the blood of human volunteers and in the liver of experimental animals. Since ethanol levels were unaffected, this reduction is believed to have been due to an increase in aldehyde dehydrogenase activity (*Watanabe - op cit*).

In vitro Experimental Study (T): Pantethine increased aldehyde dehydrogenase activity by as much as 71% (*Watanabe - op cit*).

Note: Pantethine will probably not be effective in pts. who flush after alcohol ingestion, probably due to a weak aldehyde dehydrogenase enzyme (Watanabe - op cit).

- -

COMBINED TREATMENT:

Nutritious diet plus multivitamin supplementation:
(C)

> **Experimental Controlled Study (C):** Chronic alcoholics who averaged 13 oz. alcohol daily for 15-20 years were studied. While the control gp. only received the standard hospital diet, the experimental gp. also followed a special diet plan which included foods such as wheat germ and unsweetened fruit as well as decaffeinated coffee and avoided all snacks except for nuts, cheese, peanut butter and milk. In addition, they attended a nutrition education class and were placed on a multivitamin supplement which they were asked to continue for 6 months after discharge. At the 6 month follow-up 81% of the experimental gp. was still sober compared to 38% of the control gp. *(Guenther RM. Role of nutritional therapy in alcoholism treatment. Int. J. Biosocial Res. 4(1):5-18, 1983).*

- -

OTHER FACTORS:

Rule out food sensitivities.
(C)

> Said to be a cause of alcoholism due to craving for the foods from which the alcoholic beverage is derived, since alcoholic beverages, because of their rapid absorption, "carry the activity of the foods from which they are manufactured relatively more effectively than other food fractions" *(Randolph TG. The role of specific alcoholic beverages, in Dickey LD. Clinical Ecology. Springfield, Illinois, Charles C. Thomas, 1976).*

> **Experimental Study:** The ingestion of either grain alcohol or whiskey increased the size, intensity and duration of the allergic wheal, regardless of the subjects' clinical sensitivity to alcoholic beverages. This effect was unrelated to the absolute blood alcohol level. Results suggest that, in those who are sensitive to alcohol, alcohol ingestion merely brings to a clinical level a subclinical allergic reaction, and food or inhalant allergens unrelated to the contents of the brew may become potent enough to cause symptoms, or the alcoholic medium could enhance the small quantities of allergens which it contained to a level sufficient to produce an allergic reaction *(Dees SC. An experimental study of the effect of alcohol and alcoholic beverages on allergic reactions. Ann. Allergy 7:185, 1949).*

Rule out reactive hypoglycemia.
(C)

> May be induced by alcohol.

> > **Review Article:** The increase in gastric acidity which follows alcohol ingestion might cause excessive release of gut secretagogues which augment beta-cell responsiveness to glucose fluctuations, leading to excessive insulin release *(Freinkel N, Getzger BE. Oral glucose tolerance curve and hypoglycemias in the fed state. New Engl. J. Med. 280:820-8, 1969).*

> > See Also:

> > > *Beasley JD. Managing the alcoholic: Behavioral chickens and behavioral eggs. Med. Trib. December 4, 1985, p.22*

> > > *O'Keefe SJD, Marks V. Lunchtime gin and tonic as a cause of reactive hypoglycemia. Lancet 1:1286, 1977*

> > > *Arky RA. The Biology of Alcoholism. New York, Plenum Press, 1971*

May stimulate alcohol consumption.

Animal Experimental Study (C): When insulin production was decreased by administering alloxan (which destroys pancreatic beta cells), the animals stopped drinking alcohol. Alcohol consumption resumed when insulin was administered and increased as the frequency of the insulin dose increased (*Forander et al. Quart. J. Stud. Alcohol. 19:379, 1958*).

ALLERGY
(ALTERED REACTIVITY)

OVERVIEW:

1. Plasma <u>ascorbate</u> levels are negatively correlated with blood histamine levels, and ascorbate supplementation may lower elevated blood histamine levels, but there is very little evidence that vitamin C supplementation reduces allergic reactions.

2. <u>Bioflavonoids</u> inhibit the release of histamine and other mediators of allergic response from mast cells and basophils, but further studies are needed to assess whether they benefit the clinical situation.

3. <u>Foods</u> may provoke a wide variety of symptoms by multiple mechanisms.

4. <u>MSG sensitivity</u> may possibly be reduced by nutrients. Pyridoxine was shown to do so in a double-blind study, while ascorbic acid reduced the neurotoxicity of MSG administered intra-peritoneally in an animal study.

5. <u>Sulfite sensitivity</u> may possibly be related to molybdenum deficiency, but the benefits of supplementation are unproven.

6. <u>Formaldehyde sensitivity</u> may possibly be reduced by pantethine supplementation, but clinical trials are lacking.

- -

NUTRIENTS:

Pyridoxine:

Supplementation may be beneficial for <u>MSG sensitivity</u>.

Experimental Double-blind Study: 12/27 unsupplemented students who were fasted and then challenged in sequence with either a large dose of monosodium glutamate (MSG) or placebo showed characteristic symptoms. There were no significant differences in red blood cell glutamic-oxaloacetic transaminase activity between reactive and non-reactive subjects. These 12 received pyridoxine 50 mg daily or placebo. After 12 weeks they were rechallenged with MSG. 8/9 who proved on decoding to have received pyridoxine now showed no response to MSG. Of the 3 who had received placebo, all were still MSG-responsive. A probability of less than 0.01 was calculated for a real difference in these 2 gps. of 9 and 3, respectively *(Folkers K et al. Biochemical evidence for a deficiency of vitamin B6 in subjects reacting to monosodium-L-glutamate by the chinese restaurant syndrome. Biochem. Biophys. Res. Commun. 100:972-7, 1981).*

Vitamin B12:

Supplementation may be beneficial.

Case Reports: 1000 mcg. IM once weekly for 4 weeks. Results:
Intractable asthma: 18/20 improved
Chronic urticaria: 9/10 improved
Chronic contact dermatitis: 6/6 improved.
Atopic dermatitis: 1/10 greatly improved;
5/10 moderately improved
(*Simon SW. Vitamin B12 therapy in allergy and chronic dermatoses. J.Allergy 2:183-5, 1951*)

Vitamin C:

Supplementation may reduce MSG sensitivity.

Animal Experimental Study: Injections of ascorbic acid prior to intra-peritoneal injection of MSG 2.5 g/kg in 500 chickens prevented the paralysis and convulsions that would have occurred. Similarly the adverse effects of MSG when given to guinea pigs and monkeys fed a low ascorbate diet were abolished when they were given ascorbate by intra-peritoneal injection, suggesting that the addition of ascorbic acid together with MSG to foods may prevent MSG-induced toxic reactions in man (*Ahmad K, Jahan K. Studies on the preventive and curative action of ascorbic acid on the neurological toxicity of monosodium glutamate. Food & Nutr. Bull. 7(1):51-3, 1985*).

Negatively correlated with blood histamine levels.

Observational Study: For 437 normal subjects, when the plasma-reduced ascorbic acid level was below 1 mg/100 ml, the whole blood histamine level increased exponentially as the ascorbic acid level decreased. For subjects with ascorbic acid levels below 0.7 mg/100 ml, the increase in blood histamine was highly significant (*Clemetson CA. Histamine and ascorbic acid in human blood. J. Nutr. 110(4):662-68, 1980*).

Supplementation may reduce blood histamine levels.

Experimental Study: When 11 normals with either low vitamin C levels or high blood histamine levels were given ascorbic acid 1 gm. x 3 days, blood histamine levels fell in all 11 subjects (*Clemetson CA. Histamine and ascorbic acid in human blood. J. Nutr. 110(4):662-68, 1980*).

Supplementation may be beneficial.

Negative Experimental Double-blind Study: The skin wheal and flare response to histamine and the nasal response to allergens were evaluated in 8 pts. with seasonal allergic rhinitis 3 days after receiving ascorbic acid 2 gms. daily and again after 3 days on placebo. In a second study, 6 subjects received either placebo or 1,2 or 4 gms. ascorbic acid daily. In both studies, there were no differences between placebo and ascorbic acid, which suggests that ascorbic acid in doses up to 4 gms. daily will not suppress the histamine skin response and would have no beneficial effect on symptoms resulting from allergen exposure (*Rabinowitz PS, Nelson HS. The effect of ascorbic acid on cutaneous and nasal response to histamine and allergen. J. Allergy Clin. Immunol. 69(6): 484-488, 1982*).

Experimental Controlled Study: 60 pts. with allergic rhinitis were given 1-2.25 gms. ascorbic acid along with "a few" milligrams of thiamine. 50% of pts. on the lower doses, and 75% on the higher doses improved (*Brown EA, Ruskin S. The use of cevitaminic acid in the symptomatic and coseasonal treatment of pollinosis. Ann. Allergy 7:65-70, 1949*).

Vitamin E:

Possesses antihistaminic properties.

Experimental Controlled Study: Volunteers injected with histamine showed far less swelling around the injection site when pretreated with vitamin E for 5-7 days (*Kamimura M. Antiinflammatory activity of vitamin E. J.Vitaminol., 18(4):204-9, 1972*).

- -

Molybdenum:

The trace element contained in the enzyme sulfite oxidase which detoxifies sulfite to the inert and harmless sulfate.

Deficient or absent in the majority of people with <u>sulfite sensitivity</u> (*Papaioannou R, Pfeiffer CC. Sulfite sensitivity - unrecognized threat: Is molybdenum the cause? J. Orthomol. Psychiat. 105-110, 1984*).

- -

Bioflavonoids:

Both the bioflavonoids and disodium chromoglycate possess a benzopyrone nucleus.

Inhibit histamine release from mast cells and basophils when stimulated by antigens and other ligands as well as inhibiting a number of other mediators of allergic response.

General References:

Middleton E, Drzewiecki G. Naturally occurring flavonoids and human basophil histamine release. Int. Arch. Allergy Applied Immuno. 77:155-7, 1985

Amella M et al. Inhibition of mast cell histamine release by flavonoids and bioflavonoids. Planta Medica 51:16-20, 1985

Pearce F et al. Mucosal mast cells, III. Effect of quercetin and other flavonoids on antigen induced histamine secretion from rat intestinal mast cells. J. Allergy Clin. Immunol. 73:819-23, 1984

Foreman JC. Editorial: Mast cells and the actions of flavonoids. J. Allergy Clin. Immunol. 73:769-74, 1984

- Catechin:

A naturally occurring flavonoid.

Able to inhibit histadine decarboxylase, the enzyme responsible for the conversion of histidine to histamine.

Experimental Controlled Study: Pts. with urticaria and food allergies who received catechin prior to administration of food antigens were protected from an increase of histamine in the gastric mucosa in response to the antigens (*Wendt P et al. The use of flavonoids as inhibitors of histadine decarboxylase in gastric diseases: Experimental and clinical studies. Naunyn-Schmiedeberg's Arch. Pharma (Suppl.) 313:238, 1980*).

- Quercetin:

A flavonoid believed to reduce allergic processes due to its ability to:

1. stabilize mast cells and basophils, thereby inhibiting degranulation and subsequent release of histamine and other inflammatory mediators.

In vitro Experimental Study: Quercitin exhibited a predilection to inhibit human basophil histamine release stimulated by IgE-dependent ligands (*Middleton E Jr, Drzewiecki G. Flavonoid inhibition of human basophil histamine release stimulated by various agents. Biochem. Pharmacol. 33(21):3333, 1984*).

2. inhibit several enzymes (e.g. lipoxygenase, phospholipases, cyclic nucleotide phosphodiesterase) through its interaction with calmodulin to dampen the inflammatory response (*Quercetin interacts with calmodulin, a calcium regulatory protein. Experientia 40:184-5, 1984*).

3. decrease leukotriene formation by inhibiting various steps in eicosanoid metabolism (*Yoshimoto T et al. Flavonoids: Potent inhibitors of arachidonate 5-lipoxygenase. Biochem. Biophys. Res. Commun. 116:612-18, 1983*).

Pantethine:

A metabolic intermediate which is the stable disulfide form of pantetheine, a derivative of pantethenic acid and a precursor of Coenzyme A.

May theoretically reduce the adverse effects of aldehydes by increasing the activity of aldehyde dehydrogenase, the enzyme which metabolizes it. This could be of value to pts. hypersensitive to formaldehyde.

Case Report: A man with moderately severe formaldehyde sensitivity received 300 mg pantethine twice daily. Within 1 wk. he reported a marked reduction in sensitivity (*Pantethine: possible treatment for formaldehyde sensitivity. Ecological Formulas, 1061-B Shary circle, Concord, Ca. 94518, 1986*).

Experimental Study: Administration of pantethine prior to alcohol ingestion reduced acetaldehyde levels in the blood of human volunteers and in the liver of experimental animals. Since ethanol levels were unaffected, this reduction is believed to have been due to an increase in aldehyde dehydrogenase activity (*Watanabe A et al. Lowering of blood acetaldehyde but not ethanol concentrations by pantethine following alcohol ingestion: Different effects in flushing and non-flushing subjects. Alcohol Clin. Exp. Res. 9:272, 1985*).

In vitro Experimental Study: Pantethine increased aldehyde dehydrogenase activity by as much as 71% (*Watanabe - ibid*).

Note: Pantethine will probably not be effective in pts. who flush after alcohol ingestion, probably due to a weak aldehyde dehydrogenase enzyme (Watanabe - ibid).

- -

Omega-6 Fatty Acids:

$$\text{linoleic acid} \rightarrow \text{gamma-linolenic acid} \rightarrow \text{DGLA} \rightarrow \text{PGE}_1$$

Atopic pts. may have a block in the conversion of linoleic acid to prostaglandin E_1.

Observational Study: In the plasma phospholipids of 50 pts. with atopic eczema, cis-linoleic acid was elevated and gamma-linolenic acid (GLA) as well as the prostaglandin precursors DGLA and arachidonic acid were decreased. This suggests that atopics have a defect in the functioning of delta-6-desaturase which converts linoleic acid to gamma-linolenic acid (*Manku MS et al. Reduced levels of prostaglandin precursors in the blood of atopic patients: Defective delta-6-desaturase function as a biochemical basis for atopy. Prostaglandins Leukotrienes and Med. 9(6):615-28, 1982*).

- -

OTHER FACTORS:

<u>Lactobacillus Acidophilus</u> and
<u>Bifidobacteria</u>:

Deficiency may be associated with food allergies.

Observational Study: All cases of a group of children suffering from symptoms of food allergies showed evidence of deficiencies of Lactobacillus and Bifidobacteria combined with Enterobacteriaceae overgrowth (*Kuvaeva I et al. The microecology of the gastrointestinal tract and the immunological status under food allergy. <u>Nahrung</u> 28(6-7):689-93, 1984*).

Rule out <u>food sensitivities</u>.

(See also "Rule out <u>food sensitivities</u>" in other chapters.)

Case Reports: 2 pts. with adult celiac disease and <u>bronchial asthma</u> showed improvement in asthmatic symptoms and pulmonary function studies when placed on a gluten-free diet. Since increasing bronchial hyperresponsiveness can be an occasional presenting feature of gluten gastroenteropathy, the possibility of celiac disease should be borne in mind as a possible cause of deterioration in a previously stable asthmatic (*Hosker H et al. Adult caeliac disease presenting with symptoms of worsening asthma. <u>Lancet</u> November 15, 1986, pp. 1157-58*).

Review Article: An important role for foods contributing to eczema, colitis and migraine seems very likely, although atypical food sensitivities remain controversial because the available evidence consists mainly of anecdotes and poorly controlled studies (*Podell R. Food allergy: A mainstream perspective. <u>Clin. Ecology</u> 3(2):79-84, 1985*).

Experimental Double-blind Study: For 2 wks., 21 adult pts. with active but stable <u>bronchial asthma</u> received an elemental diet (Vivasorb) along with mineral water and glucose, while 17 matched controls received regular hospital food blended to approximate the elemental diet in taste and texture. All 38 pts. also received standard medical treatment for their asthma. 9/21 pts. receiving the elemental diet improved (3 dramatically) and none deteriorated, while only 1/17 receiving hospital food clearly improved, and 5 deteriorated markedly. Outcome differences were significant both clinically and statistically. Results suggest that specific food sensitivities are likely to be important for many pts. with perennial asthma and thus they "should be tried with an antigen-free diet, preferably for 2-3 wks., even if the patients present with little or no evidence of extrinsic aetiology" (*Ho:j L et al. A double-blind controlled trial of elemental diet in severe, perennial asthma. <u>Allergy</u> 36:257-62, 1981*).

Experimental Study: 4 pts. with <u>urticaria, rhinitis and/or asthma</u> went into remission after they were placed on additive-free diets (*Freedman BJ. A diet free from additives in the management of allergic disease. <u>Clin. Allergy</u> 7:417-21, 1977*).

Experimental Study: 197 pts. with <u>perennial allergic rhinitis</u> were tested by both skin prick and IgE RAST for the main seasonal and perennial inhalant allergens in that area; if results were negative and environmental control did not relieve symptoms, they were given an elimination diet restricted to rice, olive oil, turkey, lettuce, peeled pears, salt, sugar, water and tea. Those that improved within 3 wks. were challenged with foods and received skin prick tests and IgE RAST for food allergens. When the results of skin prick tests, IgE RAST and food challenges correlated, a diagnosis of of IgE-mediated allergy was made; when such a correlation was not present, a diagnosis of "food intolerance" was made. When food challenges were negative or equivocal and skin pricks and IgE RAST were negative, chemical additive oral challenges were performed. 52/197 (26.4%) had food "intolerance," 19.8% house dust mite allergy, 18.8% seasonal or perennial inhalent allergy, 3.6% cat allergy, 1.5% mold allergy and 23% remained undiagnosed. 24 pts. (12.2%) had hypersensitivity to food additives; 25% of them to acetyl salicylic acid,

8.3% sodium salicylate, 16.6% tartrazine, 16.6% sodium bisulfite and 8% BHT-BHA. The results suggest a surprisingly high incidence of non-IgE-mediated food intolerance as well as hypersensitivity to food additives (*Pastorello E et al. Evaluation of allergic etiology in perennial rhinitis. <u>Ann. Allergy</u> 55:854-56, 1985*).

ANEMIA

See Also: CELIAC DISEASE

NUTRIENTS:

Folic Acid:

Deficiency is well-known to produce a macrocytic anemia.

Supplementation may benefit some pts. with sickle cell anemia.

Experimental Study: SCA pts. benefited from 5 mg. or more folic acid daily (*Lindenbaum J et al. New Engl. J. Med. 269:875, 1963*).

See Also:

Pierce LE, Rath CE. Evidence for folic acid deficiency in the genesis of anemic sickle cell crisis. Blood 20:19, 1962

Pantothenic Acid:

If deficient, supplementation may be beneficial.

Case Report: 53 year-old black female was admitted with anorexia, weight loss, lethargy, incontinence and hypochromic anemia with increased iron storage in the bone marrow. After an unsuccessful trial of pyridoxine, all symptoms and signs improved dramatically following administration of pantothenic acid (pantothenyl alcohol 50-200 mg IM daily). Several years later, a similar clinical picture developed and there was a clinical, but probably not a hematologic, response to a multi-vitamin preparation containing large amts. of pantothenic acid, suggesting that lethargic psychotic pts. with iron-loaded hypochromic anemia unresponsive to pyridoxine might benefit from a trial of pantothenic acid (*McCurdy PR. Is there an anemia responsive to pantothenic acid? J. Am. Geriatr. Soc. 21(2):88-91, 1973*).

Pyridoxine:

Deficiency may cause anemia despite adequate dietary intake and no other evidence of systemic B_6 deficiency (*Bernat I. Pyridoxine responsive anemias, in Iron Metabolism. New York, Plenum Press, 1983, pp. 313-14; Horrigan DL, Harris JW. Pyridoxine-responsive anemias in man. Vit. Hor. 26:549-68, 1968*).

If deficient, supplementation may be beneficial.

Experimental Study: 18/34 pts. with sideroblastic anemia unresponsive to vitamin B_6 and folate had subnormal concentrations of serum and RBC pyridoxal phosphate (PLP) and *in vitro* evidence of defective phosphorylation of pyridoxine and pyridoxal to PLP. Treatment of these pts. with parenteral PLP 25-50 mg 4 times daily for 8-10 days produced significant elevation of hemoglobin in 11 cases (*Hines JD, Love D. Abnormal vitamin B_6 metabolism in sideroblastic anemia: Effect of pyridoxal phosphate therapy. Clin. Res. 23:403A, 1975*).

Experimental Study: 3 pts. who had failed to respond to iron supplementation were given 100 mg B$_6$ daily which resolved the anemia (*Hines JD, Harris JW. Pyridoxine-responsive anemia: Description of three patients with megaloblastic erythropoiesis. Am. J. Clin. Nutr. 14:137-46, 1964*).

See Also:

Tant D. Megaloblastic anaemia due to pyridoxine deficiency associated with prolonged ingestion of an oestrogen-containing oral contraceptive. Brit. Med. J. October 23, 1976, p.979

May be of therapeutic benefit in sickle cell anemia.

Experimental Controlled Study: 16 pts. with SCA had signficantly lower plasma pyridoxal phosphate than controls while their RBC pyridoxal phosphate was significantly elevated, possibly reflecting a greater affinity of PLP to the sickle Hb beta chain than to the normal beta chain. Oral supplementation of 5 pts. with 50 mg. B$_6$ twice daily for 2 months resulted in increased plasma and red cell PLP levels and a slight, insignificant increase in erythrocyte cell number, Hb concentration and hematocrit. One subject also experienced reduction in the frequency and duration of painful crises (*Natta CL, Reynolds RD. Apparent vitamin B$_6$ deficiency in sickle cell anemia. Am. J. Clin. Nutr. 40:235-9, 1984*).

See Also:

Kark JA et al. Pyridoxal phosphate as an antisickling agent in vitro. J. Clin. Invest. 71:1224, 1983

Riboflavin:

Deficiency is associated with a normochromic, normocytic anemia and reticulocytopenia which responds to supplementation.

Experimental Study: Riboflavin deficiency was induced in 8 adult males, each of whom developed an anemia which was reversed by riboflavin administration (*Lane M, Alfrey CP, Jr. The anemia of human riboflavin deficiency. Blood 25(4):432-42, 1965*).

Thiamine:

Deficiency may cause a megaloblastic anemia.

Case Report: A 3 month-old girl presented with symptoms of severe anemia, diabetes, deafness and severe cardiac and neurological distubances which, despite normal blood transketolase, responded to 100 mg daily thiamine and reappeared when treatment was suspended, suggesting that every patient with unexplained anemia deserves a therapeutic trial with high dose thiamine (*Mangel H et al. Thiamine-dependent beriberi in the "thiamine-responsive anemia syndrome." New Engl. J. Med. 311:836-8, 1984*).

Case Report: A case of megaloblastic anemia failed to respond to B$_{12}$ or folic acid but responded to supplementation with oral thiamine 20 mg daily. When, on 2 occasions, the supplementation was stopped, the anemia recurred (*Rogers LE et al. Thiamine-responsive megaloblastic anemia. J. Pediatrics 74(4):494-504, 1969*).

See Also:

Viana MB, Carvalho RI. Thiamine-responsive megaloblastic anemia, sensorineural deafness, and diabetes mellitus: A new syndrome? J. Pediatr. 93:235, 1978

<u>Vitamin A</u>:

Deficiency is associated with anemia due to impaired hemoglobin synthesis which is reversible with supplementation.

Experimental Study: 8 middle-aged males gradually developed anemia several months after being placed on a vitamin-A deficient diet. The decline in serum hemoglobin began well before the loss of night vision or the attainment of "deficient" serum vitamin A values. Repletion with either carotene or vitamin A led to a prompt and complete hematologic recovery (*Hodges RE et al. Hematopoietic studies in vitamin A deficiency. <u>Am. J. Clin. Nutr.</u> 31:876-85, 1978*).

<u>Vitamin B$_{12}$</u>:

Deficiency is well-known to produce a macrocytic anemia.

<u>Vitamin C</u>:

Markedly enhances non-heme iron absorption for the prevention and treatment of <u>iron-deficiency anemia</u> (*Monsen ER. Ascorbic acid: An enhancing factor in iron absorption, in <u>Nutritional Bioavailability of Iron.</u> American Chemical Society, 1982, pp. 85-95*).

<u>Vitamin E</u>:

Deficiency is associated with anemia which responds to supplementation.

Review Article: Vitamin E should be viewed as a potential erythropoietic factor for humans, and it should receive trials in pts. with anemia of obscure etiology, particularly in those with erythroid hyperplasia and unexplained ineffective erythropoiesis (*Drake JR, Fitch CD. Status of vitamin E as an erythropoietic factor. <u>Am. J. Clin. Nutr.</u> 33:2386-93, 1980*).

Experimental Study: Red cell survival was studied using ^{51}Cr-tagged cells in 8 vitamin-E deficient subjects. Before vitamin E therapy, the T 1/2 for ^{51}Cr in all 8 subjects ranged from 10-28 days (mean 19.2 days). Following therapy, the values ranged from 19-30 days (mean 24.9 days), a significant difference (p less than 0.025) (*Leonard PJ, Losowsky MS. Effect of alpha-tocopherol administration on red cell survival in vitamin E-deficient human subjects. <u>Am. J. Clin. Nutr.</u> 24:388-93, 1971*).

The anemia associated with <u>cystic fibrosis</u> and other causes of <u>pancreatic insufficiency</u> may respond to vitamin E supplementation.

Experimental and Observational Study: Cystic fibrosis pts. showed a significant reduction in RBC half-life compared to controls. When treated with vitamin E, RBC survival time approached normal (*Farrell PM et al. <u>J. Clin. Inves.</u> 60:233-41, 1977*).

The anemia associated with <u>Mediterranean-type G$_6$PD deficiency</u> may respond to vitamin E supplementation.

Experimental Study: 23 pts. were treated for 90 days with 800 I.U. oral vitamin E. Compared to baseline values, RBC survival and hemoglobin concentration increased significantly, while reticulocytosis decreased significantly (*Corash L et al. Reduced chronic hemolysis during high-dose vitamin E administration in Mediterranean type glucose-6-phosphate dehydrogenase deficiency. <u>New Engl. J. Med.</u> 303:416-20, 1980*).

<u>Sickle cell anemia</u> may respond to vitamin E supplementation.

Experimental Study: Following administration of 450 IU daily oral vitamin E for 6-35 wks., 6 pts. showed an average decrease of 44% in the number of irreversibly sickled cells (*Natta CL et al. A decrease in irreversibly sickled erythrocytes in sickle cell anemia patients given vitamin E. Am. J. Clin. Nutr. 33:968-71, 1980*).

See Also:

> *Natta CL, Machlin L. Plasma levels of tocopherol in sickle cell anemia subjects. Am. J. Clin. Nutr. 32:1359, 1979*

- -

Copper:

Deficiency is associated with anemia.

Review Article: Nutritional copper deficiency is well documented in both the newborn undergoing rapid growth on a copper-poor diet and in the pt. on total parenteral nutrition for long periods without copper supplementation. In both situations, anemia and neutropenia are the most striking hematologic abnormalities (*Williams DM. Copper deficiency in humans. Semin. Hematol. 20(2):118-28, 1983*).

See Also:

> *Freycon F, Pouyau G. [Rare nutritional deficiency anemia: Deficiency of copper and vitamin E.] Sem. Hop. Paris 59(7):488-93, 1983*

> *Porter KG et al. Anemia and low serum copper during zinc therapy. Lancet October 8, 1977, p. 774*

> *Dunlap WM et al. Anemia and neutropenia caused by copper deficiency. Ann. Int. Med. 80:470, 1974*

Iron:

Deficiency is believed to be the most frequent cause of anemia and responds well to supplementation (*Bernat I. Iron deficiency, in Iron Metabolism. New York, Plenum Press, 1983, pp.215-74*).

Zinc:

May be deficient in sickle cell anemia.

Observational Study: 34 pts. with SCA in a steady state were found to have significantly lower plasma levels and higher urinary levels of zinc than 50 controls. During sickle cell crisis, the plasma zinc levels dropped to a mean value of 0.54 mcg/ml from a steady state value of 0.79 mcg/ml (*Niell HB et al. Zinc metabolism in sickle cell anemia. JAMA 242(24):2686-90, 1979*).

If deficient, supplementation may be beneficial.

Oral zinc decreased the mean number of circulating irreversibly sickled erythrocytes in 12 pts. from 28.0% to 18.6%, suggesting improved oxygenation (*Brewer GJ et al. Suppression of irreversibly sickled erythrocytes by zinc therapy in sickle cell anemia. J. Lab. Clin. Med. 90(3):549-54, 1977*).

- -

COMBINED SUPPLEMENTATION:

<u>Folic Acid,</u>
<u>Vitamin B$_{12}$</u> and
<u>Iron:</u>

Supplementation may be beneficial in <u>anemia of pregnancy</u>.

Experimental Study: Hemoglobin concentration rose in all pregnant pts. given iron, but declined in those given no iron. Those given folic acid and vitamin B$_{12}$ in addition to iron showed an even greater rise in mean hemoglobin concentration than those given iron only (*Sood SK et al. J. Trop. Med. Hyg. 77:177, 1974*).

Experimental Study: 3 gps.of pregnant pts. took daily doses of iron 100 mg, iron 100 mg and folate 300 mcg, or folate 300 mcg. 96% of the women receiving iron and folate showed a rise in hemoglobin, while only 26% of those receiving iron or folate alone showed such a rise. When a program was instituted in which iron and folate were given to all pregnant women in a selected community, anemia was reduced from over 50% to below 6% (*Izak G et al. Scand. J. Haematol. 11:236, 1973*).

- -

OTHER FACTORS:

Rule out <u>hydrochloric acid deficiency</u> in <u>iron-deficiency anemia</u>.

If deficient, iron absorption is significantly impaired.

Experimental Study: In pts. with iron-deficiency anemia, iron absorption was found to be related to the maximal acid output of the stomach following a histamine infusion (*Jacobs A et al. Gastric acidity and iron absorption. Brit. J. Haematol. 12:728-36, 1966*).

If deficient, supplementation may be beneficial.

Experimental Study: 24 pts. with histamine-fast achlorhydria were given iron 5 mg in 300 ml water or in 300 ml 0.05 N HCl. Both ferric chloride and ferrous ascorbate were better absorbed with acid, although acid failed to increase the absorption of hemoglobin iron (*Jacobs P et al. Role of hydrochloric acid in iron absorption. J. App. Physiol. 19(2):187-8, 1964*).

Experimental Study: 25 diabetic pts. with blood counts 4.2 million or less who were under good diabetic control were randomly selected to receive glutamic acid HCl 5 gr 3 times daily before meals which, at the end of 1 month, was replaced by ferrous carbonate 6 3/4 gr 3 times daily. At the end of another month, both supplements were prescribed concomitantly. Following the first month, the RBC increased significantly from 4.06 to 4.56 million, while iron supplementation failed to be followed by a significant change. Following combined supplementation, RBC again increased significantly by 1/4 million. The experiment was replicated with similar results (*Rabinowich IM. Achlorhydria and its clinical significance in diabetes mellitus. Am J. Dig. Dis. 16:322-32, 1949*).

ANOREXIA NERVOSA

NUTRIENTS:

<u>Zinc</u>: zinc sulfate 50 mg. 3 times daily with meals

Zinc deficiency is well known to be detrimental to taste and smell. Anorexia can therefore be caused by zinc deficiency which, in turn, can be caused by inadequate intake, the use of oral contraceptives or impaired absorption.

Observational Study: Zinc nutriture was evaluated in 14 hospitalized female pts. with severe AN (mean age 21.7 yrs.) and 10 controls. Although overall plasma and neutrophil zinc concentrations were comparable in the patients and controls, 3 pts. had low neutrophil zinc concentrations and 2 of these also had low plasma zinc and albumin concentrations, while 1 pt. had a low plasma zinc but normal neutrophil zinc and albumin. None of the pts. had clinical signs of zinc deficiency (*Ainley CC et al. Zinc state in anorexia nervosa. <u>Brit. Med. J.</u> Vol. 293, October 18, 1986*).

Experimental Study: Following an overnight fast and a standard meal supplemented with 50 mg zinc, serum zinc levels were lower in pts. than in normals, suggesting that pts. either have reduced zinc absorption or rapid transfer or secretion of zinc which further worsens the problem of reduced dietary intake (*Dinsmore WW et al. Zinc absorption in anorexia nervosa. Letter to the Editor. <u>Lancet</u> 1:1041-2, 1985*).

Supplementation may be beneficial, especially if deficient.

Experimental Study: 5 young female pts. were supplemented with 45-90 mg Zn^{++} (as zinc sulphate) daily. Follow-up averaged 6 months. The pt. with the longest follow-up (16 mo.) gained 10.8 kg over the first 11 mo. of zinc therapy, the total weight gain over 16 mo. being 11.5 kilogram. The remaining 4 pts. gained an ave. of 0.7 kg/month (*Safai-Kutti S, Kutti J. Zinc therapy in anorexia nervosa. Letter to the Editor. <u>Am. J. Psychiat.</u> 143(8):1059, 1986*).

Case Report: 13 year old girl was believed to have a zinc deficiency (unable to taste 0.1% zinc sulfate solution). After 2 wks. supplementation with zinc (initially 15 mg daily, then 50 mg 3 times daily), appetite and mood began to improve. After 4 months of supplementation, she gained 13 kg., her depression cleared and she became able to taste the zinc solution. 10 months after discontinuation of zinc, she had returned to her initial state which again improved after zinc was reintroduced (*Bryce-Simth D, Simpson RID. Case of anorexia nervosa responding to zinc sulphate. Letter to the Editor. <u>Lancet</u> 2:350, 1984*).

See Also:

Bryce-Smith D, Simpson RID. *Anorexia, depression and zinc deficiency. <u>Lancet</u> 2:1162, 1984*

Safai-Kutti S, Kutti J. *Zinc and anorexia nervosa. <u>Ann. Int. Med.</u> 100:317-18, 1984*

Bakan R. *The role of zinc in anorexia nervosa: Etiology and treatment. <u>Med. Hypotheses</u> 5:731-6, 1979*

Esca SA et al. *Kwashiorkor-like zinc deficiency syndrome in anorexia nervosa. <u>Acta Derm. Venereol. (Stockh.)</u> 59:361-64, 1979*

- -

<u>Essential Fatty Acids:</u>

May be deficient.

Observational Study: 17 hospitalized pts. were found to be deficient in circulating essential fatty acids as compared to normal controls, suggesting that they were at risk for developing clinical signs of essential fatty acid deficiency (*Langan SM, Farrell PM. <u>Am. J. Clin. Nutr.</u> 41:1054-60, 1985*).

ANXIETY

Associated with elevated <u>lactate</u> levels (*Buist RA. Anxiety neurosis: The lactate connection.* <u>*Int. Clin. Nutr. Rev. 5:1-4, 1985*</u>).

BASIC DIET:

Avoid <u>alcohol</u>.

Increases the lactate to pyruvate ratio (*Alberti KG, Nattrass, M.* <u>*Lancet*</u> *2:25-9, 1977*).

Avoid <u>caffeine</u>.

Increases the lactate to pyruvate ratio (*Alberti - ibid*).

Pts. with <u>panic disorder</u> are unusually sensitive.

Experimental Controlled Study: 21 pts. with either agoraphobia with panic attacks or panic disorder and 17 healthy controls ingested caffeine 10 mg/kilogram. Caffeine produced significantly greater increases in subject-rated anxiety, nervousness, fear, nausea, palpitations, restlessness and tremors in the pts. than in the controls. Only in the pts., these symptoms were significantly correlated with plasma caffeine levels. 71% of the pts. reported that the behavioral effects of caffeine were similar to those experienced during panic attacks (*Charney DS et al. Increased anxiogenic effects of caffeine in panic disorders.* <u>*Arch. Gen. Psychiat.*</u> *42:233-243, 1985*).

Experimental Double-blind Study: In response to a caffeine challenge, plasma cortisol levels, but not plasma MHPG levels, increased as did anxiety in both panic disorder pts. and controls. Two normal control subjects experienced panic attacks accompanied by a 5-fold increase in plasma cortisol after the higher of the 2 challenge doses (720 mg) (*Uhde TW et al. Caffeine and behavior: Relation to psychopathology and underlying mechanisms. Caffeine: Relationship to human anxiety, plasma MHPG and cortisol.* <u>*Psychopharm. Bull.*</u> *20(3):426-30, 1984*).

Observational Study: Pts. with panic anxiety disorder, but not affectively ill pts. or normal controls, had self-rated anxiety and depression levels that correlated with their degree of caffeine consumption (*Boulenger JP et al. Increased sensitivity to caffeine in patients with panic disorders: Preliminary evidence.* <u>*Arch. Gen. Psychiat.*</u> *41:1067-1071, 1984*).

Review Article: Not only may high caffeine intake produce symptoms which mimic anxiety disorders, but the caffeine withdrawal syndrome may also mimic anxiety (*Greden JF. Anxiety or caffeinism: A diagnostic dilemma.* <u>*Am. J. Psychiat.*</u> *Oct. 1974*).

Avoid <u>sugar</u>.

Stimulates blood sugar fluctuations by causing insulin release. Lower values of blood sugar are associated with anxiety for some people (numerous case reports) and glucose infusion can produce panic attacks in susceptible individuals (*Rainey JM et al.* <u>*Psychopharmac. Bull.*</u> *20(1):45-9, 1984*).

NUTRIENTS:

Rule out <u>vitamin B complex</u> deficiencies.

Observational Study: Of 12 agoraphobic pts., 7 were deficient in thiamine (TPP% uptake in RBC transketolase activity), 6 in pyridoxine (RBC glutamic-pyruvic transaminase), 3 in niacin (1-N-methyl-nicotinamide), 3 in vitamin B_{12} (serum B_{12} & MMA) 2 in folic acid (serum folate & FIGLU), and 1 in riboflavin (RBC glutathione reductase) (*Abbey LC. Agoraphobia. J. Orthomol. Psychiat. 11:243-259, 1982*).

Experimental Study: 23 agoraphobic pts. (including the 12 noted above) received dietary counseling, high-potency broad spectrum nutritional supplementation, and additional megavitamin supplementation for deficiencies found on laboratory testing. After 3 mo., 19/23 showed a dramatic improvement and 11/19 were free of panic attacks (*Abbey - ibid*).

-<u>Niacinamide</u>: 500 mg. twice daily

Postulated to increase conversion of lactate (associated with high levels of anxiety) to pyruvate (*Buist - op cit*).

Shown in an animal study to have anti-conflict, anti-aggressive, muscle relaxant and hypnotic actions with effectiveness similar to that of minor tranquilizers (*M:ohler H et al. Nicotinamide is a brain constituent with benzodiazepine-like actions. Nature 278:563-65, 1979*).

- <u>Pyridoxine</u>: 100 mg. daily

May diminish conversion of pyruvate to lactate by promoting transanimation reactions which produce substrate to feed the Krebs Cycle (*Buist - op cit*).

- <u>Thiamine</u>: 100 mg daily

May diminish conversion of pyruvate (from glucose) to lactate (associated with high levels of anxiety) by activating pyruvate dehydrogenase (*Buist - op cit*)

<u>Calcium:</u>

Hypocalcemia may be associated with an organic anxiety syndrome.

Case Reports:
1. 49 year-old postmenopausal vegetarian female with 30 yr. history of generalized anxiety with inability to relax, trembling, sweating, apprehensiveness, worry, insomnia, and occasional depression with worsening of symptoms associated with stress. After 1 1/2 yrs. of psychotherapy, her symptoms suddenly increased despite a lack of precipitating stresses and were unrelieved by oxazepam. 5 wks. later, she developed severe chest pain which was found to be due to 2 spontaneous rib fractures. Evaluation revealed marked osteoporosis and a serum calcium of 7.2 mg/dL (normal = 8.5-10.5 mg/dL). Her anxiety was reduced to its former level following correction of the hypocalcemia and the addition of estrogens.
2. 58 year-old insulin-dependent diabetic female with 35 yr. history of generalized anxiety disorder with worry, fear, sweating, shaking, insomnia, and mild depression. One day she reported increasing severity of all symptoms, with frequent panic attacks and a "completely different feeling." She proceeded to develop muscle spasms, stuttering, and tetany with a positive Chvostek's sign. Her serum calcium was 6.1 mg/dL. Further evaluation revealed idiopathic hypoparathyroidism. Following medical treatment her anxiety decreased to its previous level.

(Carlson RJ.   Longitudinal observations of two cases of organic anxiety syndrome.   Psychosomatics 27(7):529-31, 1986).

See Also:

Crammer JL.   Calcium metabolism and mental disorder.   Psychol. Med. 7:557-60, 1977

Houssain M.   Neurological and psychiatric manifestations in idiopathic hypoparathyroidism: Response to treatment.   J. Neurol. Neurosurg. Psychiat. 33:153-56, 1970

Denko JD, Kaelbling R.   The psychiatric aspects of hypoparathyroidism.   Acta Psychiat. Scand. 164 (suppl.):1.70, 1962

<u>Magnesium:</u>   250 - 750 mg. daily

Depletion increases the lactate to pyruvate ratio (*Buist - op cit*).

Said to be useful, especially when given with calcium, for nervousness and insomnia (*August F. Daro, professor emeritus, Stritch School of Medicine, Maywood, Illinois, 1981*).

- -

<u>L-Tryptophan:</u>

Dietary precursor to the neurotransmitter serotonin, a deficiency of which may be associated with anxiety.

- with <u>pyridoxine</u>:

Experimental Study: Pts. with <u>hyperventilation syndrome</u> were treated with tryptophan and pyridoxine. All pts. who had been found to have abnormal urinary excretion of xanthurenic acid improved, and their XA excretion following loading with pyridoxine and tryptophan normalized (*Hoes M et al. Hyperventilation syndrome, treatment with L-tryptophan and pyridoxine; Predictive values of xanthurenic acid excretion. J. Orthomol. Psychiat. 10(1):7-15, 1981*).

APHTHOUS STOMATITIS
(CANKER SORES)

NUTRIENTS:

Folic Acid,
Vitamin B$_{12}$, and/or
Iron:

Experimental and Observational Study: 47/330 (14.2%) pts were deficient in iron (#23), vitamin B$_{12}$ (#6), folic acid (#7) or 2 or more of these nutrients (#11). After 39 of these pts. with proven nutritional deficiencies received supplementation for 6 months (oral iron for 6 mo., B$_{12}$ IM every 2 mo., folic acid 5 mg 3 times daily), 23/39 had a remission, 11/39 improved, and 5/39 were not helped (*Wray DW et al. Nutritional deficiencies in recurrent aphthae. J. Oral Pathology 7:418-23, 1978*).

Zinc:

Experimental Double-blind Study: Supplementation resulted in small but statistically insignificant improvement (*Wray D. A double blind trial of systemic zinc sulfate in recurrent aphthous stomatitis. Oral Surg 53:469, 1982*).

- -

OTHER FACTORS:

Rule out food sensitivities.

Review Article: Despite the many anecdotal reports, there are no systematic studies demonstrating a causal relationship between foods and canker sores (*Bock SA. Do certain foods cause canker sores? Questions and answers. JAMA 257(3):379, 1987*).

Experimental Study: 5/12 pts. improved on a strict elimination diet and were found to be reactive to milk, cheese, wheat, tomato, vinegar, lemon, pineapple and mustard (*Hay KD, Reade PC. The use of an elimination diet in the treatment of recurrent aphthous ulceration of the oral cavity. Oral Surg., Oral Med., Oral Path. 57(5):504-7, 1984*).

Experimental Study: 25% of pts. responded to removal of gluten (*Wray D. Gluten-sensitive recurrent aphthous stomatitis. Dig. Dis. Sci. 26:737, 1981*).

Experimental Study: Gluten withdrawal resulted in complete remission of symptoms of aphthous stomatitis in pts. with celiac disease (*Ferguson R et al. Coeliac disease associated with recurrent aphthae. Gut 21:223-6, 1980*).

Observational Study: 18% of 61 pts. could associate development of the ulcers with the ingestion of specific foods (*Wilson CWM. Food sensitivities, taste changes, aphthous ulcers and atopic symptoms in allergic disease. Annals of Allergy May, 1980, pp. 302-7*).

ATHEROSCLEROSIS

See also: CARDIAC ARRHYTHMIA
CEREBROVASCULAR DISEASE

OVERVIEW:

A. To prevent the development of atherosclerosis and/or mortality from atherosclerosis.

Reduction of <u>dietary cholesterol</u> may be beneficial, but only for those whose serum cholesterol levels are affected by dietary cholesterol. Studies have suggested an association between the dietary intake of not only <u>animal fats</u>, but also <u>hydrogenated vegetable oils</u> (which have been promoted as beneficial due to their lack of cholesterol) and atherogenesis. <u>Vegetables</u> appear to be the best source of protein, and the consumption of <u>complex carbohydrates</u>, as opposed to refined sugars, should be encouraged. Epidemiologic studies suggest that <u>coffee</u> should be restricted, although it is still unclear if other atherogenic dietary factors which correlate with coffee consumption explain these findings. The contribution of <u>alcohol</u> may depend upon intake, with a maximum of 2 drinks daily being beneficial, and higher consumption having adverse effects.

Epidemiologic studies suggest that the consumption of <u>cold water fish</u> (which have a high concentration of <u>omega-3 fatty acids</u>) is beneficial, and the results of a number of experimental studies suggest that this may be due to positive effects on lipid metabolism, platelet aggregation and blood viscosity.

Marginal deficiencies of <u>pyridoxine</u>, <u>vitamin C</u>, <u>chromium</u>, <u>magnesium</u>, <u>selenium</u> or <u>linoleic acid</u> increase the risk of AS and/or the mortality from AS; thus laboratory testing to determine tissue nutriture may be of value. Supplementation with these nutrients may still be beneficial even when they are not deficient.

Dietary supplementation with certain other nutrients may also be beneficial. <u>Niacin</u> 3 gm daily (in slowly increasing doses with meals) has been shown to lower both the mortality rate and the incidence of nonfatal MI's among men with at least 1 previous MI. Supplementation with <u>condroitin sulfate A</u>, a glycosaminoglycan, reduced the incidence of MI and the mortality rate in coronary pts. compared to controls.

In animal studies, the development of AS has been prevented or retarded using <u>chromium</u>, <u>potassium iodide</u>, <u>taurine</u>, <u>eggplant</u> (along with foods rich in <u>vitamin C</u>), <u>garlic</u> or <u>onion</u>.

B. To promote regression of atherosclerotic plaques:

Scientific literature showing specific nutrients to induce plaque regression in humans is lacking. Three animal studies deserve mention: The addition of 3% <u>soya lecithin</u> to the diet for 3 mo. modified arterial lesions in rabbits with cholesterol-induced atherogenesis, supplementation with <u>bromelain</u> broke down plaque in rabbit aortas both *in vitro* and *in vivo*, and arteriosclerotic monkeys fed a diet enriched with <u>alfalfa</u> 50 gm daily showed signs of plaque regression in their coronary arteries.

C. To reduce angina pectoris:

<u>Magnesium</u> deficiency may adversely affect cardiac function and is not uncommon among angina patients; thus a leukocyte magnesium level is indicated. <u>L-carnitine</u> 750 mg - 1 gm twice daily has been

shown to be effective in several studies, some of them well-controlled. Several other nutrients may be beneficial, but the scientific evidence is not as strong.

D. To reduce intermittent claudication:

Scientific studies in this area are limited. In a 6 mo. randomized double-blind study, pts. receiving ginkgo biloba extract demonstrated significantly greater pain-free and maximum walking distance, as well as improved plethysmographic and doppler measurements in the affected limb after exercise, compared to controls. Vitamin E (D-alpha-tocopherol) 100 IU 3 times daily has been shown in a controlled study to improve walking distance and increase calf blood flow within 3 months.   Patients demonstrated arteriographic evidence of improved circulation following supplementation with vitamin C 500 mg 3 times daily for several months and, in an uncontrolled study, zinc sulfate 220 mg 3 times daily for at least 1 yr. was followed by limited symptomatic improvement in some patients.

E. To reduce cardiac arrhythymias:

Several studies have suggested that magnesium supplementation may be beneficial, perhaps because it corrects a magnesium deficiency in the myocardium (which may be evaluated with a leukocyte or lymphocyte magnesium level.) Potassium supplementation may also be beneficial, and there is preliminary evidence from animal studies that taurine may be of value.

F. To lower serum lipid levels:

A low fat, low cholesterol, high fiber diet with a high ratio of polyunsaturates to saturated fat has been well-validated. It may well be of value to avoid sugar and there are several observational studies which suggest that substantial coffee consumption is associated with higher cholesterol levels.

If nutritional supplementation is needed, the use of niacin (with the dosage raised slowly to no more than 6 gm in divided doses with meals) is well-validated (although it may have significant side-effects) and a number of controlled studies suggest that omega-3 fatty acids may be effective. Several other nutrients may be beneficial, although their validation is more limited.

G. To reduce platelet adhesiveness and/or aggregation:

Sugar has been shown to increase both adhesiveness and aggregation and should thus be restricted. A number of nutrients have been shown to have beneficial effects, including pyridoxine 50-150 mg, vitamin C 1-3 gm, vitamin E 400-1200 IU, magnesium 500-750 mg (especially if deficient), selenium 200 mcg (especially if deficient), bromelain, glycosaminoglycans, omega-3 and omega-6 fatty acids, pantethine, garlic, ginger and onions.

H. To promote fibrinolysis:

Both garlic and onion have been shown to increase fibrinolytic activity.

- -

KEY:		
	A	= concerns angina pectoris
	C	= concerns total cholesterol
	F	= concerns fibrinolysis
	G	= concerns atherogenesis
	H	= concerns HDL cholesterol
	I	= concerns intermittent claudication
	L	= concerns LDL cholesterol
	P	= concerns platelet adhesiveness and/or aggregation
	T	= concerns triglycerides

BASIC DIET:

Low <u>fat</u> diet (below 25% of calories).

Total dietary fat has been shown to be a major determinant of total serum cholesterol levels (*Keys A et al. Lessons from serum cholesterol studies in Japan, Hawaii and Los Angeles. Ann. Int. Med. 48:83, 1958*) including, the HDL cholesterol fraction (*Mensink RP, Katan MB. Effect of monunsaturated fatty acids versus complex carbohydrates on high-density lipoproteins in healthy men and women. Lancet 1:122-25, 1987*).

Fats should come mainly from <u>polyunsaturates</u> as saturated fats are twice as powerful in raising serum cholesterol as unsaturated fats are in lowering it (*Keys A, Parlin RW. Serum cholesterol response to changes in dietary lipids. Am. J. Clin. Nutr. 19:175, 1966; Hegsted DM et al. Quantitative effects of dietary fat on serum cholesterol in man. Am. J. Clin. Nutr. 17:281, 1965*).

> *Note: Olive oil, which is particularly rich in oleic acid, a <u>mono-unsaturate</u>, has a similar effect (Keys A. Lowering plasma cholesterol by diet. N. Engl. J. Med. 315(9):585, 1986; Grundy SM. N. Engl. J. Med. 314:745-48, 1986) and has been shown to <u>raise</u> HDL cholesterol (Mensink RP, Katan MB. Effect of monunsaturated fatty acids versus complex carbohydrates on high-densty lipoproteins in healthy men and women. Lancet 1:122-25, 1987), although it may stimulate malignant cell proliferation (see "<u>CANCER</u>").*

> **Experimental Study (C,H,L,T):** 22 normolipidemic women (ages 22-55) consumed the following diets consecutively for 6 wks. each:
>   1. Reference diet: P/S ratio 0.16, fat from meat, fish, poultry, milk, cheese (42% of energy) and carbohydrate (46% of energy).
>   2. Polyunsaturated diet: P/S ratio 0.1 - inclusion of sunflower oil and diet margarine.
>   3. Low fat, polyunsaturated diet: P/S ratio 0.1, fats (32% of energy) and carbohydrates (56% of energy) - less whole milk, more bread and potatoes than diet 2.
> When compared to diet 1, diet 2 caused a decrease in cholesterol and apolipoprotein B levels in VDRL without altering HDL. Diet 3 did not alter VDRL cholesterol, but caused a return of VDRL triglycerides to higher levels. VLDL lipoprotein B and apolipoprotein E both decreased in diet 3. Results suggest that polyunsaturated diets lower levels of VLDL and LDL, while HDL levels remain unchanged. Restriction of dietary fat causes a decrease in apolipoprotein E enriched VLDL levels - high levels of which in animals are associated with an accelerated development of atherosclerosis (*Weisweiler P et al. Influence of polyunsaturated fat restriction on serum lipoproteins in humans. Metabolism 34(1):83-7, 1985*).

> **Experimental Study (H):** In a study of 117 pts. aged 44-60, saturated fat intake was negatively correlated with serum HDL cholesterol (*Fehily A et al. Am. J. Clin. Nutr. 36:890-6, 1982*).

Saturated fat intake is at least as closely related to arterial and venous thrombosis as it is to atherosclerosis and is more closely related to the clotting activity of platelets and their response to thrombin than serum cholesterol (*Renaud S. Dietary fatty acids and platelet function. Proc. Nutr. Soc. Aust. 10:1-13, 1985*).

Low <u>cholesterol</u> diet.

> **Review Article:** In the usual range of dietary cholesterol (0 - 400 mg/1000 kcal), each 1 mg/1000 kcal results in approx. a 0.1 mg/dl increase in serum cholesterol (*Hagsted DM. Serum-cholesterol response to dietary cholesterol: A re-evaluation. Am. J. Clin. Nutr. 44(2):299-305, 1986*).

> *Note: Dietary cholesterol in general has less effect on plasma cholesterol than does saturated fats, although a minority will respond to a reduction in dietary cholesterol (Truswell AS. Reducing the risk of coronary heart disease. Brit. Med. J. Vol 291, July 6, 1985).*

Experimental Double-blind, Crossover Study (L): 17 college-aged lactovegetarians who usually consumed an ave. of 3 eggs/wk. were randomly assigned to either a 1 egg/ day diet or an identical-looking, egg-free diet. The egg diet was significantly correlated with raised LDL cholesterol and apolipoprotein B levels compared to the control diet, while HDL cholesterol levels were unchanged (*Sacks E et al. Ingestion of egg raises plasma low-density lipoproteins in free-living subjects.* <u>*Lancet*</u> *2:647-9, 1984*)

Observational Study (C): In a study of 912 subjects, results suggested that "differences in egg consumption usually observed in a free-living U.S. population, consuming large amounts of fats and cholesterol from other sources, are unrelated to intrapopulation differences in blood cholesterol level." The data fail to show, however, the effect of egg consumption upon people who consume negligible amounts of cholesterol from other dietary sources (*Dawber T et al. Eggs, serum cholesterol and coronary heart disease.* <u>*Am. J. Clin. Nutr.*</u> *36:617-25, 1982*).

Experimental Study (C): 1 egg a day (250 mg cholesterol) added to the diet had little effect on plasma cholesterol in 37/44 subjects (*Bronsgeest-Schoute et al.* <u>*Am. J. Clin. Nutr.*</u> *32:2193-7, 1979*).

Avoid <u>hydrogenated vegetable oils</u>.

Examples: Margarine; vegetable shortenings

Hydrogenated vegetable oils appear to be as atherogenic as animal fats; whether they are <u>more</u> atherogenic is as of yet unclear.

1. Dietary intake of hydrogenated vegetable oils is associated epidemiologically with atherosclerosis, just as is dietary intake of animal fats (*Martin W. Margarine (not butter) the culprit? Letter to the Editor.* <u>*Lancet*</u> *2:407, 1983; Kummerow FA. Nutrition imbalance and angiotoxins as dietary risk factors in coronary heart disease.* <u>*Am. J. Clin. Nutr.*</u> *32:58-83, 1979*).

2. When hydrogenated vegetable oils were tested against butter ingestion under clinically controlled conditions, the difference in serum cholesterol was insignificant (*Kummerow FA - op cit*).

3. Animal studies suggest that hydrogenated vegetable fats are at least as atherogenic as animal fats.

   Animal Experimental Study: Mature swine that had been supplemented with hydrogenated fat for 8 mo. had a greater number of atherosclerotic lesions in their aortas than swine supplemented with animal fat (*Kummerow FA et al. The influence of three sources of dietary fats and cholesterol on lipid composition of swine serum lipids and aorta tissue.* <u>*Artery*</u> *4:360, 1978*).

4. Hydrogenated vegetable oils have a high content of *trans* fatty acids which <u>elevate</u> cholesterol, perhaps because of their anti-essential fatty acid action (*Hill EG et al. Intensification of essential fatty acid deficiency in the rat by dietary trans-fatty acids.* <u>*J. Nutr.*</u> *109:1759-67, 1979*), while the natural *cis* isomer <u>lowers</u> it.

   Animal Experimental Study (C): When swine were fed a hydrogenated fat which contained 50% *trans* fatty acids, their serum cholesterol levels were 14 mg/100 ml higher than those fed animal fat even though the animal fat contained 25% more saturated fatty acids. In addition, the serum lipoproteins isolated from swine fed a basal diet that had been supplemented with animal or hydrogenated vegetable fat for 6 mo. did not differ significantly in composition (*Jackson RL et al. Influence of dietary trans-fatty acids on swine lipoprotein composition and structure.* <u>*J. Lipid Res.*</u> *18:182, 1977*).

   See Also:

   > *Anderson JT et al. Effect on serum cholesterol in man of fatty acids produced by hydrogenation of corn oil.* <u>*Fed. Proc.*</u> *20:96, 1961*

Avoid deep frying and otherwise minimize heating of fats.

Fat which has been used to deep fry chicken or fish can contain as much as 214 mg cholesterol per 100 gm (*Kummerow FA. Nutrition imbalance and angiotoxins as dietary risk factors in coronary heart disease. Am. J. Clin. Nutr. 32:58-83, 1979*).

Heating of fat is believed to oxidize cholesterol to form 25-hydroxy cholesterol which has been shown to accelerate degeneration of smooth muscle cells in arterial tissue (*Imai H et al. Angiotoxicity and arterioscleosis due to contaminants of USP-grade cholesterol. Arch. Pathol. Lab. Med., 100:565, 1976*), thus setting the stage for the development of atherosclerosis (*Alexander JC. Chemical and biological properties related to toxicity of heated fats. J. Tox. Env. Health 7:125-38, 1981; Kummerow FA - op cit*).

> *Note: Heating foods in a microwave would minimize the formation of 25-hydroxy cholesterol (Kummerow FA - op cit).*

High fiber diet (ex. oats; barley; pectin; alfalfa).

Improves lipid metabolism.

> *Note: Water-insoluble fibers (ex. wheat fiber, cellulose) are minimally effective in improving lipid metabolism compared to water-soluble fibers (ex. oat bran, guar gum, pectin) which are moderately effective due to their ability to decrease cholesterol absorption by binding dietary and biliary cholesterol.*

Experimental Study (C,H,L,T): 4 gps. of 6 healthy young men received diets providing 0, 18, 36 or 52% of calories as sucrose. Each diet was fed with both low (below 14 gm) and high (above 34 gm) levels of dietary fiber for 10 days each. Triglycerides increased during the 36% and 52% sucrose diets compared to the 0 and 18% sucrose diets, and fiber protected partially against this rise. Serum cholesterol and LDL cholesterol were lower during the 0% and 18% sucrose diets than the 36% and 52% sucrose diets, but fiber had no effect. HDL cholesterol decreased during all low fat diets, with a trend toward a greater decrease during the high sucrose diets. Results suggest that fiber protects against sucrose-induced lipemia but has no effect on cholesterol (*Albrink M, Ullrich IH. Am. J. Clin. Nutr. 43:419-28, 1986*).

Negative Experimental Crossover Study (C,H,T): 3 gps. of 10 normals received pectin 12 gm daily, cellulose 15 gm daily or lignin 12 gm daily in 8-wk. randomized crossover studies. Dietary records showed that diet was otherwise unchanged. None of the 3 fibers altered total cholesterol, HDL cholesterol, triglycerides or the ratio of HDL cholesterol to total cholesterol (*Hillman LC et al. The effects of the fiber components pectin, cellulose and lignin on serum cholesterol levels. Am. J. Clin. Nutr. 42(2):207-13, 1985*).

Experimental Study (C): Healthy volunteers received 36 gm of wheat fiber, pectin or guar gum for 2 weeks while on their normal diets. Mean serum cholesterol levels fell significantly while they received guar and pectin, but rose slightly after wheat fiber (*Jenkins DJA et al. Effect of pectin, guar gum, and wheat fiber on serum-cholesterol. Lancet May 17, 1975 pp.1116-7*).

Cereal fibers:

Negative Experimental Study (C,T): 82 male pts. with a previous MI received wheat bran 70-80 gm daily. There was no evidence of a hypolipidemic action (*Meshcheryakova A et al. Effect of wheat bran included in an anti-atherosclerotic diet on some lipid metabolism parameters in patients with coronary heart disease. Vopr. Pitan. 1985, pp. 9-13*).

Experimental Study (H): Wheat fiber (purified) 10.5 gm daily significantly increased HDL cholesterol (*Lindgarde F, Larsson L. Effects of concentrated bran fibre preparation on HDL-cholesterol in hypercholesterolemic men. Human Nutr.: Clin. Nutr. 38C:39-45, 1984*).

Experimental Controlled Study (C,H,L): Control and oat-bran diets were given in alternating sequence to 8 hypercholesterolemic men receiving standardized diets. On the experimental diet, serum total C concentration was reduced 13%, plasma LDL cholesterol was reduced 14% and HDL cholesterol was unchanged (*Kirby RW et al. Oat-bran intake selectively lowers serum low-density lipoprotein cholesterol concentrations of hypercholesterolemic men. Am. J. Clin. Nutr. 34(5):824-9, 1981*).

Guar gum:

Experimental Study (C): 13 diabetics substituted 2 rolls/day with 2.5 gm guar gum for 2 servings of their usual bread for 12 weeks. Total serum cholesterol decreased by 7.3% after 4 wks., 8.3% after 8 wks., and 13.8% after 12 weeks (*McNaughton JP et al. Changes in total serum cholesterol levels of diabetics fed 5 grams guar gum daily. Nutr. Rep. Int. 31(3):505-20, 1985*).

Experimental Single-blind Study (C,H,L,T): 19 pts. with primary hypercholesterolemia previously stabilized on diet alone received guar gum 6 gm 3 times daily with meals. 2 pts. withdrew immediately due to serious diarrhea. Of 13 pts. who completed 1 yr. of treatment, plasma cholesterol was reduced 15% (p less than 0.001) during the first 3 mo. and this effect was sustained for 12 months. The fall in plasma cholesterol was associated with a significant 20% fall in LDL cholesterol, but no change in HDL cholesterol and no significant change in triglycerides (*Simons LA et al. Long-term treatment of hypercholesterolaemia with a new palatable formulation of guar gum. Atherosclerosis 45(1):101-108, 1982*).

See Also:

> Khalsa N, Sharma PK. *Effect of guar cyamopsas-tetragonoloba on serum lipids, uric acid and proteins. Indian J. Nutr. Diet 17(8):297-301, 1980 (recd. 1981)*

Pectin:

Experimental Study (C): 2-3 apples daily (1 month trial) were effective in lowering total blood cholesterol levels for 24/30 healthy subjects whose diets were otherwise uncontrolled. Since 2-3 gm pectin-in-apple produces the same effect as 6-50 gm of purified pectin, other components of apples may also be involved (*Sable-Amplis R et al. Further studies on the cholesterol-lowering effect of apple in humans. Nutr. Res. 3:325-8, 1983*).

In vitro Experimental Study (L): Grapefruit pectin was found to interact specifically with low-density lipoprotein, suggesting a biochemical basis by which it may cause lowering of serum and/or tissue cholesterol levels (*Baig MM, Cerda JJ. Pectin: Its interaction with serum lipoproteins. Am. J. Clin. Nutr. 34:50-53, 1981*).

Experimental Study (L): After 4 wks. of pectin supplementation, 17 pts. showed a 25% reduction in ave. LDL cholesterol levels (*Richter W et al. Therapy of hypercholesterolemia with apple pectin. Dtsch. Med. Wochensche 106(19):628, 1981*).

Experimental Study (C,T): Citrus pectin 15 gm daily was added to metabolically controlled diets in 9 subjects. After 3 wks., total plasma cholesterol was reduced by a mean of 13% (p less than 0.001), fecal fat excretion increased by 44% (p less than 0.001), neutral steroids by 17% (p less than 0.001) and fecal bile acids by 33% (p less than 0.02), while plasma triglycerides did not change (*Kay RM, Truswell AS. Effect of citrus pectin on blood lipids and fecal steroid excretion. Am. J. Clin. Nutr. 30(2):171-75, 1977*).

<u>Vegetable</u> (instead of animal)<u>protein.</u>

Saponins in plants decrease cholesterol absorption by competing for cholesterol binding sites (*Potter JD, et al. Soya, saponins and plasma cholesterol. <u>Lancet</u> 1:223-4, 1979*).

Experimental Controlled Study: 39 pts. with stable angina pectoris were placed on a vegetarian diet designed to increase the polyunsaturated/saturated fat ratio to at least 2 and to decrease cholesterol intake to below 100 mg daily. After 1 yr., the P/S ratio was 2.54 (polyunsaturated fatty acid content of their diets were doubled) and cholesterol intake was 60 mg (1/2 of previous intake). Over 2 yrs., 21/39 still showed progression of their lesions. However, no progression was seen in those who maintained significantly lower values for both total cholesterol and HDL cholesterol, and higher values of HDL cholesterol (*Arntzenius AC et al. Diet lipoproteins, and the progression of coronary atherosclerosis. The Leiden Intervention Trial. <u>New Engl. J. Med.</u> 312(13):805-11, 1985*).

Negative Experimental Crossover Study (C,H,L): 8 young, healthy normolipidemic men were fed both a 100% plant protein diet and a 55% animal, 45% plant protein diet for 21 days each in a crossover design. Mean serum total cholesterol and mean plasma LDL cholesterol were not significantly different after each diet; however, mean plasma HDL cholesterol was significantly higher following the 55% animal protein diet (*Wiebe SL. <u>Am. J. Clin. Nutr.</u> 40:982-9, 1984*).

Experimental Controlled Study (C,L): Vegan diets were found to be lower in saturated fatty acids and much higher in linoleic acid compared to those of omnivores. In addition, they were devoid of arachidonic, eicosapentaenoic and docosahexaenoic acids. Plasma total cholesterol and LDL cholesterol levels were significantly lower in male vegans (*Roshanai F, Sanders TAB. Assessment of fatty acid intakes in vegans and omnivores. <u>Human Nutr.: Applied Nutr.</u> 38A:345-54, 1984*).

Review Article: Individuals consuming a diet high in animal protein whose plasma lysine to arginine ratio is 3.5 to 1 or higher have a significantly increased AS risk due to excessive dietary lysine. Compared to omnivores, individuals consuming a vegetarian diet had a significant reduction in the incidence of AS. Animal protein has a L/A ratio of 3-4/1, while plant protein has a L/A ratio of 1-1.25/1. (*Sanchez A. <u>Nutr. Reports Int.</u> 28:497-, 1983*).

Experimental Controlled Study (C,T): Subjects with elevated lipid levels showed reduction in cholesterol and triglycerides when 500 ml. of a soy product (2% butterfat) was substituted for 2% fat cow's milk (*Check W. Switch to soy protein for boring but healthful diet. <u>JAMA</u> 247:3045-6, 1982*).

Animal Experimental Study (C): After 20 days on a diet containing 400 gm casein, the serum cholesterol of a gp. of 6 rabbits was 3068 +/- 592 mg/l, while the serum cholesterol of another gp. fed a diet containing 400 gm soy protein was 800 +/- 143 mg/l. The gps. were crossed-over and, by day 10, the cholesterol levels in the 2 gps. had also crossed-over (*Terpstra AH et al. A longitudinal cross-over study of serum cholesterol and lipoproteins in rabbits fed on semi-purified diets containing either casein or soya-bean protein. <u>Br. J. Nutr.</u> 47(2):213-21, 1982*).

Experimental Controlled Study (C,H): 21 vegetarians received their usual diet for 2 wks., a diet in which 250 gm beef was added isocalorically for 4 wks., and their usual diet for 2 more weeks. HDL cholesterol was unchanged, while total cholesterol rose significantly by 19% during the meat-eating period and systolic BP increased 3% (*Sacks FM et al. Effect of ingestion of meat on plasma cholesterol of vegetarians. <u>JAMA</u> 246:640-4, 1981*).

Experimental Controlled Study (C,L): 3 different types of vegetable supplements were compared to a sucrose supplement of equal caloric content. Vegetable leaves and stalks were associated with decreased VLDL lipoprotein cholesterol and possibly LDL lipoprotein cholesterol and decreased total cholesterol. Whole grains were associated with decreased LDL cholesterol and total cholesterol (*Fraser GE et al. The effect of various vegetable supplements on serum cholesterol. <u>Am. J. Clin. Nutr.</u> 34:1272-7, 1981*).

Restrict sugar to below 10% of calories.

Sucrose may increase urinary chromium loss, and chromium deficiency is a risk factor for ASHD (*see* *"Chromium"* below).

> **Experimental Controlled Study:** 37 pts. consumed sequentially for 6 wks. each a diet containing 35% of calories from complex carbohydrates and 15% from sucrose, and a diet containing 15% of calories from complex carbohydrates and 35% from sucrose. Chromium content of each diet was 16 mcg/1000 calories. 27/37 had an increase in urinary chromium excretion during the high sucrose diet compared to the low sucrose diet ranging from 10-300%, while 10/37 had no change. Absorption of chromium did not differ between the 2 diet periods (*Kozlovsky AS et al. Effects of diets high in simple sugars on urinary chromium losses. Metabolism 35:515, 1986*).

Review Article: Long term consumption of sugars such as sucrose and fructose rather than starch and other glucose based carbohydrates has, according to many studies, enhanced risk factors associated with the development of heart disease; thus pts. known to have high triglyceride and insulin levels may benefit from reducing their intake of fructose and sucrose (*Reiser S. Effect of dietary sugars on metabolic risk factors associated with heart disease. Nutr. & Health 3:203-16, 1985*).

Theoretical Discussion: The high correlation between dietary lipid and heart disease mortality may be largely secondary to the high correlation that refined carbohydrates have with dietary lipids, on the one hand, and with CHD on the other. This becomes apparent only when examples are found of a weak or negative correlation between dietary lipids and refined carbohydrates. It is suggested that dietary lipids are only of secondary importance, while refined carbohydrate consumption is of primary importance (*Temple NJ. Coronary heart disease: Dietary lipids or refined carbohydrates? Med. Hypothesis 10(4):425-35, 1983*).

Associated with increased total cholesterol, decreased HDL cholesterol, increased triglycerides and increased platelet adhesiveness.

> **Experimental Study (C,T):** 4 healthy males were fed 3 daily meals containing 635 gm. carbohydrates, 7 gm. fats and oils, and 50 gm. proteins for 7 days. Serum triglyceride levels increased while serum cholesterol and free fatty acid levels decreased (*Miyoshi T et al. Effects of a high sugar diet on the serum constituents in healthy subjects. Igaku to Seibutsugaku 105(4):265-7, 1982*).

> **Experimental Study (H):** 14 young men increased their ave. daily sucrose intake from 115 gm to 260 gm. After 3 wks., HDL cholesterol fell significantly and it reverted to its original value when they returned to their habitual diet for 2 weeks (*Yudkin J et al. Effects of high dietary sugar. Brit. Med. J. 281:1396, 1980*).

> **Experimental Study (C,T):** When 30% of the calories consumed was in the form of sucrose rather than starch, sucrose was shown to significantly increase total serum lipids, blood cholesterol and triglyceride levels (*Reiser et al. Am. J. Clin. Nutr. 32:1659, 1979*).

Sugar may promote atherosclerosis only in people with "sucrose-induced hyperinsulinism."

> **Observational Study (P):** A gp. of 27 male pts. with peripheral vascular disease was compared to a matched control gp. consuming a similar amount of sugar (ave. 120 gm/day). Both the platelet adhesiveness and insulin level were higher in the pts. and, only in the pts., sugar intake was significantly correlated with platelet adhesiveness and insulin levels measured before and after oral glucose (*Yudkin J, Szanto S. The relationship between sucrose intake, plasma insulin and platelet adhesiveness in men with and without occlusive vascular disease. Proc. Nutr. Soc. 29(1):Suppl:2A-3A, 1970*).

> **Experimental Study (P):** A gp. of young men were given a high-sucrose diet for 10 days and their level of immuno-reactive insulin was measured before and after. Three subjects demonstrating

"sucrose-induced hyperinsulinism" (SIH) and three controls were selected to be given a high-sucrose diet while their electrophoretic platelet motility was monitored. Following 14 days, only the platelets of the 3 subjects with SIH showed a pattern of electrophoretic behavior in the presence of ADP that is characteristic of individuals with atherosclerosis. This pattern reverted towards normal 14 days after the end of the high-sucrose diet (*Szanto S, Yudkin J. Dietary sucrose and the behaviour of blood platelets. Proc. Nutr. Soc. 29(1):Suppl:3A, 1970*).

Experimental Study (P,T): 19 men ages 21-44 followed high-sucrose, no-sucrose and "normal" diets for alternating 2 wk. periods. On the high sucrose diet, there was no change in cholesterol, triglycerides rose in all 19, and 6/19 demonstrated an increase in insulin levels, platelet adhesiveness and body weight. It is suggested that the effect of sucrose in producing hyperinsulinism may be more relevant than its effect on blood lipids, and that only individuals who show sucrose-induced hyperinsulinism are susceptible to the development of ischemic heart disease by dietary sucrose (*Szanto S, Yudkin J. The effect of dietary sucrose on blood lipids, serum insulin, platelet adhesiveness and body weight in human volunteers. Postgrad. Med. J. 45:602-7, 1969*).

Observational Study (P): A positive correlation between sugar intake and platelet adhesiveness was found for men with peripheral vascular disease, but not for healthy controls (*Yudkin J, Szanto S et al. Sugar intake, serum insulin and platelet adhesiveness in men with and without peripheral vascular disease. Postgrad. Med. J. 45:608, 1969*).

Increase complex carbohydrates.

Observational Study: A prospective study analyzed the diets of 3 gps. in 1959 and surveyed subsequent mortality in 1982: men born and living in Ireland, men born in Ireland who migrated to Boston, and men born in Boston to Irish immigrants. When all gps. were combined, those who died of CHD were more likely to have significantly less total carbohydrate and fiber intake (as well as starch and vegetable protein). Cholesterol intake and the ratio of saturated to unsaturated fats were likely to be higher. The authors suggest that the nutritional change most closely linked to the increased mortality rate from ASHD (which began to rise in the 1920's) was a decrease in complex carbohydrates rather than changes in the consumption of dietary lipids (*Kushi LH et al. Diet and 20-year mortality from coronary heart disease. The Ireland-Boston Diet-Heart Study. New Eng. J. Med. 312(13):811-18, 1985*).

Avoid coffee.

Epidemiologic studies link coffee consumption with hyperlipidemia and atherosclerosis.

Observational Study: In a prospective study of 1130 male medical students followed 19-35 yrs., the relative risks of CHD for men drinking 5 or more cups of coffee per day, as compared to non-drinkers, were approx. 2.49 after adjusting for age, current smoking, hypertension status, and baseline serum cholesterol (*LaCroix AZ et al. Coffee consumption and the incidence of coronary heart disease. New Engl. J. Med. 315(16):977-82, 1986*).

Observational Study (C,L): In a study of 1007 men and 589 women, there was a significant linear association between coffee consumption in men and plasma cholesterol and LDL cholesterol. Men who drank 5 or more cups of coffee had plasma cholesterol concentrations about 0.5 mmol/l higher than non-drinkers after controlling for age, ethnicity, body mass, education, season of year, smoking, tea drinking, and dietary intake of fat and carbohydrates. In women, adjusted mean cholesterol levels were 0.34 mmol/l higher in coffee drinkers. In both sexes, the association was largely with the LDL cholesterol fractions (*Kark J et al. Coffee, tea and plasma cholesterol: The Jerusalem lipid research clinic prevalence study. Brit. Med. J. 291(6497):699-704, 1985*).

Observational Study (C,L): In a 2 year study of 381 women and 320 men, the blood levels of cholesterol (predominantly LDL) increased significantly in women but not in men with coffee intake, independent of exercise, cigarette smoking, obesity, age, alcohol intake, cream, sugar, and fat intakes. Decaf coffee did not have this effect (*Mathias S et al.   Coffee, plasma cholesterol, and lipoproteins: A population study in an adult community. Am. J. Epidemiol. 121(6):896-905, 1985*).

Observational Study (C,L): In a study of 1228 women and 923 men over 4 years, coffee (but not tea or cola) consumption was associated with increases in both total and LDL cholesterol in both men and women. Caffeine was thus not entirely responsible for this trend which, in men only, was also associated with consumption of total and saturated fats and cholesterol. Results were independent of smoking, obesity, ethnicity, age and alcohol intake (*Haffner SM et al.   Coffee consumption, diet and lipids. Am. J. Epidemiol. 122(1):1-12, 1985*).

Observational Study (C,L): In a study of 77 healthy middle-aged men, the number of cups of regular coffee consumed daily correlated positively with apolipoprotein B, total cholesterol and LDL cholesterol levels in those drinking at least 3 cups daily (*Williams PT et al.   Coffee intake and elevated cholesterol and apolipoprotein B levels in men.   JAMA 253(10):1407-11, 1985*).

Observational Study: The incidence of M.I. was found to correlate with coffee, but not tea, consumption (*Coffee drinking and acute myocardial infarction.   Lancet 2:1278-9, 1972*).

The epidemiologic link between coffee consumption, hyperlipidemia and atherosclerosis may be at least partly due to an association between coffee consumption and consumption of saturated fats, rather than to the effects of coffee.

Observational Study: Male heavy coffee drinkers were found to eat approximately 24% more saturated fats than non-coffee-drinkers (*Haffner SM et al.   Am. J. Epidemiol. July, 1985*).

Abstention may be beneficial.

Experimental Controlled Study (C): 25/33 hypercholesterolemic men abstained from coffee for 5 weeks. Compared to controls, total serum cholesterol levels fell significantly an average of 10% in all abstainers. After 10 wks., the 9 who continued to abstain showed a 13% ave. decrease, while those who returned to coffee exhibited a gradual increase to baseline levels. This effect was independent of the use of sugar, cream, tea or cigarettes (*Forde OH et al.   The Tromso heart study: Coffee consumption and serum lipid concentrations in men with hypercholesterolaemia: A randomised intervention study.   Brit. Med. J. 290:893-5, 1985*).

Drink alcoholic beverages in moderation.

The effect of alcohol on ASHD risk is controversial in regard to moderate drinking (no more than 2 drinks daily with a drink defined as 1.5 oz of 80-proof whiskey, 5 oz wine, or 12 oz beer), although heavy drinking is clearly detrimental.

A. Evidence of a beneficial effect from moderate drinking:

Observational Study: The relation of alcohol consumption to CHD was examined prospectively in 1910 men aged 38-55 years. While there was no relationship during the first follow-up period (between 1953-4 & 1971-2), men whose monthly consumption was 60 oz or more had a lower than ave. CHD incidence rate during the second follow-up period (after 1971-2) (*Gordon T, Doyle JT. Drinking and coronary heart disease: The Albany study.   Am. Heart J. 110(2):331-34, 1985*).

Review Article: In every epidemiologic study examined, the rates for cardiovascular deaths were lower for moderate drinkers than for either the low- or high-intake groups. Once alcohol intake reached 6 drinks daily, total mortality rates from all causes of death were elevated (*Turner T.   Johns Hopkins Med. J. February 1981*).

Pts. with alcoholic cirrhosis have less coronary AS than controls.

Observational Study: Postmortem cross sections of coronary arteries of pts. who had developed alcoholic cirrhosis were compared to those of matched pts. who did not have cirrhosis. Those with liver disease showed much less coronary AS (*Int. Med. News June 15-30, 1982*).

Alcohol, when taken with a meal high in saturated fat, reduces platelet aggregation.

Experimental Study (P): In a study using healthy volunteers, a 5-oz glass of white wine did not inhibit platelet aggregation unless it were taken with a meal high in saturated (but not a meal high in unsaturated) fat (*Fenn CG, Littleton JM. Interactions between ethanol and dietary fat in determining human platelet function. Thrombosis Haemostas. 51(1):50-53, 1984*).

Moderate alcohol consumption is associated with increased diameter of the coronary arteries.

Observational Study: 20/31 males aged 20-66 without angiographic evidence of coronary artery disease were non-drinkers or low alcohol consumers, while 11/31 were moderate drinkers drinking an average of 1 drink daily. Based on coronary angiography, moderate alcohol consumption was independently associated with an average 26% increase in the cross-sectional area of the left main coronary artery and an average 31% increase in the size of the left anterior descending artery (*Fried LP et al. Long-term effects of cigarette smoking and moderate alcohol consumption on coronary artery diameter. Mechanisms of coronary artery disease independent of atherosclerosis or thrombosis? Am. J. Med. 80(1):37-44, 1986*).

B. Evidence against a beneficial effect from moderate drinking:

Review Article: Epidemiologic data suggest that alcohol does not protect against coronary heart disease. Although longitudinal and cross-sectional studies have shown an association between moderate alcohol ingestion and decreased risk of coronary AS, they may be biased because the light drinkers include people who are generally more health-conscious and/or those who drink very rarely or very small amounts. Moderate alcohol ingestion, which raises HDL cholesterol, does not raise HDL_2 levels (which have been epidemiologically correlated with reduced incidence of coronary AS), but raises HDL_3 levels (which are believed to be unrelated to the incidence of coronary AS). In addition, alcohol ingestion has a detrimental effect on blood pressure, body weight and glucose tolerance, all of which relate to CHD risk. Thus the influence of alcohol is detrimental to the prevention of CHD (*Eichner ER. Alcohol versus exercise for coronary protection. Am. J. Med. 79(2):231-40, 1985*).

Observational Study: 2170 males below age 55 experiencing their first MI were compared to controls. those drinking 1-7 alcoholic drinks per week had a relative risk of 1.2 of developing MI compared to controls when age and cigarette smoking were controlled for. When personality type was controlled for, the relative risk became 1.1 (*Kaufman DW et al. Alcoholic beverages and myocardial infarction in young men. Am. J. Epidemiol. 121:548-54, 1985*).

Experimental Controlled Study: 24 healthy male non-smokers, ages 30-60, who drank at least 1 drink daily were randomly assigned to either a treatment gp. (which abstained from all alcohol for 6 wks. and then resumed normal drinking for 5 wks.) or a control gp. which made no changes. While abstention from alcohol significantly lowered HDL_3 concentrations and resumption of drinking raised these levels back to baseline, alcohol had no effect on HDL_2 levels (*Haskell W et al. The effect of cessation and resumption of moderate alcohol intake on serum high-density-lipoprotein subfractions. New Engl. J. Med. 310:805-10, 1984*).

– –

COMBINED DIETARY PROGRAM:

Experimental Study (C,T): 21 pts. followed a high-complex-carbohydrate, low fat, low cholesterol diet (the "Pritikin diet"). After 26 days, their mean serum estradiol and triglycerides fell by 50% and serum cholesterol fell by 21%. The mean estradiol/testosterone ratio was reduced 50% and mean bodyweight decreased by 5% (*Rosenthal MB et al. Effects of a high-complex-carbohydrate, low fat, low cholesterol diet on serum lipids and estradiol. Am. J. Med. 78:23-7, 1985*).

Experimental Controlled Study (C,H,T): The effects of 4 different diets (Western reference diet with 40% energy from fat & P/S ratio 0.27, low-fat diet with 27% energy from fat & P/S ratio 1.0 and reduced cholesterol content, low-fat diet supplemented with fiber and a diet with 40% energy from fat with fiber supplementation) on 12 normal males were evaluated. The effects of fat modification and fiber supplementation (reduced serum cholesterol, LDL cholesterol and serum triglycerides) were strongly additive (*Lewis B et al. Towards an improved lipid-lowering diet: Additive effects of changes in nutrient intake. Lancet December 12, 1981*).

– –

NUTRIENTS:

<u>Folic acid</u>:   5 mg daily (4 week trial)

Coenzyme in the conversion of homocysteine (toxic) to methionine. As homocysteine levels are higher in women after menopause, and as homocysteine may contribute to atherosclerosis (*see discussion under "Pyridoxine" below*), reduction in homocysteine levels may have a prophylactic effect.

Supplementation may reduce homocysteine concentrations.

Experimental Study: Folic acid 5 mg daily for 4 wks significantly reduced plasma homocysteine concentrations both before and after a methionine load in subjects with normal serum and RBC folate levels, suggesting that folic acid may have a prophylactic effect (*Brattstr:om LE et al. Folic acid responsive postmenopausal homocysteinemia. Metabolism 34(11):1073-7, 1985*).

<u>Niacin</u>:   up to 6 gm. daily in divided doses starting with 100 mg 3 times daily with meals; increase as needed
(C,H,L,T)   by 100 mg 3 times daily each week (niacinamide is ineffective)

WARNING: May have significant side-effects.

Recommended as the "first drug to be used" when dietary intervention fails to adequately reduce elevated LDL cholesterol levels (*Hoeg JM et al. Special communication: An approach to the management of hyperlipoproteinemia. JAMA 255(4):512-21, 1986*).

Review Article: Effective in decreasing triglycerides, total cholesterol and LDL cholesterol and in increasing HDL cholesterol (*The Medical Letter Vol. 27, No. 695, August 30, 1985*).

Experimental Study (C,T): Following a 1 month baseline, 12 hyperlipidemic pts. were placed on nicotinic acid for 1 month. During treatment, triglycerides decreased 52%, VDRL decreased 36%, and total cholesterol decreased 22% (*Grundy SM et al. Influence of nicotinic acid on metabolism of cholesterol and triglycerides in man. J. Lipid Res. 22:24-36, 1981*).

Experimental Study (C,T): 188 pts. with various types of hyper-lipoproteinemia were given 3 gm. nicotinic acid daily. Most responsive were pts. with Type V whose cholesterols decreased 70% and triglycerides decreased 90%, followed by Type III (50% & 60%). Both lipids were also reduced in the other types, and even pts. with "normal" lipid levels showed a 10-20% reduction in serum lipids

(Carlson LA, Oro L. Effect of treatment of nicotinic acid for one month on serum lipids in patients with different types of hyperlipidemia. Atherosclerosis 18:1-9, 1973).

Supplementation may reduce the risk of MI for pts. with a previous history of MI.

Experimental Controlled Study: Men with 1 or more MI's who took 3 gm daily had a lower incidence of nonfatal MI and, for several years after the study ended, a lower mortality rate (*Canner PL. J. Am. Coll. Cardiol. 5:442, 1985; The coronary drug project research gp., JAMA 213:360, 1975*).

Pyridoxine: 40 mg. daily
(C,P,T)

Deficiency associated with increased risk of ASHD (*Serfontein WJ et al. Plasma pyridoxal-5-phosphate level as risk index for coronary artery disease. Atherosclerosis 55:357-61, 1985*).

May inhibit platelet aggregation and prolong clotting time.

Review Article: "If thrombin and fibrin formation in addition to platelet activation are important in the pathogenesis and progress of atherosclerotic lesions, then moderate doses of vitamin B_6 (say 40 mg a day) may suffice to alter the natural history of such a process" (*Is vitamin B_6 an antithrombotic agent? Lancet 1:1299-1300, 1981*).

See Also:

> *Lam SC et al. Investigation of possible mechanisms of pyridoxal-5-phosphate inhibition of platelet reactions. Thrombosis Res. 20:633-45, 1980*

Supplementation may have an anti-hypercholesterolemic effect.

Experimental Study (C):   50 mg. of B_6 given to alcoholics along with disulfiram 500 mg daily prevented the medication's hypercholesterolemic effect (*Major LF, Goyer PF. Effects of disulfiram and pyridoxine on serum cholesterol. Ann. Int. Med. 88(1):53-56, 1978*).

Animal Experimental Study (rats) (C,T): Large doses of B_6 (5 mg/100 gm body wt.) decreased the concentrations of cholesterol and triglycerides in the serum and aortas of rats fed high-fat, high-cholesterol diets, while small doses (0.005 mg/100 gm body wt.) increased both cholesterol and triglycerides concentrations following both normal and high-fat, high-cholesterol diets (*Vijayammal PL, Kurup PA. Pyridoxine and atherosclerosis: Role of pyridoxine in the metabolism of lipids and glycosaminoglycans in rats fed normal and high fat, high cholesterol diets containing 16% casein. Austral. J. Biol. Sci. 31(1):7-20, 1978*).

Animal Exerimental Study (monkeys) (C): Animals supplemented with B_6 had lower cholesterol levels than controls (*Rhinehart JF, Greenberg LD. Vitamin B_6 deficiency in the rhesus monkey, with particular reference to the occurrence of atherosclerosis, dental caries and hepatic cirrhosis. Am. J. Clin. Nutr. 4:318, 1956*).

Promotes conversion of homocysteine (toxic) to cystathionine; thus B_6 deficiency is theorized (originally by Kilmer McCully, M.D., Professor of Pathology, Harvard Medical School) to cause arterial damage due to build-up of homocysteine. (The incidence of heterozygous homocystinuria due to cystathionine synthase deficiency is about 1 in 70.)

Note: See also "Folic acid" above and "Betaine" below - as the addition of folate and betaine to pyridoxine may increase its efficacy.

Experimental Study: 16% of 99 male pts. vs. 2% of 39 subjects with normal coronary arteries demonstrated an elevation of homocysteine following an oral methionine load, suggesting that men with mild methionine intolerance exposed to the high methionine content of the Western diet may develop intermittent homocysteinuria and may thus be at greater risk for developing coronary AS (*Murphy-Chutorian DR et al. Methionine intolerance: A possible risk factor for coronary artery disease. J. Am. Coll. Cardiol. 6:725, 1986*).

Experimental Study: Pts. developing atherosclerosis before the age of 50 were studied. Heterozygous homocystinuria was diagnosed on the basis of excessive homocysteine accumulation after methionine loading and by the presence of cystathionine synthetase deficiency in skin fibroblasts. The disorder was found in 7/25 pts. with occlusive peripheral arterial disease, 7/25 with occlusive cerebrovascular disease and 0/25 with MI. Abnormal homocysteine metabolism improved in 10/11 pts. supplemented with B$_6$ (*Boers GHJ et al. Heterozygosity for homocystinuria in premature peripheral and cerebral occlusive arterial disease. New Engl. J. Med. 313:709, 1985*).

See Also:

> *Gruberg ER, Raymond SA. Beyond cholesterol. Atlantic May 1979 - also published in book form by St. Martin's Press*

> *Levene CI, Murray JC. The aetiological role of maternal B$_6$ deficiency in the development of atherosclerosis. Lancet 1:628, 1977*

> *Bendit E. The origin of atherosclerosis. Sci. Am. 236-2:74-85, February, 1977*

> *McCully KS, Wilson RB. Homocysteine theory of atherosclerosis. Atherosclerosis 22:215, 1975*

Vitamin B Complex:

Supplementation may improve the ratio of unsaturated to saturated fatty acids in the blood.

Experimental Study: 45 pts. with coronary heart disease and hypertension received daily supplementation with thiamine diphosphate 50 mg, riboflavin 40 mg, calcium pantothenate 200 mg, nicotinic acid 200 mg and lipoic acid 50 mg. After 10 days, the content of unsaturated (linoleic and arachidonic) fatty acids in the blood increased while that of saturated (stearic and palmitic) fatty acids decreased (*Vodoevich VP, Buko VU. [Effect of the B-group vitamin complex on the blood content of saturated and unsaturated fatty acids in patients with ischemic heart disease and hypertention.] Vopr. Pitan. (2):9-11, 1986*).

Vitamin C: 1 gram three times daily (3 wk. trial)
(C,F,H,I,L,P,T)

Leukocyte and plasma concentrations of ascorbate are significantly decreased in coronary heart disease (*Horsey J et al. Ischaemic heart disease and aged patients: Effects of ascorbic acid on lipoproteins. J. Human Nutr. 35:53-58, 1981; Ramirez J, Flowers NC. Leukocyte ascorbic acid and its relationship to coronary artery disease in man. Am. J. Clin. Nutr. 33:2070-87, 1980; Vallance BD et al. Reassessment of changes in leucocyte and serum ascorbic acid after acute myocardial infaction. Br. Heart J. 4:64-68, 1978*), possibly because of increased degradation and excretion due to the greatly enhanced rates of oxidation of ascorbate in inflammation by activated neutrophils (*Roberts P et al. Vitamin C and inflammation. Med. Biol. 62:88, 1984*).

Marginal vitamin C deficiency may contribute to AS as:

1. Cholesterol-7-alpha-hydroxylase, which is utililzed in synthesizing bile acids from cholesterol, is vitamin C-dependent.

2.   Vitamin C stimulates plasma lipoprotein lipase which is required in the catabolism of triglycerides.

3.   Vitamin C is required in the hydroxylation of proline for collagen formation, and thus influences arterial wall integrity.

(*Turley S et al. Role of ascorbic acid in the regulation of cholesterol metabolism and the pathogenesis of atherosclerosis. Atherosclerosis 24:1-18, 1976*)

Supplementation may lower total cholesterol, triglycerides and total lipids, while raising HDL cholesterol levels, increasing fibrinolytic activity and decreasing platelet aggregation.

Experimental Studies (P):
1. Pts. received 1 gm vitamin C every 8 hours. After 10 days, there was a significant drop in platelet adhesiveness and aggregation.

2. The platelets of healthy males were found to have an enhanced tendency towards adhesiveness and aggregation by 4 hrs. after ingestion of 75 gm butter which was prevented by co-administration of vitamin C 1 gm.

(*Bordia A et al. Effect of vitamin C on platelet adhesiveness and platelet aggregation in coronary artery disease patients. Clin. Cardiol. 8(10):552-54, 1985*).

Experimental Controlled Study (C):   Healthy younger subjects (ages 24-34) receiving 1 gm vitamin C for 1 1/2 months decreased ave. cholesterol levels from 228 to 181 while the levels of controls were unchanged. Healthy older subjects (ages 55-61) required 12 months and an increase to 2 gms. daily during the second 6 months to achieve a significant reduction (from 270-232) (*Dobson HM et al. The effect of ascorbic acid on the seasonal variations in serum cholesterol levels. Scot. Med. J. 29(3):176-82, 1984*).

Experimental Study (P):   Ascorbic acid 2 gm. I.V.in healthy subjects significantly decreased ADP-induced platelet aggregation for from 1 - 6 hours (*Cordova C et al. Influence of ascorbic acid on platelet aggregation in vitro and in vivo. Atherosclerosis 41:15, 1982*).

Experimental Study (C,T):   79 males (ages 65-90) received 3 gm. daily. After 3 weeks there was a significant decrease in cholesterol, triglycerides and total lipids (*Fidanza A et al. Vitamin C and atherosclerosis. Aliment. Nutr. Metab. 2(3):169-182, 1981*).

Experimental Study (C,H,L):   Many pts. with ischemic heart disease were found to have low levels of both vitamin C and HDL cholesterol. When such pts. were given 1 gm daily of vitamin C for 6 wks., both HDL cholesterol levels and vitamin C levels increased while LDL cholesterol levels decreased (*Horsey J et al. Ischemic heart disease and aged patients: Effects of ascorbic acid on lipoproteins. J. Human Nutr. 35(1):53-8, 1981*).

Experimental Double-blind Study (C,F,P): 1 gm. daily had no effect on blood measures for 40 pts. (ages 40-60) with a MI within the last 18 months, but 2 gm. daily increased fibrinolytic activity 45%, decreased platelet aggregation 27% and decreased serum cholesterol 12% while pts. receiving placebo had no changes (*Bordia AK. The effect of vitamin C on blood lipids, fibrinolytic activity and platelet adhesiveness in patients with coronary artery disease. Atherosclerosis 35:181-187, 1980*).

- with Pectin:

   Experimental Study: 21 healthy subjects with mild hypercholesterolemia received 15 gms. pectin and 450 mg. ascorbic acid. After 6 wks., total serum cholesterol dropped significantly by 24 mg./100 ml., while high density lipoproteins were unchanged. In 11 hyperlipemic pts. (types IIa, IIb & IV), the same regime was followed by a 68 mg./ 100 ml. (19%) drop in total serum cholesterol (*Ginter E et al. Natural hypocholesterolemic agent: Pectin plus ascorbic acid. Int. J. Vit. Nutr. Res. 52:55-9, 1982*).

Although vitamin C lowers elevated cholesterol levels, the maximum drop is after about 6 mo. and sometimes it may rise again - probably because, as it accelerates the conversion of cholesterol to bile acids recycling through the liver, a feedback system slows down the reaction. However, if a cholesterol-binding agent is given along with vitamin C, the decline in cholesterol is striking and sustained (*Ginter, Emil - 1981*).

Supplementation may improve peripheral arterial circulation.

> **Experimental Study (I):** 10 pts. with intermittent claudication received baseline arteriograms prior to supplementation with ascorbic acid 500 mg 3 times daily.   After several months, repeat arteriograms revealed definite improvement in some of the involved arteries for 6/10 pts. (*Willis GC. The reversibility of atherosclerosis. Canad. Med. Assoc. J. July 15, 1957, pp. 106-09; Willis GC et al. Serial arteriography in atherosclerosis. Canad. Med. Assoc. J. December, 1954, pp. 562-68*).

Vitamin D:

WARNING: Animal studies suggest that excess intake may accelerate the frequency of degenerated smooth muscle cell death in the intima of arterial tissue. The resulting lesions appear under electron microscopy to be identical to those in thoracic aortic tissue obtained during coronary bypass surgery (*Kummerow FA. Nutrition imbalance and angiotoxins as dietary risk factors in coronary heart disease. Am. J. Clin. Nutr. 32:58-83, 1979*).

> **Animal Experimental Study:** Grossly normal areas of the aorta from weanling swine fed vitamin D_3 25,000 IU/lb. of basal ration for 3 mo. had a higher frequency of degenerated smooth muscle cells under electron microscopy than similar areas of control swine. Similarly,weanling piglets fed 12,500 IU/lb. developed identical lesions and developed extensive lipid deposits and coronary occlusion by age 6 months (*Taura M et al. Coronary atherosclerosis in normo-cholesterolemic swine artery. Arter. Wall 4:395, 1978; Huang WY et al. The influence of vitamin D on plasma and tissue lipids and atherosclerosis in swine. Artery 3:439, 1977*).

Vitamin E: 600 I.U. three times daily
(C,H,I,L,P,T)

WARNING: High dosages are not recommended for people with hypertension, rheumatic heart disease or ischemic heart disease except under close medical supervision.

May affect platelet function.

> **Experimental Study (P):**   400- 1200 IU daily produced a small but significant reduction of collagen-induced platelet aggregation and a highly significant reduction in platelet adhesiveness to collagen when given with aspirin (300 mg. every other day), while aspirin alone was ineffective (*Steiner M. Effect of alpha-tocopherol administration on platelet function in man. Thromb. Haemost. 49(2): 73-7, 1983*).

> **Experimental Study (P):**   Supplementation was effective in inhibiting ADP-induced but not arachidonic acid-induced platelet aggregation (*Creter D et al. Effect of vitamin E on platelet aggregation in diabetic retinopathy. Acta Hematol. 62:74, 1979*).

> **Negative Experimental Study (P):** 1000 IU x 8 days was ineffective for 10 pts., 5 with coronary artery disease and 5 with nonspecific non-coronary chest pain (*Gomes JAC et al. The effect of vitamin E on platelet aggregation. Am. Heart J. April, 1976*).

> **Experimental Study (P):**   Up to 1800 IU daily, increasing concentrations increased vitamin concentrations in platelets and plasma as it inhibited platelet aggregation (*Steiner M, Anastasi J. Vitamin E: An inhibitor of the platelet release reaction. J. Clin. Inves. 57:732-7, 1976*).

May affect lipid metabolism.

Negative Experimental Double-blind Study (H): 78 volunteers received alpha tocopherol 728 mg or placebo. No consistent effect on HDL cholesterol levels was observed either at 4 wks. or at 6 months. Further analysis indicated that there were no significant changes in HDL cholesterol in subjects with low initial levels (*Kalbfleisch JH et al. Alpha-tocopherol supplements and high-density-lipoprotein-cholesterol levels. Br. J. Nutr. 55(1):71-78, 1986*).

Negative Experimental Double-blind Study (H): 36 60-year-old subjects received 800 IU vitamin E daily without a significant increase in HDL cholesterol after 16 weeks (*Stampfer MJ et al. Effect of vitamin E on lipids. Am. J. Clin. Path. 79(6):714-6, 1983*).

Experimental Study (H): 43 subjects receiving 800 IU vitamin E daily increased HDL cholesterol significantly, with the greatest increases in those with the lowest initial HDL levels (*Barboriak JJ et al. Vitamin E supplements and plasma high-density lipoprotein cholesterol. Letter to the Editor. Am. J. Clin. Path. 77(3):371, 1982*).

Negative Experimental Study: (H): 39 volunteers received vitamin E 600 IU daily. After 30 days, no significant change in serum HDL cholesterol could be documented (*Howard DR et al. Vitamin E does not modify HDL-cholesterol. Am. J. Clin. Pathol. 77(1):86-89, 1982*).

Experimental Study (C,H,L): 17 young women with mammary dysplasia and 6 age-matched controls received alpha tocopherol 600 IU for 4 months. While total serum cholesterol was unchanged, ratios of serum cholesterol to HDL cholesterol decreased in the pt. gp. whose ratios were higher than those of controls. HDL_3 cholesterol concentrations increased significantly only in the pts., while VLDL plus LDL free cholesterol increased significantly in both pts. and controls (*Sundaram GS et al. Serum hormones and lipoproteins in benign breast disease. Cancer Res. 41:3814-16, 1981*).

Experimental Study (C,H,T): 5 subjects with average HDL cholesterol levels and 5 with low HDL cholesterol levels received 600 IU daily. Within 7 weeks, 9/10 showed increased HDL cholesterol and all 5 with low levels showed major increases, with HDL cholesterol levels increasing from 220-483%, while VDRL decreased 25% and triglycerides decreased 20% (*Hermann WJ et al. The effect of tocopherol on high-density lipoprotein cholesterol: A clinical observation. Am. J. Clin. Path. 72:848-52, 1979*).

See Also:

> **Negative Experimental Study (C,H):** *Hatam LJ, Kayden HJ. The failure of alpha-tocopherol supplementation to alter the distribution of lipoprotein cholesterol in normal and hyper-lipoproteinemic persons. Am. J. Clin. Path. 76:122-4, 1981*

May reduce intermittent claudication.

Experimental Controlled Study (I): 32/47 men with severe symptoms received 100 IU D-alpha-tocopherol 3 times daily while the control gp. received drugs. After about 3 months, 54% of the men on vitamin E vs. 23% of the controls could walk 1 kilometer. After about 18 mo., 29/32 men on vitamin E demonstrated increased calf blood flow while 10/14 of the men in the control gp. demonstrated a decrease (*Haeger K. Long-time treatment of intermittent claudication with vitamin E. Am. J. Clin. Nutr. 27(10):1179-81, 1974*).

Review Article: Numerous studies and 4 controlled trials give a positive result for tocopherol at doses of at least 400 mg for periods of greater than 12 weeks. By contrast, only 1 study had negative results, and this study is open to question because (1) wheat germ oil was given so that the actual daily dose of tocopherol appears to have been only 40 mg, and (2) supplementation was only provided for 12 wks. while the positive studies lasted longer (*Marks J. Critical appraisal of the therapeutic value of alpha-tocopherol. Vitam. Hormones 20:573-98, 1962*).

See Also:

Reilly CP. Are vitamin E supplements beneficial? Med. J. Australia 2(21):795, 1974

Haeger K. Walking distance and arterial flow during long term treatment of intermittent claudication with d-alpha-tocopherol. Vasa 2:280-7, 1973

Williams HTG et al. Alpha tocopherol in the treatment of intermittent claudication. Surg. Gyn. & Obst. April, 1971, pp. 662-6.

- -

Calcium: 1.5 gram daily
(C,P,T)

Combines with fatty acids in the gut to cause excretion of calcium soaps.

Supplementation may decrease total cholesterol and triglycerides and inhibit platelet aggregation.

Animal Experimental Study (C,P,T): Rabbits were fed a high (45%) saturated fat diet containing either a basic amount of calcium and magnesium (group I) or increased calcium (group II). After 6 months, gp. II rabbits demonstrated significant prolongation of clotting time, decrease in platelet aggregation, and decrease in plasma total cholesterol, with a less significant decrease in plasma triglycerides. In addition the excretion of fecal lipids and saturated fatty acids was greatly increased. Compared to gp. I, rabbits in gp. II demonstrated significantly less severe atherosclerosis and significantly less accumulation of cholesterol in the aorta (*Renaud S et al. Protective effects of dietary calcium and magnesium on platelet function and atherosclerosis in rabbits fed saturated fat. Atherosclerosis 47:187-98, 1983*).

Experimental Controlled Study (C): Healthy elderly women received 1025-1200 mg calcium daily. Total serum cholesterol significantly decreased in the supplemented gp. but not in controls (*Albanese AA. Nutrition Reports Int. August 1973*).

Experimental Study (C): 10 hyperlipemic pts. with 1 year baseline cholesterol levels between 3-500 mg received 1 gm calcium carbonate twice daily for 1 year with an average decrease in total cholesterol of 25% by 6 mo. (*Bierenbaum ML et al. Long term human studies on the lipid effects of oral calcium. Lipids 7:202-6, 1972*).

Experimental Single-blind Study (C): 16 hyperlipidemic pts. received 2 gm. calcium daily for 8 weeks following 4 wks. on placebo. While serum triglycerides were unchanged, serum cholesterol decreased significantly when compared to the mean value during placebo therapy (*Carlson LA et al. Effects of oral calcium upon serum cholesterol and triglycerides in patients with hyperlipidemia. Atherosclerosis 14:391-400, 1971*).

Animal Experimental Study: Rabbits fed a low-calcium atherogenic diet developed pronounced aortic AS, while 2 out of 3 rabbits fed the same diet supplemented with calcium showed no signs of AS and exhibited greatly reduced cholesterol in their aortas (*Yacowitz H. Trans. N.Y. Acad. Sci. vol. 33, 1971*).

Experimental Study (C,T): Subjects received 1.6 gm calcium daily for 3 weeks. Both triglyceride and cholesterol levels decreased significantly, with the major decrease in the first week (*Yacowitz H. Brit. Med. J. May, 1965*).

Chromium:
(C,G,H,T)

Chromium deficiency is a risk factor for ASHD.

Observational Study: Coronary arteriography revealed coronary AS in 67/109 pts. with extreme, un-provoked anxiety. All of these pts. were found to be low in chromium, while the levels were higher in 80% of pts. found to be free of disease, suggesting that, above the critical level of 6 mg/ml of blood chromium, coronary artery disease is extremely unlikely (*Simonoff M et al. Low plasma chromium in patients with coronary artery and heart diseases. Biological Trace Element Res. 6:431, 1984*).

Review Article: Studies strongly suggest that chromium has an effect on lipid metabolism and that chromium deficiency could be a risk factor in ASHD (*Nutr. Rev. 41:307-10, 1983*).

Chromium supplementation may reduce total cholesterol and triglycerides and raise HDL cholesterol (*see also: "Brewer's Yeast" below*).

Negative Experimental Double-blind Crossover Study (C,H,L,T): 10 noninsulin-dependent diabetics (aged 37-68) received trivalent chromium 200 mcg daily. After 6 wks., serum total cholesterol and triglycerides and their high-density, low-density and very low-density lipoprotein fractions showed no change as compared to the placebo period (*Uusitupa MI et al. Effect of inorganic chromium supplementation on glucose tolerance, insulin response, and serum lipids in noninsulin-dependent diabetics. Am. J. Clin. Nutr. 38(3):404-10, 1983*).

Experimental Double-blind Study (C,H,T): 13/23 healthy adult men received 200 mcg daily of chromium as chromic chloride while the rest received placebo. After 12 wks., the experimental subjects demonstrated decreased serum triglycerides and total cholesterol, increased HDL cholesterol and improved glucose tolerance (*Railes R, Albrink MJ. Effect of chromium chloride supplementation on glucose tolerance and serum lipids including high density lipoprotein of adult men. Am. J. Clin. Nutr. 34:2670-8, 1981*).

Chromium supplementation retards the development of experimental atherosclerosis and may result in plaque regression in experimental animals.

Animal Experimental Study (G): Chromium supplements reduced coronary artery plaques 50% in rabbits fed a high-cholesterol diet compared to unsupplemented rabbits (*Abraham AS et al. The effect of chromium on cholesterol-induced atherosclerosis in rabbits. Atherosclerosis 41:371-79, 1982*).

Animal Experimental Study (G): Rabbits with established atherosclerotic plaques who were supplemented with chromium showed evidence of significant plaque regression (*Abraham AS et al. The effect of chromium on established atherosclerotic plaques in rabbits. Am. J. Clin. Nutr. 33:2294-98, 1980*).

See Also:

Abraham AS et al. The action of chromium on serum lipids and on atherosclerosis in cholesterol-fed rabbits. Atherosclerosis 42:185-95, 1982

Copper: 2-4 mg daily
(C)

Copper deficiency is associated with increased total cholesterol levels.

Experimental Study (C): Individuals depleted of copper responded with an increase in total serum cholesterol. After copper repletion, cholesterol returned to normal (*Klevey LM et al. Clin. Res. 28:758A, 1980*).

<u>Magnesium:</u>   500 mg. daily
(A,C,H,P)

May be deficient.

Observational Study: During the first 32 hrs., 13 pts. with acute MI had significant reductions in serum Mg level, while no increase in urinary Mg was seen, suggesting that hypomagnesemia during acute MI is caused by a shift of the mineral from the extracellular to the intracellular space (*Rasmussen HS. Magnesium and acute myocardial infarction. Arch. Int. Med. 146:872, 1986*).

Observational Study: 5 pts. with acute MI and 5 controls received a magnesium retention test and a muscle biopsy. Magnesium retention was 42% in the MI gp. and 22% in the controls (p less than 0.01), and muscle magnesium content was lower in the MI gp. compared to controls (*Jeppesen BB. Magnesium status in patients with acute myocardial infarction: A pilot study. Magnesium 5:95, 1986*).

Observational Study: Out of 102 consecutive pts. admitted to a medical ICU, 20% had hypomagnesemia (*Reinhart R et al. Hypomagnesemia in patients entering the ICU. Critical Care Med. 13(6):506, 1985*).

Review Article: "Chronic, low grade magnesium deficiency may be much more common than is conventionally considered since magnesium is not studied regularly in clinical medicine, as are sodium, potassium, and chloride....The need in clinical medicine to measure serum concentration of magnesium in all patients with heart disease ... cannot be overemphasized" (*Burch GE, Giles TD. The importance of magnesium deficiency in cardiovascular disease. Am. Heart J. 94:649-57, 1977*).

Observational Study: Plasma magnesium levels of 40 men with recent MI were significantly lower than those of healthy controls (2.3 vs. 2.6 mg/100 ml)(p less than 0.001) (*Hughes A, Tonks RS. Platelets, magnesium, and myocardial infarction. Lancet 1:1044-6, 1965*).

See Also:

> *Abrahams S et al. Serum magnesium levels in patients with acute myocardial infarction. New Engl. J. Med. 296:862-63, 1977*

Magnesium deficiency is associated with increased risk of coronary artery disease, sudden cardiac death, myocardial infarction and ventricular tachyarrhythmias (*Manthey J. Magnesium and trace metals: Risk factors for CHD. Circulation 64:722-9, October, 1981; Burch GE, Giles TD. The importance of magnesium deficiency in cardiovascular disease. Am. Heart J. November, 1977*).

Supplementation may reduce risk of:
1. cardiac arrhythmias
2. vasospastic angina
3. death following myocardial infarction.

Experimental Double-blind Study: Based on 6 reports documenting a rapid drop in serum magnesium levels after acute MI, 273 pts. with suspected MI's received either IV magnesium or placebo immediately upon arrival at a CCU. MI was confirmed in 130 pts., 56 of whom had received magnesium chloride. 4-week mortality for the magnesium-treated pts. was 7%, compared to 19% for the controls. 12/56 pts. (21%) given magnesium developed arrhythmias compared to 35/74 (47%) of the placebo-treated patients. No evidence of Mg toxicity was seen (*Rasmussen HS et al. Intravenous magnesium in acute myocardial infarction. Lancet 1:234, 1986*).

Experimental Double-blind Study: Pts. with acute MI received IV magnesium sulfate 2.7 mmol/hr. or placebo during the 24 hrs. following the MI starting within 1 hr. of entering a CCU. In the first 24 hrs., there were 2 deaths in the Mg gp. compared to 7 in the control gp. (p less than 0.1). Ventricular tachycardia or fibrillation occurred in 5.4% and 9.7% of the Mg and placebo gps., respectively (p less than 0.1), and total cardiac events (arrhythmias and death) were 56% lower in the Mg-treated gp. (p less than 0.02). No evidence of Mg toxicity was seen (*Smith L et al. Magnesium sulphate infusion after acute myocardial infarction: Effects on arrhythmias and mortality. Clin. Sci. 68 (Suppl. 11):56, 1985*).

Case Report: 71 year-old female with previous MI, chest pain and chronic diarrhea since a small-bowel resection was found to be magnesium-deficient. The author suggests that hypomagnesemia precipitated her MI's and notes that cellular magnesium deficiency may co-exist with normal serum Mg levels. He advises magnesium therapy in any pt. with vasospastic cardiac ischemia not treated successfully with calcium channel-blocking drugs (*Hanline M. Hypomagnesemia causes coronary artery spasm. JAMA 253:342, 1985*).

Experimental Study (A): 15 pts. with variant angina were injected IV with 10 ml of 20% magnesium sulfate during each anginal episode. While, untreated, each episode lasted 5-15 minutes, treated attacks lasted 1/2 - 2 minutes. Pretreatment with parenteral Mg sulfate in 4 of these pts. prevented further attacks (*Cohen L, Kitzes R. Magnesium sulfate in the treatment of variant angina. Magnesium 3:46-49, 1984*).

Observational Study: Cardiac Mg levels were significantly lower (p less than 0.01) in 54 cases of accidental death in cities with relatively soft water than in 29 cases in cities with relatively hard water, while there were no significant differences in myocardial calcium, zinc, copper, chromium, lead or cadmium levels, suggesting that the relatively high death rates in some soft water areas may be due to a suboptimal intake of magnesium (*Anderson TN et al. Letter: Ischemic heart disease, water hardness and myocardial magnesium. Can. Med. Assoc. J. 113(3):199-203, 1975*).

See Also:

> *Fredman HS. Coronary vasospasm and its relationship to Mg deficiency. Magnesium 1:81-83, 1982*

> *Turlapaty PDMV, Altura BM. Magnesium deficiency produces spasms of coronary arteries: Relationship to etiology of sudden death IHD. Science 208(11): 199-200, 1980*

Supplementation may prevent calcification of blood vessels and the development of atherosclerosis (*Seelig MS, Heggtveit HA. Magnesium interrelationships in ischemic heart disease: A review. Am. J. Clin. Nutr. 27(1):59-79, 1974*).

Experimental Study: Reductions in the magnesium content of aortas were associated with higher calcium contents (which may lead to atherosclerosis and hypertension), while elevations in magnesium were associated with lower calcium contents (*Altura BM, Altura BT. Magnesium ions and contraction of vascular smooth muscles: Relationship to some vascular diseases. Fed. Proc. 40(12):2672-9, 1981*).

Supplementation may reduce total cholesterol, raise HDL cholesterol and inhibit platelet aggregation.

Experimental Study (C,H,L): 16 pts. with abnormally low HDL cholesterol levels (also elevated LDL and VLDL cholesterol) received enteric coated magnesium chloride (400 mg. elemental Mg) for a mean of 4 months. Total plasma cholesterol significantly decreased from 297 to 257; HDL cholesterol significantly increased from 35.2 to 46.7; and VLDL and LDL cholesterol significantly decreased from 262 to 210 mg/dl, suggesting that magnesium therapy should be considered a first-choice option in the treatment of lipid abnormalities since it is safer than drugs in current use (*Davis*

WH et al. Monotherapy with magnesium increases abnormally low high density lipoprotein cholesterol: A clinical essay. Curr. Ther. Res. 36:341, 1984).

Animal Experimental Study (C,P,T): Rabbits were fed a high (45%) saturated fat diet containing either a basic amount of calcium and magnesium (group I), increased calcium (group II), or increased magnesium (group III). After 6 months, gp. II rabbits demonstrated significant prolongation of clotting time, decrease in platelet aggregation, and decrease in plasma total cholesterol, with a less significant decrease in plasma triglycerides. In addition the excretion of fecal lipids and saturated fatty acids was greatly increased. Compared to gp. I, rabbits in gp. II demonstrated significantly less severe atherosclerosis and significantly less accumulation of cholesterol in the aorta. The results in group III were similar to those of group II, but less significant (*Renaud S et al. Protective effects of dietary calcium and magnesium on platelet function and atherosclerosis in rabbits fed saturated fat. Atherosclerosis 47:187-98, 1983*).

In vitro Experimental Study (P): While sodium and potassium failed to affect platelet clumping and blood-clotting, these effects were both highly correlated with the concentration of added magnesium (*Hughes A, Tonks RS. Platelets, magnesium, and myocardial infarction. Lancet 1:1044-6, 1965*).

See Also:

> *Sachdeva JR et al. Serum magnesium levels and platelet adhesiveness in acute myocardial infarction. J. Indian Med. Assoc. 71(7):165-67, 1978*

Potassium:

Deficiency (which may exist despite normal serum potassium levels) is associated with arrhythmias as well as decreased tolerance to cardiac medications and EKG alterations.

Observational Study: Serum potassium concentration was an inverse predictor of ventricular tachycardia and frequent unifocal PVC's early in acute myocardial infarction (*Nordrehaug J et al. Serum potassium concentration as a risk factor of ventricular arrhythmias early in acute myocardial infarction. Circulation 71(4):645-9, 1985*).

Experimental and Observational Study: Serum and red blood cell potassium was measured in 17 pts. with EKG abnormalities. Although some of the abnormalities were typical of potassium deficiency, most were non-specific T wave changes which are commonly attributed (without substantiation) to ischemia. Serum potassium levels were normal but RBC potassium levels were below normal in all cases and returned to normal (as did the EKG abnormalities) after treatment with potassium salts (*Sangiori GB et al. Serum potassium levels, red-blood-cell potassium and alterations of the repolarization phase of electrocardiography in old subjects. Age Aging 13:309, 1984*).

Potassium and Magnesium:

May be more effective when administered together when the level of either is deficient due to the inability of the heart muscle to hold on to potassium in the absence of magnesium (*Dychner T, Wester PO. Magnesium and potassium in serum and muscle in relation to disturbances of cardiac rhythm, in Magnesium in Health and Disease. Spectrum Publishing Company, 1980, pp. 551-7; Shils ME. Experimental human magnesium depletion. Medicine 48(1):61-85, 1969*).

Potassium Iodide:
(G)
May inhibit atherogenesis.

Animal Experimental Study (G):   Rabbits were placed on a high cholesterol diet plus various amounts of potassium iodide. After 10 wks. no significant atheroma was seen in the aorta of rabbits that had consumed high doses, while those that had consumed none or low doses developed severe atheroma (*Fani K, Weissman M. Inhibition of dietary atherosclerosis by iodide. Res. Commun. Chem. Pathol. Pharmacol. 1(2):169-84, 1970*).

Selenium:
(C,P)

Serum selenium levels are negatively correlated with AS.

Observational Study (C): In a sample of 1110 men aged 55-74, serum selenium levels were negatively correlated with age and positively correlated with HGb levels and serum cholesterol. Men with coronary heart disease or claudication significantly more frequently exhibited levels below 45 mcg/l. Levels below 45 mcg/l were significantly associated with increased risk of death from all causes including cardiovascular disease, but only in individuals with evidence of coronary heart disease. In the entire population, death from stroke was responsible for more than half of the increased mortality associated with low selenium levels (*Virtamo J et al. Serum selenium and the risk of coronary heart disease and stroke. Am. J. Epidemiology 122:276-282, 1985*).

Observational Study: Plasma selenium levels were measured in 106 hospitalized pts. undergoing coronary angiography for suspected coronary disease. The highest ave. level (136 mcg/l) was seen in those with normal findings and the lowest level (105 mcg/l) in those with atheromatous blockage of all 3 coronary arteries. Pts. with 1-2 occluded arteries had intermediate selenium levels (*Moore JA et al. Selenium concentrations in plasma of patients with arteriographically defined coronary atherosclerosis. Clin. Chem. 30:1171, 1984*).

Observational Study: 8113 Finnish people provided both baseline and follow-up data. Over 7 yrs., 367 people developed CVD and were compared with matched controls. Baseline serum selenium samples demonstrated a significant negative correlation with both the development of coronary disease and coronary mortality. For males, the relative risk of CHD death for selenium levels below 45 mcg/l was 3.6; for CVD death, 2.7; for MI 2.2. It is possible that, since nutrient levels are associated with dietary fat, a low selenium diet may merely be a marker for a high fat diet, or one inadequate in polyunsaturates, with fat being the atherogenic factor (*Salonen JT et al. Association between cardiovascular death and myocardial infarction and serum selenium in a matched-pair longitudinal study. Lancet 2:175-9, 1982*).

May reduce platelet aggregation (by increasing prostacyclin production).

Experimental Study (P): Elderly nursing home residents received high selenium yeast containing 200 mcg selenium daily. After 5 wks., plasma levels of both platelet factor 4 and thromboglobulin had fallen significantly, indicating a reduction of platelet aggregation (*Stead NW et al. Selenium (Se) balance in the dependent elderly. Am. J. Clin. Nutr. 39:677, 1984*).

Experimental Study: In 6 human volunteers given supplementary selenium 10 mcg/kg for 6 wks., bleeding time nearly doubled. (*Schiavon R et al. Selenium enhances prostacyclin production by cultured epithelial cells: Possible explanation for increased bleeding times in volunteers taking selenium as a dietary supplement. Thrombosis Res. 34:389, 1984*).

See Also:

   Schone NW et al. Effects of selenium deficiency on aggregation and thromboxane formation in rat platelets. Fed. Proc. 43:477, 1984

<u>Zinc</u>:
(C,H,I)

The association of zinc with serum cholesterol is complex:

1. Animal studies suggest that zinc and HDL cholesterol levels are <u>positively</u> correlated.

> **Animal Experimental Study (rats) (H):** Rats received either a 1% cholesterol or a no cholesterol isocaloric diet, both of which had equal and adequate zinc levels. Cholesterol feeding significantly decreased HDL cholesterol and increased VLDL cholesterol, while serum zinc levels were significantly decreased and copper levels were unchanged. There was a significant positive correlation between serum HDL and zinc, suggesting that there may be a specific metabolic link between zinc and HDL cholesterol (*Koo S, Ramlet J. Am. J. Clin. Nutr. 37:918-23, 1983*).

> **Animal Experimental Study (rats) (C,H,L):** Total serum cholesterol significantly decreased on a zinc-deficient diet; however, this decrease was almost entirely due to a decrease in HDL cholesterol as there were no alterations in LDL or VLDL cholesterol levels. Serum HDL cholesterol levels were positively correlated with serum zinc levels, suggesting an adverse effect of marginal zinc intake on cardiovascular health (*Koo SI, Williams DA. Relationship between the nutritional status of zinc and cholesterol concentration of serum lipoproteins in adult male rats. Am. J. Clin. Nutr. 34(11):2376-81, 1981*).

2. However, supplementation of 160 mg daily has been shown to be followed by a marked <u>decrease</u> in HDL cholesterol in humans without a change in total cholesterol, LDL cholesterol or triglycerides.

> **Experimental Single-blind Study (C,H,L):** 12 healthy young men received zinc sulphate containing 80 mg. elemental zinc twice daily for 5 weeks and the results were compared with those of 8 matched controls who received placebo capsules. Zinc supplementation was associated with a marked decrease in HDL cholesterol by the seventh week which returned to normal by 11 weeks after zinc was stopped. Cholesterol, triglyceride and LDL cholesterol were unchanged (*Hooper PL et al. Zinc lowers high-density lipoprotein-cholesterol levels. JAMA 244:1960, 1980*).

3. In addition, minimal zinc supplementation (over 15 mg daily) in humans has been shown to prevent the exercise-related increase in HDL cholesterol.

> **Experimental Study (H):** Healthy elderly volunteers failed to experience an increase in HDL cholesterol from exercise so long as they supplemented their diets with over 15 mg zinc daily. Cessation of zinc supplementation for 8 wks. resulted in an exercise-related increase in HDL cholesterol (*Goodwin JS et al. Relationship between zinc intake, physical activity and blood levels of high density lipoprotein cholesterol in a healthy elderly population. Metabolism 34(6):519-23, 1985*).

> **Experimental Study (C,H,L,T):** 21 men engaged in endurance exercises and 23 sedentary men took zinc sulphate 50 mg daily. After 8 wks., while plasma zinc increased 15%, there were no significant changes in fasting HDL cholesterol, LDL cholesterol, total cholesterol or triglycerides (*Crouse SF et al. Zinc ingestion and lipoprotein values in sedentary and endurance-trained men. JAMA 252:755-87, 1984*).

4. It has been suggested that these contradictory findings are due to the fact that, while improved zinc nutriture has a beneficial effect on HDL cholesterol, higher levels of zinc supplementation may lower body copper levels, and the resultant copper deficiency could account for the adverse effects on cholesterol metabolism. If so, copper supplementation may sometimes be indicated when supplemental zinc is provided (*Klevay LM. Interactions of copper and zinc in cardiovascular disease. Ann. N.Y. Acad. Sci. 355:140-151, 1980; Fischer P et al. The effect of dietary copper and zinc on cholesterol metabolism. Am. J. Clin. Nutr. 33:1019-25, 1980*).

Animal Experimental Study (rats) (C): Plasma cholesterol levels were 50% higher after 7 mo. of consuming a diet supplemented with 200 mg/kg zinc compared to an unsupplemented control group. Differences in cholesterol levels became significant at 3 months. Although the increased cholesterol may be due directly to zinc supplementation, copper levels dropped in both liver and plasma; thus secondary depletion in copper levels could indirectly cause the increase in cholesterol (*Katya-Katya M et al. The effect of zinc supplementation on plasma cholesterol levels. Nutr. Res. 4:633-38, 1984*).

Supplementation may reduce intermittent claudication.

Experimental Study (I): 24 pts. with severe intermittent claudication received 220 mg. zinc sulfate 3 times daily for 1 yr. or longer. 8 became able to live independently but continued to have limited exercise tolerance (*Henzel JH, U. of Missouri School of Med. - reported in Med. Trib. 10/26/70; Henzel JH et al. Trace elements in atherosclerosis: Efficacy of zinc medication as a therapeutic modality. Proc. 2nd Ann. Conf. Trace Substances in Environ. Health 1968, pp. 83-9*).

— —

Arginine and
Lysine:

Lowering the lysine/arginine ratio may be beneficial.

Review Article: Individuals consuming a diet high in animal protein whose plasma lysine to arginine ratio is 3.5 to 1 or higher have a significantly increased AS risk due to excessive dietary lysine. Compared to omnivores, individuals consuming a vegetarian diet have a significant reduction in the incidence of AS. Animal protein has a L/A ratio of 3-4/1, while plant protein has a L/A ratio of 1-1.25/1. (*Sanchez A. Nutr. Reports Int. 28:497, 1983*).

Animal Study: The effect of varying the compositions of dietary proteins on the relative cholesterolemic effects of animal and vegetable proteins was investigated in rabbits. It was concluded that the lysine/arginine ratio is not the major determinant of the cholesterolemic properties of proteins, but that the overall amino acid composition is primarily concerned (*Gibney MJ. The effect of dietary lysine to arginine ratio on cholesterol kinetics in rabbits. Atherosclerosis 47(3):263-70, 1983*).

Betaine:

- with folic acid and pyridoxine:

Supplementation may be beneficial for pts. with homocysteinuria.

Note: See "Pyridoxine" above for a discussion of homocysteinuria.

Experimental Study: The effects on plasma amino acids of a methionine load were assessed for 6 pyridoxine-responsive homocysteinuric patients both before and after adding betaine 6 gm daily to the treatment regimen of pyridoxine and folic acid. Prior to betaine, all pts. had higher plasma methionine and homocysteine and lower cysteine than 17 controls during the 24 hrs. after challenge. After betaine, these responses were reduced to near normal (*Wilcken DE et al. Homocystinuria due to cystathionine beta-synthase deficiency -- the effects of betaine treatment in pyridoxine-responsive patients. Metabolism 34(12):1115-21, 1985*).

Bromelain:
(A,G,P)

The proteolytic enzyme derived from the pineapple plant.

Said to inhibit platelet aggregation *in vitro* and *in vivo*, relieve angina pectoris and break down arteriosclerotic plaques.

General Ref.: *Taussig SJ, Heper HA. Bromelain: Its use in prevention and treatment of cardiovascular disease: Present status. J. Int. Acad. Prev. Med. Vol. 6, No. 1, 1979*

Experimental Study (A):   14 pts. with angina pectoris received 400-1000 mg daily with disappearance of symptoms in all pts. within 4 - 90 days depending upon the severity of the coronary sclerosis (*Nieper HA. Effect of bromelain on coronary heart disease and angina pectoris. Acta Med. Empirica 5:274-75, 1978*).

Animal Experimental Study (G): Bromelain broke down arteriosclerotic plaque in rabbit aorta both *in vivo* and *in vitro* (*Chen JR. In vivo and in vitro studies of the effect of bromelain on cholesterol-protein binding. Dissert. Abstr. B 1975 35 (2 Pt) 6013, Ord. No. 75-13, 735*).

Experimental Study (P): 2 tablets reduced platelet aggregability in 2 hours in 8/9 pts. with hyper-aggregable platelets and 8/11 pts. with normal platelet sensitivity (*Heinicke RM et al. Effect of bromelain (Ananase) on human platelet aggregation. Experientia 28:844, 1972*).

Carnitine: DL: 1500 mg. twice daily (1 month trial)
(A,C,H,T)   L: 750 mg. twice daily

Supplementation may allow the ischemic heart increased energy expenditure before coronary insufficiency develops by increasing its ability to oxidize fatty acids.

Experimental Double-blind Crossover Study (A):   44 men with chronic stable effort-induced angina randomly received either L-carnitine 1 gm twice daily or placebo.   After 4 wks., the exercise workload was increased, onset of angina was delayed, and ST segment depression at maximum workload was reduced in the pts. receiving L-carnitine compared to controls (*Cherchi A et al. Effects of L-carnitine on exercise tolerance in chronic, stable angina: A multicenter, double-blind, randomized, placebo controlled crossover study. Int. J. Clin. Pharmacol. Ther. Toxicol. 23(10):569-72, 1985*).

Experimental Study (A): IV infusions of L-carnitine in 18 coronary artery disease pts. improved free fatty acid metabolism and prevented lactate accumulation during atrial pacing, suggesting that L-carnitine may improve myocardial metabolism in such pts. (*Ferrari R et al. The metabolical effects of L-carnitine in angina pectoris. Int. J. Cardiol. 5:213, 1984*).

Experimental Placebo-controlled Study (A): 18 pts. with angina or coronary ischemia received injections or either carnitine or placebo and their treadmill performance was evaluated.   Compared to controls, pts. receiving carnitine exercised with less strain on the heart, maintained a lower heart rate and worked out longer before experiencing angina (*Kosolcharoen P et al. Improved exercise tolerance after administration of carnitine. Curr. Ther. Res. November, 1981, pp. 753-64*).

See Also:

Suzuki Y et al. Effect of L-carnitine on cardiac hemodynamics. Jap. Heart J. March, 1981, pp. 219-25

Thomsen JH et al. Improved pacing tolerance of the ischemic human myocardium after administration of carnitine. Am. J. Cardiol. 42:300-5, February, 1979

Folts JD et al. Protection of the ischemic dog myocardium with carnitine. Am. J. Cardiol. June, 1978, pp. 1209-14

May improve lipid metabolism.

Experimental Study (C,T): 20 diabetics received 1 mg/kg DL-carnitine for 10 days. There was a significant reduction of total serum lipids, triglycerides and cholesterol (*Abdel-Aziz MT et al. Effect of carnitine on blood lipid pattern in diabetic patients. Nutr. Rep. Internat. 29:1071, 1984*).

Experimental Study (H,T): 2 pts. with low HDL cholesterol but otherwise normal levels of cholesterol and triglycerides received 1 gm carnitine daily. HDL cholesterol substantially increased along with an increase in the HDL/total cholesterol ratio, while triglycerides decreased (*Rossi CS, Silliprandi N. Effect of carnitine on serum HDL cholesterol: Report of two cases. Johns Hopkins Med. J. 150:51-4, 1982*).

Experimental Study (T): 6 uremic pts. with type IV hypertriglyceridemia received 2400 mg carnitine daily for 6-24 months. In all 6, triglycerides fell to normal levels in 14 days and remained normal so long as carnitine was given. VLDL and free fatty acids also decreased (*Bougneres PF et al. Hypolipaemic effect of carnitine in uraemic patients. Lancet June, 1979, pp. 1401-2*).

Experimental Study (T): 18 pts. with type IV hyper-triglyceridemia were found to have significant reductions in triglycerides after 900 mg D,L carnitine daily (*Maebashi M et al. Lipid-lowering effect of carnitine in patients with Type IV hyper-lipoproteinemia. Lancet October 14, 1978, pp 805-7*).

See Also:

Pola P et al. *Carnitine in the therapy of dyslipidemic patients. Curr. Ther. Res. February, 1980, pp. 208-16*

Opie LH. *Role of carnitine in fatty acid metabolism of normal and ischemic myocardium. Am. Heart J. March, 1979, pp. 375-88*

Coenzyme A:
(C,H,T)

Derived from pantethine which, at doses of 300 mg 3 times daily, has been shown in several controlled studies to improve lipid metabolism (*see "Pantethine" below*).

Injections may improve lipid metabolism.

Experimental Study (C,H,T): 14 pts. with type II or type IV hyperlipidemia received injections of coenzyme A daily. After 20, days, mean total serum cholesterol fell about 10%, triglycerides fell 36.5%, and HDL cholesterol increased by 23% (*Ghidini O et al. Effects of short-term treatment with coenzyme A or sulodexide on plasma lipids in patients with hypertriglyceridemia (type IV) or mixed hyperlipemia (type IIb). Int. J. Clin. Pharmacol. Ther. Toxicol. 24:390, 1986*).

Coenzyme Q: 30 mg. daily in divided doses
(A)

Supplementation may reduce anginal episodes and improve cardiac function.

Experimental Double-blind Study: 10 men and women with stable angina pectoris received in random order 150 mg CoQ_{10} daily or placebo. After 4 weeks, subjects as compared to controls experienced a 53% reduction in the frequency of anginal episodes (1.25 vs. 2.65/wk; not statistically significant). Treadmill tolerance time (i.e. before angina) was significantly increased from 345 to 406 seconds, and the time until 1 mm of ST-segment depression occurred increased significantly from 196-284 seconds (*Kamikawa T et al. Effects of coenzyme Q_{10} on exercise tolerance in chronic stable angina pectoris. Am. J. Cardiol. 56:247, 1985*).

Experimental Controlled Study: After 3 mo. of supplementation, 22 pts. showed improvement vs. controls in functional class, exercise-induced S-T segment depression and exercise tolerance (*Biomed. & Clin. Aspects of Coenzyme Q* Vol. 2. *Amsterdam, Elsevier Science Publishers, 1980, p. 247*).

Glycosaminoglycans: 1200 mg. three times daily
(C,P,T)

Chondroitin sulphate is a constituent of acidic glycosaminoglycans found in arterial walls. These substances have anti-coagulant, anti-lipemic and anti-thrombogenic properties in addition to facilitating wound healing. They appear to form complexes with VLDL and LDL lipoproteins *in vitro* and *in vivo*. It has been suggested that the binding of LDL to glycosaminoglycans plays a significant role in the promotion of atheroma by causing a breakdown in the integrity of the extracellular collagen matrix components and an increased affinity for cholesterol (*Kostner GM et al. The interaction of human plasma low density lipoproteins with glycosamino-glycans: Influence of the chemical composition. Lipids 21:24-8, 1985*).

Experimental Controlled Study (C,T): Half of 46 elderly pts. received 3 gm chondroitin polysulphate daily while the other half received placebo. After 6-64 mo., serum cholesterol in the treated gp. fell to 10-20% lower and serum triglycerides fell to 27% lower than controls. After 3 mo., mean clotting time was prolonged by 50%. It is suggested that CPS acts similarly to heparin, but is much safer as no side-effects were reported (*Nakazawa K, Murata K. The therapeutic effect of chondroitin polysulphate in elderly atherosclerotic patients. J. Int. Med. Res. 6(3):217-25, 1978*).

Experimental Controlled Study (C): Of 120 EKG-demonstrated CHD pts. followed for 6 years, those receiving chondroitin-4-sulfate showed significantly fewer abnormal cardiac events (10%) vs. those in the control gp. (70%). There was also a highly significant difference in the death rate (7% vs. 23%) and treated pts. showed significant prolongation of thrombus formation time and reduced serum cholesterol levels. 10 gm. pure C-4-S was given 3 times daily for 3 months, then 1.5-3 gms. daily for 4.5 years, and 0.75-1.5 gm. daily for the rest of the study (*Izuka K, Murata K. Experientia 29:255-7, 1973*).

Experimental Controlled Study: 60/120 pts. with proven CHD were randomly selected to receive chondroitin sulfate A daily for 6 yrs. in addition to conventional treatment, while 60 received only conventional treatment. Whereas 42 controls experienced coronary incidents, only 6 pts. receiving CSA experienced incidents (p less than 0.001). Similarly, whereas 14 controls died of MI, only 4 pts. receiving CSA died of MI (p less than 0.001) (*Morrison LM, Enrick L. Coronary heart disease: Reduction of death rate by chondroitin sulfate A. Angiology 24:269-87, 1973*).

Omega-3 Fatty Acids:
(A,C,H,L,P,T)

Highest in cold water fish. Available in a refined form as "MaxEPA" (18% eicosapentaenoic acid)

Suggested MaxEPA dosage: 3 - 10 grams daily in divided doses (or10 ml. concentrate twice daily)

Tissue levels may be inversely correlated with the risk of ASHD.

Observational Study: In a study of several hundred randomly selected middle-aged men, platelet eicosapentaenoic acid made a significant and independent contribution to the explanation of angina pectoris but not to acute myocardial infarction, while platelet levels of docosahexaenoic acid did not differ between cases and controls. Omega-3 fatty acids were not found in adipose tissue (*Wood DA et al. Linoleic and eicosapentaenoic acids in adipose tissue and platelets and risk of coronary heart disease. Lancet 1:176-82, 1987*).

Observational Study: The fish consumption and mortality from coronary heart disease were studied over 20 years regarding 872 men residing in a town in the Netherlands. An inverse dose-response relation was observed between fish consumption in 1960 and CHD during 20 years of follow-up, with mortality more than 50% lower among those who consumed at least 30 gms. of fish daily. As little as 1-2 fish dishes per week may help to prevent CHD (*Kromhout D et al. The inverse relation between fish consumption and 20-year mortality from coronary heart disease. New Eng. J. Med. 312:1205-9, 1985*).

May decrease blood viscosity.

Experimental Study: Normal subjects receiving 3 gm. daily of MaxEPA for 3 wks. showed evidence of increased lipid fluidity and red cell deformability and reduced whole blood viscosity (*Cartwright IJ et al. The effects of dietary w-3 polyunsaturated fatty acids on erythrocyte membrane phospholipids, erythrocyte deformability and blood viscosity in healthy volunteers. Atherosclerosis 55:267-81, 1985*).

Experimental Study (T): 19 pts.with intermittent claudication decreased both whole blood viscosity and triglycerides after receiving 1.8 gm. fish oil for 7 weeks (*Woodcock BE et al. Beneficial effects of fish oil on blood viscosity in peripheral vascular disease. Brit. Med. J. 288:592-4, 1984*).

In addition to possibly reducing total cholesterol and increasing HDL cholesterol, it is the only polyunsaturated oil which may lower triglycerides.

Experimental Study (C,H,L,T): 6 subjects were given either a habitual diet (P/S 0.47, cholesterol 710 mg/d), a fish oil diet (MaxEPA 40 gm/day, P/S 1.62, cholesterol 190 mg/d), or a fish oil & egg yolk diet (P/S 1.62, cholesterol 940 mg/d). Changing from habitual to fish oil significantly lowered cholesterol and triglyceride levels in plasma, VLDL, LDL & HDL and in plasma apol-A$_1$ and apo-B. However, the addition of 750 mg/day of cholesterol failed to significantly raise lipoprotein cholesterol or apoprotein levels, although plasma cholesterol rose slightly. Results suggest that omega-3 fatty acids can lower lipoprotein cholesterol when dietary cholesterol is high (*Nestel P. Am. J. Clin. Nutr. 43:752-57, 1986*).

Experimental Controlled Study (C,T): 10 pts. with Type IIb hyperlipidemia and 10 with Type V were put on 3 diets for 4 wks. each: a control diet, a fish oil diet and a vegetable oil diet. The control diet contained a fatty acid mixture typical of a low-fat therapeutic diet (ratio of polyunsaturates to saturates = 1.4). The fish oil diet led to marked decreases in total cholesterol, triglycerides and VDRL's in both the Type IIb and the Type V groups as compared to the control diet. The vegetable oil diet produced a rapid rise in plasma triglyceride levels and a much smaller reduction in total cholesterol and VDRL's (*Phillipson BE et al. Reduction of plasma lipids, lipoproteins, and apoproteins by dietary fish oils in patients with hypertriglyceridemia. New Eng. J. Med. 312:1210-6, 1985*).

Experimental Crossover Study (C,H,T): 8 pts. with type IV and V hyperlipoproteinemia were put on a mackerel and herring diet for 2 weeks each. After mackerel, serum triglycerides and total cholesterol were significantly lower, returning to basal levels 3 mo. later, while HDL cholesterol was slightly increased. After herring (which contained half as much EPA) the differences were minor (*Singer P et al. Influence on serum lipids, lipoproteins and blood pressure of mackerel and herring diet in patients with type IV and V hyperlipoproteinemia. Athero. 56(1):111-18, 1985*).

Experimental Double-blind Crossover Study (C,H,T): 16 male pts. consumed MaxEPA 5 gms. daily for 2 months. Compared to baseline fasting lipid levels, total triglycerides and total cholesterol significantly decreased while HDL cholesterol significantly increased. By contrast, consumption of omega-6 rich vegetable oil (5 gm. twice daily) only slightly decreased total triglycerides and slightly increased HDL cholesterol (*Saynor R. Effects of omega-3 fatty acids on serum lipids. Lancet 2:696-7, 1984*).

Experimental Controlled Study (C,T): 7 subjects were placed on 3 consecutive diets, each containing equal amts. of cholesterol and 40% fat. Fat in the control diet was saturated, while fat from the second diet came from unsaturated safflower and corn oil (sources of omega-6 EFA) and fat from the third diet came from salmon and salmon oil (sources of omega-3 EFA). Compared to the control diet, both experimental diets reduced cholesterol by 11%; however, only the fish oil diet reduced triglycerides (by 33%). In addition, gram for gram, the omega-3 EFA were far more potent than the omega-6 EFA in reducing cholesterol (*Harris WS et al. Metabolism 32:179, 1983*).

Experimental Double-blind Study (C,H,P,T): 10 healthy subjects were given 10 gm. MaxEPA or vegetable oil for 2 weeks. Following either supplement, there was a lower response to one of the platelet aggregating agents and no change in plasma cholesterol. Only the MaxEPA lowered plasma triglyceride concentrations and increased HDL cholesterol (*Sanders TAB et al. A comparison of the influence on plasma lipids and platelet function of supplements of w3 and w6 polyunsaturated fatty acids. Brit. J. Nutr. 50:521-30, 1983*).

See Also:

(C,T) *Simons LA et al. On the effects of dietary n-3 fatty acids (MaxEPA) on plasma lipids and lipoproteins in patients with hyperlipidemia. Atherosclerosis 54:75-88, 1985*

May reduce tissue damage from acute ischemia.

Animal Experimental Study: When dogs had coronary arteries tied off, 25% of the left ventricle was damaged in controls compared to only 3% damage in dogs fed omega-3 fatty acids (*Culp BR et al. Prostaglandins 20:1021, 1980*).

May reduce anginal pain and improve exercise tolerance.

Experimental Study (A,C,H,L,T): 107 subjects with either heart disease, hyperlipidemia or no symptoms received 3.6 gm. daily of Max-EPA for up to 2 years. At the end, those with angina reported fewer episodes of pain and needed less nitroglycerin. Triglycerides, cholesterol, bleeding times and VLDL and LDL lipoproteins decreased, while HDL increased significantly (*Saynor R et al. The long-term effect of dietary supplementation with fish lipid concentrate on serum lipids, bleeding time, platelets and angina. Atherosclerosis 50:3-10, 1984*).

Experimental Study (A,C,H,T): 150 ASHD pts. and normal volunteers were supplemented with MaxEPA for up to 3 years. Long term patients were able to reduce nitrate therapy and exhibited increased exercise tolerance while taking the supplement. After 2 years, triglycerides, which fell sharply during the first few weeks, remained low. Total cholesterol was significantly lower and HDL cholesterol was significantly higher. Bleeding time increased when the daily dose was 20 ml. (3.6 gm.) but not when it was 10 ml. (1.8 gm) (*Saynor R, Verel D. Lancet 1:1335, 1983*).

May play a very important role in the treatment of thrombotic disorders by reducing platelet aggregation and improving blood flow dynamics.

Experimental Study (P): 8 healthy volunteers received 3.5 gm. daily of highly purified EPA for 4 weeks, after which platelet aggregation was decreased, whole blood viscosity was reduced and erythrocyte deformability was increased (*Terano T et al. Effects of eicosapentaenoic acid on platelet function, blood viscosity and red cell deformity in humans. Atherosclerosis 46:321-31, 1983*).

Experimental Study (C,P,T): 12 men and women received 2 gms. of 67% pure eicosapentaenoic ester daily for 4 weeks. Cholesterol, triglycerides and platelet aggregation were significantly decreased (*Nagakawa Y. Effects of eicosapentaenoic acid on the platelet aggregation and composition of fatty acids in man. Atherosclerosis 47(1):71-5, 1983*).

<u>Omega-6 Fatty Acids:</u>
(C,P)

$$\text{Linoleic acid} \rightarrow \text{GLA} \rightarrow \text{DGLA} \rightarrow \text{Prostaglandin E}_1$$

Several oils are rich in linoleic acid, while evening primrose oil is one of the richest sources of gammalinolenic acid (GLA). When, due to such factors as aging, the intake of *trans* fatty acids, pyridoxine, magnesium or zinc deficiencies, excessive alcohol consumption, etc., the conversion of linoleic acid to GLA is inhibited, primrose oil is superior to most oils as a PGE_1 precursor (*Horrobin DF. The importance of gamma-linolenic acid and prostaglandin E_1 in human nutrition and medicine. J. Holistic Med. 3:118-139, 1981*).

Tissue levels of prostaglandin E_1 precursors may be inversely correlated with the risk of ASHD.

Observational Study: In a study of several hundred randomly selected middle-aged men, there was a progressive inverse relationship between adipose linoleic acid and the estimated relative risk of angina pectoris. This relationship was independent of traditional risk factors. There was also a progressive inverse relationship between adipose tissue linoleic acid and the estimated relative risk of acute myocardial infarction, but it was confounded by smoking habit as smokers consumed less linoleic acid than non-smokers (*Wood DA et al. Linoleic and eicosapentaenoic acids in adipose tissue and platelets and risk of coronary heart diseae. Lancet 1:176-82, 1987*).

Observational Study: Stepwise regression analysis found that, for post-infarction middle-aged men, low linoleic acid levels correlated most strongly with cardiovascular death, followed by previous MI, heart volume index, and hyperlipoproteinemia (*Valek J et al. Serum linoleic acid and cardiovascular death in postinfarction middle-aged men. Atherosclerosis 54:11-8, 1985*).

Observational Study: Men with previously diagnosed CHD have a significantly lower level of linoleic and dihomogammalinolenic acids in their adipose tissue than other men, including those with newly diagnosed CHD (*Wood DA et al. Adipose tissue and platelet fatty acids and coronary heart disease in Scottish men. Lancet 2:117-121, 1984*).

Observational Study: 32 men who had recently sustained a MI were matched with healthy controls. Pts. had a significantly lower proportion of linoleic acid in their plasma fatty acids. Their red-cell membrane phosphatidylcholine (which reflects long-term fat intake) also showed a significantly lower proportion of linoleic acid (*Simpson H et al. Low dietary intake of linoleic acid predisposes to myocardial infarction. Br. Med. J. 285:684, 1982*).

See Also:

Review Article: *Willis AL. Dihomo-gamma-linolenic acid as the endogenous protective agent for myocardial infarction. Lancet 2:697, 1984*

May lower plasma cholesterol.

Experimental Placebo-controlled Study (C):   84 pts. received 4 gm. evening primrose oil daily x 12 weeks. Afterwards, cholesterol was significantly decreased in pts. whose cholesterols had been above 192 mg% (*Horrobin DF, Manku MS. How do poly-unsaturated fatty acids lower plasma cholesterol levels? Lipids 18:558-62, 1983*).

May decrease platelet aggregability.

Experimental Study (C,P): 6 healthy volunteers received safflower oil 60 mg. daily as a source of linoleic acid. After 2 wks., there was decreased platelet aggregation to ADP in addition to decreased cholesterol. Fibrinolysis and bleeding times were unaltered (*Challen AD et al. The effect* *of aspirin and linoleic on platelet aggregation, platelet fatty acid composition and haemostatis in man. Hum. Nutr.: Clin. Nutr. 37(3):197-208, 1983).*

Experimental Study (P): Most subjects receiving 0.1-2 gm. DGLA demonstrated decreases in plasma heparin neutralizing activity and in ADP-induced platelet aggregation, especially when the dose was 1 gm. or higher (*Kernoff PBA et al. Antithrombotic potential of dihomo-gamma-linolenic acid in man. Brit.Med. 2:1441, 1977*).

Pantethine: 300 mg 2-4 times daily with food
(C,H,L,P,T)   Changes in cholesterol may take 1-2 months and maximal effect may require 4 or more months

The active form of pantothenic acid (the fundamental moiety of coenzyme A). (*see "Coenzyme A" above*)

May decrease serum triglyceride and cholesterol levels.

Experimental Study (C,H,T): 24 pts. (mean age 51 yrs.) with Types IIA, IIB or IV hyperlipidemia received pantethine 300 mg 3 times daily. After 1 yr., there was a highly significant (p less than 0.001) reduction of about 17% in mean serum cholesterol levels which had become evident within 1 month and persisted thereafter. Mean HDL cholesterol levels increased by about 15% (results not significant) and mean triglyceride levels fell by 48% (p less than 0.01). There were no significant side effects (*Pantethine treatment of hyperlipidemia. Clin. Ther. 8:537, 1986*).

Experimental Study (C): In an open randomized study of hypercholesterolemic pts., pantethine was as effective as fenofibrate in lowering total and LDL cholesterol levels but without the side effects of the drug, suggesting that it is the therapy of choice for hypercholesterolemia (*Cattin L et al. Treatment of hypercholesterolemia with pantethine and fenofibrate: An open randomized study on 43 subjects. Current Ther. Res. 38(3):386-95, 1985*).

Negative Experimental Double-blind Study (C): Supplementation was ineffective for pts. who had previously failed to respond to a combined drug/diet regime (*Da Col PG et al. Pantethine in the treatment of hyper-cholesterolemia: A randomized double-blind trial versus tiadenol. Curr. Ther. Res. 36:314, 1984*).

Experimental Study (C,T): Following supplementation, normal values were obtained in 83% of hypercholesterolemic pts. and 35.7% of hyper-triglyceridemic pts. (*Galeone F et al. The lipid lowering effect of pantethine in hyperlipidemic patients: A clinical investigation. Curr. Ther. Res. 34:383-90, 1983*).

See Also:

> **Experimental Study (H):** *Maioli M et al. Effect of pantethine on the subfractions of HDL in dislipemic patients. Curr. Ther. Res. 35:307, 1984*

> **Experimental Crossover Double-blind Study** (C,T): *Angelico M et al. Improvement in serum lipid profile in hyper-lipoproteinaemic patients after treatment with pantethine: a crossover, double-blind trial versus placebo. Curr. Ther. Res. 33:1091, 1983*

May increase microsomal lipoprotein lipase which is positively correlated with HDL cholesterol levels.

> **Animal Experimental Study:** *Noma A et al. Effect of pantethine on post-heparin plasma lipolytic activities and adipose tissue lipoprotein lipase in rats. Horm. Met. Res. 16:233-6, 1984*

May have anti-arrhythmic activity during hypoxia.

> **Animal Experimental Study:** *Hayashi H et al. Effects of pantethine on action potential of canine papillary muscle during hypoxic infusion. Jap. Heart J. 26:289-96, 1985*

May inhibit platelet aggregation.

> **Experimental Study (P):** Following 28 days of supplementation with pantethine 300 mg 4 times daily, hyperlipidemic pts. demonstrated inhibition of platelet aggregation and thromboxane A$_2$ production (*Prisco D et al. Effect of pantethine treatment on platelet aggregation and thromboxane A$_2$ production. Curr. Ther. Res. 35:700, 1984*).

Phosphatidyl Choline:
(C,G,H,L,T)

Supplementation may not only improve lipoprotein metabolism, but may cause regression of plaques.

> **Animal Experimental Study (C,G,T):** The addition of 3% soya lecithin for 3 months successfully restored a healthy distribution of plasma lipoproteins and modified arterial lesions in rabbits with cholesterol-induced atherogenesis (*Hunt C et al. Hyperlipoproteinaemia and atherosclerosis in rabbits fed low-level cholesterol and lecithin. Brit. J. Exp. Path. 66:35-46, 1985*).

> **Experimental Double-blind Crossover Study (C,H,L):** 35 gm. daily of lecithin (53% phosphatidyl choline) significantly lowered total cholesterol and LDL cholesterol and raised HDL cholesterol after 2-3 mo. in 10 Alzheimer's pts. (*Vroulis G et al. Reduction of cholesterol risk factors by lecithin in patients with Alzheimer's disease. Am. J. Psychiat. 139:1633-4, 1982*).

> **Experimental Controlled Study (C,H,L,T):** Raised HDL cholesterol while lowering LDL cholesterol and triglycerides (*Childs MT et al. The contrasting effects of a dietary soya-lecithin product and corn oil on lipoprotein lipids in normolipidemic and familial hypercholesterolemic subjects. Atherosclerosis 38:217-28, 1981*).

Phytosterols: 300 mg daily (based on beta-sitosterol content)
(C)   immediately before or after meals (2 wk. trial)

Cholesterol analogs found in vegetables which may lower serum cholesterol.

May decrease cholesterol absorption.

> **Experimental Study:** Ingestion of phytosterols with a meal decreased cholesterol absorption by as much as 64% (*Mattson FH et al. Optimizing the effect of plant sterols on cholesterol absorption in man. Am. J. Clin. Nutr. 35:697-700, 1982*).

May reduce serum cholesterol even in the total absence of dietary cholesterol (*Beveridge et al. Can. J. Biochem. Physiol. 36:895, 1958*).

See Also:

> *Drexel H et al. Lowering plasma cholesterol with beta sitosterol and diet. Lancet 1:157, 1981*

> *Vahouny GV, Kritchevsky D. Plant and marine sterols and cholesterol metabolism. Nutritional Pharmacol. 32-72, 1981*

> *Lees RS, Lees AM. Effects of sitosterol therapy on plasma lipid and lipoprotein concentrations. Lipoprotein Metab. 119-24, 1976*

Taurine:
(G)

Arrhythmias characteristic of acute myocardial ischemia may be partly due to loss of intracellular taurine (*Crass MF, Lombardini JB. Release of tissue taurine from the oxygen-deficient perfused rat heart. Proc. Soc. Exp. Biol. & Med. 157:486-8, 1978*)

Observational Study: Blood samples from 97 consecutive pts. admitted for chest pains were analyzed for taurine concentrations. The mean maximum taurine concentrations in whole blood from acute MI pts. were greater than that of pts. without acute MI. By contrast, there was no difference in plasma taurine in the 2 gps., indicating that a cellular component(s) of whole blood was sequestering taurine. A myocardial source for the blood taurine rise is probable, and there is evidence that the myocardium selectively leaks taurine but not other amino acids (*Lombardini JB, Cooper MW. Elevated blood taurine levels in acute and evolving myocardial infarction. J. Lab. Clin. Med. 98(6):849-59, 1981*).

Much like magnesium, taurine affects membrane excitability by normalizing potassium flux in and out of the heart muscle cell (*Chazov EL et al. Taurine and electrical activity of the heart. Circ. Res. 35 Suppl. 3:11-21, 1974*).

Experimental Animal Study: After the balanced electrolytic state in rat myocardium was impaired by adrenaline administration at arrhythmogenic doses, taurine normalized the content of potassium and calcium ions both *in vivo* and *in vitro* (*Shustova TI et al. [Effect of taurine on potassium, calcium and sodium levels in the blood and tissues of rats.] Vopr. Med. Khim. 32(4):113-116, 1986*).

In vitro Experimental Animal Study: In isolated guinea-pig heart submitted to hypoxia and subsequent oxygenation, taurine decreased LDH release and ventricular arrhythmias and increased the recovery of normal electrical and mechanical activity (*Franconi F et al. The protective effect of taurine on hypoxia (performed in the absence of glucose) and on reoxygenation (in the presence of glucose) in guinea-pig heart. Biochem. Pharmacol. 34(15):2611-15, 1985*).

See Also:

Huxtable RJ, Sebring LA. Cardiovascular actions of taurine. Prog. Clin. Biol. Res. 125:5-37, 1983

Supplementation may prevent atherogenesis.

Animal Experimental Study (G): Mice receiving nicotine along with vitamin D3 developed severe myocardial and aortic calcinosis within 4 days. Treatment with taurine increased the survival rate and reduced the elevation of calcium content in both aorta and myocardium, suggesting that taurine, which is capable of regulating calcium flux, may also prevent the progression of arteriosclerosis (*Yamauchi-Takihara K et al. Taurine protection against experimental arterial calcinosis in mice. Biochem. Biophys. Res. Commun. 140(2):679-83, 1986*).

- -

Alfalfa:
(C,G,H,L)

Rich in saponins which are capable of binding to cholesterol and bile salts in the gut to prevent absorption. In addition, the interaction of other components with bile acids may be equally important (*Story JA et al. Am. J. Clin. Nutr. 39:917-29, 1984*).

Experimental Study (C,H,L): Following 3 wks. on a diet enriched with 10 tsp. alfalfa seed powder daily, blood cholesterol levels declined as much as 20% and HDL/LDL ratios improved by up to 40% (*Malinow MR et al. Alfalfa. Am. J. Clin. Nutr. 1810-12, 1979*).

May cause regression and dissolution of plaque.

Animal Experimental Study (G): Arteriosclerotic monkeys on a diet enriched with 50 gm. alfalfa daily showed considerable reduction in blood cholesterol along with signs of regression of atherosclerotic plaques in the coronary arteries that were present at the start of the study (*Malinow MR et al. Atherosclerosis 30:27-43,1973*).

Beans: 1/2 cup daily (3 week trial)
(C,L)

Supplementation may lower LDL cholesterol levels.

Experimental Study (C,H,L): 8 hypercholesterolemic men ate balanced diets for 1 wk. followed by diets that included 115 gm. (1/2 cup dry) common beans (pinto, navy, kidney, etc.). After 3 wks., total cholesterol levels dropped an ave. of 20%. While HDL cholesterol levels were unchanged, LDL lipoprotein cholesterol decreased 24% (*Anderson JW, Chen WL. Effects of legumes and their soluble fibers on cholesterol-rich lipoproteins. Am. Chem. Soc. Abstracts AGFD #39, 1982*).

Brewer's Yeast: 20 gm. daily (8 week trial)
(C,H,L,T)

Supplementation may lower LDL cholesterol while raising HDL cholesterol.

Experimental Study (C,H): 46 healthy volunteers were classified as either normolipidemic or hyper-lipidemic and supplemented with brewer's yeast. After 8 wks., triglycerides were unchanged but serum cholesterol was reduced for 8/15 hyperlipidemic subjects and 10/11 normolipidemic subjects, while HDL cholesterol increased for both groups (*Elwood JC et al. Effect of high-chromium brewer's yeast on human serum lipids. J. Am. Coll. Nutr. 1:263-74, 1982*).

Experimental Single-blind Study (C):   24 elderly pts. (4 of whom were hypercholesterolemic) who received chromium-rich brewer's yeast for 8 wks improved glucose tolerance and significantly decreased serum cholesterol (especially in the hypercholesterolemic pts.) and total lipids, while the findings on controls who received chromium-poor tortula yeast were unchanged (*Offenbachaer EG, Pi-Sunyer FX. Beneficial effect of chromium-rich yeast on glucose tolerance and blood lipids in elderly subjects. Diabetes 29:919-25, 1980*).

Experimental Study (H,L): Subjects received 7 gm GTF-rich brewer's yeast (15 mcg chromium). After 6 wks. there was a significant increase (ave. 17.6%) in HDL cholesterol levels. HDL to LDL ratios improved from an ave. of 0.413 to 0.596, an improvement of 44% (*Riales R. Chromium in Nutrition and Metabolism. North-Holland Biomedical Press, 1979, pp. 199-212*).

Eggplant:
(G)

- with vitamin C:

May protect against the development of plaques.

Animal Experimental Study (G): Animals fed eggplant along with vitamin C-rich foods were protected from developing fatty plaques (*Mitschek GHA. Experimentelle Pathologie vol. 10, 1975*).

Garlic and
Onion:
(C,F,G,P,T)

Garlic may reduce cholesterol by inhibiting its synthesis.

Experimental Controlled Study (C,T): 10 hypercholesterolemic pts. were treated with 600 mg garlic powder daily (equivalent to 1800 gm fresh garlic) and showed a 10% mean decrease in cholesterol levels and a significant decrease in plasma viscosity, levels of triglycerides and low density lipoproteins compared to controls (*Ernst E et al. Garlic and blood lipids. Brit. Med. J. 291:139, 1985*).

Supplementation may protect against atherogenesis.

Experimental Studies (C,H,T): 1. 20 healthy volunteers were fed garlic for 6 mo. and then followed for another 2 mo. without garlic. Garlic significantly lowered serum cholesterol and triglycerides while raising high density lipoproteins. 2. 62 pts. with CHD and elevated serum cholesterol were randomly divided so that one gp. received garlic for 10 mo. while the other gp. served as a control. Garlic decreased serum cholesterol (p less than 0.05), triglycerides (p less than 0.05) and low-density lipoprotein (p less than 0.05) while increasing the high-density fraction (p less than 0.001) (*Bordia A. Effect of garlic on blood lipids in patients with coronary heart disease. Am. J. Clin. Nutr. 34:2100-03, 1981*).

Animal Experimental Study (C,G): Garlic fed to rabbits on a high cholesterol diet prevented a rise in blood cholesterol and inhibited development of atherosclerosis in the aorta (*Jain RC. Am. J. Clin. Nutr. 31:1982, 1978*).

Animal Experimental Study (G): The administration of garlic and onion prevented the formation of experimental AS in rabbits (*Bordia A et al. Effect of essential oil of onion and garlic on experimental atherosclerosis in rabbits. Atherosclerosis 26:379-82, 1977*).

Both onions and garlic inhibit platelet aggregation by blocking thromboxane synthesis for several hours (*Makheja AN. Lancet April 7, 1979*).

In vitro Experimental Study: Aqueous extracts of onion and garlic inhibited platelet aggregation induced by several aggregation agents, including arachidonate, in a dose-dependent manner (*Srivastava KC. Aqueous extracts of onion, garlic and ginger inhibit platelet aggregation and alter arachidonic acid metabolism. Biomed. Biochim. Acta 43(8/9):S335-S346, 1984*).

Experimental Study (P): 100-150 mg./kg. fresh garlic completely inhibited platelet aggregation to 5-hydroxytryptamine for 1-2 1/2 hours after ingestion (*Doullin DJ. Garlic as a platelet inhibitor. Lancet 1:776-7, 1981*).

Experimental Study (P): 6 healthy subjects took 25 mg. of garlic oil daily. After 5 days, platelet aggregation induced by 3 different aggregating agents was inhibited (*Bordia A. Effect of garlic on human platelet aggregation in vitro. Atherosclerosis 30:355, 1978*).

See Also:

Baghurst KI et al. Onions and platelet aggregation. Lancet January 8, 1977

Supplementation may increase fibrinolytic activity.

Experimental Study (F): Onion increased fibrinolytic activity (*Baghurst KI et al. - ibid*).

Experimental Study (F): When garlic (equivalent to the essential oil of garlic extracted from 1 gm of raw garlic per kgm of body weight) was given within 24 hours after a M.I., fibrinolytic activity increased 63% after 10 days and 95% after 20 days. When given to normals, fibrinolytic activity rose 130% (*Bordia AK et al. Effect of garlic oil on fibrinolytic activity in patients with CHD. Atherosclerosis 28:155-9, 1977*).

Ginger:
(C,P)

Supplementation may inhibit platelet aggregation.

Review Article (P): Ginger is a potent inhibitor of thromboxane synthetase as is aspirin and other inhibitors of platelet aggregation. In contrast to other platelet aggregation inhibitors, however, it raises levels of prostacyclin without a concomitant rise in inflammatory prostaglandins; thus it should cause substantially fewer side-effects (*Backon J. Ginger: Inhibition of thromboxane synthetase and stimulation of prostacyclin: Relevance for medicine and psychiatry. Med. Hypotheses 20:271, 1986*).

In vitro Experimental Study (P): Ginger inhibited platelet aggregation *in vitro* more than either onion or garlic (*Srivastava KC. Effects of aqueous extracts of onion, garlic and ginger on platelet aggregation and metabolism of arachidonic acid in the blood vascular system: In vitro study. Prostagl. Med. 13:227, 1984*).

In vitro Experimental Study (P): Platelet-rich plasma was preincubated for 1-60 min. with an ethanol extract of ground ginger. The extract completely inhibited arachidonate-induced platelet aggregation, whereas the ethanol vehicle was without effect (*Dorso CR et al. Chinese food and platelets. Letter to the Editor. New Engl. J. Med. 303:756-57, 1980*

Supplementation may reduce cholesterol levels.

Animal Experimental Study (C): *Gujaral S et al. Effect of ginger (zinger officinale roscoe) oleoresin on serum and hepatic cholesterol levels in cholesterol fed rats. Nutr. Rep. Int. 17:183-9, 1978*

Ginkgo biloba:
(C,I)

Supplementation may protect against arterial hypoxia.

Experimental Double-blind Study: *Schaffler VK, Reeh PW. Double-blind study of the hypoxia-protective effect of a standardized ginkgo bilobae preparation after repeated administration in healthy volunteers. Arzneim-Forsch 35:1283-6, 1985*

Supplementation may relieve symptoms of peripheral arterial insufficiency.

Experimental Double-blind Study (I): Pts. receiving the supplement demonstrated significantly greater pain-free and maximum walking distance, as well as improved plethysmographic and doppler measurements in the affected limb after exercise (*Bauer U. 6-month double-blind randomized clinical trial of ginkgo biloba extract versus placebo in two parallel groups in patients suffering from peripheral arterial insufficiency. Arzneim-Forsch 34:716-21, 1984*).

Sardine Oil:

Rich in eicosapentaenoic acid (omega-3 fatty acid) and vitamin E.

Supplementation may increase RBC membrane fluidity, thus potentially reducing symptoms due to impaired red cell deformability (such as intermittent claudication).

Experimental Controlled Study: Dietary sardine oil 2.7 gm daily was given to diabetic and control subjects. Compared to controls, RBC membrane fluidity was lower in the diabetics prior to supplementation. After 4 wks., membrane fluidity was increased in both diabetics and controls, and remained elevated for the entire 8 wk. study, with disappearance of the difference in RBC membrane fluidity between diabetics and controls (*Kamada T et al. Dietary sardine oil increases erythrocyte membrane fluidity in diabetic patients. Diabetes 35:604, 1986*).

Yogurt: 3 cups daily (1 week trial)
(C)

Supplementation may reduce total cholesterol levels.

Experimental Study (C): 5 men and 6 women ate 3 cups yogurt daily. After the first week, their average cholesterol level had decreased from 252-230 where it stayed for the remaining 11 wks. of the study (*Hepner B et al. Hypocholesterolemic effect of yogurt and milk. Am. J. Clin. Nutr. 32:19-24, 1979*).

- -

OTHER FACTORS:

Activated Charcoal:
(C,H,L,T)

Supplementation may reduce triglycerides and may reduce LDL cholesterol while raising HDL cholesterol.

Experimental Study (C,H,L): 7 pts. with hypercholesterolemia who had responded only marginally to 10 yrs. of treatment with clofibrate, gemfibrozil and/or nicotinic acid received activated charcoal 8 gm 3 times daily. After 4 wks., plasma total cholesterol decreased by 41%, LDL cholesterol decreased by 25%, and HDL cholesterol increased by 8%. Except for black stools, there were no side effects (*Kuusisto R et al. Effect of activated charcoal on hypercholesterolaemia. Lancet 2:366-67, 1986*).

Experimental Study (C,T): 6 uremic pts. received 35 gms. daily of activated charcoal. After 24 wks., cholesterol levels had dropped as much as 43%, and triglyceride levels had fallen as much as 76% (*Friedman EA et al. Charcoal-induced lipid reduction in uremia. Kidney Int. 13(suppl 8):170-76, 1978*).

AUTISM

NUTRIENTS:

<u>Pyridoxine:</u>   350 mg. (small child) - 1 gm. (adult) daily

Supplementation may be beneficial.

> **Experimental Study:** Vitamin B6 supplementation   changed electrophysiological and biochemical values of autistic children to more normal values (*Lelord G et al. Electrophysiological and biochemical studies in autistic children treated with vitamin B6 in Lehmann D, Callaway E. <u>Human Evoked Potentials: Applications and Problems</u>. New York, Plenum Press, 1979*).

> **Experimental Study:** Vitamin B6 supplementation improved behavior in 15/37 autistic children. In addition, B6 reduced homovanillic acid (the principal derivative of dopamine) levels in the urines of 33/37 autistic children and increased it in 11/11 normal controls (*Lelord G et al. Modifications in urinary homovanillic acid after ingestion of vitamin B6: Functional study in autistic children. <u>Rev. Neuro. (Paris)</u> 134(12):797-801*).

> **Experimental Double-blind Crossover Study:** 16 autistic-type children who appeared to benefit from B6 in a non-blind study had their B6 supplements replaced during 2 separate experimental periods by another B6 supplement or a matched placebo. Behavior was rated as deteriorating significantly during the B6 withdrawal (*Rimland B et al. The effect of high doses of vitamin B6 on autistic children: A double-blind crossover study. <u>Am. J. Psychiat.</u> 135:472-475, 1978*).

- with <u>Magnesium:</u>

The addition of magnesium to pyridoxine is said to prevent the irritability, sound hypersensitivity and enuresis sometimes caused by pyridoxine supplementation (which can create a relative deficiency of magnesium) when given at 1/2 the dosage of pyridoxine (*Rimland B. An Orthomolecular study of psychotic children. <u>J. Orthomol. Psychiat.</u> 3:371-7, 1974*).

> **Experimental Crossed-sequential Double-blind Study:**   60 autistic children were given trials of vitamin B6 alone, magnesium alone, or B6 plus magnesium. A behavioral improvement was only observed with the vitamin B6-magnesium combination; this improvement was associated with decreased urinary homovanillic acid excretion and normalization of evoked potential amplitude and morphology (*Martineau J et al. Vitamin B6, magnesium, and combined B6-Mg: Therapeutic effects in childhood autism. <u>Biol. Psychiat.</u> 20:467-78, 1985*).

> **Experimental Double-blind Crossover Study:** 44 autistic children (34 of whom were on psychotropic medications) were treated with B6 and magnesium lactate. 15/44 (34%) improved during the trial and 14/15 regressed 3 wks. after terminating supplementation. During treatment, 3/44 became nauseated, 3 showed increased excitability, and 4 increased autistic symptoms. Later, 13 responders and 8 nonresponders were restudied in a 4 wk. double-blind crossover trial with B6 and placebo, each being provided for 2 weeks. Only 3/13 responders failed to improve during supplementation while only 2/8 nonresponders improved during supplementation, suggesting that the effects of B6 and magnesium in the responders represented a repeatable response to their treatment (*Lelord G et al. Effects of pyridoxine and magnesium on autistic symptoms - Initial observations. <u>J. Autism Dev. Disord.</u> 11:219-230, 1981*).

Experimental Study: 11 normal children and 12 autistic children received 30 mg/kg B_6 daily with magnesium lactate. Although the level of urinary homovanillic acid (the main metabolite of dopamine) was higher in the autistic than in the control children before treatment, B_6 produced a decrease in HVA in the autistic children and a slight insignificant increase in the normal children. Auditory evoked potential amplitudes, found to be lower in the autistic children, tended to increase with B_6 in the autistic children, and the correlation between changes in AEP and HVA for autistic children showed a significant inverse relationship. 6/12 autistic children showed marked clinical improvement during B_6 therapy, and the tendency towards clinical normalization was accompanied by a tendency towards normalization of AEP and HVA levels (*Martineau J et al. Effects of vitamin B_6 on averaged evoked potentials in infantile autism. Biol. Psychiat. 16:627-41, 1981*).

Magnesium:

May be deficient.

Observational Study: Hair magnesium levels of 28 autistic children were lower than those of 18 controls including 14 siblings, and magnesium was the main element that statistically distinguished the two groups (*Marlow M et al. Decreased magnesium in the hair of autistic children. J. Orthomol. Psychiat. 13(2):117-122, 1984*).

OTHER FACTORS:

Rule out food sensitivities.

Observational Study: Parents of autistic children rated their impressions of the effectiveness of various treatments:

Treatment	# Cases	Some Improvement or Definitely Helped
(Operant Conditioning)	603	82%
(Day School)	1703	70%
(Patterning)	211	53%
Remove SUGAR	202	52%
Remove MILK	250	44%
Remove WHEAT	148	44%
(Psychotherapy)	656	34%

(*Rimland, Bernard. Comparative effects of treatment on child's behavior. Publication 34, Institute for Child Behavior Research, 4157 Adams Avenue, San Diego, California 92116, June, 1977*)

AUTO-IMMUNE DISORDERS
(GENERAL)

See Also: LUPUS   RAYNAUD'S SYNDROME
     MULTIPLE SCLEROSIS   RHEUMATOID ARTHRITIS
     MUSCULAR DYSTROPHY   SCLERODERMA
     NEUROMUSCULAR DEGENERATION VASCULITIS

NUTRIENTS:

Vitamin E:

Supplementation may be beneficial.

Case Reports: Pts. are described with various autoimmune diseases who improved following months of supplementation with D-alpha-tocopherol acetate or succinate, 800-1600 IU daily (*Ayres S, Mihan R. Is vitamin E involved in the autoimmune mechanism? Cutis 21:321-25, 1978*).

Animal Experimental Study (dogs): Estrogen administration produced thrombocytopenic purpura which was cured by large doses of vitamin E and could be prevented by prior administration of vitamin E (*Skelton F et al. Science 163:762, 1946*).

- -

Omega-3 Fatty Acids:

("MaxEPA" is a refined source with 18% eicosapentaenoic acid.)

May change the balance of prostaglandins and leukotrienes (which are powerful mediators of inflammation and immune responses).

Experimental Study: The diets of 7 normal subjects were supplemented with 3.2 gm EPA or 1.8 gm MaxEPA daily for 6 weeks. EPA in neutrophils was increased 7 fold without any increase in arachidonic acid. When the neutrophils were activated, there was a 37% reduction in the release of arachidonic acid and a 48% reduction in the inflammatory products of this pathway. In addition, the adherence of neutrophils to bovine epithelial cells as monolayers treated with leukotriene B-4 was completely inhibited. The results suggest that diets enriched with fish oil-derived fatty acids have anti-inflammatory effects by inhibiting the 5-lipoxygenase pathway, thus causing a reduction in the release of leukotrienes along with a reduction in the release of superoxide from neutrophils (*Lee TH et al. New Eng. J. Med. 312:1217, 1985*).

Shown in animal models of autoimmune disease to help prevent kidney destruction and prolong life.

Animal Experimental Study: Dietary supplementation of fish oil as the exclusive source of lipid was found to suppress autoimmune lupus in mice, delaying the onset of renal disease and prolonging survival (*Kelley VE et al. A fish oil diet rich in eicosapentaenoic acid reduces cyclooxygenase metabolites, and suppresses lupus in MRL-lpr mice. J. Immunol. 134(3):1914-19, 1985*).

Animal Experimental Study: 98% of mice fed the control diet (beef tallow) had died of severe renal disease by 19 months of age compared to only 15% of the fish oil-treated group. Mice started on the fish oil diet as late as 4-5 months of age (instead of at weaning) were similarly protected (*Prickett JD et al. Effects of dietary enrichment with eicosapentaenoic acid upon autoimmune nephritis in female NZBxNZW/F$_1$ mice. Arth. Rheumat. 26:133-39, 1983*).

Omega-6 Fatty Acids: (Example: evening primrose oil 1 gm. 4 times daily)

Prostaglandin E$_1$ is said to be a key determinant of T-suppressor cell activity and thus excessive PGE$_1$ formation would be associated with excess suppressor function in the immune system. However, since stores of PGE$_1$ precursor dihomo-gammalinolenic acid are limited, excess PGE$_1$ formation may be followed by depletion of DGLA and a fall in PGE$_1$ leading to failure of T-suppressor function with autoimmune attack. Evening primrose oil, a source of gamma linolenic acid (the DGLA precursor) may thus be beneficial in recurrent and relapsing auto-immune disorders such as multiple sclerosis, rheumatoid arthritis, familial Mediterranean fever, asthma, migraine and inflammatory disorders of the skin and bowel (*Horrobin DF. A biochemical basis for the actions of lithium on behavior and on relapsing and remitting disorders of inflammation and immunity. Med. Hypotheses 7(7):891-906, 1981*).

Animal Experimental Study: PGE$_1$ successfully controlled the auto-immune inflammatory disease, including kidney damage, which develops spontaneously in NZB/W mice (*Zurier RB et al. Prostaglandin E treatment in NZB/W mice, I. Arthritis Rheum. 20:723-8, 1977; Krakauer K et al. Prostaglandin E$_1$ treatment of NZB/W mice, III. Clin. Immunol. Immunopathol. 11:256, 1978*).

See Also:

> *McCormick JN et al. Immunosuppressive effect of linoleic acid. Letter to the Editor. Lancet 2:508, 1977*

BENIGN PROSTATIC HYPERPLASIA

NUTRIENTS:

Zinc:

Supplementation may be beneficial.

Experimental Study: Zinc supplementation reduced the size of the prostate and BPH symptomatology in the majority of patients (*Fahim M et al. Zinc treatment for the reduction of hyperplasia of the prostate. Fed. Proc. 35:361, 1976*).

Experimental Study: 19 pts. took zinc sulphate 150 mg daily for 2 mo. followed by 50-100 mg daily. 14/19 had shrinkage of the prostate, as determined by rectal palpation, X-ray and endoscopy (*Bush IM et al. Zinc and the prostate. Presented at the annual meeting of the Am. Med. Association. Chicago, 1974*).

- -

Amino Acids:

Supplementation with the combination of L-glutamic acid, L-alanine and glycine (two 6-gr caps 3 times daily for 2 wks. following by 1 cap 3 times daily) may be beneficial.

Experimental Study: 17 pts. either with or without residual urine were treated with a mixture of L-glutamic acid, L-alanine and glycine. The residual urine was reduced in 8/13 and dysuria in 14/17. There were no side effects (*Aito K, Iwatsubo E. [The conservative treatment of prostatic hypertrophy with Paraprost.] Hinyokika Kiyo 18(1):41-44, 1972*).

Experimental Double-blind Study: Pts. randomly received either (1) L-glutamic acid, L-alanine and glycine, (2) L-glutamic acid and L-alanine, or (3) L-glutamic acid alone. Outcomes showed a significant difference between the reduction in subjective symptoms in the gp. receiving all 3 agents versus the 2 control groups. However, in none of the pts. was satisfactory improvement observed on rectal palpation or x-ray examination (*Shimaya M, Sugiura H. [Double blind test of PPC for prostatic hyperplasia.] Hinyokika Kiyo 16(5):231-36, 1970*).

Experimental Controlled Study: In a study of 45 pts. supplemented with glutamic acid, alanine and glycine, nocturia was relieved or reduced in 95%, urgency reduced in 81%, frequency reduced in 73%, and delayed micturition alleviated in 70% (*Dumrau F. Benign prostatic hyperplasia: Amino acid therapy for symptomatic relief. Am. J. Ger. 10:426-30, 1962*).

See Also:

Experimental Controlled Study: *Feinblatt HM, Gant JC. Palliative treatment of benign prostatic hypertrophy: Value of glycine, alanine, glutamic acid combination. J. Maine Med. Assoc. 46:99-102, 1958*

Essential Fatty Acids:

Nutritional precursors to prostaglandins.

A prostaglandin deficiency may be a cause of BPH.

Theoretical Discussion: Experimental data suggest that, when testosterone enters the prostate cell, it both converts to dihydrotestosterone (which enters the cell nucleus and stimulates protein synthesis and growth), and stimulates prostaglandin synthesis and release. The released prostaglandins, in addition to their role in male reproductive physiology, inhibit further testosterone binding to the prostate. With aging, PG synthesis may become less efficient, resulting in a decline of the putative inhibitory effect of PG on cell growth and an increase in testosterone binding to prostatic cells. The combined effects might produce unrestrained protein synthesis and cell growth resulting in BPH (*Klein LA, Stoff JS. Prostaglandins and the prostate: An hypothesis on the etiology of benign prostatic hyperplasia. Prostate 4(3):247-51, 1983*).

Review Article: "The importance of PGs in inflammatory changes in the prostate gland and the therapeutic possibilities for these clinical symptoms which may result from influencing PGs can be seen from some studies, but it is not yet possible to draw a final conclusion at this point in time" (*Bach D, Walker H. How important are prostaglandins in the urology of man? Urol. int. 37(3):160-71, 1982*).

See Also:

> *Narayan JP et al. Prostaglandins in benign prostatic hypertrophy. Indian J. Physiol. Pharmacol. 29(3):183-84, 1985*

Supplementation may reduce residual urine.

Experimental Study: 19/19 pts. showed diminution of residual urine following supplementation with an essential fatty acid complex containing linoleic, linolenic, and arachidonic acids. Following several wks. of treatment, 12/19 no longer had any residual urine (*Hart JP, Cooper WL. Vitamin F in the treatment of prostatic hyperplasia. Report Number 1, Lee Foundation for Nutritional Research, Milwaukee, Wi., 1941*).

- -

OTHER FACTORS:

Rule out cadmium toxicity.

Cadmium exposure may result in BPH.

Animal Experimental Study: Cadmium chloride was injected into the rt. ventral prostatic lobe of 100 12-mo.-old male rats. 270 days after the injection, simple hyperplasia was found in 38, atypical hyperplasia in 29, atypical hyperplasia with severe dysplasia in 11 and invasive prostatic carcinoma in 5 (*Hoffman L et al. Carcinogenic effects of cadmium on the prostate of the rat. J. Cancer Res. Clin. Oncol. 109(3):193-99, 1985*).

Prostatic cadmium levels may be elevated in BPH.

Negative Observational Study: In a study of cadmium levels of prostatic tissue, there was no evidence of high cadmium concentrations in hypertrophic and cacinomatous prostatic tissue (*Lahtonen R. Zinc and cadmium concentrations in whole tissue and in separated epithelium and stroma from human benign prostatic hypertrophic glands. Prostate 6(2):177-83, 1985*).

Observational Study: Prostatic cadmium concentrations in BPH were measured by atomic absorption spectroscopy and were found to be considerably higher than in normal tissue (23.11 +/- 3.28 vs. 5.25 +/- 0.62 nmol/g). Prostatic dihydrotestosterone levels were directly proportional to the cadmium concentrations (*Habib FK et al. Metal-androgen interrelationships in carcinoma and hyperplasia of the human prostate. J. Endocrinol. 71(1):133-41, 1976*).

Selenium:

May protect against cadmium-induced growth stimulation of prostatic tissue.

In vitro Experimental Study: While cadmium was found to stimulate the growth of human prostatic epithelium, selenium (at proper concentrations) inhibited the growth stimulation induced by cadmium *(Webber MM. Selenium prevents the growth stimulatory effects of cadmium on human prostatic epithelium. Biochem. Biophy. Res. Commun. 127(3):871-77, 1985).*

BIPOLAR DISORDER

See Also: DEPRESSION

OVERVIEW:

1. Deficiencies of folic acid, vitamin B$_{12}$ or vitamin C are associated with bipolar disorder.

2. Lithium carbonate can cause a folic acid deficiency, and one study suggests that the side-effects of lithium may sometimes be ameliorated by supplementation with safflower oil, a rich source of omega-6 fatty acids.

3. Mania may be caused of excessive body loads of vanadium and it is theorized that drug treatments (as well as ascorbic acid supplementation) may work by antagonizing its effects. Excessive ingestion of L-glutamine, an excitatory amino acid, has also been shown to cause mania.

4. Early studies suggest that supplementation with nutritional precursors of major neurotransmitters may be effective. These nutrients include L-phenylalanine (precursor to dopamine and nor-epinephrine), phosphatidyl choline (precursor to acetyl choline) and L-tryptophan (precursor to serotonin).

- -

NUTRIENTS:

Folic Acid:

May be deficient.

> **Review Article:** Folate deficiency is the most common nutrient deficiency and may be found in over 1/4 of hospitalized psychiatric patients (*Lipton M et al. Vitamins, megavitamin therapy and the nervous system, in Wurtman R, Wurtman J, Ed. Nutrition and the Brain Volume 33. New York, Raven Press, 1979, pp. 183-264; Kallstrom B et al. Vitamin B$_{12}$ and folate concentrations in mental patients. Acta Psychiat. Scand. 45:137-52, 1969; Hunter R et al. Serum B$_{12}$ and folate concentration in mental patients. Brit. J. Psychiat. 113:1291-5, 1967*)

Folate deficiency is associated with a wide variety of psychiatric symptoms including psychosis, depression, confusion, disorientation, and dementia as well as with neurologic symptoms of weakness, numbness, stiffness and spasticity, both with and without muscular atrophy (*Howard JS. Folate deficiency in psychiatric practice. Psychosomatics 16:112-15, 1975*).

Lithium carbonate can cause a folate deficiency.

> **Case Report:** *Prakash R et al. A case report of megaloblastic anemia secondary to lithium. Am. J. Psychiat. 138:849, 1981*

Required for the synthesis of brain 5-hydroxytryptamine which is involved in mood regulation (*Botez MI et al. Relapsing neuropathy, cerebral atrophy and folate deficiency. A close association. Appl. Neurophysiol.42(3):171-83, 1979*).

Supplementation may be beneficial.

Experimental Double-blind Study: 42 pts. with affective disorders on lithium therapy received either folic acid 200 mcg or placebo.   After 1 yr., there was a small but insignificant change in the affective morbidity index (AMI) in both groups; however, when the supplemented pts. were divided into 2 gps. according to their AMI scores, those with lower AMI scores had a significantly higher mean end-of-trial folate concentration than those with higher scores.   Also, when the pts. were divided into 2 gps. according to their end-of-trial folate concentration, those with the higher folate concentrations had lower mean AMI scores than those with lower concentrations (results not significant).   A similar trend was found when Beck depression scores were used (*Coppen A.   Folic acid enhances lithium prophylaxis. J. Affective Disord. 10:9-13, 1986*).

See Also:

> *Coppen A.   Plasma folate and affective morbidity during long term lithium therapy.   Br. J. Psychiat. 141:87-89, 1982*

Vitamin B$_{12}$:

Deficiency may cause a secondary mania (even in the absence of clinical features of pernicious anemia) which responds to supplementation.

Case Report: Pt. presented with a full manic syndrome and low serum B$_{12}$ in the absence of clinical features of pernicious anemia, but with a positive Schilling test and antibodies to parietal cells and intrinsic factor. Mental status normalized with B$_{12}$ replacement (*Goggans FC.   A case of mania secondary to vitamin B$_{12}$ deficiency. Am. J. Psychiat. 141(2):300-1, 1984*).

Vitamin C:

Certain bipolar pts. may be in a state of "subscurvy."

Observational Study: The ave. plasma vitamin C level in 885 psychiatric pts. was 0.51/100 ml compared to 0.87/100 ml in 110 healthy controls.   32% of the pts. had levels below 0.35 mg/100 ml, the threshold which has been associated with detrimental effects on immune responses and behavior (*Schorah CJ et al. Human Nutr.: Clin. Nutr. 37C:447-52, 1983*).

Observational Study: Anxiety and excitement were found to increase the rate of breakdown of ascorbic acid (*Maas JW. Arch. Gen. Psychiat. 4:109, 1961*).

See Also:

> *Leitner ZA, Church IC. Lancet 1:565, 1956*

If deficient, supplementation may be beneficial.

Experimental Double-blind Study: 40 chronic male psychiatric pts. including 4 with Bipolar Disorder randomly received either ascorbic acid 1 gm daily or placebo.   After 3 wks., there was a significant decrease in the MMPI "D" (depression) scale (p less than 0.01) only for the experimental group.   The nurse felt that 5 pts. had obviously improved and the doctor agreed in regard to 4 of them; all 5 turned out to be in the experimental group.   The Wittenborn Psychiatric Rating Scale rating the manic state showed significant improvement (p less than 0.02) only in the experimental gp., while the scale rating the depressed state showed significant improvement in both the experimental gp. (p less than 0.01) and the control gp. (p less than 0.05).   The 24 hr. ascorbic acid urinary excretion in the control gp. was at the very lowest limit of normal.   While normal subjects can be saturated with ascorbic acid after 1-2 days of supplementation with 1 gm daily, pts. with borderline or frank scurvy require 7-10 days and the pts. in this study required an ave. of 6 days.   These findings suggest that chronic psychiatric pts. may be in a state of "subscurvy" and thus could benefit from ascorbic acid supplementation (*Milner G. Ascorbic acid in chronic psychiatric patients: A controlled trial. Brit. J. Psychiat. 109:294-99, 1963*).

Vitamin C may possibly reduce symptoms of bipolar disorder due to its ability to reduce the detrimental effects of vanadium on RBC Na^+-K^+-ATPase activity by reducing vanadate ($+5$) to the vanadyl ion ($+4$), the latter being a much less effective inhibitor of Na^+-K^+-ATPase activity than the former (*Vanadium, vitamin C and depression. Nutr. Rev. 40(10):293-5, 1981*).

(See also "Vanadium" below.)

Experimental Double-blind Crossover Study: 23 hospitalized bipolar pts. (11 manic, 12 depressed) were rated as to symptoms, given ascorbic acid 3 gm or placebo, and rated hourly for the next 6 hours. The next day, the procedure was repeated except that ascorbic acid and placebo were switched. The severity of illness fell slowly during the day in the placebo gp. but much more rapidly in the treated gp. with significant differences at 3,4 and 5 hours post-ingestion. (*Naylor GJ, Smith AHW. Vanadium: A possible aetiological factor in manic-depressive illness. Psychol. Med. 11:249-56, 1981*).

- with EDTA:

Experimental Double-blind Study: The combination of ascorbic acid and EDTA was compared to recognized treatment regimes. Depressed pts. responded similarly to amitriptyline and the experimental regime, while manic pts. responded better to lithium than the experimental regime, suggesting that vanadium may be of etiological importance in depressive psychosis, but not for mania (*Kay DS et al. The therapeutic effect of ascorbic acid and EDTA in manic-depressive psychosis: Double-blind comparisons with standard treatments. Psychol. Med. 14(3):533-38, 1984*).

- -

Vanadium:

Elevated vanadium has been reported in the plasma of pts. with mania and depression and in the hair of pts. with mania (*Naylor GJ. Vanadium and manic depressive psychosis. Nutr. & Health 3(1-2):79-85, 1984*).

Observational Study: Plasma vanadium concentrations from 8 manic-depressives and 9 normals were compared. Manic-depressives were found to have significantly higher mean vanadium levels than normals (*Dick DA et al. Psych. Med. 12:533-7, 1982*).

Observational Study: Plasma vanadium concentrations from 26 bipolar manic subjects, 20 bipolar depressed subjects, and 32 bipolar subjects who had recovered from episodes of either mania or depression were compared. The difference between manic and control subjects was significant (*Dick DA et al. Plasma vanadium concentrations in manic-depressive illness. J. Physiol. 310:27, 1981*).

Vanadium toxicity is known to be associated with depression and melancholia (*Witkowska D, Brzezinski, J. Alteration of brain noradrenaline, dopamine and 5-hydroxy-tryptamine levels during vanadium poisoning. Pol. J. Pharacol. Pharm. 31:393-8, 1979*).

Vanadium has been shown to be a powerful inhibitor of Na^+-K^+-ATPase activity (*Cantley LC et al. Vanadate is a potent (Na,K)-ATPase inhibitor found in ATP derived from muscle. J. Biol. Chem. 252:7421-3, 1977*).

Increased plasma vanadium is negatively correlated with Na^+-K^+-ATPase activity in manic-depressives, but not in normals.

Observational Study: Increased vanadium levels correlated significantly with low Na^+-K^+-ATPase levels in 4 M-D subjects, but not in 3 normal controls (*Dick DA et al. Psych. Med. 12:533-7, 1982*).

Observational Study: There was a significant negative correlation between vanadium concentration and the ratio of Na^+-K^+-ATPase to Mg ATPase levels in 72 MD subjects but not in 23 normal controls (*Dick DA et al. Plasma vanadium concentrations in manic-depressive illness. J. Physiol. 310:27, 1981*).

Lymphocytes from manic-depressives show impairment in the ability to produce new Na^+-K^+-ATPase pump sites in response to challenges.

In vitro Experimental Study: Lymphocytes from manic-depressives were found to have a significantly reduced ability to produce new Na^+-K^+-ATPase pump sites in response to challenges, perhaps due to an underlying genetic flaw (*Naylor GJ, Smith AHW. Defective genetic control of sodium-pump density in manic-depressive psychosis. Psychol. Med. 11:257-63, 1981*).

Na^+-K^+-ATPase activity is reduced in depressive illness (*Vanadium, vitamin C and depression. Nutr. Rev. 40(10):293-5, 1981*).

Medications utilized in the treatment of bipolar disorder may antagonize the effects of vanadium:
1. Phenothiazines and monamine oxidase inhibitors catalyze the reduction of vanadate to the less active vanadyl ion.
2. Lithium is known to increase Na^+-K^+-ATPase activity as clinical response occurs (*Naylor, 1984 - op cit*).

Therapies based on decreasing vanadate levels in the body (e.g. ascorbic acid, EDTA, methylene blue) have been reported to be effective in both depression and mania (*Naylor, 1984, - op cit*).

Decreased dietary vanadium may be beneficial.

- with EDTA:

Experimental Double-blind Crossover Study: 23 pts. (10 depressed, 13 manic) subjects consumed a diet of normal vanadium content (1-2 mg daily) for 4 days followed by 10 days of a low vanadium diet along with supplements of either vanadium 0.7 mg or EDTA 3 gm for 5 days each. 7/10 depressed subjects were better during the period of low vanadium intake (p less than 0.05) and 10/11 manic subjects were better (p less than 0.005) and 10/13 slept 1-2 hrs. more nightly (p less than 0.05) (*Naylor GJ, Smith AHW. Vanadium: A possible aetiological factor in manic-depressive illness. Psychol. Med. 11:249-56, 1981*).

- with ascorbic acid and EDTA:

Case Reports:
1. 28 year-old female with 15 yr. history bipolar disorder with 8-10 wk. cycle unresponsive to lithium and other treatments. She was placed on a low vanadium diet for 21 wks., supplemented with EDTA 1 gm 3 times daily and ascorbic acid 1 gm 3 times daily. Although her mania did not change, she skipped a depressive period for the first time in the 10 yrs. she had been under observation.
2. 82 year-old female with severe bipolar disorder unresponsive to lithium and other treatments. Within 2 wks. after starting the low vanadium, high EDTA, high ascorbate regime, she settled into a mild hypomanic state and showed no depressive phases for 8 weeks. 5 days after withdrawal of the supplements, she became severely depressed, but returned to the hypomanic condition upon their resumption (*Naylor GJ, Smith AHW - ibid*).

- -

L-Glutamine:

WARNING: Megadoses may <u>cause</u> mania.

Case Reports:
1. Pt. with no prior psychiatric history was hospitalized with a 1 wk. history of increasing motor and verbal activity culminating in grandiose delusions, hypersexuality, and insomnia. Two wks. earlier, he had begun to ingest up to 4 gm L-glutamine daily. Symptoms ceased within 1 wk. of stopping the supplement.
2. Pt. in psychotherapy with dysthymic disorder began to experience increasing sleep loss, unusually high energy and increased mental acuity and became unusually outgoing and talkative following 1 wk. of ingesting up to 2 gm daily of L-glutamine.
(*Mebane AH. L-Glutamine and Mania. 'Letter to the Editor. <u>Am. J. Psychiat.</u> 141(10), October, 1984*).

Omega-6 Fatty Acids:

Example: <u>Evening Primrose Oil</u> which contains 8-10% GLA (500 mg. - 1 gram 3-4 times daily)

To prevent neurotoxic side effects from lithium carbonate (<u>not</u> to be taken without lithium during manic phase).

Negative Experimental Study: 6 pts. with lithium-induced tremor were treated with evening primrose oil 1 gm 4 times daily for 4 days without benefit (*Schou M. Linoleic acid in the treatment of lithium-induced tremor: A pilot study with negative outcome. <u>Prostaglandins Med.</u> 5:343-44, 1980*).

Case Reports: 5 pts. are described with lithium-induced neurotoxicity whose symptoms quickly remitted with safflower oil 3-5000 ml twice daily (*Lieb J. Linoleic acid in the treatment of lithium toxicity and familial tremor. <u>Prostaglandins Med.</u> 4:275-9, 1980*).

L-Phenylalanine: Start with 500 mg. daily and increase dosage as needed (average of 3-4 gms. daily)
        (2-6 month trial)

Precursor of L-tyrosine.

Can be decarboxylated to phenylethylamine (PEA), an amphetamine-like neurotransmitter which is found in high quantities in chocolate.

- with pyridoxine 100-200 mg.:

(Pyridoxine is necessary to convert L-phenylalanine to phenylethylamine (PEA).)

Experimental Study: 40 pts. with major depression (8 bipolar depressives) were supplemented with L-phenylalanine and vitamin B_6. Treatment was initiated with 500 mg L-PA in the morning and at noon along with B_6 100 mg twice daily, and the L-PA dosage was increased by 500 mg daily until therapeutic or side effects developed, or to a limit of 2-3 gm over the previous dose at 1 wk. intervals (gp. mean = 3-4 gm daily). 31/40 improved "almost immediately" and 10 of the responders were completely relieved of depression. 7/8 (88%) of the bipolar depressives responded and most of the 24/32 (75%) unipolar depressives who responded had "soft" signs of bipolarity (strong impulsive tendencies, hypersomnia, and family histories of bipolar illness), suggesting that supplementation is effective primarily for <u>bipolar</u> depressions. Side effects were slight, transient headaches, constipation, transient nausea, insomnia and increased anxiety. Prior to supplementation, the 23 drug-free depressives were found to have significantly lower PAA urinary excretion than normals (PAA is a PEA metabolite). During supplementation, urinary PAA excretion rose in tandem with their spirits

(Sabelli HC et al. Clinical studies on the phenylethylamine hypothesis of affective disorder: Urine and blood phenylacetic acid and phenylalanine dietary supplements. J. Clin. Psychiat. 47(2):66-70, 1986; Phenylalanine: A psychoactive nutrient for some depressives? Med. World News October 27, 1983).

<u>Phosphatidyl Choline:</u>

The active ingredient in lecithin.

Increases brain acetylcholine stores *(Hirsch MJ, Wurtman RJ. Lecithin consumption increases acetylcholine concentrations in rat brain and adrenal gland. Science 202:223-5, 1978).*

Supplementation may be beneficial.

> **Experimental Double-blind Study:** Improvement with 90% pure phosphatidyl choline 10 gm three times daily was significantly greater than with placebo in 5/6 patients by 1 week *(Cohen BM et al. Lecithin in the treatment of mania: Double-blind, placebo-controlled trials. Am. J. Psychiat. 139:1162-4, 1982).*

> **Case Report:** A 13 year-old girl with stress-related, early-onset bipolar illness responded poorly to neuroleptics and not at all to lithium but responded well to lecithin (15-23 gm. daily of 90% pure phosphatidyl choline) over several weeks *(Schreier HA. Mania responsive to lecithin in a 13-year old girl. Am. J. Psychiat. 139:108-110, 1982).*

> **Case Reports:** 4/8 bipolar pts. in the manic phase on lithium and/or neuroleptics who received 15-30 gm daily of 90% pure phosphatidyl choline showed marked improvement *(Cohen BM et al. Lecithin in mania: A preliminary report. Am. J. Psychiat. 137:242-3, 1980).*

<u>L-Tryptophan:</u>   6-12 grams in divided doses (2wk. trial)
  Avoid protein for 90 minutes before & after.
  Take with sugar (insulin improves absorption by lowering levels of competing amino acids).

Review Article: Published studies suggest that doses above 6 gms daily appear to be indicated for bipolar patients *(Walinder J. Combination of tryptophan with MAO inhibitors, tricyclic antidepressants and selective 5-HT reuptake inhibitors. Adv. Biol. Psychiat. 10:82-93, 1983; Chouinard G et al. Tryptophan-nicotinamide, imipramine and their combination in depression: A controlled study. Acta Psychiat. Scand. 59:395-414, 1979).*

Possible indications:

1. For treatment of mania.

> **Experimental Double-blind Study:** 24 newly-admitted manic pts. were treated for 1 wk. with 12 gm daily; then 1/2 the pts. (chosen at random) continued on tryptophan while the other 1/2 received placebo. In the open phase, there was a clinically and statistically significant reduction in manic symptom scores. During the second wk., only pts. switched to placebo tended to show an increase in manic symptom scores *(Chouinard G et al. A controlled clinical trial of L-Tryptophan in acute mania. Biol. Psychiat. 20:546-57, 1985).*

> **Review Article:** 2/3 studies have found some therapeutic effect. The negative study *(Chambers CA, Naylor GJ. A controlled trial of L-tryptophan in mania. Brit. J. Psychiat. 132:555-59, 1978)* was carried out in only a small number of female pts. (5 in each treatment gp.) and included concomitant use of chlorpromazine and nitrazepam, all factors which decrease the likelihood of seeing a treatment difference *(Chouinard G et al. Tryptophan in the treatment of depression and mania. Adv. Biol. Psychiat. 10:47-66, 1983).*

2. Potentiates effects of lithium in bipolar patients.

> **Experimental Double-blind Study:** Compared to 5 bipolar pts. who received lithium alone, the combination of lithium and L-tryptophan (3 gm 3 times daily) resulted in significantly greater improvement in 4 bipolar patients (*Brewerton TD, Reus VI. Lithium carbonate and L-tryptophan in the treatment of bipolar and schizoaffective disorders. Am. J. Psychiat. 140:757-60, 1983*).

3. Treatment for patients with bipolarII illness.

> **Case Report:** A 63 year-old female failed to respond to imipramine and lithium but responded well to a trial of L-tryptophan alone for 11 months (*Beitman BD, Dunner DL. L-tryptophan in the maintenance treatment of bipolar II manic-depressive illness. Am. J. Psychiat. 139:1498-9, 1982*).

4. Treatment of bipolar depression.

> **Review Article:** Of 9 studies reviewed, only a total of 16/44 pts. (36%) responded, which may only represent a placebo response. On the other hand, the study of Murphy et al. (*Murphy DL et al. L-tryptophan in affective disorders: Indoleamine changes and differential clinical effects. Psychopharmacologia 34:11-20, 1974*), which found a response in 3/8, all of whom relapsed on placebo, might indicate a therapeutic effect in some bipolar patients (*Chouinard G et al. Tryptophan in the treatment of depression and mania. Adv. Biol. Psychiat. 10:47-66, 1983*).

- with <u>niacinamide</u>:

> **Review Article:** The rationale for the addition of niacinamide is that the high rate of catabolism of tryptophan by the liver suggested by animal work can be inhibited with niacinamide (*Young SN, Sourkes TL. The antidepressant effect of tryptophan. Lancet 2:897-98, 1974*). Recent data, however, indicate that niacinamide will not inhibit breakdown of tryptophan in humans at clinical doses following an acute loading (*Green AR et al. Metabolism of an oral tryptophan load: Effect of pretreatment with the putative tryptophan pyrrolase inhibitors nicotinamide or allopurinol. Brit. J. Clin. Pharmacol. 10:611-15, 1980*). In addition, in pts. receiving up to 6 gm tryptophan daily along with niacinamide, tryptophan metabolism was still highly variable. Thus it is unlikely that niacinamide is a useful adjunct (*Chouinard G et al. Tryptophan in the treatment of depression and mania. Adv. Biol. Psychiat. 10:47-66, 1983*).

- with <u>pyridoxine</u>:

Tryptophan pyrrolase in the liver can degrade tryptophan to kynurenine which is taken up in the brain and transferred by the same transport carrier as tryptophan. The competitively inhibitory effect of kynurenine on tryptophan transport is of the same order as that of the competing essential amino acids (*Moller SE et al. Tryptophan availability in endogenous depression - relation to efficacy of L-tryptophan treatment. Adv. Biol. Psychiat. 10:30-46, 1983*).

Supplementation with tryptophan increases the plasma concentration of kynurenine in proportion to the dose given and, after longer-term administration, there is a marked increase in basal kynurenine with a further substantial increase following a further dose of tryptophan. This large increase in kynurenine concentration might reflect a relative saturation of the kynurenine pathway, possibly because of vitamin B_6 depletion since many of the degradative enzymes down the pathway are B_6-dependent. Consistent with this hypothesis are findings that, when tryptophan is given for 7 days with pyridoxine, the basal plasma kynurenine is half that seen in subjects given tryptophan alone and the peak concentration following a single load is the same after long-term pre-treatment with tryptophan plus pyridoxine as after no pre-treatment and only half that seen in subjects who have taken longer-term tryptophan without pyridoxine (*Green AR, Aronson JK. The pharmacokinetics of oral L-tryptophan: Effects of dose and concomitant pyridoxine, allopurinol or nicotinamide administration. Adv. Biol. Psychiat. 10:67-81, 1983*).

BRONCHIAL ASTHMA

See Also: ALLERGY

OVERVIEW:

1. Preliminary evidence suggests that certain asthmatics may be provoked by specific food challenges, although further confirmation is needed. In one uncontrolled study, pts. showed an excellent response to a vegan diet, possibly due to the removal of provoking foods.

2. Early studies suggest that asthmatics may be deficient in pyridoxine, ascorbic acid or magnesium. There is also early evidence that supplementation with these nutrients may be effective. Perhaps supplementation is beneficial when it remedies a pre-existing deficiency, but this hypothesis remains to be validated.

3. Caffeine appears to be as effective a bronchodilator as theophylline although, due to its adverse effects, its use should be limited to acute situations.

- -

BASIC DIET:

Vegan diet.

> **Experimental Study:** 25 treated pts. followed a pure vegetarian diet which prohibited meat, fish, eggs, dairy products, coffee, ordinary tea, chocolate, sugar, salt, tap water, apples, citrus, soybeans and peas. Grains were either very restricted or eliminated and potatoes were restricted. 71% improved within 4 months and 92% improved by 1 year as determined by a number of both clinical and laboratory variables (*Lindahl O et al. Vegan diet regimen with reduced medication in the treatment of bronchial asthma. J. Asthma 22:45-55, 1985*).

- -

NUTRIENTS:

Pyridoxine:

> May be deficient.

> > **Observational Study:** 15 pts. had significantly lower levels of plasma and erythrocyte pyridoxal-5-phosphate than nonasthmatics (*Reynolds RD, Natta CL. Depressed plasma pyridoxal phosphate concentrations in adult asthmatics. Am. J. Clin. Nutr. 41:684-8, 1985*).

> Supplementation may be beneficial.

> > **Experimental Controlled Study:** 7 pts. and 6 controls received 50 mg pyridoxine twice daily. Both plasma and erythrocyte pyridoxal phosphate levels only increased significantly in the controls; however, all asthmatics reported a dramatic decrease in the frequency, duration and severity of asthmatic attacks and wheezing ceased in about 1 week (*Reynolds RD - ibid*).

> > **Experimental Study:** 76 asthmatic children who received pyridoxine 200 mg daily demonstrated significant symptom improvement and a reduction in dosage of bronchodilators and cortisone required

to relieve symptoms (*Collip PJ et al. Pyridoxine treatment of childhood bronchial asthma. Ann. Allergy 35:93-7, 1975*).

Vitamin B$_{12}$:

Supplementation by injection may be beneficial.

Experimental Study: When given preceeding a sulfite challenge, vitamin B$_{12}$ was more effective than pharmacologic agents in blocking asthmatic reactions and was effective over a longer period of time (*Simon RA et al. Sulfite-sensitive asthma. Res. Instit. of Scripps Clinic Scientific Report 39:57-58, 1982-83*).

Case Reports: 18/20 pts. improved following IM injections of vitamin B$_{12}$ 1000 mcg. once weekly for 4 weeks (*Simon SW. Vitamin B$_{12}$ therapy in allergy and chronic dermatoses. J.Allergy 2:183-5, 1951*)

See also:

Caruselli M. *Upon therapy for asthma using vitamin B$_{12}$. Riforma Medica August 2, 1952, pp. 849-51*

Vitamin C: 2 grams daily; 4 -8 grams during reactions

Negatively correlated with blood histamine levels.

Observational Study: For 437 normal subjects, when the plasma-reduced ascorbic acid level was below 1 mg/100 ml, the whole blood histamine level increased exponentially as the ascorbic acid level decreased. For subjects with ascorbic acid levels below 0.7 mg/100 ml, the increase in blood histamine was highly significant (*Clemetson CA. Histamine and ascorbic acid in human blood. J. Nutr. 110(4):662-68, 1980*).

Levels may be reduced in bronchial asthma.

Observational Study: Compared to a matched control gp., plasma ascorbic acid was significantly lower in 51 asthmatic children, suggesting that routine vitamin C supplementation may be necessary (*Aderele WI et al. Plasma vitamin C (ascorbic acid) levels in asthmatic children. Afr. J. Med. Sci. 14:115, 1985*).

Observational Study: Compared to controls, both treated and untreated asthmatics had significantly lower levels of ascorbic acid in both serum and leukocytes (*Olusi SO et al. Plasma and white blood cell ascorbic acid concentrations in patients with bronchial asthma. Clinica Chimica Acta 92:161-6, 1979*).

Supplementation may reduce histamine levels.

Experimental Study: When 11 normals with either low vitamin C levels or high blood histamine levels were given ascorbic acid 1 gm. x 3 days, blood histamine levels fell in all 11 subjects (*Clemetson CA. Histamine and ascorbic acid in human blood. J. Nutr. 110(4):662-68, 1980*).

Supplementation may be beneficial.

Experimental Study: Broncho-constriction brought on by methacholine challenge in 14 mild asthmatics was inhibited by 1 gram oral ascorbic acid. The effects of ascorbic acid were blocked by indocin, suggesting that ascorbic acid exerts its effect via alteration of arachidonic acid metabolism (*Mohsenin V et al. Effect of ascorbic acid on response to methacholine challenge in asthmatic subjects. Am. Rev. Respir. Dis. 127:143-7, 1983*).

Experimental Double-blind Study: 1 gram daily was effective in preventing attacks for some pts. (*Anah CO et al. High dose ascorbic acid in Nigerian asthmatics. Tropical Geograph. Med. 32:132-7, 1980*).

Experimental Study: Large doses of ascorbic acid successfully inhibited histamine-induced airway constriction (*Zuskin E et al. Inhibition of histamine-induced airway constriction by ascorbic acid. J. Allergy Immunol. 51:218-26, 1973*).

See Also:

Schacter EN, Schlesinger A. *The attenuation of exercise-induced bronchospasm by ascorbic acid. Ann. Allergy 49:146-50, 1982*

Kordansky DW et al. *Effect of vitamin C on antigen induced bronchospasm. J. Allergy Clin. Immunol. 63:61-4, 1979*

- -

Magnesium:

Supplementation may be beneficial.

Experimental Study: Bronchoconstriction in 10 pts. with mild attacks and 3 pts. with severe attacks was successfully relieved with an infusion of IV magnesium sulfate (*Okayama H et al. JAMA February 27, 1987*).

Experimental Double-blind Study: Parenterally-administered magnesium significantly improved pulmonary function of asthmatic patients. The degree of improvement was positively correlated with serum magnesium levels (*Brunner EH et al. Effect of parenteral magnesium on pulmonary function, plasma cAMP, and histamine in bronchial asthma. J. Asthma 22:3-11, 1985*).

Experimental Study: Supplementation was beneficial for pts. with acute attacks (*Haury VG. Blood serum magnesium in bronchial asthma and its treatment by the administration of magnesium sulfate. J. Lab. Clin. Med. 26:340-4, 1940*).

- -

Omega-3 Fatty Acids:

Supplementation may be beneficial.

Experimental Study: 6 pts. with chronic disease received EPA 4 gm daily. After 8 wks., there was no clinical improvement, although their immune cells showed a positive response and results suggested that a subset of pts. may benefit (*Payan Donald G - reported in Med. World News July 14, 1986*).

See Also:

Review Article: *Lee TH, Arm JP. Prospects for modifying the allergic response by fish oil diets. Clin. Allergy 16(2):89-100, 1986*

Omega-6 Fatty Acids:

Example: Evening Primrose Oil   2 - 3 gms. twice daily (3 month trial)

Supplementation may be beneficial.

Experimental Study: *Stenius-Aarniala B et al. Symptomatic effect of evening primrose oil, fish oil and olive oil in patients with bronchial asthma (abstract). Ann. Allergy 55(2):490-94, 1985*

L-Tryptophan.

WARNING: May aggravate bronchial asthma.

Experimental Double-blind Study: Pts. on a low-tryptophan diet improved (*Urge G et al. Effect of dietary tryptophan restrictions on clinical symptoms in patients with endogenous asthma. Allergy 38:211-2, 1983*).

- -

OTHER FACTORS:

Caffeine:

Theophylline is a metabolic product of caffeine.

WARNING: May be toxic when combined with theophylline.

Effective as a bronchodilator (but is not recommended on a regular basis due to its potential for side-effects).

Experimental Double-blind Study: Pts. received 3 6-oz cups of brewed coffee, each containing 150 mg caffeine. Even a single cup was found to produce as much as a 15% increase in FEV_1. The effect was 40% as potent as that of theophylline (*Gong H Jr et al. Chest March, 1986*).

Experimental Double-blind Study: 23 pts. on continuous bronchodilator therapy whose forced expiratory flow from 25-75% of vital capacity (FEF 25-75) was less than 50% of normal received either caffeine 10 mg/kg (equivalent to 2 strong cups of coffee for a 50 kg person) or theophylline 5 mg/kg. The effects of the 2 drugs were very similar and minor side effects of headache, dizziness and tremor were noted with both (*Becker AJ et al. The bronchodilator effects and pharmacokinetics of caffeine in asthma. N. Engl. J. Med. 310(12):743-46, 1984*).

Rule out food sensitivities.

Experimental Study: 118 pts. (most without known histories of food sensitivities) were challenged with foods and bronchial responses were followed by spirometry. 93% (110/118) experienced a distinct decrease in asthmatic symptoms after avoiding test-positive foods for 6-12 months. Responses to challenges ranged from as soon as 20 minutes to as late as 56 hours (*Peliken Z et al. Bronchial asthma due to food allergy. Paper presented at the XII International Congress of Allergy and Clinical Immunology, Washington, D.C., October, 1985*).

Experimental Double-blind Study: 41 hospitalized pts. were fed either a hypoallergenic defined elemental formula diet or the normal hospital diet, both liquified and sweetened so as to be similar in appearance and taste. Outcomes were assessed by a predetermined formula based on pulmonary functions and medications taken during the last versus the first 4 days of the 2 wk. trial period. 9/21 completing the elemental diet improved and none deteriorated, while only 1/16 controls improved and 5 deteriorated. The difference was significant (p = .05). The 9 elemental diet pts. who improved had no higher frequency of positive skin prick tests to common foods than did the 12 whose condition remained stable, suggesting that a trial of the elemental diet is justified for all perennial asthmatics even without evidence of extrinsic etiology (*Hoj L et al. A double-blind controlled trial elemental diet for severe perennial asthma. Allergy 36:257-62, 1981*).

Negative Experimental Double-blind Study: 38 children whose parents and physicians believed that specific foods worsened their asthma were fed the suspected foods or a placebo, both hidden in opaque capsules.   Positive reactions after feeding the suspect food occurred in only 11 children and for only 14/70 suspect foods, with G.I. symptoms being the most common.   In every case where food challenge was positive, skin prick was also positive, although skin prick was also positive when challenge was negative (*May C.   Objective clinical and laboratory studies of immediate hypersensitivity reactions to foods in asthmatic children.   J. Allergy. Clin. Immunol. 58:500-12, 1978*).

See Also:

> Oehling A.   *Importance of food allergy in childhood asthma.   Allergol. Immunopathol. Suppl. IX:71-3, 1981*

> Ogle KA, Bullocks JD.   *Children with allergic rhinitis and/or bronchial asthma treated with elimination diet: A five-year follow-up.   Ann. Allergy 44:273-8, 1980*

Rule out <u>hydrochloric acid deficiency</u>.

Diminished HCl may impair digestion and thus increase the potential allergenicity of foods.

Observational Study: 80% of 200 asthmatic children had sub-normal levels of gastric acidity (*Bray GW.   The hypochlorhydria of asthma of childhood.   Quart. J. Med. 24:181-97, 1931*).

See Also:

> Gillespie M.   *Hypochlorhydria in asthma with special reference to the age incidence.   Quart. J. Med. 4:397-405, 1935*

BURSITIS

NUTRIENTS:

<u>Vitamin B$_{12}$</u>:   Intramuscular injection

Supplementation may be beneficial.

> **Experimental Study:**   40 acute pts. (mostly sub-deltoid bursitis) received vitamin B$_{12}$ 1000 micrograms I.M. daily for 7-10 days; then 3 times weekly for 2-3 weeks; then 1-2 times weekly for 2-3 weeks (depending upon their rate of progress). All but 2 or 3 improved with rapid relief of pain and subjective symptoms, sometimes within a few hours. Complete relief was often noted in several days. Follow-up x-rays of cases of calcific bursitis showed considerable resorption of calcium deposits (*Klemes IS. Vitamin B$_{12}$ in acute subdeltoid bursitis.* <u>*Indust. Med. & Surg.*</u> *26:290-2, 1957*).

<u>Vitamin C</u> and
<u>Bioflavonoids</u>:

Supplementation may be beneficial.

> **Case Report:** 38 year-old male presented with severe subpatellar bursitis with extensive local swelling and heat, extreme tenderness, severe pain and limitation of motion. He was treated with vitamin C along with citrus bioflavonoids 200 mg 3 times daily. Within 24 hrs. there was noticable diminuation in swelling and pain, and in 72 hrs. the lesion had subsided almost completely, leaving only slight local tenderness (*Biskind MS, Martin WC. l The use of citrus flavonoids in infection. II.* <u>*Am. J. Digest. Dis.*</u> *22:41-45, 1955*).

CANCER

See Also: CERVICAL DYSPLASIA
FIBROCYSTIC BREAST DISEASE
"HYPERESTROGENISM"

OVERVIEW:

The National Academy of Sciences estimates that 60% of women's cancers and 40% of men's cancers are related to nutritional factors (*The National Academy of Sciences. Nutrition, Diet and Cancer, 1982*). The cancers most closely associated with nutritional factors are breast and endometrial cancer in women, prostate cancer in men, and gastrointestinal cancer (*Silverberg E. Cancer statistics, 1985. Ca - J. for Clinicians 35(1):19, 1985*).

The value of a low fat, high fiber diet in cancer prevention is well-documented. Avoidance of smoked, pickled and salt-cured foods (due to their nitrosamine content) has been shown in both epidemiologic and animal studies to be beneficial in preventing cancers of the GI tract.

Although epidemiologic studies have established that many nutrients are lower in cancer patients than in healthy controls (selenium is probably the best documented), it remains unclear whether these differences have causal implications. Missing are human studies linking nutritional supplementation with an improved prognosis once cancer is established.

On the other hand, there is early evidence that certain precancerous changes may be reversible with supplementation. Cervical dysplasia, for example, may possibly be reversed with folic acid supplementation, especially if folic acid levels are deficient, and calcium supplementation may reduce the number of rapidly proliferating cells in the colonic epithelium in pts. with family histories of colon cancer and elevated numbers of such cells compared to controls. Vitamin A or beta-carotene reduce the percent of genetically-damaged cells inside the cheek when betel quid, a tobacco-like plant mixture, is chewed regularly, while vitamin C 1 gm daily reduces nitrosamine levels in the stomach.

- -

BASIC DIET:

Low fat diet.

Review Article: "Of all the dietary factors that have been associated epidemiologically with cancers of various sites, fat has probably been studied most thoroughly and produced the greatest frequency of direct associations" (*U.S. Academy of Sciences. Diet, Nutrition and Cancer. Washington, D.C., National Academy Press, 1982*).

Breast Cancer:

Negative Observational Study: In a 4-year prospective study of 601 cases of breast cancer diagnosed among almost 90,000 nurses, there was no evidence of a positive relation between dietary total or saturated fat, linoleic acid, or cholesterol and the risk of breast cancer, suggesting that a moderate reduction in fat intake by adult women is unlikely to result in a substantial reduction in the incidence of breast cancer (*Willett WC et al. Dietary fat and the risk of breast cancer. New Engl. J. Med. 316:22-28, 1987*).

Negative Animal Experimental Study: Different gps. of rats were force-fed a mammary-cancer inducer and fed a high-fat unrestricted diet, a low-fat unrestricted diet, or a high fat restricted diet. After 24 wks., the tumor incidence in the high-fat unrestricted diet was 73%; low-fat unrestricted, 43%; and high-fat restricted, 7%, suggesting that the proportion of fat in the diet is not nearly as important as the energy balance of the subject. The authors note that, while obesity and excess calorie intake have now been linked to carcinogenesis in animal research and human epidemiologic studies, fat per se has not (*Boisson-neault GA et al. J. Nat. Cancer Instit. 76:335-38, 1986*).

Review Article: Numerous studies have associated the development of mammary tumors with dietary fat intake. In rodents, diets high in polyunsaturates were associated with carcinogen-induced mammary tumors more than high saturated fat diets (*Erickson KL, Thomas IK. The role of dietary fat in mammary tumorigenesis. Food Technology February, 1985, pp. 69-73*).

Review Article: Epidemiologic and experimental evidence over the past 40 years suggests that dietary fat is an important determinant of breast cancer risk and probability of survival after surgery (*Wynder EL, Cohen LA. A rationale for dietary intervention in the treatment of post-menopausal breast cancer patients. Nutr.& Cancer 3(4):195-199, 1982*).

Observational Study: The incidence of breast cancer was positively associated with consumption of animal fat (*Lubin JH et al. Int. J. Cancer 28:685-9, 1981*).

Observational Study: In a comparison of cancer patients with non-cancer pts., the incidence of breast cancer was associated with high fat consumption (*Phillips RL. Role of life-style and dietary habits among Seventh-Day Adventists. Cancer Res. 35:3513-22, 1975*).

Intestinal Cancer:

Intake of dietary fat is strongly correlated with mortality from intestinal cancer (except rectal) (*Carroll KK, Khor HT. Prog. Biochem. Pharmacol. 10:308-53, 1975*).

Observational Study: In comparing the diets of 50 colorectal cancer pts. with those of 50 healthy controls, the cancer pts. were found to consume 16% more energy than controls, mainly in the form of carbohydrate (largely in the form of fiber-depleted sugars) and fat (as combinations of fat and fiber-depleted sugars) (*Bristol JB. Sugar, fat and the risk of colorectal cancer. Brit. Med. J. 291:1457, 1985*).

Frequent consumption of high saturated fat foods among blacks is directly associated with the incidence of colon cancer (*Dales LG et al. Am. J. Epidemio. 109:132-44, 1978; Jain M et al. Int. J. Cancer 26:757-68, 1980*).

Ovarian Cancer:

Observational Study: Dietary histories of 215 women with recently diagnosed ovarian cancer were compared with those of 215 matched healthy controls. Coffee and alcohol consumption did not affect risk but pts. were found to consume 7% more animal fat than controls in the form of butter, whole milk and red meat (*Cramer DW et al. Dietary animal fat in relation to ovarian cancer risk. Obstet. Gyn. 63(6):833-8, 1984*).

Prostatic Cancer:

High fat intake has been shown to be a risk factor for cancer of the prostate (*Armstrong B, Doll R. Int. J. Cancer 15:617-31, 1975; Kolonel LN et al. Brit. J. Cancer 44:332-9, 1981*).

Low cholesterol diet.

Risk of lung cancer is associated with dietary cholesterol.

Observational Study: Data from 188 males with lung cancer and 294 controls were adjusted for age, ethnicity, cigarette smoking and exposure to lung carcinogens. Dietary cholesterol was found to be positively and significantly associated with lung cancer risk (*Hinds MW et al. Am. J. Clin. Nutr. 37:192-3, 1983*).

High fiber diet.

Protects against colorectal and breast cancer, possibly by removing carcinogens and excess estrogen.

Review Article: For Western women, dietary fiber may be important in the prevention of breast cancer, and both the early onset of menarche and a high fat diet are risk factors in breast cancer. Breast cancer may be estrogen-dependent and dietary fiber may increase the fecal excretion of estrogen. Perhaps high fat diets are necessarily low in fiber and low fiber intake rather than high fat intake is the reason why high dietary fat is a risk factor (*Hughes RE. Hypothesis: A new look at dietary fiber. Human Nutr.: Clin. Nutr. 40C:81-86, 1986*).

Review Article: The international studies and most of the epidemiologic case-control studies show a protective benefit of foods containing fiber and none shows harm, suggesting that a variety of fiber-containing foods be eaten to protect against colon cancer (*Greenward P, Lanza E. Dietary fiber and colon cancer. Contemp. Nutr. 11(1), 1986*).

Review Article: Epidemiologic studies examining various dietary components and colon cancer incidence and mortality show a correlation between risk for colon cancer and a high fat, low cereal, low fiber diet, which is typical of Westernized nations (*American Cancer Society. Ca 34(2):121-6, 1984*).

Observational Study: Dietary fiber was more highly correlated (inversely) than crude fiber with colon cancer. Cereals were the only source of fiber that showed an association with lower colon cancer mortality (*McKeoun-Eyssen G, Bright-See E. Nutr. & Cancer 6:160, 1984*).

Observational Study: It is known that, while the fat intake and risk of heart disease in Finland is among the highest in the world, the incidence of colon cancer is less than 1/3 that of the United States. This study found a strong inverse correlation between whole grain cereal intake and colon cancer. Consumption of the popular coarse rye bread results in fecal bulk 3 times that of most Westernized nations and a significant reduction in fecal bile acid concentration (*Englyst HN et al. Nutr. & Cancer 4:50-60, 1982*).

Observational Study: The fiber intake of colon cancer pts. prior to diagnosis compared to that of control subjects was estimated from a frequency questionnaire listing foods rich in fiber. High fat and low fiber were associated with colon cancer (*Modan B et al. J. National Cancer Instit. 55:15-18, 1975*).

Observational Studies: Marked inverse international correlations of colon cancer and cereal consumption were found (*Armstrong B, Doll R. Int. J. Cancer 15:617, 1975; Irving D, Drasar BS. Brit. J. Cancer 28:462, 1973*).

May protect against prostate cancer.

Observational Study: The relationship between crude and dietary fiber ingestion and hormone levels was investigated in 30 men. Plasma levels of testosterone and estradiol-17 beta had a significant inverse relationship with both crude and dietary fiber intakes, suggesting that increasing fiber ingestion may modify the risk of prostate cancer (*Howie BJ, Schultz TD. Am. J. Clin. Nutr. 432:127-34, 1985*).

<u>Vegetarian</u> diet.

Benefits may be due to its low fat and high fiber content.

May decrease the risk of <u>breast cancer</u> by lowering estrogen levels.

Observational Study: 10 vegetarian premenopausal women were found to excrete 2-3 times as much estrogen as 10 non-vegetarian controls and have lower serum estrogen levels, suggesting that the fiber present in a whole-grain, whole-vegetable diet absorbs estrogen and removes it via fecal excretion (*Goldin BR et al. Estrogen excretion patterns and plasma levels in vegetarian and omnivorous women. New Eng. J. Med. 307:1542-47, 1982*).

See Also:

Barale R et al. Vegetables inhibit, in vivo, the mutagenicity of nitrite combined with nitrosable compounds. Mutation Res. 120:145, 1983

Eat plenty of <u>fruits and vegetables</u>.

Consumption negatively correlated with cancer mortality.

Observational Study: The association between consumption of carotene-containing vegetables and subsequent 5 year mortality from cancer was examined for 1271 subjects 66 years of age or older. After controlling for age and smoking, those in the highest quintile of intake had a cancer mortality risk of 30% that of those in the lowest quintile. However, since salads, carrots and squash consumption was unrelated to risk of cancer mortality, and consumption of tomatoes or strawberries was most strongly correlated with low cancer risk, some other factor besides beta-carotene may be responsible (*Colditz GA et al. Am. J. Clin. Nutr. 41:32-6, 1985*).

Observational Study: A large scale, 20-year study found a negative correlation between eating green-yellow vegetables daily and the risk of <u>lung, stomach and other cancers</u>. Ex-smokers who ate green-yellow vegetables daily also decreased their risk of lung cancer. Among those who increased their vegetable consumption, there was a more than 25% reduction in the number of deaths from <u>stomach cancer</u> (*Dietary Aspects of Carcinogenesis September, 1983*).

Avoid <u>alcohol</u>.

Associated with increased cancer risk, especially <u>upper respiratory</u> cancers and <u>gastrointestinal cancers</u> (*Sandler RS. Nutrition and Cancer 4:273-8, 1983*).

See Also:

Beer drinking and the risk of rectal cancer. Nutr. Rev. 42:244, 1984

Potter JD, McMichael AJ. Alcohol, beer and lung cancer: A meaningful relationship? Internat. J. Epidemiol. 13:240, 1984

Rosenberg L et al. Breast cancer and alcoholic beverage consumption. Lancet 1:267, 1982

Avoid <u>smoked, pickled and salt-cured foods</u>.

Contain nitrosamines and polycyclic aromatic hydrocarbons which cause cancer in animals; also linked in epidemiologic studies with cancers of the <u>stomach</u> and <u>esophagus</u> (*The National Academy of Sciences. Nutrition, Diet and Cancer, 1982*).

Negative Observational Study: Nitrates and nitrites were measured in the saliva of 2 populations who differed in their risk of developing <u>gastric cancer</u>. The levels of both ions were significantly <u>higher</u> in the low-risk group, suggesting that, at least in Great Britain, nitrates are not an important cause of gastric cancer (*Forman D et al. Nitrates, nitrites and gastric cancer in Great Britain. <u>Nature</u> 313(6004):620-25, 1985*).

Observational Study: Decreasing <u>stomach cancer</u> rates have been linked to decreasing consumption of nitrates and nitrites, since americans now eat 1/4 the nitrates and nitrites they did in 1925 and there has been a three-fold decrease in stomach cancer mortality since that year. In addition, other countries where more nitrates are eaten have a higher stomach cancer rate (*<u>Environmental Med.</u> vol. 5, 1983*).

Avoid <u>eggs</u> and <u>fried foods</u>.

Observational Study: In a study of over 16,000 Seventh-Day Adventist women, those who ate eggs (fried or otherwise) at least 3 times weekly had a 3 times greater risk of fatal <u>ovarian cancer</u> than did women who ate eggs less than once weekly, while fish, chicken and potatoes were also positively associated with fatal ovarian cancer when they were fried. Consumption of fried eggs showed the strongest association with fatal ovarian cancer, perhaps due to interference with cholesterol biosynthesis and consequently the manufacture of ovarian hormones from the production of cytotoxic oxidation products of cholesterol (*Snowdon DA. Letter to the Editor. <u>JAMA</u> 254(3):356-7, 1985*).

Avoid <u>sugar</u>.

Harmful effects may be either direct or indirect (for example, high sucrose intake is associated with a low intake of fiber).

Observational Study: In comparing the diets of 50 <u>colorectal cancer</u> pts. with those of 50 very closely matched healthy controls, the cancer pts. were found to ingest 14% more energy (p less than 0.001), mostly in the form of carbohydrate (21% increase; p less than 0.001) and fat (14% increase; p less than 0.001). The extra carbohydrate was largely in the form of fiber-depleted sugar (40% increase; p less than 0.005) and the extra fat as fat/sugar combinations (36% increase; p less than 0.02). No difference was found in daily intakes of total dietary fiber, cereal fiber, vegetable fiber, natural sugar, or vitamins A,C and D. Energy intake per gm. of dietary fiber was 23% higher in cancer pts. (p less than 0.0005), suggesting a more refined diet. Thus fiber-depleted foods, especially sugar, may predispose to the development of large bowel cancer (*Bristol JB et al. Colorectal cancer and diet: A case-control study with special reference to dietary fibre and sugar. <u>Proc. Am. Assoc. of Cancer Res.</u> 26:206, March, 1985*).

Observational Study: In comparing the diets of 50 <u>colorectal cancer</u> pts. with those of 50 healthy controls, the cancer pts. were found to consume 16% more energy than controls, mainly in the form of carbohydrate (largely in the form of fiber-depleted sugars) and fat (as combinations of fat and fiber-depleted sugars) (*Bristol JB. Sugar, fat and the risk of colorectal cancer. <u>Brit. Med. J.</u> 291:1457, 1985*).

Observational Study: An epidemiologic survey of 21 countries has suggested that high sucrose intake is a major risk factor for the development of <u>breast cancer</u> in women over 45 years of age (*Seely S, Horrobin DF. Diet and breast cancer: The possible connection with sugar consumption. <u>Med. Hypo.</u> 11(3):319-27, 1983*).

Animal Experimental Study: Rats on high sugar diets developed significantly more <u>mammary tumors</u> than those on a high starch diet (*Hoehn SK, Carroll KK. Effects of dietary carbohydrate on the incidence of mammary tumors induced in rats by 7,12-dimethylbenz(a)-anthracene. <u>Nutri. Cancer,</u> 1(3):27-30, Spring, 1979*).

Review Article: Human breast cancer mortality shows a positive correlation with dietary sugar, and a negative correlation with complex carbohydrates in the diet (*Carroll KK. Dietary factors in hormone-dependent cancers, in Winick M, Ed. Current Concepts in Nutrition, Volume 6, Nutrition and Cancer. New York, John Wiley & Sons, 1977, pp. 25-40*).

Avoid partially hydrogenated oils.

The un-natural *trans* form of fatty acids (up to 17% of processed vegetable oils, 47% of margarines and 58% of vegetable shortening) may be a major contributor to the carcinogenic effect of fats (*Enig MG et al. Dietary fat and cancer trends. Fed. Proc. 37:2215-20, 1978*).

Avoid olive oil.

May stimulate malignant cell proliferation.

Review Article: Oleic acid, a mono-unsaturated non-essential fatty acid present in vegetable oils and abundant in olive oil, has been shown to stimulate malignant cell proliferation *in vitro*, while the essential fatty acids of both the omega-3 and omega-6 series appear to have a protective effect. Recent findings that polyunsaturated fatty acids may be tumorigenic are most likely due to their oleic acid content (*Booyens J et al. Dietary fats and cancer. Med. Hypotheses 17:351-62, 1985*).

Observational Study: The ratio of stearic to oleic acid (reflecting the degree of desaturation of stearic acid) in the RBC cell membranes was calculated for 60 cancer pts., 41 pts. with other diseases, and 40 healthy subjects. The mean desaturation ratio for cancer pts. was 0.69 compared to 1.45 for the pts. with other diseases and 1.5 for the healthy subjects. The desaturation ratio was also significantly lower for the cancer pts. with recurrent tumors compared to those without recurrence (*Wood CB et al. Increase of oleic acid in erythrocytes associated with malignancies. Brit. Med. J. 291:163, 1985*).

- -

NUTRIENTS:

Beta Carotene:

Intake is negatively correlated with the risk of certain cancers - independent of the effect of vitamin A (*see also "Vitamin A" and "Beta-Carotene" below*).

Note: Only a small percentage of beta-carotene is converted into vitamin A, and this conversion is impaired in liver disease and hypothyroidism.

Cervical Cancer:

Observational Study: In a study comparing 78 women with untreated cervical cancer with controls, plasma beta-carotene was significantly lower in cancer pts. (*Orr JW et al. Am. J. Obstet. & Gyn. 151:632-5, 1985*).

Observational Study: In a case-control study of 191 pts. and 191 age-matched controls, intake of dietary beta-carotene (in carrots and green vegetables) was inversely and strongly related to the risk of cervical cancer. However, consumption of retinoids (in milk, liver and meats) had no effect on cervical cancer risk, suggesting that either dietary beta-carotene or some related aspect of a vegetable-rich diet is protective (*La Vecchia C et al. Dietary vitamin A and the risk of invasive cervical cancer. Int. J. Cancer vol. 34:319-22, 1984*).

Lung Cancer:

Observational Study: Levels of beta-carotene in serum collected from 99 individuals who were subsequently found to have lung cancer as compared to 196 matched controls showed a strong inverse correlation between beta-carotene levels and the risk of squamous-cell carcinoma of the lung (*Menkes MS et al. Serum beta-carotene, vitamins A and E, selenium and the risk of lung cancer. New Engl. J. Med. 315:1250, 1986*).

Observational Study: In a survey of over 6000 people, low beta-carotene levels were correlated with lung cancer mortality (*Stahelin HB et al. J. Nat. Cancer Instit. 73:1463-8, 1984*).

Observational Study: In a study of 763 cancer pts. and 900 controls, vitamin A and retinol intake had no demonstrable effect on cancer risk, but the 25% of the sample who consumed the least carotene had a 30% greater risk of lung cancer than the 25% whose carotene intake was the highest (*Ziegler RG et al. J. Nat. Cancer Instit. 73:1429-35, 1984*).

Observational Study: In a 19-year prospective study of 1954 middle-aged men, the intake of beta-carotene was inversely related to the incidence of lung cancer(*Shekelle RB et al. Dietary vitamin A and risk of cancer in the Western Electric study. Lancet November 28, 1981, pp. 1185-90*).

Oral Cancer:

Experimental Controlled Study: Inuits using smokeless tobacco eat a diet rich in meat including liver, but low in vegetables, leading to normal serum vitamin A levels but low beta-carotene levels. Supplementation with beta-carotene 90 mg twice weekly for 10 wks. significantly decreased the frequency of exfoliated cells from the oral mucosa with micronuclei, while placebo and untreated controls showed no change (*Stich HF et al. A pilot beta-carotene intervention trial with Inuits using smokeless tobacco. Int. J. Cancer 36:321, 1985*).

Folic Acid:

Localized deficiency in cervical epithelial cells may promote cervical dysplasia and eventually carcinoma of the cervix.

Observational Study: 78 women with untreated cervical cancer, when compared to 240 healthy controls, were found to have lower mean values of plasma folate (*Orr JW. Am. J. Obstet. & Gyn. 151:632-5, 1985*).

Experimental Double-blind Study: 47 young women on combination-type birth control pills with mild or moderate dysplasia received either 10 mg oral folate daily or placebo. After 3 months, cervical biopsies showed significant improvement only in the women receiving folate. Pre-treatment folate levels were lowest in subjects on the pill without dysplasia and subjects not on the pill and without dysplasia (whose levels were highest). The dysplasia completely disappeared in 7 women receiving folate, while 4 women on placebo showed progression to carcinoma in situ (*Butterworth CE et al. Improvement in cervical dysplasia associated with folic acid therapy in users of oral contraceptives. Am. J. Clin. Nutr. 35:73-82, 1982*).

Experimental and Observational Study: Cervical epithelial cells of women using steroid hormones as oral contraceptive agents showed megaloblastic features. Despite the lack of evidence of systemic folate deficiency, they disappeared with oral folate supplementation (*Whitehead N et al. Megaloblastic changes in the cervical epithelium: Association with oral contraceptive therapy and reversal with folic acid. JAMA 226:1421-1424, 1973*).

Pyridoxine:

Theoretical Discussion: Since B_6 is a co-enzyme in the biosynthesis of thymidine, a deficiency of which can increase mutagenesis, a B_6 deficiency along with contact with carcinogens could lead to tumor initiation (*Prior F. Theoretical involvement of vitamin B_6 in tumor initiation. Med. Hypotheses 16:421-8, 1985*).

Deficiency may be associated with cervical cancer.

Observational Study: RBC transaminase, a measure of B_6 status, was decreased in 1/3 of pts. with cervical cancer (*Ramaswamy P, Natarajan R. Vitamin B_6 status in patients with cancer of the uterine cervix. Nutr. Cancer 6:176-80, 1984*).

Vitamin A:

May inhibit carcinogenesis in certain cancers (*see also "Vitamin A and Beta-Carotene" below*).

Review Article: The association of high retinoid intake with decreased cancer risk may be due to immuno-suppression during vitamin A deficiency or immuno-enhancement during extremely high intakes. High dietary vitamin A enhances macrophage functioning, while retinol suppresses T-lymphocyte function *in vitro* (*Watson R et al. Cancer prevention by retinoids: Role of immunological modification. Nutr. Res. 5:663-75, 1985*).

Breast Cancer:

Low serum retinol levels are associated with a diminished response to chemotherapy.

Observational Study: Serum alpha-tocopherol and retinol levels of 37 women with breast cancer who were to undergo initial chemotherapy and of 35 controls were analyzed. Among the pts. with serum retinol levels equal to or greater than the control mean, 83% responded to chemotherapy, 17% remained stable and none progressed. Among the pts. with serum retinol levels below the control mean, 36% responded, 24% remained stable and 40% progressed. There were no differences in tocopherol levels between gps. suggesting that differences in retinol are not the result of general nutritional debilitation and that specific nutritional or metabolic differences relating to vitamin A may exist (*Brown RR et al. Correlation of serum retinol levels with response to chemotherapy in breast cancer. Meeting Abstract. Proc. Am. Assoc. Cancer Res. 22:184, 1981*).

Cervical Cancer:

Observational Study: Compared to controls, women with cervical intraepithelial neoplasia had a statistically lower level of serum vitamin A (p = 0.1), although dietary profiles did not reveal a significant difference (*Bernstein A, Harris B. The relationship of dietary and serum vitamin A to the occurrence of cervical intraepithelial neoplasia in sexually active women. Am. J. Obstet. Gynecol. 148(3):309-12, 1984*).

Laryngeal Cancer:

Observational Study: In a study of 374 males with cancer of the larynx and 381 controls, those ingesting low amounts of vitamin A in their diets had twice the risk of those ingesting large amounts, even when controlling for smoking and drinking (*Graham S et al. Dietary factors in the epidemiology of cancer of the larynx. Am. J. Epidemiol. 113(6):675-80, 1981*).

Lung Cancer:

Negative Observational Study: There was no significant correlation between serum retinol or retinol-binding protein levels and subsequent risk of lung cancer (*Friedman GD et al. Am. J. Epidemiol. 123(5):781-89, 1986*).

Prostate Cancer:

Observational Study: In 19 pts. with prostate cancer, serum zinc was significantly lower than in 27 pts. with benign prostatic hyperplasia and there was a significant zinc/vitamin A correlation (p less than 0.05) (*Whelen P et al. Zinc, vitamin A and prostatic cancer. Brit. J. Urology. 55(5):525-8, 1983*).

Stomach Cancer:

Observational Study: All pts. dying of stomach cancer over 2 yrs. in 4 Pennsylvania counties were matched to controls dying of heart disease. People with stomach cancer tended to have lower levels of vitamin A intake compared to controls, with the greatest risk associated with the lowest vitamin A levels. This increased risk of stomach cancer due to vitamin A deficiency was relatively low (about twofold), suggesting that the degenerative effects of vitamin A deficiencies on the stomach's epithelium may play only a weak, permissive role in the carcinogenic process (*Stehr PA et al. Am. J. Epidemiol. 121:65-70, 1985*).

Observational Study: In a survey of over 6000 people, low vitamin A levels were associated with death from stomach cancer (*Stahelin HB et al. J. Nat. Cancer Instit. 73:1463-6, 1984*).

Vitamin A and
Beta-Carotene:

May reduce the risk of certain cancers.

Cervical Cancer:

Observational Study: The vitamin A and beta carotene intake as well as cellular retinol binding protein (CRBP) levels were assessed for 49 women with dysplastic changes or carcinoma in situ (CIS) and 49 matched controls. Women consuming less than average vitamin A and beta carotene were 3 times as likely to develop severe dysplasia and 2 3/4 times as likely to develop CIS. CRBP levels in the cervical tissue samples were inversely correlated with the severity of the dysplasia (*Wylie-Rosett JA et al. Influence of vitamin A on cervical dysplasia and carcinoma in situ. Nutrition and Cancer 6(1):49-57, 1984*).

Oral Cancer:

Experimental Double-blind Study: Members of the Phillipine Ifugao tribe who chew betel quid, a tobacco-like plant mixture that promotes cellular damage, received weekly doses of vitamin A, beta-carotene, canthaxanthin or placebo. Both at baseline and after 9 weeks, 3-5% of the cells from inside the cheek had genetic damage in both the placebo and canthaxanthin groups, while the percentage of damaged cells decreased in the vitamin A gp. from 4% to 2% and in the beta-carotene group from 3.5% to 1% (*Stich HF. Int. J. Cancer 34:745-50, 1984*).

Vitamin C:

May be protective against a variety of cancers.

Observational Study: In a survey of cancer mortality among 6000 people, vitamin C levels were lower in all cancer groups, and especially low in those dying from gastric cancer (*Stahelin HB et al. J. Nat. Cancer Instit. 73:1463-8, 1984*).

Cervical Cancer:

Observational Study: In a study comparing 78 women with untreated cervical cancer to healthy controls, plasma vitamin C levels were significantly lower in cancer patients (*Orr JW et al. Am. J. Obstet. & Gyn. 151:632-5, 1985*).

Observational Study: Serum vitamin C levels were examined in 46 women with either 2 consecutive suspicious Pap smears or 1 positive Pap smear and compared to normal controls. The mean plasma vitamin C level in cases was about 1/2 that of the controls. While plasma vitamin C was low in women with severe dysplasia or cervical cancer, it was even lower in women with severe dysplasia and lowest in women with inflammatory cervical disease (*Romney SL et al. Am. J. Obstet. & Gyn. 151:976-80, 1985*).

Laryngeal Cancer:

Observational Study: In a study of 374 males with cancer of the larynx and 381 controls, those ingesting low amounts of vitamin C in their diets had twice the risk of those ingesting large amounts, even when controlling for smoking and drinking (*Graham S et al. Dietary factors in the epidemiology of cancer of the larynx. Am. J. Epidemiol. 113(6):675-80, 1981*).

Supplementation may increase survival time of terminal patients.

Negative Experimental Double-blind Study: 100 advanced large bowel cancer pts. who had received no chemotherapy were treated with either vitamin C 10 gms daily for a median of 2.5 months or placebo. There were no differences in survival rates between the 2 groups, although none of the pts. on vitamin C died while taking vitamin C (*Moertel CG et al. High-dose vitamin C versus placebo in the treatment of patients with advanced cancer who have had no prior chemotherapy: A randomized double-blind comparison. New Engl. J. Med. 312:137-141, 1985*).

> *Note: In rebuttal, Linus Pauling Ph.D. claims that the negative results were due to premature discontinuation of vitamin C after 2.5 months which, in addition to not providing sufficient time for vitamin C to demonstrate its effectiveness, caused a rebound effect which may have worsened the patients' status. He concludes that the Moertel study only shows that vitamin C should not be given to cancer pts. for a short time and then withdrawn (Int. Clin. Nutr. Rev. 5(4):163-5, 1985).*

Negative Experimental Double-blind Study: 150 pts. with advanced cancer received ascorbic acid 10 gm or placebo. Sixty "evaluable" pts. received vitamin C and 63 similar randomized pts. received a lactose placebo, while 27 of the randomized pts. elected not to participate. All but 9 of the 123 pts. had previously received radiation, chemotherapy, or both. Neither vitamin C nor placebo improved survival times which averaged 51 days; however those who withdrew only survived 25 days, raising the question as to how the decision to withdraw may have influenced survival. The authors note that, in contrast to the earlier Pauling and Cameron study, a larger proportion of pts. in this study had received radiation and/or chemotherapy (*Creagan ET et al. New Engl. J. Med. 301:687-90, 1979*).

Experimental Controlled Study: Vitamin C 10 gm daily in divided doses was given orally to "hopelessly ill" patients. Mean survival times were 300 days longer when they were compared to historical controls. Survival for longer than 1 yr. after the "date of untreatability" was observed in 22% of the experimental gp. but only 0.4% of historical controls. In addition, 370 non-random concurrent controls showed the same survival statistics (*Cameron E, Pauling L. Supplemental ascorbate in the supportive treatment of cancer: Reevaluation of prolongation of survival times in terminal human cancer.*

Proc. Nat. Acad. Sci. USA 75:4538-42, 1978; Cameron E, Pauling L. Supplemental ascorbate in the supportive treatment or cancer: Prolongation of survival times in terminal human cancer. Proc. Nat. Acad. Sci. USA 73:3685-9, 1976).

> *Note: This study has been criticized on the following grounds:*
> *1. Lack of a prospective random double-blind study.*
> *2. Lack of rigidly-defined criteria for untreatability.*
> *3. Failure to match pts. by histological identification of type and origin of cancer cells.*
> *4. Failure to ensure that cases and controls adhere to their medication schedules.*
> *(Comroe J Jr. Proc. Natl. Acad. Sci. USA 75:4543, 1978).*

May enhance the effect of cytotoxic drugs in certain cancers.

In vitro Experimental Study: Sodium L-ascorbate and sodium D-ascorbate at nonlethal concentrations potentiated the effect of 5-FU, x-radiation, bleomycin, prostaglandin E_1, and sodium butyrate on mouse neuroblastoma cells but not on rat glioma cells (*Prasad KN et al. Sodium ascorbate potentiates the growth inhibitory effect of certain agents on neuroblastoma cells in culture. Proc. Natl. Acad. Sci. USA 76(2):829-32, 1979*).

See Also:

> *Prasad KN. Modulation of the effects of tumor therapeutic agents by vitamin C. Life Sci. 21(2):275-80, 1980*

May block the formation of carcinogenic nitrosamines to protect against stomach cancer.

Experimental Study: 8 volunteers received ascorbic acid 1 gm daily. In 7/8, levels of mutagenic activity in the gastric juice were significantly lower after 1 wk. than at baseline, suggesting that vitamin C supplementation may significantly reduce the levels of genotoxic chemicals in gastric juice (*O'Connor HJ et al. Effect of increased intake of vitamin C on the mutagenic activity of gastric juice and intragastric concentrations of ascorbic acid. Carcinogenesis 6(11):1675-76, 1985*).

Experimental Study: Vitamin C 2 gm daily was effective in blocking the formation of nitrosoamines in 10 students fed nitrate and proline (*Wagner DA et al. Cancer Res. 45:6519-22, 1985*).

Observational Study: Gastric cancer incidence among Japanese who migrated to Hawaii, Caucasians who migrated to Hawaii from the U.S., Hawaiian-born Caucasians and Japanese in Japan were compared. The rates for Japanese were higher than those for Caucasians and highest for Japanese in Japan. Dietary analyses revealed a positive correlation between gastric cancer incidence and consumption of dried, salted fish, pickled vegetables and rice, and a negative correlation with fresh fruits and vitamin C. Results are consistent with the hypothesis that stomach cancer is caused by endogenous nitrosamine formation from dietary precursors, and that vitamin C may protect against the disease (*Kolonel LN et al. Association of diet and place of birth with stomach cancer incidence in Hawaii Japanese and Caucasians. Am. J. Clin. Nutr. 34(11):2478-85, 1981*).

Animal Experimental Study: A characteristic nitrosamine-caused form of liver damage was produced in mice by feeding them nitrite and amines. When their diet was supplemented with ascorbic acid, no liver damage occurred, suggesting that the addition of ascorbic acid prevented the nitrosamines from being formed (*Greenblatt M. Brief communication: Ascorbic acid blocking of aminopyrine nitrosation in NZO-B1 mice. J. Natl. Cancer Inst. 50(4):1055-56, 1973*).

In vitro Experimental Study: Vitamin C blocked the formation of nitrosamines from nitrite by successfully competing with amines for the nitrite (*Mirvish S et al. Science July 7, 1972*).

Vitamin B$_{12}$ and
Vitamin C:

May inhibit carcinogenesis when given together.

Animal Experimental Study: Inhibited the mitotic activity of transplantable mouse tumors and produced a 100% survival rate, while neither vitamin alone at the same dosage had any effect on mitosis or morphology of the cells studied. Microscopic exam of ascites fluid from treated mice showed a few tumor cells in various stages of disintegration which later disappeared (*Poydock ME et al. Inhibiting effect of vitamins C and B$_{12}$ on the mitotic activity of ascites tumors. Exp. Cell. Biol. 47(3):210-17, 1979*).

Vitamin E:

May reduce the level of mutagens in stool.

Experimental Study: Vitamin E supplements reduced stool mutagen levels by as much as 79% (*Bruce WR, Dion PW. Studies relating to a fecal mutagen. Am. J. Clin. Nutr. 33:2511-12, 1980*).

May block the formation of nitrosamines.

Experimental Study: Vitamin E 400 IU daily was effective in blocking the formation of nitrosoamines in 10 students fed nitrate and proline (*Wagner DA et al. Cancer Res. 45:6519-22, 1985*).

Blood levels may be negatively correlated with the risk of certain cancers.

Bowel Cancer:

Observational Study: In a survey of over 6000 people, low vitamin E and lipid levels were correlated with mortality from bowel cancer (*Stahelin HB et al. J. Nat. Cancer Instit. 73:1463-8, 1984*).

Breast Cancer:

Observational Study: In a study of 5004 women, those who developed breast cancer had a mean plasma vitamin E level of 4.7 mg/l. This was significantly lower than in control subjects (6 mg/l) matched for age, menopausal status, parity and family history of breast disease (*Wald NJ et al. Plasma retinol, beta-carotene and vitamin E levels in relation to the future risk of breast cancer. Brit. J. Cancer 49:321-4, 1984*).

Lung Cancer:

Observational Study: Mean levels of vitamin E in serum collected from 99 individuals who were subsequently found to have lung cancer were lower than those of 196 matched controls (*Menkes MS et al. Serum beta-carotene, vitamins A and E, selenium and the risk of lung cancer. New Engl. J. Med. 315:1250, 1986*).

May enhance the effect of cytotoxic drugs, permitting a reduction in drug dosage, and reduce their toxicity.

In vitro Experimental Study: Vitamin E inhibited the growth of mouse neuroblastoma and rat glioma cells in culture and induced reversion of these cells towards normal morphology. It also enhanced the growth inhibitory effect of vincristine on mouse melanoma cells and enhanced the differentiating effect of prostaglandin E$_1$ on neuroblastoma cells in culture. In animal studies, it reduced adriamycin-induced cardiac and skin toxicity and bleomycin-induced lung fibrosis (*Prasad

KN et al. Vitamin E increases the growth inhibitory and differentiating effects of tumor therapeutic agents on neuroblastoma and glioma cells in culture. <u>Proc. Soc. Exp. Biol. Med.</u> 164(2):158-63, 1980).

May protect against the toxic side-effects of doxorubicin (Adriamycin) such as cardiac toxicity and hair loss.

Experimental Study: 69% of pts. on doxorubicin receiving 1600 IU dl-alpha tocopherol acetate daily did not develop alopecia. Those who did develop alopecia were believed to have received vitamin E too late before chemotherapy, as it should be started 5-7 days prior to commencement (*Wood L. Possible prevention of Adriamycin-induced alopecia by tocopherol. <u>New Engl. J. Med.</u> 312:1060, 1985*).

- -

<u>Calcium:</u>

Intake is negatively associated with <u>colon cancer</u>.

Negative Observational Study: In a prospective cohort study, 8006 men of Japanese ancestry were examined. There was no significant association between dietary calcium intake and colon cancer risk (*Heibrun LK et al. Colon cancer and dietary fat, phosphorus, and calcium in Hawaiian-Japanese men. <u>Am. J. Clin. Nutr.</u> 43(2):306-9, 1986*).

Experimental Study: Patterns of proliferation of the epithelial cells lining colonic crypts in rectal mucosal biopsies of 10 pts. with family histories of colon cancer were examined and found to be characteristic of pts. with familial colon cancer. They were given 1.25 gm calcium daily and, after 2-3 months, the number of rapidly proliferating cells in their colonic epithelium had significantly decreased and was almost the same as in people at low risk for colon cancer (*Lipkin M, Newmark H. Effect of added dietary calcium on colonic epithelial-cell proliferation in subjects at high risk for familial colonic cancer. <u>New Engl. J. Med.</u> 313:1381-4, 1985*).

Observational Study: People drinking soft water (low in calcium) have a higher incidence of colon cancer, while those eating high calcium diets have a lower incidence of colon cancer (<u>Science News</u> *3/2/85 p. 141 and 9/21/85 p. 187*).

May reduce the adverse effects of bile acids and free ionized fatty acids in the colon by forming insoluble soaps.

Theoretical Discussion: Increased dietary fat may promote colon cancer by increasing the levels of free ionized fatty acids and bile acids in the colon contents. In the presence of calcium ions, the irritating and toxic effects of these acids could be reduced by being converted to insoluble calcium soaps (*Newmark HL et al. Colon cancer and dietary fat, phosphate, and calcium: A hypothesis. <u>JNCI</u> 72(6):1323-25, 1984*).

Animal Experimental Study: Part of a gp. of deoxycholic acid-treated mice received oral supplements of calcium lactate. Those mice also receiving the supplements showed minimal tissue necrosis due to DCA administration and the frequency of mitotic events and cellular proliferative activity remained similar to levels seen in untreated controls, suggesting that sequestration of bile acids by calcium salts may inhibit the untoward effects of bile acids on the colonic epithelium (*Wargovich MJ et al. Calcium ameliorates the toxic effect of deoxycholic acid on colonic epithelium. <u>Carcinogenesis</u> 4(9):1205-7, 1983*).

Calcium and
Phosphorus:

Low dietary calcium to phosphorus ratios are associated with <u>colorectal cancer</u> (*Lipkin M, Newmark MS. - op cit*).

Calcium and
Vitamin D:

Intake is negatively correlated with risk of colorectal cancer.

> **Observational Study:** In a prospective study of 1954 men, those who had the lowest combined index of calcium and vitamin D were 2 1/2 times as likely to develop colorectal cancer as men who had the highest index, even after age, cigarette and alcohol consumption, body mass index, and fat intake were taken into account (*Garland C et al. Dietary vitamin D and calcium and risk of colorectal cancer: A 19-year prospective study in men. <u>Lancet</u> 1:307-9, 1985*).

Fluoride:

WARNING: May be carcinogenic.

> **In vitro Experimental Study:** 45-135 ppm fluoride (as NaF) caused a dose-dependent unscheduled DNA synthesis in human oral keratinocytes within 4 hours (*Tsutsui T et al. Induction of unscheduled DNA synthesis in cultured human oral keratinocytes by sodium fluoride. <u>Mutation Res.</u> 140:43-48, 1984*).

> *Note: The concentration of NaF in toothpaste and mouthwash is 23 times this high, suggesting that they may be carcinogenic (Sutton PRN. Letter to the Editor. <u>N.Z. Med. J.</u> 98(775):207, 1985).*

Iodine:

Intake is negatively correlated with risk of <u>breast</u>, <u>endometrial</u> and <u>ovarian</u> cancer.

> **Review Article (<u>breast cancer</u>):** Women with low iodine levels often have symptoms relating to severe hyperplasia and fibrocystic disease of the breast, precancerous lesions which have been corrected by iodine replacement in clinical trials (*Eskin BA. <u>Biol. Trace Element Res.</u> 5:399-412, 1983*).

> See Also:

> *Stadel VV. Dietary iodine and the risk of breast, endometrial, and ovarian cancer. <u>Lancet</u> April 24, 1976, pp. 890-1*

Magnesium:

Intake is negatively correlated with cancer incidence and mortality.

> **Review Article:** Animal studies report increased cancer in magnesium-deficient diets and a preventive effect in animals fed excess magnesium. Epidemiologic studies suggest that magnesium levels in water, soil, food and air are inversely related to cancer mortality (*Blondell JM. The anticarcinogenic effect of magnesium. <u>Med. Hypotheses</u> 6:863-871, 1980*).

Selenium:

Deficiency is associated with increased cancer risk.

It has been estimated that 250-300 mcg daily can prevent most cancers, while typical selenium consumption in the U.S. is about 100 mcg (*Schrauzer, Gerhard, Ph.D. - 1981*).

General:

Review Article: Recent research has failed to substantiate earlier claims that selenium was carcinogenic. A large proportion of animal studies showing a positive effect of selenium found at least a 35% reduction in tumor incidence, suggesting that a dietary deficiency of selenium may increase carcinogenesis in certain circumstances. Epidemiologic studies have confirmed that cancer pts. tend to have lower blood or plasma selenium levels than controls. Prospective studies suggest that it is unlikely that this correlation is due to an effect of cancer upon selenium metabolism (*Combs GF, Clark LC. Can dietary selenium modify cancer risk? Nutr. Rev. 43:325-31, 1985*).

Observational Study: In a 4 year case-control study of 51 cancer patients investigating the relationship between serum concentrations of selenium and vitamins A and E, fatal cancer corresponded to selenium deficiency, vitamin E contributed to this effect and, among smoking men with low serum selenium, inadequate vitamin A or beta-carotene intake was associated with an increased incidence of lung cancer (*Salonen J et al. Risk of cancer in relation to serum concentrations of selenium and vitamin A and E: Matched case-control analysis of prospective data. Brit. Med. J. 290:417, 1985*).

Review Article: Past epidemiological studies suggesting an association of selenium nutrition or blood levels and cancer incidence and mortality are reviewed. In a re-analysis of data indicating an inverse association between cancer incidence and selenium forage crop levels in the U.S., results confirmed an inverse association between selenium availability and total cancer mortality in both males and females (*Clark LC. The epidemiology of selenium and cancer. Fed. Proceed. 44:2584, 1985*).

Observational Study: Age-adjusted cancer mortality showed a strong inverse correlation with selenium levels in pooled blood from 24 regions in China. A similar pattern was seen for cancers of the esophagus, stomach and liver (*Yu S-Y et al. Regional variation of cancer mortality incidence and its relation to selenium levels in China. Biological Trace Element Res. 7:21, 1985*).

Observational Study: In a study of 4480 adults, the subsequent risk of developing cancer appears to be predicted by the serum selenium level, but not by the vitamin A, carotenoid or vitamin E level (*Serum vitamin and provitamin A levels and the risk of cancer. Nutr. Rev. 42(6):214-5, 1984*).

Observational Study: In a case-control study of over 800 adults, those whose blood selenium levels were below 45 mcg/l had an excess cancer risk at the 6 year follow-up (*Salonen JT et al. Association between serum selenium and the risk of cancer. Am. J. Epidemiol. 120:342, 1984*).

Observational Study: Serum samples were collected and stored for up to 5 years when selenium levels in those who developed cancer during this time were compared to those who did not. The overall risk of cancer for those with selenium levels in the lowest fifth was twice that of people with levels in the highest fifth (*Willett WC, MacMahon B. Diet and cancer: An overview. New Engl. J. Med. 310(11):697-703, 1984*).

Observational Study: Serum selenium levels from 111 subjects who developed cancer in the subsequent 5 years were compared with controls. Subjects had significantly lower selenium levels and lower levels of the vitamins A and E, suggesting that low selenium intake increases cancer risk and that supplementation could benefit those with low selenium levels (*Willett WC et al. Prediagnostic serum selenium and the risk of cancer. Lancet 2:130-3, 1983*).

Observational Study: Age-adjusted cancer mortalities were correlated with estimated selenium intakes in the states of the U.S. and in other nations calculated from food-consumption data or by measuring selenium content of pooled blood. Significant inverse correlations were found for cancers of the colon, rectum, prostate, breast, ovary and for leukemia (*Schrauzer GN et al. Cancer mor-*

tality correlation studies - III: Statistical associations with dietary selenium intakes. Bioinorganic Chem. 7:23, 1977).

Breast Cancer:

Animal Experimental Study: Selenium prevented or delayed the appearance of breast tumors in mice infected with a carcinogenic virus (*Schrauzer GN et al. Effects of temporary selenium supplementation on the genesis of spontaneous mammary tumors in inbred female C₃H/St mice. Carcinogenesis 1:199, 1980*).

Observational Study: 35 breast cancer pts. had significantly lower mean serum selenium levels than healthy controls (*McConnell KP et al. The relationship between dietary selenium and breast cancer. J. Surg. Oncol. 15(1):67-70, 1980*).

Skin Cancer:

Observational Study: This case-control study found lower plasma selenium in skin cancer patients (basal cell or squamous cell carcinoma) than in matched controls. The relative risk of cancer for subjects with plasma selenium in the lowest decile was at least two-fold that of subjects with plasma selenium in the highest decile (*Clark LC et al. Plasma selenium and skin neoplasms: A case control study. Nutr. Cancer 6:13, 1985*).

<u>Zinc</u>:

Serum levels in <u>prostatic cancer</u> are low compared to pts. with benign prostatic hypertrophy.

Observational Study: 19 pts. with prostatic carcinoma had a significantly lower level of serum zinc than 27 pts. with benign prostatic hypertrophy (p less than 0.05) and there was a significant zinc/vitamin A correlation (p less than 0.05) (*Whelen P et al. Zinc, vitamin A and prostatic cancer. Brit. J. Urology 55(5):525-8, 1983*).

Prostatic tissue levels are low in <u>prostatic cancer</u> compared to normals.

Observational Study: Compared to normal prostatic tissue, zinc concentrations in neoplastic tissue as measured by atomic absorption spectroscopy were significantly lower (6.84 +/- 1.19 vs. 2.61 +/- 0.45 mumol/g). The concentrations of testosterone and dihydrotestosterone in neoplastic tissue were inversely proportional to the zinc levels (*Habib FK et al. Metal-androgen interrelationships in carcinoma and hyperplasia of the human prostate. J. Endocrinol. 71(1):133-41, 1976*).

Prostatic tissue levels are low in <u>prostatic cancer</u> compared to pts. with prostatic hyperplasia.

Observational Study: As measured by a spectrographic method, the ash from neoplastic prostatic tissue contained less zinc than that from adenomatous prostatic tissue (*Romics I, Katchalova L. Spectrographic determination of zinc in the tissues of adenoma and carcinoma of the prostate. Int. Urol. Nephrol. 15(2):171-76, 1983*).

Cadmium may stimulate the growth of prostatic epithelium by replacing zinc *(see also: "<u>Cadmium</u>" below)*.

In vitro Experimental Study: Cadmium, a known antagonist of zinc, was found to have the ability to stimulate the growth of human prostatic epithelium at low concentrations, suggesting that cadmium may promote carcinogenesis by replacing zinc in the prostate (*Webber MM. Effects of zinc and cadmium on the growth of human prostatic epithelium in vitro. Nutr. Res. 6:35-40, 1986*).

Observational Study: As measured by atomic absorption spectrometry, there were distinct differences in Zn and Cd content in the nuclear fractions of malignant tissues in comparison with BPH and normal tissues. The highest values of Cd were obtained in the nuclear fractions of poorly-differentiated carcinomas, along with the lowest levels of Zn (*Feustel A, Wennrich R. Determination of the distribution of zinc and cadmium in cellular fractions of BPH, normal prostate and prostatic cancers of different histologies by atomic and laser absorption spectrometry in tissue slices. Urol. Res. 12(5):253-56, 1984*).

- -

Omega-3 Fatty Acids:

Example: "MaxEPA," a fish oil concentrate which contains 18% eicosapentaenoic acid.

Indomethacin, a chemical cyclooxygenase inhibitor, has been shown to inhibit carcinogenesis in animal models (*McCormick DL et al. Cancer Res. 45:1803-8, 1985*). Since EPA is also a cyclooxygenase inhibitor, it may have a similar effect.

Dietary fish oil may inhibit the development of breast cancer.

Animal Studies:

Jurkowski JJ, Cave WT. *J. Natl. Cancer Inst.* 74:1145-50, 1985

Karmali RS et al. *J. Natl. Cancer Inst.* 73:457-61, 1984

Carroll KK, Braden LM. *Nutr. and Cancer* 6:254-9, 1984

Omega-6 Fatty Acids:

Linoleic acid → gammalinolenic acid → DGLA → PGE_1

Evening Primrose Oil is relatively high in GLA, production of which from linoleic acid is sometimes blocked.

May reverse carcinogenesis by restoring normal prostaglandin E series metabolism (*Horrobin D. Med. Hypotheses 6:469-86, 1980*).

Animal Experimental Study: Benzo(a)pyrene (a mutagen with carcinogenic metabolites) or gamma-radiation (250r) was administered with or without gamma-linolenic acid to mice. Bone marrow smears showed significant genetic damage only to the mice not receiving gamma-linolenic acid. Administration of arachidonic acid had no such protective effect (*Das UN et al. Benzo(a)pyrene and gamma-radiation-induced genetic damage in mice can be prevented by gamma-linolenic acid but not by arachidonic acid. Nutr. Res. 5:101-5, 1985*).

In vitro Experimental Studies: GLA was added to 3 different malignant cell lines (human hepatoma, human esophageal carcinoma and mouse melanoma). Growth rate of hepatoma and mouse melanoma cells was markedly inhibited, while GLA produced marked morphologic changes in esophageal carcinoma cells culminating in cell death. No growth inhibition or toxicity occurred when GLA was added to normal, benign cells (*Dippenaar N et al. S. Afr. Med. J. 62:505 & 683, 1982; Leary WP et al. S. Afr. Med. J. 62:681, 1982*).

Phytosterols:

Cholesterol analogs found in plants which may be protective against colon cancer.

Observational Study: 3-day composite diets of 4 study gps. of 18 Seventh-day Adventist (SDA) pure vegetarians, 50 SDA lacto-ovo-vegetarians, 50 SDA nonvegetarians, and 50 general population nonvegetarians were analyzed for their sterol composition and the plant sterol/cholesterol ratios were calculated. Results suggest that the absolute amts. of cholesterol consumed as a factor by itself might not be as significant in colon carcinogenesis as its relationship to total plant sterols in the diet (*Nair PP et al. Diet, nutrition intake, and metabolism in populations at high and low risk for colon cancer: Dietary cholesterol, beta-sitosterol, and stigmasterol. Am. J. Clin. Nutr. 40(4 suppl.):927-30, 1984*).

See Also:

> *Deschner EE et al. The kinetics of the protective effect of beta sitosterol against MNU-induced colonic neoplasia. J. Can. Res. Clin. Oncol. 103:49-54, 1982*

> *Raicht RF et al. Protective effect of plant sterols against chemically induced colon tumors in rats. Cancer Res. 40:403-5, 1980*

- -

Garlic or Onion:

Supplementation may inhibit tumor growth.

> **Experimental Study:** Garlic oil 1 mg/kg and onion oil 10 mg/kg were equally effective in decreasing the number and incidence of skin tumors (*Belman S. Onion and garlic oil inhibit tumor growth. Carcinogenesis 4(8):1063-5, 1983*).

> **Animal Experimental Study:** Raw garlic was effective in preventing certain tumors in predisposed mice (*Kroning F. Garlic as an inhibitor for spontaneous tumors in mice. Acta Unio. Intern. Contra Cancrum 20(3):855, 1964*).

- -

OTHER FACTORS:

Avoid obesity.

> **Observational Study:** Both males and females who were at least 25% overweight had an increased risk of fatal rectal cancer, while only males at least 25% overwieght had an increased risk of colon cancer (*Phillips RL, Snowdon DA. Dietary Relationships with fatal colorectal cancer among Seventh-Day Adventists. J. Natl. Cancer Inst. 74:307-17, 1985*).

> **Observational Study:** The relationship between cancer mortality and obesity was examined among 750,000 men and women. It was found that cancer mortality was significantly increased only in the gp. that was 40% or more overweight (*Lew EA, Garfinkle L. J. Chronic Dis. 32:563-576, 1979*).

See Also:

> *Snowdon DA et al. Diet, obesity, and the risk of fatal prostate cancer. Am. J. Epidemiol. 120:244, 1984*

Rule out cadmium toxicity.

Cadmium exposure is associated with increased cancer risk.

> **Review Article:** A combination of all available data from the most recent follow up of causes of deaths among cadmium workers in 6 different cohorts suggests that long-term, high-level exposure to cadmium is associated with an increased risk of prostatic and lung cancer (*Elinder CG et al. Cancer mortality of cadmium workers. Br. J. Ind. Med. 42(10):651-55, 1985*).

Increased in prostatic tissue in prostatic cancer.

Observational Study: As measured by atomic absorption spectrometry, there were distinct differences in the Cd content in the nuclear fractions of malignant tissues in comparison with BPH and normal prostatic tissue, with the highest Cd levels being in the nuclear fractions of poorly-differentiated carcinomas (*Feustel A, Wennrich R. Zinc and cadmium in cell fractions of prostatic cancer tissues of different histological grading in comparison to BPH and normal prostate. Urol. Res. 12(2):147-50, 1984*).

Observational Study: As measured by atomic absorption spectroscopy, cadmium levels in carinomatous prostatic tissue were markedly increased compared to normal controls (129.79 +/- 22.22 vs. 5.15 +/- 0.62 nmol/g). Dihydrotestosterone levels in the malignant tissue were proportional to the cadmium concentrations (*Habib FK et al. Metal-androgen interrelationships in carcinoma and hyperplasia of the human prostate. J. Endocrinol. 71(1):133-41, 1976*).

Lactobacillus Acidophilus:

Supplementation may help to prevent cancer of the colon.

Experimental Crossover Study: 21 healthy young subjects were fed viable lactobacillus acidophilus cultures with milk in concentrations similar to those in commercial acidophilus milk and LA yogurt cultures. The fecal concentrations of bacterial enzymes known to catalyze the conversion of procarcinogens to proximal carcinogens were significantly reduced by the end of one month, but not when milk was given without the LA, suggesting that LA in milk may help to prevent cancer of the colon (*Goldin BR, Gorbach SL. The effect of milk and lactobacillus feeding on human intestinal bacterial enzyme activity. Am. J. Clin. Nutr. 39:756-61, 1984*).

Review article: The link between diet and colon cancer can be explained, in part, by the alterations in fecal bacterial enzyme activity induced by the Western-style high beef, high fat, low fiber diet. These alterations can be normalized in experimental animals by the addition of lactobacillus acidophilus to the diet (*Gorbach SL. The intestinal microflora and its colon cancer connection. Infection 10(6):379-84, 1982*).

CARDIAC ARRHYTHMIA

See Also: ATHEROSCLEROSIS

BASIC DIET:

Avoid <u>caffeine</u>.

> **Experimental Study:** 7 normal volunteers and 12 pts. received oral coffee or IV caffeine citrate. 7 pts. had mitral valve prolapse, 1 had cardiomyopathy, 7 had symptoms of syncope or near syncope and 4 had palpitations. Cardioactive drugs were stopped 24 hrs. and caffeine 48 hrs. before the procedure. Atrial and ventricular pacing were accomplished with a digital stimulator. Although there was no significant change in conduction intervals, caffeine significantly shortened the effective refractory period of the high and low rt. atrium, the AV node and the rt. ventricle while increasing the effective refractory period of the left atrium. 2 pts. had unsustained ventricular tachycardia in response to programmed ventricular stimulation after caffeine; 3 controls had sustained atrial flutter-fibrillation in response to atrial extra-stimuli only after caffeine; before caffeine, only 1 pt. had sustained tachycardia whereas 6 had sustained atrial flutter-fibrillation afterwards; 1 pt. had sustained atrioventricular nodal-reentry tachycardia only after caffeine (*Dobmeyer DJ et al. The arrhythmogenic effects of caffeine in human beings. <u>New Engl. J. Med.</u> 308(14):814-16, 1983*).

- -

NUTRIENTS:

<u>Copper</u> and
<u>Zinc</u>:

Excessive zinc and/or deficient copper may cause premature ventricular contractions.

> **Case Reports:** 3 pts. are described (*Spencer JC. Direct relationship between the body's copper/zinc ratio, ventricular premature beats and sudden cardiac death. Letter to the Editor. <u>Am. J. Clin. Nutr.</u> June, 1979, pp. 1184-5*).

<u>Magnesium</u>:

May be deficient.

> **Observational Study:** 20% of 45 consecutive pts. with symptomatic <u>atrial fibrillation</u> had deficient serum magnesium levels (*DeCarli C et al. Serum magnesium levels in symptomatic atrial fibrillation and their relation to rhythm control by intravenous digoxin. <u>Am. J. Cardiol.</u> 57:956, 1986*).

> **Observational Study:** Out of 102 consecutive pts. admitted to a medical ICU, 20% had hypomagnesemia (*Reinhart R et al. Hypomagnesemia in patients entering the ICU. <u>Critical Care Med.</u> 13(6):506, 1985*).

> **Review Article:** "Chronic, low grade magnesium deficiency may be much more common than is conventionally considered since magnesium is not studied regularly in clinical medicine, as are sodium, potassium, and chloride....The need in clinical medicine to measure serum concentration of mag-

nesium in all patients with heart disease ... cannot be overemphasized" (*Burch GE, Giles TD. The importance of magnesium deficiency in cardiovascular disease. Am. Heart J. 94:649-57, 1977*).

> *Note: Leukocyte Mg levels are better correlated with myocardial Mg levels than are serum levels (Peter WF et al. Leucocyte magnesium concentration as an indicator of myocardial magnesium. Nutr. Reports Int. 26:105, July 1982; Juan D. Clinical review: The clinical importance of hypomagnesemia. Surgery 5:510-16, 1982).*

Arrhythmias may respond to supplementation.

Experimental Blinded Study: 9 pts. with symptomatic atrial fibrillation and deficient serum magnesium levels required twice as much digoxin as did normomagnesemic patients (*DeCarli C et al. Serum magnesium levels in symptomatic atrial fibrillation and their relation to rhythm control by intravenous digoxin. Am. J. Cardiol. 57:956, 1986*).

Review Article: Despite the fact that some pts. improve shortly after magnesium infusion and animal experiments which explain why magnesium depletion might be expected to promote arrhythmia, cause and effect has yet to be really demonstrated. The number of subjects has been small, there have rarely been comparable controls, there have been no placebo infusions and clinical details such as the duration of arrhythmia before magnesium infusion and the frequency of nonresponsivness to magnesium have not been included. In addition, if pts. are being considered magnesium deficient on the basis of low lymphocyte magnesium despite normal serum magnesium, why is it that serum magnesium appears to decrease early during experimental magnesium depletion? However, since magnesium supplementation is usually safe, inexpensive, and easy, and the potential risks of inadequately treating arrhythmia are catastrophic, magnesium treatment can be rational and desirable as a clinical intervention (*Podell RN. The magnesium mavens: Much ado about something. Postgrad. Med. 78(5):219, 1985*).

Experimental Study: 3 consecutive pts. with torsades de pointes, a type of ventricular tachycardia, responded to I.V. magnesium sulfate (*Tzivoni D et al. Magnesium therapy for torsades de pointes. Am. J. Cardiol. 53:528, 1984*).

Experimental Study: 2 elderly pts. with ventricular tachycardia received magnesium infusions which resulted in magnesium retention and cessation of the attacks (*Dyckner T, Wester PO. Magnesium deficiency contributing to ventricular tachycardia. Two case reports. Acta Medica Scandinav. 212:89-91, 1982*).

Experimental Study: 2 cases in which serious ventricular arrhythmias were associated with hypomagnesemia are described. It is suggested that magnesium is very useful, not only in hypomagnesemic tachyarrhythmias, but also in digitalis-toxic tachyarrhythmias and normo-magnesemic tachyarrhythmias (*Iseri LT et al. Magnesium deficiency and cardiac disorders. Am. J. Med. 58:837-46, 1975*).

Case Report: A paroxysmal supraventricular tachycardia in a pt. who was not receiving digitalis was abolished by the administration of IV magnesium sulfate (*Chadda KD et al. Hypomagnesemia and refractory cardiac arrhythmia in a nondigitalized patient. Am. J. Cardiol. 31:98, 1973*).

May prevent toxic arrhythmias caused by digitalis, perhaps because they tend to produce a loss of intracellular potassium (*Cohen L, Kitzes R. Magnesium deficiency and digitalis toxicity. JAMA 251:730, 1984; Cohen L, Kitzes R. Magnesium sulfate and digitalis-toxic arrhythmias. JAMA 249:2808-10, 1983*).

Potassium:

Deficiency (which may exist despite normal serum potassium levels) is associated with arrhythmias as well as decreased tolerance to cardiac medications and EKG alterations.

Experimental and Observational Study: Serum and red blood cell potassium was measured in 17 pts. with EKG abnormalities. Although some of the abnormalities were typical of potassium deficiency, most were non-specific T wave changes which are commonly attributed (without substantiation) to ischemia. Serum potassium levels were normal but RBC potassium levels were below normal in all cases and returned to normal (as did the EKG abnormalities) after treatment with potassium salts (*Sangiori GB et al. Serum potassium levels, red-blood-cell potassium and alterations of the repolarization phase of electrocardiography in old subjects. Age Aging 13:309, 1984*).

Magnesium and
Potassium:

May be more effective when administered together when the level of either is deficient due to the inability of the heart muscle to hold on to potassium in the absence of magnesium (*Dychner T, Wester PO. Magnesium and potassium in serum and muscle in relation to disturbances of cardiac rhythm, in Magnesium in Health and Disease. Spectrum Publishing Company, 1980, pp. 551-7; Shils ME. Experimental human magnesium depletion. Medicine 48(1):61-85, 1969*).

- -

Carnitine:

Supplementation may be beneficial.

Animal Experimental Study: Carnitine 100 mg/kg IV had much less of an antiarrhythmic effect than quinidine 5 mg/kg, but after atropinization, it was similar in effect to quinidine without causing the BP depression seen with quinidine (*DiPalma JR et al. Cardiovascular and antiarrhythmic effects of carnitine. Arch. Int. Pharmacdynamie Ther. 217:246-50, 1975*).

Coenzyme Q_{10}:

Supplementation may be beneficial.

Experimental Study: 27 pts. with ventricular premature beats (VPBs) and no clinical findings of organic cardiopathies received coenzyme Q_{10}. Results were beneficial in 6/27 (22%), consisting of 1 pt. with hypertension and 5 pts. with diabetes mellitus. In the remaining 2 pts. with diabetes, the frequency of VPBs was reduced by 50% or more during treatment. The mean reduction of VPBs frequency in the 5 responders plus the additional 2 diabetic pts. was 85.7%, suggesting that CoQ_{10} exhibits an effective antiarrhythmic action not merely on organic heart disease but also on VPBs supervening in diabetes mellitus (*Fujioka T et al. Clinical study of cardiac arrhythmias using a 24-hour continuous electrocardiographic recorder (5th report): Antiarrhythmic action of conenzyme Q_{10} in diabetics. Tohoku J. Exp. Med. 141(suppl.):453-63, 1983*).

Taurine:

Much like magnesium, taurine affects membrane excitability by normalizing potassium flux in and out of the heart muscle cell (*Chazov EL et al. Taurine and electrical activity of the heart. Cir. Res. 34-5, Suppl. III, pp. 11-21, 1974*).

- -

OTHER FACTORS:

Rule out food and chemical sensitivities.

Case Reports:
1. 60 year-old male truck driver was resuscitated following ventricular fibrillation. When fed he immediately developed bloating, PVC's and hypotension on 3 occasions. He noted that milk or eggs usually precipitated these symptoms as well as gasoline fumes.
2. 65 year-old female presented with an 8 year history of recurrent atrial fibrillation along with arthritis, blurring of vision, coughing spells and generalized muscle pain. Challenge with various chemicals would produce her symptoms.
(Rea WJ, Suits CW. *Cardiovascular disease triggered by foods and chemicals, in Gerrard JW, Ed. Food Allergy: New Perspectives. Springfield, Illinois, Charles C. Thomas, 1980).*

See Also:

Rea EJ et al. *Recurrent environmentally triggered thrombophlebitis: A five-year follow-up. Ann. Allergy 47:338-44, 1981*

Spizer FE et al. *Palpitation rate associated with fluorocarbon exposure in a hospital setting. New Engl. J. Med. 292:624, 1975*

Taylor GS, Hern WS. *Cardiac arrhythmias to aerosol propellants. JAMA 219:8, 1970*

CARDIOMYOPATHY

BASIC DIET:

Avoid <u>alcoholic beverages</u>.

Excessive intake is known to be associated with the development of cardiomyopathy due to 1 or more of the following:
1. direct toxic injury by alcohol to the myocardium
2. nutritional disturbances (beri-beri)
3. toxic effects of substances contained in alcoholic beverages (e.g. cobalt)
(*Burch GE, Giles TD. Alcoholic cardiomyopathy, in Kissin B, Begleiter H, Eds. <u>The Biology of Alcoholism: Vol. 3: Clinical Pathology.</u> New York, Plenum, 1974*).

- -

NUTRIENTS:

<u>Selenium:</u>

Deficiency associated with cardiomyopathy.

Review Article: The possibility of selenium deficiency should be thought of in cases of alcoholic cardiomyopathy (*Goldman IS, Kantrowitz NE. Cardiomyopathy associated with selenium deficiency. Letter to the Editor. <u>New Eng. J. Med.</u> 305:701, 1982*).

Case Report: 2 year-old girl with dyspnea, cardiomegaly and CHF was found to have minimal selenium in her diet and a low serum selenium and improved with supplementation (*Collipp PJ, Chen SY. Cardiomyopathy and selenium deficiency in a two-year-old girl. Letter to the Editor. <u>New Engl. J. Med.</u> 304:1304-5, 1981*).

See Also:

Johnson RA et al. An Occidental case of cardiomyopathy and selenium deficiency. <u>New Engl. J. Med.</u> 304:1210-2, 1981

Aaseth J et al. Decreased serum selenium in alcoholic cirrhosis. <u>New Engl. J. Med.</u> 303:844-5, 1980).

- -

<u>L-Carnitine:</u>

Deficiency may cause cardiomyopathy.

Experimental Study: 5 pts. with endocardial fibroelastosis were found to have systemic carnitine deficiency which responded to supplementation (*Tripp ME et al. Systemic carnitine deficiency presenting as familial endocardial fibroelastosis: A treatable cardiomyopathy. <u>New Engl. J. Med.</u> 305:385, 1982*).

<u>Coenzyme Q</u>:

May be deficient (*Folkers K et al. Biochemical rationale and myocardial tissue data on the effective therapy of cardiomyopathy with coenzyme Q$_{10}$. <u>Proc. Natl. Acad. Sci.</u> 82:901, 1985*).

Supplementation may be beneficial.

Experimental Double-blind Study: Daily administration of CoQ$_{10}$ for 12 wks. increased cardiac ejection fraction significantly, reduced shortness of breath and increased muscle strength. These improvements lasted as long as 3 yrs. in pts. treated continuously, but cardiac function deteriorated when CoQ$_{10}$ was discontinued. Of the 80 pts. treated, 89% improved with supplementation (*Folkers K et al. Biochemical rationale and myocardial tissue data on the effective therapy of cardiomyopathy with coenzyme Q$_{10}$. <u>Proc. Natl. Acad. Sci.</u> 82:901, 1985*).

Experimental Study: 34 pts. with severe (N.Y. Heart Assoc. Class IV) congestive cardiomyopathy received 100 mg CoQ$_{10}$ daily. 82% improved as shown by increased stroke volume and cardiac index. Mean ejection fraction increased from about 25% to about 40%. Two year survival rate was 62%, compared to 25% for a similar series of pts. treated by conventional methods alone (*Judy WV et al. Myocardial effects of Co-enzyme Q$_{10}$ in primary heart failure, in Folkers K, Yamamura Y, Eds., <u>Biomed. and Clin. Aspects of Coenzyme Q</u>. Vol. 4. Amsterdam, Elsevier/North Holland Biomedical Press, 1984, pp. 353-67*).

See Also:

Langsjoen PH et al. Response of patients in classes III and IV of cardiomyopathy to therapy in a blind and crossover trial with coenzyme Q$_{10}$. <u>Proc. Natl. Acad. Sci.</u> 82:4240, 1985

Coenzyme aids cardiomyopathy. <u>Med. World News</u>, August 12, 1985, p. 69

CARPAL TUNNEL SYNDROME

See Also: NEURALGIA AND NEUROPATHY

SIGNS AND SYMPTOMS:

1. Pains in hands, elbows, shoulders or knees
2. Morning stiffness of fingers
3. Impaired finger flexion
4. Transitory nocturnal paralysis of arm and hand
5. Paresthesias of hands - possibly also of face
6. Painful adduction rotation of the thumb at metacarpophalangeal joint
7. Weakness of hand grip
8. Fluctuating edema in hands, feet or ankles
9. Impaired tactile sensations in fingers
10. Tenderness over carpal tunnel
11. Dropping of objects
12. Nocturnal muscle spasms in extremities

OFFICE EVALUATION:

1. Hold the hands out with palms up.
2. Bend the fingers at the 2 outer joints only, leaving the metacarpophalangeal joints in a straight line with the wrists.
3. Bring the tips of the fingers down to the palms of the hands, right to the crease that separates fingers from hands.
4. If any of these 16 joints cannot be bent completely and without pain, carpal tunnel syndrome is suspected.

(*Ellis, John M. and Presley, James. <u>Vitamin B6: The Doctor's Report</u>. New York, Harper & Row, 1973*).

- -

NUTRIENT:

<u>Pyridoxine</u>: 100 mg. daily (3 month trial)

WARNING: Pyridoxine supplementation may <u>cause</u> a sensory neuropathy in doses as low as 200 mg daily over 3 years (usually 2-5 gm daily). The neurotoxicity is believed to due to exceeding the liver's ability to phosphorylate pyridoxine to the active coenzyme, pyridoxal phosphate. The resulting high pyridoxine blood level could be directly neurotoxic or may compete for binding sites with pyridoxal phosphate resulting in a relative deficiency of the active metabolite (*Parry GJ, Bredesen DE. Sensory neuropathy with low-dose pyridoxine. <u>Neurology</u> 35:1466-68, 1985*). Supplementation in the form of pyridoxal phosphate should thus avoid this danger.

Improvement from supplementation is said to start in a few weeks with complete cure in 8-12 weeks for 85% of patients (many of the others are said to benefit from <u>pyridoxal-5-phosphate</u> or from the addition of <u>magnesium</u>).

> **Experimental Study:** 19 pts. were treated with pyridoxine. Two-thirds of the pts. who specifically presented symptoms of median neuropathy eventually required surgical release suggesting that, al-

though pyridoxine may have a place alongside other nonsurgical modalities in the treatment of CTS, surgical release continues to be indicated in many pts. (*Amadio PC. Pyridoxine as an adjunct in the treatment of carpal tunnel syndrome. J. Hand Surg. [Am.] 10(2):237-41, 1985*).

Experimental Study: Using electrodiagnostic criteria, pts. with carpal tunnel syndrome (CTS) were categorized into 4 groups of at least 7 subjects each: CTS, peripheral neuropathy (PN), CTS and PN, and normal. Based on RBC glutamine oxaloacetic acid transaminase (EGOT) activity with vs. without pyridoxal phosphate, a significant difference in pyridoxine metabolic activity (PMA) was found between gps. by both chi square (p less than 0.05) and analysis of variance (p less than 0.05) which was associated with the presence or absence of PN. There was no difference in PMA when gps. were separated on the basis of CTS, suggesting that a PMA abnormality is highly correlated, not with CTS, but with PN, and that pts. with CTS responding to pyridoxine may have an unrecognized PN (*Byers CM et al. Pyridoxine metabolism in carpal tunnel syndrome with and without peripheral neuropathy. Arch Phys. Med. Rehabil. 65(11):712-16, 1984*).

Negative Experimental Study: 13 pts. failed to improve after receiving pyridoxine 300 mg daily for 6 wks. followed by 100 mg daily (*Scheyer RD, Haas DS. Pyridoxine in carpal tunnel syndrome. Lancet 2:42, 1985*).

Negative Experimental Study: 6 pts. were studied before and after receiving pyridoxine 100 mg daily for 9-26 weeks. Based on plasma pyridoxal phosphate levels and *in vitro* stimulation of EAA, there was no evidence of B_6 deficiency. 4/6 pts. claimed partial symptom relief during B_6 therapy; however the authors conclude that this was probably a placebo effect (*Smith GP et al. Biochemical studies of pyridoxal and pyridoxal phosphate status and therapeutic trial of pyridoxine in patients with carpal tunnel syndrome. Ann. Neurol. 15:104, 1984*).

> *Note:*
> *1. Without controls, the conclusion that symptom relief was a placebo effect is subject to question.*
> *2. The specific activity of EAA doubled in most pts. during B6 therapy, suggesting that supplementation improved B6 nutriture.*
> *3. Clinical experience by Ellis and his group suggests that those subjects who received supplementation for less than 11 weeks may not have had an adequate trial. (Gaby, Alan - 1984)*

Case Report: A man being treated with tranylcypromine for depression (which may interfere with B_6 metabolism) developed bilateral CTS in association with laboratory evidence of B_6 deficiency. After treatment with 300 mg pyridoxine daily for 8 wks., symptoms of CTS almost completely disappeared. Nerve conduction studies after 12 wks. of B_6 therapy were significantly improved (*Harrison W et al. Case report of carpal tunnel syndrome associated with tranylcypromine. Am. J. Psychiat. 140:1229, 1983*).

Observational Study: The specific activities and % deficiencies of RBC glutamic oxaloacetic transaminase (EGOT) were found to suggest severe pyridoxine deficiencies in 4 pts. evaluated at the time of surgery to relieve the compression of CTS (*Ellis J et al. Therapy with vitamin B6 with and without surgery for treatment of patients having the idiopathic carpal tunnel syndrome. Res. Comm. Chem. Path. Pharm. 33(2):331, 1981*).

Experimental Single-blind Crossover Case Study: A pt. with severe CTS and a significant B_6 deficiency (low EGOT) was treated with B_6 2 mg daily (the RDA) for 11 wks., then 100 mg daily for 12 wks., then placebo for 9 wks., and again B_6 100 mg daily for 11 weeks. 2 mg B_6 daily reduced the EGOT activity deficiency, maintained a pyridoxal phosphate deficiency, and relieved all but marginal symptoms. 100 mg B_6 daily nearly achieved a ceiling EGOT level and eliminated the pyridoxyl phosphate deficiency. Placebo administration led to reappearance of the EGOT and pyridoxal phosphate deficiencies and clinical symptoms worsened. Re-administration of B_6 100 mg daily eliminated the deficiencies and the pt. became asymptomatic (*Ellis J et al. Clinical results of a crossover treatment with pyridoxine and placebo of the carpal tunnel syndrome. Am. J. Clin. Nutr. 32:2040-*

6, 1979; Folkers K et al. Biochemical evidence for a deficiency of vitamin B6 in the carpal tunnel syndrome based on a crossover clinical study. Proc. Natl. Acad. Sci. USA 75(7):3410-2, July 1978).

See Also:

Ellis JM et al. Response of vitamin B6 deficiency and the carpal tunnel syndrome to pyridoxine. Proc. Natl. Acad. Sci. U.S.A. 79:7494-98, 1982

Hamfelt A. Carpal tunnel syndrome and vitamin B6 deficiency. Clin. Chem. 28:721, 1982

Ellis JM et al. Survey and new data on treatment with pyridoxine of patients having a clinical syndrome including the carpal tunnel and other defects. Res. Comm. Clin. Path. Pharm. 17:165-67, 1977

CATARACT

See Also: DIABETES MELLITUS

BASIC DIET:

Restrict <u>sugar</u>.

The monosaccharides D-glucose, D-galactose, D-xylose and L-arabinose enter the lens through diffusion from the aqueous humor and are known to be cataractogenic. When they are excessive in the diet, sugar alcohol products accumulate in the lens as they are not efficiently metabolized and have slower rates of diffusion out of the lens than the parent sugars. Accumulation causes hypertonicity and osmotic swelling which can cause rupture of the fiber cells (*Kinoshita JH. Invest. Ophthalmol. 4:786-99, 1965*). In addition, alteration of lens crystallins may occur leading to gradual deterioration (*Stevens VJ et al. Proc. Natl. Acad. Sci. USA 71:4164-68, 1974*).

- -

NUTRIENTS:

<u>Riboflavin</u>:

WARNING: Cataract pts. should not receive more than 10 mg of riboflavin supplementation daily since the combination of light, ambient oxygen and riboflavin/FAD can generate free radicals and induce cataracts (*Varma S et al. Light-induced damage to ocular lens cation pump: Prevention by vitamin C. Proc. Natl. Acad. Sci. 76:3504-06, 1979; Varma S et al. Protection against superoxide radicals in rat lens. Ophthal. Res. 9:421-31, 1977*).

Deficiency may cause cataracts.

Observational Study: In a study of 173 cataract pts., 20% of those under age 50 were deficient in riboflavin, as were 34% of those over age 50, while none of 16 normals over age 50 was riboflavin-deficient (*Skalka HW et al. Riboflavin deficiency and cataract formation. Metabol. & Ped. Ophthal. 5(1):17-20, 1981*).

Observational Study: 8/22 pts. were deficient in riboflavin, suggesting that riboflavin deficiency may play a role in cataract formation (*Prchal J et al. Association of pre-senile cataracts with hetero-zygousity for galactosemic states and riboflavin deficiency. Lancet 1:12-13, 1978*).

Animal Experimental Study: Kittens given a riboflavin-deficient diet developed cataracts (*Gershoff SN et al. J. Nutr. 68:75-88, 1959*).

Animal Experimental Study: Pigs given a riboflavin-deficient diet developed cataracts (*Miller ER et al. J. Nutr. 52:405-13, 1954*).

See Also:

Skalka H, Prchal J. Cataracts and riboflavin deficiency. Am. J. Clin. Nutr. 34:861-63, 1981

Vitamin C:

Supplementation may be effective in preventing cataracts.

In vitro Experimental Study: Since excessive free radical oxidation is thought to be a cause of cataracts, rat lenses were maintained in a special solution that caused free-radical damage. When vitamin C, an anti-oxidant, was added to the solution, the lenses were significantly protected. The researchers theorize that the anti-oxidant action of vitamin C may explain why the level of this vitamin in the aqueous humor is among the highest of the various body fluids (*Varma SD, Richards RD. Light-induced damage to ocular lens cation pump: Prevention by vitamin C. Proc. Nat. Acad. Sci. 76:3504-06, 1979*).

Experimental Study: 450 pts. with incipient cataracts were placed in a nutritional program that included ascorbic acid 1 gm daily, resulting in a reduction in cataract devlopment (*Atkinson D. Malnutrition as an etiological factor in senile cataract. Eye, Ear, Nose & Throat Monthly 31:79-83, 1952*).

See Also:

Bouton S. Vitamin C and the aging eye. *Arch. Int. Med. 63:930-45, 1939*

Vitamin E:

Supplementation may be effective in preventing cataracts.

Animal Experimental Study: Adult rats, some pretreated for 2 wks. with daily injections of vitamin E, were made diabetic by an IV streptozotocin injection. In the animals that had not received vitamin E, changes appeared in the lenses as the hyperglycemia continued, while the lenses of the vitamin E-treated animals showed minimal changes (*Ross WM et al. Modelling cortical cataractogenesis: III. In vivo effects of vitamin E on cataractogenesis in diabetic rats. Can. J. Ophthalmol. 17(2):61-66, 1982*).

In vitro Animal Experimental Study: Since excessive free radical oxidation is thought to be a cause of cataracts, rat lenses were maintained in a special solution that caused free-radical damage when exposed to daylight. When vitamin E, an anti-oxidant, was added to the solution, the lenses suffered only 1/5 as much damage (*Varma SD, Richards RD. Photochem. & Photobiol. vol. 36, no. 6, 1982*).

See Also:

Creighton MO et al. *Modelling cortical cataractogenesis: V. Steroid cataracts induced by solumedrol partially prevented by vitamin E in vitro. Exp. Eye Res. 37(1):65-76, 1983*

Ross WM et al. *Radiation cataract formation diminished by vitamin E in rat lenses in vitro. Exp. Eye Res. 36(5):645-53, 1983*

Selenium:

Required for the functioning of glutathione peroxidase, an important anti-oxidant in the lens (*Whanger P, Weswig P. Effects of selenium, chromium and antioxidants on growth, eye cataracts, plasma cholesterol and blood glucose in selenium deficient, vitamin E supplemented rats. Nutr. Rep. Int. 12:345-58, 1975*).

May be deficient in cataractous lenses.

Observational Study: The selenium content of human cataractous lenses is only 15% of normal levels (*Swanson A, Truesdale A.   Elemental analysis in normal and cataractous human lens tissue.   Biochem. Biophys. Res. Comm. 45:1488-96, 1971*).

Zinc:

Deficiency may cause cataracts.

Observational Study: A child with acrodermatitis enteropathica, a zinc-deficiency disease, developed bilateral cataracts, suggesting that zinc deficiency may have an etiologic role (*Racz P et al.   Bilateral cataract in acrodermatitis enteropathica.   J. Pediatr. Ophthalmol. Strabismus 16(3):180-82, 1979*).

Animal Experimental Study: Most trout fed a zinc-deficient diet developed cataracts, while no trout on the same diet supplemented with zinc developed them (*Ketola HG. J. Nutr. 109:965-69, 1979*).

See Also:

Cataract as an outcome of zinc deficiency in salmon.   *Nutr. Rev. 44(3):118-20, 1986*

Supplementation may be beneficial.

Review Article: In senile cataract glucose utilization is disturbed due to loss of activity of some key zinc-dependent enzymes in the lens.   Zinc supplementation improves the impaired glucose metabolism occurring in old age, and prolonged administration of zinc aspartate is indicated for the prophylaxis and therapy of senile cataract.   In the presence of magnesium deficiency, magnesium salts should also be given.   Also, cation eliminating exogenous or endogenous factors must be taken into consideration (*Heinitz M.   [Clinical and biochemical aspects of the prophylaxis and therapy of senile cataract with zinc aspartate.]   Klin. Monatsbl. Augenheilkd. 172(5):778-83, 1978*).

See Also:

Tiekert CG.   *More on the medical "cure" for cataracts.   Letter to the Editor.   J. Am. Vet. Med. Assoc. 188(12):1364, 1986*

Chuistova IP et al.   *[Experimental morphological basis for using zinc in treating senile cataract.]   Oftalmol. Zh. (7):394-96, 1985*

- -

Cysteine or
Methionine:

Supplementation may retard cataract formation.

Theoretical Discussion: Glutathione protects the lens from the destructive effects of ultraviolet light but its concentration diminishes with age due to a decrease in the activity of the enzyme necessary for its synthesis.   Perhaps a diet higher in cysteine or methionine, the rate-limiting amino acids in glutathione synthesis, would retard the age-related decline in glutathione levels and thus prevent cataract formation (*Cole H.   Enzyme activity may hold the key to cataract activity.   JAMA 254(8):1008, 1985*).

CELIAC DISEASE

See Also: DERMITITIS HERPETIFORMIS

NUTRIENTS:

Folic Acid:

Plasma levels usually indicate deficiency, and megaloblastic anemia is frequently present in adults, but uncommon in children. While correction occurs coincidentally with the improvement in absorption resulting from a gluten-free diet, folic acid should be given orally until recovery is complete (*Passmore R, Eastwood MA. Davidson and Passmore: Human Nutrition and Dietetics. Edinburgh, Churchill Livingstone, 1986, p. 440*).

Pyridoxine:

Absorption may be impaired.

> **Experimental Controlled Study:** The increase in pyridoxal phosphate of children with acute celiac disease after loading orally with 5 mg pyridoxine hydrochloride/kg was significantly decreased when compared to that of control subjects (*Reinken L, Zieglauer H. Vitamin B6 absorption in children with acute celiac disease and in control subjects. J. Nutr. 108:1562, 1978*).

Depression, which is common in adult patients, may be treated successfully with pyridoxine.

> **Experimental Study:** 12 depressed adult celiacs who had been on a gluten-free diet for years received supplementation with 80 mg pyridoxine daily. After 6 months, depression had significantly improved in all patients (*Hallert C, Astrom J, Walan A. Reversal of psychopathology in adult celiac disease with the aid of pyridoxine (vitamin B6). Scand. J. Gastroenterol. 18:299, 1983*).

Vitamin A:

May be deficient due to malabsorption of fats (*Passmore R, Eastwood MA. Davidson and Passmore: Human Nutrition and Dietetics. Edinburgh, Churchill Livingstone, 1986, p. 141*).

Vitamin B12:

May be deficient.

> **Observational Study:** Compared to controls, the absorption of vitamin B12 in pediatric pts. was significantly decreased, especially in infants, while the serum B12 level was decreased only in the oldest children, suggesting that the absorption defect becomes clnically significant only after a long duration of the disease (*Kokkonen J, Simil:a S. Gastric function and absorption of vitamin B12 in children with celiac disease. Eur. J. Pediatr. 132(2):71-75, 1979*).

Vitamin D:

May be deficient due to malabsorption of fats (*Passmore R, Eastwood MA. Davidson and Passmore: Human Nutrition and Dietetics. Edinburgh, Churchill Livingstone, 1986, p. 141*).

<u>Vitamin E:</u>

May be deficient due to malabsorption of fats (*Passmore R, Eastwood MA. <u>Davidson and Passmore: Human Nutrition and Dietetics</u>. Edinburgh, Churchill Livingstone, 1986, p. 141*).

<u>Vitamin K:</u>

May be deficient due to malabsorption of fats (*Passmore R, Eastwood MA. <u>Davidson and Passmore: Human Nutrition and Dietetics</u>. Edinburgh, Churchill Livingstone, 1986, p. 141*).

- -

<u>Copper:</u>

May be deficient.

> **Observational Study:** Compared to normal controls, copper uptake during 3 hrs. from an oral test dose of copper sulphate solution giving 3 mg Cu^{++} was significantly reduced in pts. with proximal intestinal disease. 3/10 pts. had abnormal and otherwise unexplained blood counts compatible with the known hematological effects of copper deficiency and were restored to normal levels on a gluten-free diet. Copper deficiency and proximal intestinal disease should be suspected in pts. with otherwise unexplained anemia or neutropenia (*Jameson S et al. Copper malabsorption in coeliac disease. <u>Sci. Total Environ.</u> 42(1-2):29-36, 1985*).

> **Observational Study:** 2 infants aged 7 and 7.5 mo. with celiac disease and severe malnutrition had severe hypocupremia and persistent neutropenia; bone radiographs were also compatible with copper deficiency. Rapid and complete correction of these anomalies could only be obtained after addition of copper sulfate to the gluten-free diet; thus it is suggested that young children with severe celiac disease be monitored for their copper status (*Goyens P et al. Copper deficiency in infants with active celiac disease. <u>J. Pediatr. Gastroenterol. Nutr.</u> 4(4):677-80, 1985*).

<u>Iron:</u>

Deficiency causes over 90% of the anemia which is usually present in patients. Correction of the anemia occurs coincidentally with the improvement in absorption which results from a gluten-free diet but, until recovery is complete, it is advisable to give iron to pts. with hypochromic anemia (*Passmore R, Eastwood MA. <u>Davidson and Passmore: Human Nutrition and Dietetics</u>. Edinburgh, Churchill Livingstone, 1986, p. 440*).

<u>Selenium:</u>

May be deficient.

> **Observational Study:** The selenium concentration in whole blood, plasma and leucocytes of 16 pts. on gluten free diets was significantly lower than that of 32 controls. This may either be because the gluten-free diet was selenium-deficient or because of impaired selenium absorption which occurs primarily in the duodenum. Since selenium deficiency increases the risk of malignancy, it may explain the high incidence of cancer among pts. with this disorder (*Hinks LJ et al. <u>Brit. Med. J.</u> 288:1862-3, 1984*).

- -

OTHER FACTORS:

Avoid <u>gluten</u>.

Gluten is found in wheat, rye, oats, barley (including malt) and buckwheat.

Experimental Study: 314 infants and children were diagnosed on the basis of a flat proximal small bowel mucosa when untreated and an unequivocal response and remission on a gluten-free diet (GFD). In 91 pts., interruptions of the GFD were documented by repeated intestinal biopsies. 81% had a flat mucosa after 0.25-14.67 yrs. off the diet, while in 12% a successive deterioration of the mucosa occurred during 0.5-6.67 yrs. after interruption of the GFD without becoming flat. 6.6% had a normal intestinal mucosa after 2.24-6.92 yrs. off the diet, while 3 pts. were off the diet less than 2 yrs. and are thus still under study. A mucosal relapse within 2 yrs. after stopping the GFD was observed in 21/24 (87.5%) pts. studied longitudinally during planned challenges. It is concluded that only a minority (6.6%) will not relapse after an interruption of the GFD, while another small gp. (12%) will deteriorate very slowly; thus routine gluten challenges are not justifiable (*Shmerling DH, Franckx J. Childhood celiac disease: A long-term analysis of relapses in 91 pts.* J. Pediatr. Gastroenterol. Nutr. *5(4):565-69, 1986*).

Observational Study: Of 71 children suspected of having malabsorption, 16/17 diagnosed histologically as having childhood celiac disease had elevated antibodies to the alpha-gliadin fraction of wheat gluten (94% sensitivity). Of the 54 with normal biopsies, 48 had normal levels of alpha-gliadin antibodies (88% specificity) (*Kelly J et al. Alpha-gliadin antibodies in childhood celiac disease. Letter to the Editor.* Lancet *September 7, 1985, p. 558*).

Rule out lactase deficiency.

Many adult celiacs have low levels of intestinal lactase which is secondary to the disease process, probably due to reduced epithelial cells and alterations in the function of individual cells (*Plotkin GR, Isselbacher KJ. Secondary disaccharidase deficiency in adult celiac disease.* New Engl. J. Med. *271:1033-7, 1964*).

CEREBROVASCULAR DISEASE

See Also: ATHEROSCLEROSIS
                    HYPERTENSION

BASIC DIET:

Eat fresh <u>fruits and vegetables</u>.

Observational Study: A low incidence of cerebrovascular disease was associated with geographical regions where fresh fruit and vegetable consumption was high (*Acheson R, Williams D. <u>Lancet</u> 1191-93, 1983*).

Limit consumption of plants high in <u>phyto-estrogens</u>.

Theoretical Discussion: While coronary disease is correlated with consumption of foods of animal origin, cerebrovascular disease correlates with consumption of plant proteins. The author proposes that steroidal estrogens and plant metabolites which mimic estrogens (phyto-estrogens) are atherogenic and suggests that digestion products of phyto-estrogens pass through the blood/brain barrier while steroidal estrogens cannot. Rich sources of phyto-estrogens include soybeans and peanuts (*Seely S. Diet and cerebrovascular disease. <u>Nutr. & Health</u> 2:173-9, 1983*).

Avoid <u>alcoholic beverages</u>.

Alcohol, when taken with a meal high in saturated fats, reduces platelet aggregation and thus may increase the chance of cerebral hemorrhage.

Experimental Study: In a study using healthy volunteers, a 5-oz glass of wine did not inhibit platelet aggregation unless taken with a meal high in saturated fats, when it had a significant inhibitory effect compared to the meal alone (*Littleton JM. Interactions between ethanol and dietary fat in determining human platelet function. <u>Thromb. Haemost.</u> 51(1):50-53, 1984*).

Regular alcohol ingestion is associated with an increased risk of hemorrhagic, but not thromboembolic, strokes, perhaps because of alcohol's effect on platelet aggregation.

Observational Study: In a study of the 12-yr. incidence of stroke in 8000 males of Japanese ancestry, hemorrhagic stroke incidence increased steadily with the amount of alcohol consumed. 2-3 drinks weekly was associated with more than double the risk, while heavy drinking was associated with almost triple the risk, independent of other risk factors. The differences in risk of thromboembolic stroke between abstainers and heavy drinkers, however, were insignificant (*Donahue RP et al. Alcohol and hemorrhagic stroke. The Honolulu Heart Program. <u>JAMA</u> 255(17):2311-14, 1986*).

Alcoholic binges may acutely cause stroke.

Case Reports: 2 males, ages 30 and 36, are described who suffered debilitating strokes after single episodes of excessive alcoholic intake (*Wilkins MR, Kendall MJ. Stroke affecting young men after alcoholic binges. <u>Brit. Med. J.</u> 291:1342, 1985*).

- -

NUTRIENTS:

Vitamin E:

May protect against cerebral thrombosis.

Animal Experimental Study: The platelet survival time was shortened in stroke-prone spontaneously hypertensive rats at 10 wks. of age fed a regular diet but was normalized with a vitamin E-supplemented diet. Conversely, platelet survival time was normal in stroke-resistent spontaneously hypertensive rats at 10 wks. of age fed a regular diet, but was shortened with a vitamin E-free diet (*Koganemaru S, Kuramoto A. The effect of vitamin E on platelet kinetics of stroke-prone spontaneously hypertensive rats. J. Nutr. Sci. & Vitaminology 28:1-10, 1982*).

- -

Omega-3 Fatty Acids:

May protect against decreases in cerebral blood flow and cerebral edema in the presence of an acute carotid occlusion.

Animal Experimental Study: Gerbils were fed either a standard diet or a diet supplemented with menhaden fish oil (high in eicosapentaenoic acid) for 2 months. Ischemia was produced by bilateral carotid occlusion for 10 min., followed by reperfusion for 60 minutes. In control animals, cerebral blood flow was decreased 30 and 60 min. after reperfusion and brain water was increased, while in experimental animals cerebral blood flow did not fall during reperfusion and edema did not appear (*Black KL et al. Eicosapentaenoic acid: Effect on brain prostaglandins, cerebral blood flow and edema in ischemic gerbils. Stroke 15(1):65-69, 1984*).

- -

Ginkgo Biloba:

May relieve symptoms of chronic cerebrovascular insufficiency.

Experimental Study: 112 geriatric pts. received ginkgo bilboa extract 120 mg daily. Symptoms (including vertigo, headache, tinnitus, short-term memory loss, lack-of-vigilance and depression) were significantly reduced (p less than 0.001) and there were no side-effects (*Vorberg G. Ginkgo-biloba extract (GBE): A long-term study of chronic cerebral insufficiency in geriatric patients. Clin. Trials J. 22:149-57, 1985*).

CERVICAL DYSPLASIA

See Also: CANCER

NUTRIENTS:

<u>Folic Acid</u>:   5 mg. twice daily (3 month trial)

Deficiency (best measured by RBC folate as serum folate may be normal) may be associated with the use of oral contraceptives (*Steiff R. Folate deficiency and oral contraceptives. <u>JAMA</u> 214:105-08, 1970*) and may be correlated with cervical dysplastic changes (*Lindenbaum J et al. Oral contraceptive hormones, folate metabolism, and the cervical epithelium. <u>Am. J. Clin. Nutr.</u> April, 1975, pp. 346-53*).

Supplementation may be beneficial.

Experimental Double-blind Study: 47 young women with mild or moderate dysplasia who had been on combination-type oral contraceptive agents (OCA's) for at least 6 months received either 10 mg oral folate daily or placebo. Pre-treatment red cell folate levels were lower in subjects on OCA's (189 ng/ml) than in those not on OCA's (269 ng/ml), and lowest in subjects on OCA's with cervical dysplasia (162 ng/ml). After 3 months, cervical biopsies showed significant improvement only in the women receiving folate. The dysplasia completely disappeared in 7 women receiving folate, while 4 women on placebo showed progression to carcinoma in situ (*Butterworth CE et al. Improvement in cervical dysplasia associated with folic acid therapy in users of oral contraceptives. <u>Am. J. Clin. Nutr.</u> 35:73-82, 1982*).

Experimental Study: Following treatment with folic acid 10 mg daily, 100% of cases reverted to normal as determined by colposcopy/biopsy examination (*Whitehead N et al. Megaloblastic changes in the cervical epithelium. Association with oral contraceptive therapy and reversal with folic acid. <u>JAMA</u> 226:1421-4, 1973*).

<u>Vitamin A</u>:   60,000 I.U. daily for 2 months; then 25,000 I.U. daily

Deficiency associated with cervical dysplasia.

Observational Study: The vitamin A and beta carotene intake as well as cellular retinol binding protein (CRBP) levels were assessed for 87 women with dysplastic changes or carcinoma in situ (CIS). Women consuming less than average vitamin A and beta carotene were 3 times as likely to develop severe dysplasia and 2 3/4 times as likely to develop CIS. CRBP levels in the cervical tissue samples were inversely correlated with the severity of the dysplasia (*Wilie-Rosett JA et al. Influence of vitamin A on cervical dysplasia and carcinoma in situ. <u>Nutrition and Cancer</u> 6(1):49-57, 1984*).

Observational Study: From a gp. of 87 cases with abnormal uterocervical cytology and 82 controls, a subset of cases were matched to controls for age, ethnicity, socioeconomic status, and parity. Those cases with severe dysplasia or carcinoma in situ were more likely to have a total dietary vitamin A intake below the pooled median and/or a beta-carotene intake below the pooled median than were normal matched controls (p less than 0.05; p less than 0.025). Odds ratios revealed approx. a 3-fold greater risk for severe dysplasia or CIS in women with lowered vitamin A or beta-carotene intake. In addition, retinol binding protein was either absent or undetectable in 78.8% of the dysplastic tissue samples, versus 23.5% of the normal tissue samples (p less than 0.005) (*Wylie-*

Rosett JA et al.   Influence of vitamin A on cervical dysplasia and carcinoma in situ.   Nutr. Cancer 6(1):49-57, 1984).

Observational Study: Women with abnormal cytology were matched with normal control subjects for age, parity, ethnicity, and socioeconomic class. A nutritional survey revealed statistically significant differences for vitamins A and C and beta carotene. Sucrose gradient ultracentrifugation studies of colposcopic biopsy tissue specimens revealed that retinol binding protein was absent or minimally detectable and inversely related to the severity of the dysplasia (*Romney SL et al. Retinoids and the prevention of cervical dysplasias. Am. J. Obs. & Gyn. 141(8):890-4, 1981).*

See Also:

Vitamin A, tumor initiation and tumor promotion.   Nutr. Rev. May, 1979, pp. 153-6

Basu TK.   Vitamin A and cancer of epithelial origin.   J. Human Nutr. 33:24-31, 1979

Vitamin C: 300 mg. daily

Intake is negatively correlated with cervical dysplasia.

Observational Study: 46 pts. with 1 positive or 2 consecutive suspicious Pap smears for cervical dysplasia were found to have significantly lower vitamin C levels (0.36 mg/dl) than 34 controls with no gynecological dysfunction (0.75 mg/ml) (*Romney SL et al. Plasma vitamin C and uterine cervical dysplasia. Am. J. Obstet. & Gyn. 151(7):976-80, 1985).*

Observational Study: The dietary habits of 49 women with cervical abnormalities were compared to those of 49 matched negative controls. Mean daily vitamin C intake was 80 mg for cases compared to 107 mg for controls (p less than 0.01). Similarly, 29% of cases compared to 3% of controls had a vitamin C intake less than 50% of the RDA, yielding a 10-fold increase in risk of cervical dysplasia as estimated by odds ratio (p less than 0.05). Multiple logistic analysis indicated that low vitamin C intake is an independent contributor to risk of severe cervical dysplasia when age and sexual activity variables are controlled (*Wassertheil-Smoller S et al.   Dietary vitamin C and uterine cervical dysplasia. Am. J. Epidemiol. 114(5):714-24, 1981).*

Observational Study: Women with abnormal cytology were matched with normal control subjects for age, parity, ethnicity, and socioeconomic class. A nutritional survey revealed statistically significant differences for vitamins A and C and beta carotene (*Romney SL et al. Retinoids and the prevention of cervical dysplasias. Am. J. Obs. & Gyn. 141(8):890-4, 1981).*

- -

Selenium:

Deficiency is correlated with increased risk of epithelial cancers (*Prasad K, Ed.   Vitamins, Nutrition and Cancer.   New York, Karger, 1984).*

May be deficient.

Observational Study: Serum selenium levels were significantly lower in pts. with cervical dysplasia (*Dawson E et al.   Serum vitamin and selenium changes in cervical dysplasia.   Fed. Proc. 43:612, 1984).*

CONGESTIVE HEART FAILURE

See Also: ATHEROSCLEROSIS
CARDIOMYOPATHY
HYPERTENSION

NUTRIENTS:

Calcium:

Increasing myocardial muscle cell calcium may be beneficial.

Review Article: Positively inotropic interventions aim to increase the cytosolic calcium ion concentration in the myocardium, including the use of digitalis glycosides, beta-agonists and amrinone (*Opie LH. Principles of therapy for congestive heart failure. Eur. Heart J. 4 Suppl. A:199-208, 1983*).

Reducing vascular smooth muscle calcium may be beneficial.

Experimental Study: Intercellular vascular smooth muscle calcium results in vasoconstriction and may thus potentially increase afterload in chronic CHF. In a study of the response to nifedipine, a calcium channel blocking agent, calcium antagonism resulted in significant afterload reduction and hemodynamic improvement in chronic CHF (*Prida XE et al. Evaluation of calcium-mediated vasoconstriction in chronic congestive heart failure. Am. J. Med. 75(5):795-800, 1983*).

Magnesium:

Myocardial and serum magnesium may be deficient.

Review Article and Observational Study: In CHF there is a loss of magnesium (along with elevation of intracellular sodium and reduction of intracellular potassium) due to activation of the renin-angiotensin-aldosterone system. This deficiency may, in turn, add to the elevation of intracellular sodium and reduction of intracellular potassium since magnesium is necessary for the function of the Na-K pump. In 297 pts. with diuretic-treated CHF, 37% had hypomagnesemia and 43% had low muscle magnesium (*Wester PO, Dyckner T. Intracellular electrolytes in cardiac failure. Acta Med. Scand. [Suppl.] 707:33-36, 1986*).

Review Article: CHF is often associated with hypomagnesemia as well as magnesium tissue deficits. Cardiac glycosides and diuretics (loop and distal types) often exacerbate, or result in, hypomagnesemia, which may lead to cardiac arrhythmias and sudden cardiac death. Deficits in extracellular and vascular tissue magnesium lead to peripheral vasoconstriction which may contribute to the increase in peripheral vascular resistence commonly noted. More attention must be paid to monitoring magnesium levels in tissues (possibly using lymphocytes) and in plasma, and deficits must be corrected. The nonspecific vasodilator properties of Mg^{++} together with its ability to unload the heart should be considered as an important adjunctive tool in CHF management (*Altura BM, Altura BT. Biochemistry and pathophysiology of congestive heart failure: Is there a role for magnesium? Magnesium 5(3-4):134-43, 1986*).

Supplementation may assist in the correction of muscle potassium deficiencies as well as in correction of the disturbed relation between extra- and intracellular electrolytes.

Experimental Study: It was found that, for pts. with CHF, a deficiency of muscle potassium could not be corrected when there was also a concomitant magnesium deficiency. In addition, magnesium infusions changed the disturbed relation between extra- and intracellular electrolytes towards normal (*Wester & Dyckner - op cit*).

Potassium:

Myocardial and serum potassium may be deficient.

Review Article and Observational Study: In CHF the activation of the renin-angiotension-aldosterone system causes potassium losses, while the secondary hyperaldosteronism may give rise to low intracellular potassium through a direct permeability effect on the cell membrane. In addition, magnesium loss (which is also due to activation of the renin-angiotension-aldosterone system) leads to further loss of intracellular potassium as magnesium is necessary for the function of the Na-K pump. In 297 pts. with diuretic-treated CHF, 42% had hypokalemia and 52% had depletion of muscle potassium (*Wester & Dyckner - op cit*).

Review Article: CHF is often associated with hypokalemia as well as potassium tissue deficits. Cardiac glycosides and diuretics (loop and distal types) often exacerbate, or result in, hypokalemia, which may lead to cardiac arrhythmias and sudden cardiac death. Potassium deficits may contribute to the increase in peripheral vascular resistence commonly noted. More attention must be paid to monitoring potassium levels in tissues (possibly using lymphocytes) and in plasma, and deficits must be corrected (*Altura BM, Altura BT - op cit*).

Sodium:

Myocardial sodium may be elevated, while serum sodium may be deficient.

Review Article and Observational Study: In CHF the activation of the renin-angiotension-aldosterone system causes sodium retention, while the secondary hyperaldosteronism may give rise to elevated intracellular sodium through a direct permeability effect on the cell membrane. In addition, magnesium loss (which is also due to activation of the renin-angiotension-aldosterone system) leads to further retention of intracellular sodium as magnesium is necessary for the function of the Na-K pump. In 297 pts. with diuretic-treated CHF, 12% had hyponatremia and 57% had excessive muscle sodium (*Wester & Dyckner - op cit*).

Coenzyme Q10:

Deficiency in myocardial tissues is common in CHF (*Kitamura N et al. Myocardial tissue level of coenzyme Q10 in patients with cardiac failure, in Folkers K, Yamamura Y, Eds., Biomed. & Clin. Aspects of Coenzyme Q. Vol. 4. Amsterdam, Elsevier/North Holland Biomedical Press, 1984, pp. 243-252*).

Supplementation may be beneficial.

Experimental Study: 12 pts. with advanced CHF and an insufficient response to therapy with diuretics and digitalis received coenzyme Q10 100 mg daily and were followed for a mean period of 7 months. With a mean latency period of 30 days, 8/12 showed definite clinical improvement. Subjectively, they felt less tired, their general activity tolerance increased and dyspnea at rest disappeared. There were obvious signs of decreased right-sided stasis (hepatic congestion). Their heart rate fell significantly, and the heart volume decreased (result n.s.). There was a significant reduction in left atrial size and a significant decline in the PEP/LVET ratio (STI) indicative of improved myocardial performance. Preliminary results of withdrawal of the supplement were severe clinical relapse with improvement upon resumption (*Mortensen SA et al. Long-term conenzyme Q10 therapy: A major advance in the management of resistant myocardial failure. Drugs Exp. Clin. Res. 11(8):581-93, 1985*).

Experimental Study: Subjective improvements following coenzyme Q_{10} supplementation were confirmed by tests showing increased cardiac output, stroke volume, cardiac index, and ejection fraction (*Judy WV et al. Myocardial effects of Co-enzyme Q_{10} in primary heart failure, in Folkers K, Yamamura Y, Eds. Biomed. & Clin. Aspects of Coenzyme Q. Vol. 4. Amsterdam, Elsevier/North Holland Biomedical Press, 1984, pp. 353-67; Vanfraechem JHP et al. Coenzyme Q_{10} and physical performance in myocardial failure, in Folkers K, Yamamura Y, Eds. Biomed. & Clin. Aspects of Coenzyme Q. Vol. 4. Amsterdam, Elsevier/North Holland Biomedical Press, 1984, pp. 281-90*).

Experimental Study: 20 pts. with CHF due either to ischemic or hypertensive heart disease were treated with coenzyme Q_{10} 30 mg daily for 1-2 months. 55% reported subjective improvement, 50% showed a decrease in New York Heart Association functional class, and 30% showed a "remarkable" decrease in chest congestion on chest x-ray. CoQ_{10} also prevented the negative inotropic effect of beta-blocker therapy without apparently reducing the beneficial effect of beta-blockers on myocardial oxygen consumption. Its positive inotropic effect was not as potent as that of digitalis (*Tsuyusaki T et al. Mechanocardiography of ischemic or hypertensive heart failure, in Yamamura Y et al., Ed. Biomed. & Clin. Aspects of Coenzyme Q. Vol. 2. Amsterdam, Elsevier/North Holland Biomedical Press, 1980, pp. 273-88*).

Experimental Study: 17 pts. with mild CHF received CoQ_{10} 30 mg daily. All improved and 9 (53%) became asymptomatic after 4 weeks (*Ishiyama T et al. A clinical study of the effect of coenzyme Q on congestive heart failure. Jpn. Heart J. 17:32, 1976*).

See Also:

Colucci WS et al. New positive inotropic agents in the treatment of congestive heart failure. Mechanisms of action and recent clinical developments. 2. N. Engl. J. Med. 314(6):349-58, 1986

Taurine: 2 gm two-three times daily

Supplementation may be beneficial.

Experimental Double-blind Crossover Study: Taurine 6 gm daily in divided doses or placebo was given to 14 pts. in addition to conventional treatment in a randomized crossover design for 4 wks. each with a 2-wk. wash-out period in between. 11/14 (79%) improved on taurine compared to 3/14 (21%) on placebo. Compared to placebo, taurine significantly improved New York Heart Association functional class, pulmonary crackles, and chest film abnormalities. While heart-failure scorces failed to change significantly on placebo, their decrease was highly significant on taurine (p less than 0.001) during which pre-injection period (corrected for heart rate) and the quotient of pre-ejection period/left ventricular ejection time decreased. No pt. worsened during taurine administration, but 4 pts. did during placebo (*Azuma J et al. Therapeutic effect of taurine in congestive heart failure: A double-blind crossover trial. Clin. Cardiol. 8:276-82, 1985; Azuma J et al. Taurine and failing heart: Experimental and clinical aspects. Prog. Clin. Biol. Res. 179:195-213, 1985*).

Animal Experimental Study: Congestive heart failure was produced in rabbits with surgically-induced aortic regurgitation. Mortality after 8 wks. in the untreated gp. was 52% compared to 11% in the taurine treated group. Taurine (100 mg/kg) maintained cardiac function, while cardiac function deteriorated significantly in untreated rabbits (*Azuma J et al. Beneficial effect of taurine on congestive heart failure induced by chronic aortic regurgitation in rabbits. Res. Comm. Chem. Pathol. Pharmacol. 435:261, 1984*).

Experimental Double-blind Crossover Study: Taurine 2 gm 3 times daily or placebo was given to 62 pts. in a randomized crossover design for 4 wks. each. After 4 wks. of taurine, there was a highly significant improvement in dyspnea, palpitations, crackles, edema, cardiothoracic ratio on x-ray and New York Heart Association functional class. Taurine was significantly more effective than placebo (p less than 0.05), suggesting that it is clinically beneficial (*Azuma J et al. Double-blind randomized crossover trial of taurine in congestive heart failure. Current Therapeu. Res. 34(4):543-57, 1983*).

Experimental Study: 24 pts. received taurine 2 gm twice daily. After 4-8 wks., taurine was effective in 19/24 patients as based on reduction in clinical signs and symptoms and x-ray data. 13 out of the 15 pts. who formerly were designated as N.Y. Heart Association functional class III or IV could be designated as class II (*Azuma J et al. Therapy of congestive heart failure with orally administered taurine. Clin. Ther. 5(4):398-408, 1983*).

CONSTIPATION

BASIC DIET:

High fiber diet or supplementation with bran (ex. 1 1/2 tablespoons twice daily), or psyllium.

Review Article: For the treatment of chronic constipation, the author recommends that pts. be started with 1/2 cup of 100% bran cereal (9 gm of dietary fiber) daily with increases by 1/2 cup increments to the equivalent of 27 gm daily which should result in satisfactory stool frequency and volume. The major side effect will be increased flatus which tends to diminish as tolerance develops (*Franklin JF. Treatment of chronic constipation. Questions and Answers. JAMA 256(5):652, 1986*).

Experimental Controlled Study: Bran consumption was positively associated with increased fecal weight, increased bowel movement frequency and decreased intestinal transit time. Corn bran was more effective than wheat bran, possibly due to its higher total fiber content or its greater resistence to degradation (*Graham DY et al. The effect of bran on bowel function in constipation. Am.J.Gastroenterol. 77:599-603, 1982*).

Experimental Controlled Study: Bran (10 gm twice daily) was significantly superior to a bulk laxative for 10 geriatric pts. (mean transit times: 89 vs. 126 hrs.) (*Andersson H et al. Transit time in constipated geriatric patients during treatment with a bulk laxative and bran: A comparison. Scandinavian J. Gastroenterol. 14:821-26, 1979*).

See Also:

Hull C et al. Alleviation of constipation in the elderly by dietary fiber supplementation. J. Am. Geriat. Soc. 28:410, 1980

- -

NUTRIENTS:

Folic Acid: up to 60 mg. daily as needed

May be effective in cases of deficiency.

Experimental Study: 3 women with folate deficiency presented with chronic constipation along with restless legs, depression, tiredness, depressed ankle jerks and impaired vibratory sensation and recovered with supplementation (*Botez MI et al. Neurologic disorders responsive to folic acid therapy. Can. Med. Assoc. J. 15:217, 1976*).

- -

OTHER FACTORS:

Rule out food sensitivities.

Observational Study: 40 pts. with G.I. "allergy." Constipation as well as gas, bloating and pain were the most common complaints. All showed physical evidence of hypothyroidism and had lowered basal metabolic rates. X-rays most frequently showed disharmonic or spastic colon (*Gay LP. Gastrointestinal Allergy. J. Missouri Med. Assoc. 29:7-10, 1932*).

Lactobacillus Acidophilus: may require weeks to months

Supplementation may be beneficial.

Experimental Studies (compilation of previous studies):
305/356 cases of chronic constipation responded (_Lancet General Advertiser_ September 21, 1957).

Experimental Study: Successful implantation of LA was followed by symptom relief in mucous colitis, irritable colon, idiopathic ulcerative colitis, and various other disorders causing constipation (_Rettger LF et al._ _Lactobacillus acidophilus._ _Its therapeutic application._ _New Haven, Yale U. Press, 1935_).

See Also:

Experimental Study: _Weinstein L et al._ _Therapeutic application of acidophilus milk in simple constipation._ _Arch. Int. Med._ 52:384, 1933

Experimental Study: _Kopeloff N._ _Clinical results obtained with bacillus acidophilus._ _Arch. Int. Med._ 33:47, 1924

CROHN'S DISEASE

See Also: ULCERATIVE COLITIS

BASIC DIET:

Consider an <u>elemental diet</u> for very active disease.

(Note: The benefits of this diet may be due to better alimentation, its hypoallergenicity, or both.)

Experimental Controlled Study: 10 pts. were given 0.75 mg. prednisone daily for 14 days, while 11 pts. were given a protein free elemental diet. At the end of 4 wks., 8/10 steroid pts. and 9/11 diet pts. were in remission. At 3 months, 1 pt. in each gp. was a treatment failure. Thus a hypoallergic diet was as effective as prednisone without the danger of its side-effects (*Nutri. Res. Newsletter October, 1984*).

Experimental Study: 15 pts. aged 6-20 were followed for up to 3 years on a hypoallergenic elemental diet. The diet was associated with remissions in the 14 pts. who tolerated it (*O'Morain C et al. Elemental diet in acute Crohn's disease. Arch. Dis. Childhood 53:44, 1983*).

See Also:

> Ferguson A et al. *Treatment of jejunal Crohn's disease with an elemental (antigen-free) diet. Clin. Allergy 10:349, 1980*

Restrict <u>refined carbohydrates</u>, especially <u>refined sugar</u>.

Review Article: Therapeutic regimes with reduction of synthetic carbohydrates as well as increase in crude fiber content of the diet have demonstrated a positive influence on the disease (*Riemann JF, Kolb S. Zuckerarme und faserreiche Kost bei Morbus Crohn. Fortschr. Med. 102(4):67-70, 1984*).

Observational Study: 70 pts. with Crohn's, 50 with ulcerative colitis, and 58 control subjects were questioned about sugar consumption which was found to be significantly increased only in Crohn's patients compared to controls. No relationship was found between sugar consumption, taste acuity and plasma zinc (*Penny WJ et al. Relationship between trace elements, sugar consumption, and taste in Crohn's disease. Gut 24(4):288-92, 1983*).

Experimental Controlled Study: 80% of pts.on a low carbohydrate diet which excluded all refined sugar had symptom relief within 18 months,while 40% of pts.on a high carbohydrate diet which was high in refined sugar had to discontinue the diet due to flare-ups (*Brandes JW, Lorenz-Meyer H. [Sugar free diet: A new perspective in the treatment of Crohn disease? Randomized, control study.] Z. Gastroenterol. 19(1):1-12, 1981*).

Observational Study: A questionnaire revealed that 32 pts. with recently diagnosed Crohn's consumed significantly greater amounts of sugar and sugar-containing foods than did matched controls. When all food eaten over 5 days was weighed and recorded for 16 pts., only the consumption of added sugars was greater than controls. This added sugar consumption appears unrelated to other dietary abnormalities and may reflect a deficiency in the perception of sweetness by Crohn's patients (*Mayberry JF et al. Diet in Crohn's disease: Two studies of current and previous habits in newly diagnosed patients. Dig. Dis. Sci. 26(5):444-8, 1981*).

Observational Study: The current intake of refined carbohydrate and added sugar was significantly greater for 27 Crohn's pts. than for matched controls. It is suggested that there is a secondary rather than a causal relationship between sugar consumption and Crohn's (*Silkoff K et al. Consumption of refined carbohydrate by patients with Crohn's disease in Tel-Aviv-Yafo. Postgrad. Med. J. 56:842-6, 1980*).

Observational Study: 120 pts. with Crohn's, 100 with ulcerative colitis and matched controls were interviewed by questionnaire. Crohn's pts. ate significantly more sugar than either controls or pts. with ulcerative colitis (*Mayberry JF et al. Increased sugar consumption in Crohn's disease. Digestion 20:323-6, 1980*).

Experimental Controlled Study: 32 Crohn's pts. were treated with a fiber-rich unrefined carbohydrate diet in addition to conventional management and followed for a mean of 4 years and 4 months. Their course was compared retrospectively with that of 32 matched pts. who had received no dietary instruction. Hospital admissions were significantly fewer and shorter in the diet-treated pts. (111 vs. 533 days). Whereas 5 of the controls required intestinal surgery, only 1 diet-treated pt. required it. There were no cases of intestinal obstruction among the diet-treated patients. (*Heaton KW et al. Treatment of Crohn's disease with an unrefined-carbohydrate, fibre-rich diet. Brit. Med. J. 2:764-6, 1979*).

Observational Study: 32 newly diagnosed Crohn's pts. were compared to 30 matched controls. The pts. ate substantially more refined sugar, slightly less dietary fiber, and considerably less raw fruit and vegetables than the controls, suggesting that a diet high in refined sugar and low in raw fruit and vegetables precedes and may favor the development of Crohn's (*Thornton JR et al. Diet and Crohn's disease: Characteristics of the pre-illness diet. Brit. Med. J. 2:762-4, 1979*).

- -

NUTRIENTS:

General:

Observational Study: For 23 male and 24 female patients, the mean daily intake of vitamin B6 and folate by both men and women and iron by women was below the RDA. 50% of the women had inadequate intakes of iron, 13% of riboflavin, 21% of thiamin and 21% of vitamin A (*Hodges P et al. Vitamin and iron intake in patients with Crohn's disease. J. Am. Diet. Assoc. 84(1):52-8, 1984*).

Experimental Crossover Study: 28 malnourished pts. spent 2 months on an ordinary diet followed by 2 months on the same diet with the addition of a low-residue liquid nutritional supplement. All anthropometric measurements, serum proteins, creatinine height index and circulating T lymphocytes increased significantly, while serum orosomucoid levels dropped significantly - suggesting that disease activity was reduced. The benefits appeared to be due to the higher calorie intake with the oral supplement (*Harries AD et al. Controlled trial of supplemented oral nutrition in Crohn's disease. Lancet 1:8330, 1983*).

Review Article: A wide range of nutritional disturbances may be found in Crohn's patients which need to be recognized early on and treated (*Harries AD, Heatley RV. Nutritional disturbances in Crohn's disease. Postgrad. Med. J. 50:690-7, 1983*).

Folic Acid:

May be deficient due to inadequate intake and/or poor absorption.

Observational Study: The mean daily intake of folate was below the RDA for 23 male and 24 female patients. Serum folate was low in 21% of the men and 26% of the women. Of several nutrients studied, serum folate was the only one which correlated with nutrient intake, with low serum folate being predictive of potential risk of deficiencies of vitamins B6, B12 and C (*Hodges P et al. Vitamin and iron intake in patients with Crohn's disease. J. Am. Diet. Assoc. 84(1):52-8, 1984*).

Observational Study: Of 216 pts. with chronic inflammatory bowel disease, low serum folate levels were found in 59% and low RBC levels in 26%. It is suggested that folate deficiency is of multiple origin: inadequate diet, malabsorption and chronic drug-induced low-grade hemolysis (*Elsborg L, Larsen L. Folate deficiency in chronic inflammatory bowel disease. Scand. J. Gastroenterol. 14:1019-24, 1979*).

See Also:

Elsborg L. Vitamin B_{12} and folic acid in Crohn's disease. Dan. Med. Bull. 29(7):362-5, 1982

Gerson CD, Cohen N. Folic acid absorption in regional enteritis. Am. J. Clin. Nutr. 29:182, 1976

Folate deficiency may be due to the use of sulfasalazine.

In vitro Experimental Study: Studies on rat lymphocytes demonstrate that sulfasalazine acts as a folate antagonist (*Baum CL et al. Antifolate actions of sulfasalazine on intact lymphocytes. J. Lab. Clin. Med. 97(6):779-84, 1981*).

See Also:

Halsted CH et al. Sulfasalazine inhibits the absorption of folates in ulcerative colitis. New Eng. J. Med. 305(25):1513, 1981

Folate supplementation may reduce diarrhea (*Carruthers LB. Chronic diarrhea treated with folic acid. Lancet 1:849, 1946*).

Vitamin A: 50,000 - 75,000 IU daily

May be deficient.

Observational Study: Compared to controls, 54 pts. had significantly lower serum vitamin A. There was a marked correlation between vitamin A and the activity of the disease, but no correlation with B_{12} absorption, the localization of the disease or previous ileal resection, suggesting that the deficiency is not primarily caused by absorption abnormalities (*Schoelmerich J et al. Zinc and vitamin A deficiency in patients with Crohn's disease is correlated with activity but not with localization or extent of the disease. Hepatogastroentero. 32(1):34-8, 1985*).

Observational Study: 52 pts. were investigated for vitamin A deficiency. Results suggest that pts. with extensive disease who weigh less than 80% of ideal weight merit measurement of plama retinol concentration. Those with plasma retinol below 0.8 micromol. per liter (below 22.9 microgram %) run a high risk of night blindness and are likely to be protein-depleted (*Main ANH et al. Vitamin A deficiency in Crohn's disease. Gut 24(12):1169-1175, 1983*).

See Also:

Skogh M et al. Vitamin A in Crohn's disease. Lancet 1:766, 1980

Dvorak AM. Vitamin A in Crohn's disease. Lancet 1:1303-4, 1980

Supplementation has not been shown to be beneficial in long-term controlled trials.

Negative Experimental Double-blind Study: 86 pts. in remission failed to benefit from 50,000 I.U. twice daily (*Wright JP et al. Gastroenterol. 88(2):512-14, 1985*).

See Also:

> Norrby S et al. *Ineffectiveness of vitamin A therapy in severe Crohn's disease.* Acta Chir. Scand. 151:465-68, 1985

Vitamin B_{12}:   intramuscular injections (if deficient)

May be deficient.

> **Review Article:** Vitamin B_{12} is absorbed in the terminal ileum, and thus may not be properly absorbed in pts (*Elsborg L. Vitamin B_{12} and folic acid in Crohn's disease.* Dan. Med. Bull. 29(7):362-5, 1982).

Vitamin C:

May be deficient.

> **Observational Study:** Crohn's pts. had 32% lower vitamin C levels than normals (*Hughes RG, Williams N. Leukocyte ascorbic acid in Crohn's disease.* Digestion 17:272, 1978).

> **Observational Study:** Crohn's pts. with fistulas had 54% lower vitamin C levels than those without (*Gerson CD, Fabry EM. Ascorbic acid deficiency and fistula formation in regional enteritis.* Gastroenterology 67:428, 1974).

Vitamin D:

May be deficient.

> **Observational Study:** Mild deficiency was common and severe deficiency (25-OHD levels less than 8 nmol/l) was encountered. Deficiency was more common in pts. with active vs. inactive disease. Plasma 25-OHD levels were significantly correlated with hemoglobin and ESR. Evidence of secondary hyperparathyroidism and osteomalacia was noted (*Dibble JB et al. A survey of vitamin D deficiency in gastrointestinal and liver disorders.* Quart. J. Med. 53:119-34, 1984).

See Also:

> Harries AD et al. *Vitamin D status in Crohn's disease: Association with nutrition and disease activity.* Gut 26:1197-1203, 1985

Vitamin K:

May be deficient, especially when the disease occurs in the terminal ileum.

> **Experimental and Observatonal Study:** 18/58 (31%) pts. with chronic G.I. disorders were found to have evidence of vitamin K deficiency; all pts. with deficiency had either Crohn's of the terminal ileum or ulcerative colitis treated with sulfasalazine or antibiotics.   The mean vitamin E level was lower in pts. with vitamin K deficiency than in those without it. Abnormal prothrombin levels returned toward normal in pts. treated with vitamin K (*Krasinski SD et al. The prevalence of vitamin K deficiency in chronic gastrointestinal disorders.* Am. J. Clin. Nutr. 41(3):639-43, 1985).

– –

Calcium:

May be deficient due to loss of absorptive surfaces, steatorrhea, corticosteroid treatment, and vitamin D deficiency (*Rosenberg IH et al. Nutritional aspects of inflammatory bowel disease. Ann. Rev. Nutr. 5:463-84, 1985*).

Magnesium:

May be deficient.

> **Observational Study:** Mg depletion as judged by serum and 24 hr. urine concentrations was present in 21/25 pts. with severe disease, 15 of whom required IV nutrition. Mg deficient was statistically more likely to occur in pts. on IV nutrition taking less than 5 mmol IV Mg/ 24 hr. After discharge, 5 pts. who had received IV nutrition frequently complained of muscle cramps, tetany and bone pain and were found to have recurrent low serum Mg levels over some months (*Russell RI. Magnesium requirements in patients with chronic inflammatory disease receiving intravenous nutrition. J. Am. Coll. Nutr. 4(5):553-58, 1985*).

> **Observational Study:** The Mg status of 87 Crohn's pts. with various lengths of small bowel resection was studied. Serum Mg was not abnormally low; however, both urinary and muscle Mg concentration decreased with increasing resection length and muscular fatigue was positively correlated to a pathologically low muscle Mg concentration. Results suggest that clinically important Mg deficiency occurs in pts. with resections exceeding 75 cm. (*Hessov I et al. Magnesium deficiency after ileal resections for Crohn's disease. Scand. J. Gastroenterol. 18:643-49, 1983*).

While serum levels are rarely decreased, intracellular levels are frequently low and may be associated with weakness, anorexia, hypotension, confusion, hyperirritability, tetany, convulsions, and EKG or EEG abnormalities (*Rosenberg IH et al. Nutritional aspects of inflammatory bowel disease. Ann. Rev. Nutr. 5:463-84, 1985*).

Selenium:

May be deficient.

> **Observational Study:** Compared to controls, whole blood selenium was reduced in Crohn's pts. (*Penny WJ et al. Relationship between trace elements, sugar consumption, and taste in Crohn's disease. Gut 24(4):288-92, 1983*).

Zinc:

May be deficient.

> **Observational Study:** Compared to controls, 54 pts. had significantly lower serum zinc. Zinc levels correlated markedly with the activity of the disease. Since there was no correlation between zinc levels, B_{12} absorption, localization of the disease or previous ileal resection, the deficiency does not appear to be primarily caused by absorption abnormalities (*Schoelmerich J et al. Zinc and vitamin A deficiency in patients with Crohn's disease is correlated with activity but not with localization or extent of the disease. Hepatogastroenterol.. 32(1):34-8, 1985*).

> **Observational Study:** 17/50 pts. (34%) had low serum zinc levels. Compared to pts. without fistulas, zinc levels were significantly lower in pts. with fistulas, and were found in 11/17 (65%). Thus zinc deficiency may play a role in the formation and clinical course of fistulas (*Kruis W et al. Zinc*

deficiency as a problem in patients with Crohn's disease and fistula formation. Hepatogastroenterol.. 32(3):133-4, 1985).

Review Article: Diarrhea is one of the clinical manifestations of zinc deficiency; thus chronic diarrhea may be due to malabsorption of zinc which may, in turn, be due to excessive intake of fiber or phytates (*Giorgi PL et al. Zinco ed eteropatie croniche. Pediatr. Med. Chir. 6(5):625-36, 1984*).

Observational Study: Compared to controls, plasma zinc was reduced in Crohn's pts. (*Penny WJ et al. Relationship between trace elements, sugar consumption, and taste in Crohn's disease. Gut 24(4):288-92, 1983*).

Observational Study: Compared to controls, plasma zinc was reduced and the sense of taste was 65% duller (*Solomons NW et al. Zinc deficiency in Crohn's disease. Digestion 16:87, 1977*).

See Also:

> *Nishida K et al. [A study on a low serum zinc level in Crohn's disease.] Nippon Shok. Gakkai Zasshi 82(3):424-33, 1985*

> *McClain CJ et al. Zinc-deficiency-induced retinal dysfunction in Crohn's disease. Dig. Dis. Sci. 28:85, 1983*

> *Zinc deficiency in Crohn's Disease. Nutr. Rev. 40:109, 1982*

Glycosaminoglycans:

Supplementation may be beneficial.

Experimental Study: 4 pts. with inadequate results from traditional treatments received sub-cut. injections of an activated acid-pepsin-digested calf tracheal cartilege preparation ("Catrix-S") over 10-35 days followed by booster injections every 3-4 weeks. 3/4 had an excellent response, while 1/4 had a good response (*Prudden JF, Balassa LL. The biological activity of bovine cartilage preparations. Sem. Arthritis & Rheum. 3(4):287-321, 1974*).

OTHER FACTORS:

Rule out food sensitivities.

Experimental Controlled Study: 20 pts. with active disease received either an unrefined carbohydrate fibre-rich diet or a diet which excluded specific foods to which a pt. was intolerant (as determined by a prior water fast followed by single food provocations). 7/10 pts. on the exclusion diet remained in remission for 6 months compared with 0/10 on the unrefined CH diet. In an uncontrolled study, an exclusion diet allowed 51/77 pts. to remain well on the diet alone for periods of up to 51 months, and with an annual relapse rate of less than 10% (*Jones VA et al. Crohn's disease: Maintenance of remission by diet. Lancet July 27, 1985, pp. 177-180*).

Experimental Study: 33 pts. became-symptom free by following an elimination diet, elemental diet or total parenteral nutrition. 29/33 reported specific food intolerances and 21/29 remained in remission on diet alone. Foods provoking symptoms most commonly were wheat (69%), dairy products (48%), yeast (31%), corn (24%), potato and tap water (17%) and banana, tomato, wine, eggs (14%) (*Workman EM et al. Diet in the management of Crohn's disease. Human Nutrition: Applied Nutrition 38A:469-73, 1985*).

Experimental and Observational Study: Based on a symptom survey listing atopic allergic symptoms, 61/91 (67%) pts. were judged to be possibly allergic. In addition, over 50 IBD pts. treated with inhalent allergy hyposensitization and dietary changes consisting of rotation and diversification of allergic foods were considerably improved in both their respiratory and abdominal symptoms, suggesting an allergic diathesis (*Siegel J. Inflammatory bowel disease: Another possible facet of the allergic diathesis. <u>Ann. Allergy</u> 47:92-94, 1981*).

DEMENTIA

NUTRIENTS:

General:

Pts. with dementia are more likely than controls to be nutritionally deficient, although it is unclear if the deficiency is secondary to the effect of the disease on eating behavior.

Observational Study: 29 pts. with senile dementia were compared to 35 healthy elderly controls. Dietary intakes were below recommended levels for 1/3 of the controls and for a greater proportion of the patients. Few in either gp. received sufficient vitamin D or folic acid. A higher proportion of pts. displayed evidence of vitamin deficiency than controls - especially re: ascorbic acid and folic acid. Total fasting tryptophan concentrations were significantly lower in demented pts. (*Shaw DM et al. Senile dementia and nutrition. Letter to the Editor. Brit. Med. J. 288:792-93, 1984*).

Nutritional supplementation may be beneficial.

Experimental Study: 10 pts. and 10 controls (from the above study) were given vitamin supplements daily for 2 months. Some of these pts. showed clinical improvement. Although vitamin concentration differences disappeared, differences in fasting tryptophan concentrations remained the same (*Shaw DM - ibid*).

Folic acid: If deficient: 10-20 mg. daily for 1 wk.; then 2.5-10 mg. daily as needed

Deficiency is associated with apathy, disorientation, poor concentration and memory deficits in addition to pyramidal tract damage (*Strachan RW, Henderson JG. Dementia and folate deficiency. Quart. J. Med. 36:189-204, 1967*).

Deficiency is not uncommon among elderly psychiatric patients.

Observational Study: 255 consecutive referrals to a psychogeriatric assessment unit were classified as "organic" if they suffered from dementia or confusional states, "functional" if suffering from neurosis or psychosis, and "mixed" if functional and organic symptoms were both present. There was also a small miscellaneous group. Low folic acid concentrations were found in 20/114 (18%) of the "organic" pts., 14/62 (23%) of the "functional" pts., and 8/35 (23%) of the "mixed" pts., suggesting that low folate is widely distributed among more severely mentally ill old people (*Bober MJ. Senile dementia and nutrition. Letter to the Editor. Brit. Med. J. 288:1234, 1984*).

Deficiency may be correlated with the presence of an organic brain syndrome.

Observational Study: A statistical correlation was found between low serum folate levels and organic brain syndrome (*Sneath P et al. Folate status in a geriatric population and its relation to dementia. Age Ageing 2:177-182, 1973*).

If deficient, supplementation may be beneficial.

Case Report: A 75 year-old epileptic female with severe dementia demonstrated reversal of the dementia, regression of the spastic tetraparesis, normalization of extensor plantar responses, and improvement in serial EEG's following folate supplementation (*Melamed E et al. Reversible central nervous system dysfunction in folate deficiency.* J. Neurol. Sci. *25:93-98, 1975*).

Case Reports: 2 elderly widows with advanced dementia and nutritional folate deficiency with anemia were supplemented with folic acid, following which both the intellectual and personality deterioration and the anemia were corrected. In addition, their abnormal EEG's were normalized over a period of several weeks (*Strachan & Henderson - op cit*).

Note: This study has been criticized as:
1. any anemia in the elderly may cause an organic brain syndrome.
2. it is possible that the social intervention that brought them to the hospital and to a caring environment was responsible for their improvement (Shulman R. An overview of folic acid deficiency and psychiatric illness, in Botez MI, Reynolds EH. Folic Acid in Neurology, Psychiatry, and Internal Medicine. New York, Raven Press, 1979).

See Also:

Enk C et al. Reversible dementia and neuropathy associated with folate deficiency 16 years after partial gastrectomy. Scand. J. Haematol. *25:63, 1980*

Pyridoxine:

Often deficient in elderly Alzheimer pts. as compared to healthy elderly controls (*Keatinge AMB et al. Vitamin B$_1$, B$_2$, B$_6$ and C status in the elderly.* Irish Med. J. *76:488-90, 1983*)

There is an age-related fall in dopamine receptors which parallels a decline in plasma vitamin B$_6$ levels (*Wagner HN Jr. - interviewed in* Psychology Today *July 1985*).

Functional recovery of damaged dopamine receptors in the elderly may be impaired by a pyridoxine deficiency.

Animal Experimental Study: The rate of return of damaged dopamine receptors in older rats made B$_6$-deficient was slower than that of controls (*Wagner HN et al.* Science *226(4681)*).

Vitamin B$_{12}$:   If deficient: 100 mcg. I.M. daily for 1 wk. initially; then continued as needed

Deficiency is associated with depression, confusion, memory deficits and mental slowness along with neurologic deficits.

Often deficient despite the lack of hematologic findings suggestive of pernicious anemia.

Experimental and Observational Study: 4 pts. with presenile dementia for over 4 yrs. failed to show hematologic findings suggesting vitamin B$_{12}$ deficiency, yet their serum B$_{12}$ levels were clearly deficient. B$_{12}$ supplementation did not improve their mental status (*Abalan F, Delile JM. B$_{12}$ deficiency in presenile dementia. Letter to the Editor.* Biol. Psychiat. *20(11):1251, 1985*).

Observational Study: Alzheimer pts. had lower serum B$_{12}$ levels at all ages compared to normals and pts. with other forms of dementia, but demonstrated no hematological changes suggestive of B$_{12}$ deficiency (*Cole MG, Prchal JF. Low serum B$_{12}$ in Alzheimer-type dementia.* Age & Aging *13:101-5, 1984*).

Supplementation may be effective.

Case Report: 35 year-old man with a 3 year history of mental illness suggestive of an organic brain syndrome with suicidal behavior. Because of an earlier history of a partial gastrectomy, serum B$_{12}$

was evaluated but found to be normal. After medication and ECT were ineffective, an injection of B12 was tried which was so effective that he was discharged symptom-free after 8 days and remained so on 1000 mcg B12 IM every few weeks (*Geagea K, Ananth J. Response of a psychiatric patient to vitamin B12 therapy. Dis. Nerv. Syst. 36(6):343-44, 1975*).

Vitamin C:

Deficiency is not uncommon among elderly psychiatric patients.

Observational Study: 255 consecutive referrals to a psychogeriatric assessment unit were classified as "organic" if they suffered from dementia or confusional states, "functional" if suffering from neurosis or psychosis, and "mixed" if functional and organic symptoms were both present. There was also a small miscellaneous group. Low ascorbic acid concentrations were found in 57/102 (56%) of the "organic" pts., 22/44 (50%) of the "functional" pts., and 18/32 (57%) of the "mixed" pts., suggesting that low ascorbate is widely distributed among more severely mentally ill old people (*Bober MJ. Senile dementia and nutrition. Letter to the Editor. Brit. Med. J. 288:1234, 1984*).

Among a psychiatric population, deficiency is particularly marked in patients with senile dementia.

Observational Study: The ave. plasma vitamin C level in 885 psychiatric pts. was 0.51/100 ml compared to 0.87/100 ml in 110 healthy controls. The lowest values were found in pts. with senile dementia and in females on iron therapy. 32% of the pts. had levels below 0.35 mg/100 ml, the threshold which has been associated with detrimental effects on immune responses and behavior (*Schorah CJ et al. Human Nutr.: Clin. Nutr. 37C:447-52, 1983*).

Vitamin E:

May be deficient.

Observational Study: Nearly 60% of Alzheimer pts. had serum vitamin E levels below the accepted normal range. A 3-day dietary survey showed that the mean intake of vitamin E was only about 1/3 of what the British Dept. of Health estimates an average diet should contain (*Burns A, Holland T. Vitamin E deficiency. Letter to the Editor. Lancet April 5, 1986, pp. 805-6*).

People with Down's Syndrome, who are prone to Alzheimer-like neuropathological change in middle age and are at high risk of clinical dementia (*Wisniewski KE et al. Occurrence of neuropathological changes and dementia of Alzheimer's disease in Down's sundrome. Ann. Neurol. 17:270-82, 1985*), have increased superoxide dismutase activity which may damage cell membranes because of increased hydroxyl radicals. Since vitamin E is a free-radical scavenger, supplementation may theoretically reduce the damage (*Sylverster PE. Ageing in the mentally retarded, in Dobbing J et al., Eds. Scientific Studies in Mental Retardation. London, Macmillian, for the Royal Society of Medicine, 1984, pp. 259-77*). If the same events occur in other groups predisposed to AD, vitamin E deficiency could lower the age of onset or increase the rate of progression of the disease (*Burns A, Holland T - op cit*).

On the other hand, circulating blood concentrations are not always reflective of tissue content as studies have shown that the ave. alpha tocopherol content of the cerebral cortex of Alzheimer's pts. and fetuses with Down's Syndrome did not differ significantly from controls (*Muller D et al. Vitamin E in brains of patients with Alzheimer's disease and Down's syndrome. Lancet 1:1093-94, 1986*).

May protect against lipid peroxidative damage in the cerebrum.

Animal Experimental Study: After 8 wks., blood vitamin E levels of 1 mo. old rats supplemented daily with vitamin E 200 IU/kg were 32 fold higher than vitamin E-deficient animals and 3 fold higher in the brain cerebrum. In older (15 mo. old) rats, vitamin E blood levels were 1.8 fold higher and cerebral levels 1.5 fold higher, which increased to 8 fold and 2 fold differences after an additional 12 weeks. Selenium deficiency had a slight sparing effect on blood vitamin E levels in vitamin E-deficient animals. While an indicator of *in vivo* peroxidation in the cerebrum was not significantly affected by vitamin E supplementation, when all age gps. were analyzed together, the vitamin E-deficient diet supplemented with selenium 0.2 ppm had a significant effect on increasing brain peroxide levels. Incubation of cerebrum homogenates showed an inverse relationship between ex-vivo peroxidation levels and brain vitamin E content. In the old animals, relatively long-term supplementation (20 wks.) was required to inhibit peroxidation capacity in the brain. Results suggest that vitamin E has a major role in protecting against *in vitro* and possibly *in vivo* lipid peroxidation in the cerebrum while dietary selenium has a minimal effect (*Meydani M et al. Effect of vitamin E, selenium and age on lipid peroxidation events in rat cerebrum. Nutr. Res. 5:1227-36, 1985*).

- -

Copper:

Excess copper accumulation is known to cause brain injury.

Wilson's Disease (hepatolenticular degeneration) is an inborn error of metabolism characterized by abnormal copper accumulation causing mental deterioration (*Wilson SA. Progressive lenticular degeneration: A familial nervous disease associated with cirrhosis of the liver. Brain 34:296, 1912*).

Manganese:

Chronically excessive exposure is associated with an increased risk of dementia (*Mena I. Manganese, in Bronner F, Coburn JW, Eds. Disorders of Mineral Metabolism. I. Trace Minerals. New York, Academic Press, 1981, pp. 233-70*).

Zinc:

May be deficient.

> **Observational Study:** Of 1200 pts. over 65, the 220 senile pts. had significantly lower zinc levels than those who were not senile. Results with a younger gp. (under 65) who were just starting to show signs of senility were similar (*Hullin RP. Serum zinc in psychiatric patients. Prog. Clin. Biol. Res. 129:197-206, 1983*).

Supplementation may be beneficial in Wilson's Disease to prevent the intestinal absorption of copper (*Brewer GJ et al. Oral zinc therapy for Wilson's disease. Ann. Intern. Med. 99:314-20, 1983*).

- -

Phosphatidyl choline: 10-20 gm. daily (95% PC) (minimum 6 mo. trial)
                          (Note: The percentage of phosphatidyl choline varies between 10% and 95% in commercial "phosphatidyl choline" and "lecithin.")

Deficiency may be associated with Alzheimer's Disease.

> **Observational Study:** Among AD pts., the theoretical choline uptake into choline-depleted RBC's was strongly correlated with the severity of the dementia (*Kanof P. Red blood cell choline. Biol. Psychiat. 20:375-83, 1985*).

Supplementation may be beneficial.

> **Review Article:** Recent short-term lecithin studies and a single dose study failed to demonstrate clinically significant improvement in cognitive functioning and are consistent with earlier trials with choline and lecithin. The 6-month studies, however, suggest that lecithin may be useful in retarding the rate of disease progression. These results are preliminary and need to be replicated in even

longer term clinical trials (*Dysken M. A review of recent clinical trials in the treatment of Alzheimer's dementia. Psychiatric Annals 17(3):178, 1987*).

Experimental Double-blind Study: 51 pts. with early AD received either the maximal tolerated daily dose of 90% pure phosphatidyl choline (20-25 gm) or placebo. After 6 months, there was only a "tendency" in favor of better outcome among the experimental gp.; however, those who took less than the prescribed dose did the best (with moderate improvements in orientation, learning and memory at 4 months), suggesting that (as with physostigmine) there may be a narrow therapeutic window. In addition, these poor compliers were an ave. of 79 years old compared to an average of 69 years of age for the good compliers. This is consistent with reports that AD involves multiple neurotransmitter defects in younger pts., but is limited to cholinergic dysfunction in older pts. (*Little A et al. A double-blind, placebo controlled trial of high-dose lecithin in Alzheimer's Disease J. Neurol. Neurosurg. & Psychiat. 48:736-42, 1985*).

Experimental Double-blind Crossover Study: 13 AD pts. received placebo and 95% phosphatidyl choline in a 6 month trial, with the dose of phosphatidyl choline ranging from 10-20 gm. per day. Although the PC did not reduce symptoms, 12/13 pts. showed no evidence of deterioration over the study period; thus PC may delay the rate of progression of the disease (*Weintraub S et al. Lecithin in the treatment of Alzheimer's disease. Arch. Neurol. 40:527, 1983*).

Negative Double-blind Experimental Study: 21 pts. received lecithin 25 gm daily or placebo. Equal improvement was noted in both groups, and serum lecithin levels 12-14 hrs. after administration were not increased with supplementation (*Fisman M et al. Double blind study of lecithin in patients with Alzheimer's disease. Can. J. Psychiat. 26:426-28, 1981*).

Double-blind Experimental Study: 10 pts. who met DSM-III criteria for primary degenerative dementia received lecithin (95% phosphatidyl choline) mixed with milk and flavoring in doses of 4, 12, and 20 gm/day. Pts. received all 3 doses plus placebo for 1 wk. each. After the 4 wks., the best dose was chosen for each pt. and a replication phase was conducted in which pts. received both the best dose and placebo in a counterbalanced order for 1 week. Despite increases in plasma and RBC choline levels, there was no improvement in memory test performance with lecithin. One pt., however, did have considerably better performance with 20 gm daily of lecithin (the least impaired pt. in the sample). During the replication phase this patient's level of performance improved again on 20 gm/day of lecithin compared to a second placebo trial (*Brinkman SD et al. A dose-ranging study of lecithin in the treatment of primary degenerative dementia (Alzheimer disease). Brief Reports 2:281-85, 1982*).

Animal Experimental Study: Marked behavioral differences were found between elderly mice placed on choline-enriched versus choline-deficient diets for 4 1/2 months, with the choline-enriched mice performing as well as young mice and the choline-deficient mice performing as poorly as senescent mice (*Bartus R et al. Age related changes in passive avoidance retention: modulation with dietary choline. Science 209:301-3, 1980*).

See Also:

> *Etienne P et al. Alzheimer disease: Lack of effect of lecithin treatment for 3 months. Neurology 31:1552, 1981*

- -

OTHER FACTORS:

Avoid aluminum exposure.

The causative role of aluminum is currently controversial.

Positive evidence:

Animal Experimental Study (rabbits):   Aluminum exposure caused neurofibrillary tangles (*King RG. Do raised aluminum levels in Alzheimer's Dementia contribute to cholinergic neuronal deficits? Med. Hypoth. 14:301-6, 1984*).

Observational Study: 18 adults with memory loss were found to have elevated serum aluminum levels (*Howard JMH. Clinical import of small increases in serum aluminum. Clin. Chem. 30(10):1722-3, 1984*).

Experimental Controlled Study: 6 AD pts. received injections of the aluminum-chelating agent desferoxamine for 4-24 months. While 11 controls showed continued deterioration, the experimental pts. had slower deterioration, and even improved in some cases (*McLachlan DR et al. Aluminum and neurodegenerative disease: Therapeutic implications. Am. J. Kidney Dis. 6(5):322-29, 1985*).

Review Article: The level of tetrahydrobiopterin, the rate-limiting co-factor in the synthesis of many neurotransmitters, is significantly reduced in AD and aluminum is known to inhibit its production at levels commonly found in pts. (*Leeming RJ, Pheasant AE. The role of tetrahydrobiopterin in neurological disease: A review. J. Ment. Defic. Res. 25:231-41, 1981*).

Negative evidence:

Although it concentrates in the senile plaques and NFT of AD pts., aluminum is not consistently elevated in the brain, the hair, the serum or the cerebrospinal fluid. In addition, the nuclei of neurons in the brains of both AD pts. and healthy elderly controls may contain focal aluminum concentrations (*Hershey CO et al. Cerebrospinal fluid trace element content in dementia: Clinical, radiologic, and pathologic correlations. Neurol. 33:1350-3, 1983; Shore D, Wyatt RJ. J. Nerv. Ment. Dis. 171:553-8, 1983*).

No experimental antialuminum therapy has shown any effect on the rate of progression or degree of AD symptoms (*Shore & Wyatt - ibid*).

Note: see Mclachlan D (op cit) which claims success for such an experimental antialuminum therapy.

Many medical conditions increase brain aluminum without producing senile dementia or neuronal degeneration typical of AD (*Shore & Wyatt - ibid*).

DEPRESSION

See Also: BIPOLAR DISORDER
"HYPOGLYCEMIA"
INSOMNIA
ORGANIC MENTAL DISORDER
PREMENSTRUAL SYNDROME

OVERVIEW:

1. Deficiencies of biotin, folic acid, pyridoxine, riboflavin, thiamine, vitamin B_{12} and vitamin C are associated with depression.

2. Deficiencies of calcium, iron, magnesium and potassium are associated with depression.

3. Excesses of magnesium and vanadium are associated with depression.

4. Supplementation with the amino acids phenylalanine, tryptophan and tyrosine, which are nutritional precursors of the neurotransmitters nor-epinephrine and serotonin, may be beneficial.

- -

NUTRIENTS:

Biotin:

Deficiency may cause depression as part of a syndrome.

Case Report: Pt. on total parenteral nutrition developed depression along with nausea and vomiting, insomnia, paresthesias, headaches and lethargy. Within 5 days after being supplemented with biotin 300 mcg daily, he began to improve and quickly returned to his previous state (*Levenson JL. J. Parenteral & Enteral Nutr. 7(2):181-3, 1983*).

Experimental Study: 4 normal subjects received a diet deficient only in biotin. After 10 wks., they were depressed, fatigued, sleepy and complained of nausea, anorexia and muscular pains. Also noted were dry skin, anemia, hypercholesterolemia, hyperaesthesiae and paresthesiae. The findings were identical to those of thiamine deficiency. All signs and symptoms were relieved by biotin supplementation (*Sydenstricker VP et al. Observations on the 'egg white' injury in man. JAMA 118:1199-1200, 1940*).

Folic Acid:

Depression is a common symptom of folate deficiency (*Abou-Saleh MT, Coppen A. The biology of folate in depression; Implications for nutritional hypotheses of the psychoses. J. Psychiat. Res. 20(2):91-101, 1986*).

Observational Study: In a series of 48 in-patients, serum folate levels in depressed pts. were significantly lower than in non-depressed pts. who were either medically or psychiatrically ill, and they were negatively correlated with the degree of depression (*Ghadirian AM et al. Folic acid deficiency and depression. Psychosomatics 21(11):926-9, 1980*).

Observational Study: Epileptic children on anti-convulsants who showed evidence of depression and neurotic disturbances had significantly lower red cell folate values than the rest of the population (*Trimble MR. J. Neurol. Neurosurg. & Psychiat. vol. 43, no. 11, 1980*).

See Also:

> *Reynolds EH et al. Folate deficiency in depressive illness. Brit. J. Psychiat. 117:287-92, 1970*

Supplementation may be beneficial, especially if deficient.

Experimental Double-blind Study: 42 pts. with affective disorders on lithium therapy received either folic acid 200 mcg or placebo. After 1 yr., there was a small but insignificant change in the affective morbidity index (AMI) in both groups, and unipolar pts. receiving folate showed a small but significant reduction in their average Beck depression scores. When the supplemented pts. were divided into 2 gps. according to their AMI scores, those with lower AMI scores had significantly higher mean end-of-trial folate concentrations than those with higher scores. Also, when the pts. were divided into 2 gps. according to their end-of-trial folate concentrations, those with the higher folate concentrations had lower mean AMI scores than those with lower concentrations (results not significant). A similar trend was found when Beck depression scores were used. Analysis of the combined results of both placebo and active treatment gps. for unipolar pts. revealed that those with high folate concentrations had a significant reduction (over 40%) in their AMI scores over the trial period (*Coppen A. Folic acid enhances lithium prophylaxis. J. Affective Disord. 10:9-13, 1986*).

Review Article: The authors' studies suggest that the only cases of depression associated with folate deficiency which will respond to supplementation are those which are secondary to easy fatigability (*Botez MI et al. Neuropsychological correlates of folic acid deficiency: Facts and hypotheses, in Botez MI, Reynolds, Eds. Folic Acid in Neurology, Psychiatry, and Internal Medicine. New York, Raven Press, 1979*).

Pyridoxine: 100 - 500 mg. daily

An important coenzyme in the production of monoamine neurotransmitters (MAO inhibitors may cause deficiency).

Necessary for the conversion of tryptophan into serotonin, a neurotransmitter which, when deficient, may cause depression (*see "L-Tryptophan" below*).

May be deficient, especially in depressed patients.

Observational Study: Pyridoxine deficiency was found in 21/101 medically cleared, depressed patients. 14/101 also had mild neurologic symptoms (numbness, paresthesias, and "electric shock" sensations) which were associated with deficient pyridoxine levels (*Stewart JW et al. Low B6 levels in depressed outpatients. Biol. Psychiat. 19(4):613-616, 1984*).

Observational Study: In a study of 172 successive psychiatric hospital admissions, pyridoxine deficiency (red cell aspartate transaminase) and riboflavin deficiency (glutathione reductase) were associated with a diagnosis of affective disorder, suggesting that affective changes are characteristic of these deficiencies (*Carney MW et al. Thiamine, riboflavin and pyridoxine deficiency in psychiatric in-patients. Br. J. Psychiat. 141:271-72, 1982*).

Observational Study: Deficiency (raised red cell aspartate transaminase) correlated specificially with endogenous depression versus other psychiatric diagnoses among hospitalized psychiatric patients (*Carney M et al. Thiamin and pyridoxine lack in newly-admitted psychiatric patients. Br. J. Psychiat. 135:249-254, 1979*).

Observational Study: Compared to normal controls, 1/23 pts. had conclusive evidence of pyridoxal phosphate deficiency, while 3/23 had suggestive evidence (*Nobbs B. Pyridoxal phosphate status in clinical depression. Letter to the Editor. Lancet 1:405, 1974*).

See Also:

> Russ C et al. *Vitamin B₆ status of depressed and obsessive-compulsive patients.* *Nutr. Rep. Intl.* 27:867-73, 1983

By blocking the activity of pyridoxine (required for the synthesis of serotonin) and accelerating the metabolism of tryptophan (making it less available for conversion into serotonin), estrogens can cause depression due to their effects on serotonin metabolism. Supplementation with pyridoxine may thus be beneficial for depressed women whose pyridoxine deficiencies are due to birth control pills or other causes of relative estrogen excess.

Review Article: Studies carried out over the last 15 yrs. have provided evidence that supplementation with estro-progestational hormones may be accompanied by increased urinary excretion of tryptophan metabolites, as happens in pyridoxine deficiency. Evaluation of pyridoxine levels in humans have confirmed an impaired status in women using hormonal contraception, and disturbances in tryptophan metabolism have been shown to be responsible for depression, anxiety, decrease in libido and impairment of glucose tolerance in some of the oral contraceptive users. Administration of 40 mg of vitamin B_6 daily not only restores normal biochemical values but also relieves the clinical symptoms in those vitamin B_6 deficiency women taking oral contraceptives (*Bermond P. Therapy of side effects of oral contraceptive agents with vitamin B₆. Acta Vitaminol. Enzymol. 4(1-2):45-54, 1982*).

Experimental Placebo-controlled Study: 19/39 depressed women on oral contraceptives had an absolute deficiency of pyridoxine. When they were given pyridoxine supplements, 16 of the 19 pyridoxine-deficient women improved in mood (as demonstrated by Beck depression scores) compared to only 8/20 depressed controls, while there was no difference in response to placebo between depressed pyridoxine-deficient women vs. depressed controls (*Adams PW et al. Vitamin B₆, depression, and oral contraception. Letter to the Editor. Lancet 2:516-17, 1974*).

Riboflavin:

Deficiency may be asssociated with depression.

Observational Study: In a study of 172 successive psychiatric hospital admissions, pyridoxine deficiency (red cell aspartate transaminase) and riboflavin deficiency (glutathione reductase) were associated with a diagnosis of affective disorder, suggesting that affective changes are characteristic of these deficiencies (*Carney MW et al. Thiamine, riboflavin and pyridoxine deficiency in psychiatric in-patients. Br. J. Psychiat. 141:271-72, 1982*).

Thiamine:

Depression and irritability are common in thiamine deficiency.

Experimental Study: 5/9 normal subjects placed on thiamine-deficient diets developed marked depression and irritability (*Brozek J. Psychologic effects of thiamine restriction and deprivation in normal young men. Am. J. Clin. Nutr. 5(2):109-20, 1957*).

Vitamin B₁₂:

A vitamin B_{12} deficiency may cause depression, even in the absence of anemia (*Zucker DK et al. B_{12} deficiency and psychiatric disorders: Case report and literature review. Biol. Psychiat. 16:197-205, 1981*).

<u>Vitamin C</u>:   1000 mg. daily

Chronic depression, tiredness, irritability and vague ill-health can be part of a sub-scorbutic state.

> **Observational Study:** In a study of 885 psychiatric pts., the ave. plasma vitamin C level was 0.51 mg/100 ml compared to 0.87/100 ml in 110 healthy controls. 32% of the psychiatric pts. had levels below the threshold (0.35 mg/100 ml) which has been associated with detrimental effects on immune responses and behavior (*Schorah CJ et al. Human Nutr.:Clin. Nutr. 37C:447-52, 1983*).

> **Experimental Double-blind Study:** 40 chronic male psychiatric pts. (4 with Bipolar Disorder, 2 with Tertiary Syphillis and 34 with Schizophrenia) randomly received either ascorbic acid 1 gm daily or placebo. After 3 wks., there was a significant decrease in the MMPI "D" (depression) scale (p less than 0.01) only for the experimental group. The nurse felt that 5 pts. had obviously improved and the doctor agreed in regard to 4 of them; all 5 turned out to be in the experimental group. The 24-hour ascorbic acid urinary excretion in the control gp. was at the very lowest limit of normal. While normal subjects can be saturated with ascorbic acid after 1-2 days of supplementation with 1 gm daily, pts. with borderline or frank scurvy require 7-10 days and the pts. in this study required an ave. of 6 days. These findings suggest that chronic psychiatric pts. may be in a state of "subscurvy" and thus could benefit from ascorbic acid supplementation (*Milner G. Ascorbic acid in chronic psychiatric patients: A controlled trial. Brit. J. Psychiat. 109:294-99, 1963*).

> **Observational Study:** Over 10% of 465 hospitalized psychiatric pts. in Essex, England showed delayed ascorbic acid saturation (seventh day of loading or later) which indicates borderline or actual scurvy. Most of these pts. had obvious clinical signs of the scorbutic state (*Leitner ZA, Church IC. Nutritional studies in a mental hospital. Lancet 1:565-67, 1956*).

- -

<u>Calcium</u>:

For the treatment of depression, supplementation may be especially effective for post-menopausal and puerperal depressions and the elderly (*Crammer J. Lithium, calcium, and mental illness. Letter to the Editor. Lancet 1:215-16, 1975*).

<u>Iron</u>:

Depression is part of the deficiency syndrome.

> **Review Article:** Chronic deficiency (most commonly in women due to menstruation) is known to be associated with depression which is one of the last signs to resolve months after hemoglobin levels have normalized and appears to be associated with a marked depression of monamine oxidase activity (*Parker SD. Depression and nutrition: Anemia and glucose imbalances. Anabolism Jan.-Feb., 1984*).

<u>Magnesium</u>:

Deficiency is associated with depression.

> **Observational Study:** In a study of CSF calcium and magnesium concentrations in 41 hospitalized pts. with major depression, schizophrenic disorder or adjustment disorder and 15 neurological controls, CSF magnesium (but not calcium) was significantly lower in pts. who had made suicide attempts irrespective of the diagnosis and significantly correlated with CSF 5-HIAA, suggesting that magnesium may be necessary in maintaining normal serotonergic activity in the CNS (*Banki CM et al. Cerebrospinal fluid magnesium and calcium related to amine metabolites, diagnosis, and suicide attempts. Biol. Psychiat. 20:163-171, 1985*).

Observational Study: Many pts. with depression of unknown cause were found to have reduced total plasma magnesium levels (*Hall RCW, Joffe JR. Hypomagnesemia: Physical and psychiatric-symptoms. JAMA 224:1749-51, 1973*).

Observational Study: Plasma magnesium was significantly lower in depressed pts. than in 12 controls (*Frizel D et al. Plasma calcium and magnesium in depression. Br. J. Psychiat. 115:1375-77, 1969*).

Elevation in plasma levels may be associated with depression.

Observational Study: Mean plasma magnesium levels in depressed pts. was higher than in controls (*Bj:orum N. Electrolytes in blood in endogenous depression. Acta Psychiatr. Scand. 48:59-68, 1972*).

Observational Study: 8 depressed pts. had raised plasma magnesium levels both before and after recovery compared to 15 controls (*Cade JFJA. A significant elevation of plasma magnesium levels in schizophrenia and depressive states. Med. J. Austr. 1:195-96, 1964*).

Potassium:

Hypokalemia is frequently associated with a dysphoric mood, tearfulness, weakness, and fatigue. Not uncommonly, a frank organic brain syndrome may also be noted. Decreased intracellar potassium has been noted in depressed pts. compared to controls and pts. who have suicided have been found to have decreased cerebral potassium (*Webb WL, Gehi M. Electrolyte and fluid imbalance: Neuropsychiatric manifestations. Psychosomatics 22(3):199-203, 1981*).

Depressed pts. may have decreased intracellular potassium despite normal plasma levels.

Observational Study: Even though plasma potassium and sodium levels were normal, depressed pts. were found to demonstrate a loss of intracellular potassium and a retention of intracellular sodium (*Cox JR et al. Changes in sodium, potassium and fluid spaces in depression and dementia. Gerontology Clin. 13:232-245, 1971*).

Vanadium:

Vanadium toxicity is known to be associated with depression and melancholia.

Experimental Study: *Witkowska D, Brzezinski, J. Alteration of brain noradrenaline, dopamine and 5-hydroxy-tryptamine levels during vanadium poisoning. Pol. J. Pharacol. Pharm. 31:393-8, 1979*).

Vanadium has been shown to be a powerful inhibitor of Na^+-K^+-ATPase activity (*Cantley LC et al. Vanadate is a potent (Na,K)-ATPase inhibitor found in ATP derived from muscle. J. Biol. Chem. 252:7421-3, 1977*) which is reduced in depressive illness (*Vanadium, vitamin C and depression. Nutr. Rev. 40(10):293-5, 1981*).

- -

Omega-6 Fatty Acids:

Evening Primrose Oil is a rich source of GLA, a precursor to prostaglandin E_1 (dosage: 1 gm 3 times daily)

Prostaglandin E_1 may be deficient in depression.

Observational Study: 29/30 pts. had increased PGE_2 levels and 30/30 had increased TXB_2 levels compared to normal controls. Based on this study and other literature, the authors suggest that depression may be partly caused by decreased levels of PGE$_1$ and increased levels of PGE$_2$ (*Lieb J et al. Prostagl. Leukotrienes & Med. 10:361-7, 1983*).

D-Phenylalanine:

Can be decarboxylated to phenylethylamine (PEA) which has amphetamine-like stimulatory properties (found in high quantities in chocolate).

Supplementation may be beneficial.

> **Review Article:** There is some evidence from published studies on D-phenylalanine that it is active in a substantial part of pts. with affective disorders (*Beckmann H. Phenylalanine in affective disorders. Adv. Biol. Psychiat. 10:137-47, 1983*).

D,L-Phenylalanine: 150-200 mg. daily (1 month trial)

Supplementation may be beneficial.

> **Review Article:** There is some evidence from published studies on D,L-phenylalanine that it is active in a substantial part of pts. with affective disorders (*Beckmann H. Phenylalanine in affective disorders. Adv. Biol. Psychiat. 10:137-47, 1983*).

> **Experimental Double-blind Study:** 14 depressed pts. received D,L phenylalanine 150-200 mg daily, while 13 received imipramine 150-200 mg daily. After 30 days no significant difference could be found between the 2 groups   (*Beckmann H et al. DL-phenylalanine versus imipramine: A double-blind controlled study. Arch. Psychiat. Nervenkr. 227:49-58, 1979*).

> **Experimental Study:** 20 pts. received D,L-phenylalanine 75-200 mg daily. After 20 days, 8 pts. had a complete recovery, 4 had a good response, 4 with partially untypical depressions experienced mild-moderate response, and 4 failed to respond (*Beckmann H et al. DL-phenylalanine in depressed patients: An open study. J. Neural Transm. 41(2-3):123-34, 1977*).

L-Phenylalanine: Start with 500 mg. daily and increase dosage as needed (average of 3-4 gms. daily)
                              (2-6 month trial)

Precursor of L-tyrosine.

Can be decarboxylated to phenylethylamine (PEA) an amphetamine-like neurotransmitter which is found in high quantities in chocolate.

- with pyridoxine 200 mg.:

Pyridoxine is necessary to convert L-phenylalanine to phenylethylamine(PEA).

Supplementation may be beneficial.

> **Experimental Study:** 40 pts. with major depression (32 unipolar depressives) were supplemented with L-phenylalanine and vitamin B$_6$. Treatment was initiated with 500 mg L-PA in the morning and at noon along with B$_6$ 100 mg twice daily, and the L-PA dosage was increased by 500 mg daily until therapeutic or side effects developed, or to a limit of 2-3 gm over the previous dose at 1 wk. intervals (gp. mean = 3-4 gm daily). 31/40 improved "almost immediately" and 10 of the responders were completely relieved of depression. 7/8 (88%) of the bipolar depressives responded and most of the 24/32 (75%) unipolar depressives who responded had "soft" signs of bipolarity (strong impulsive tendencies, hypersomnia, and family histories of bipolar illness), suggesting that supplementation is effective primarily for bipolar depressions.

Side effects were slight, transient headaches, constipation, transient nausea, insomnia and increased anxiety. Prior to supplementation, the 23 drug-free depressives were found to have significantly lower PAA urinary excretion than normals (PAA is a PEA metabolite). During supplementation, urinary PAA excretion rose in tandem with their spirits (*Sabelli HC et al. Clinical studies on the phenylethylamine hypothesis of affective disorder: Urine and blood phenylacetic acid and phenylalanine dietary supplements. J. Clin. Psychiat. 47(2):66-70, 1986; Phenylalanine: A psychoactive nutrient for some depressives? Med. World News October 27, 1983*).

L-Tryptophan: 4 - 6 gms daily
Avoid protein for 90 minutes before & after.
Take with sugar (insulin improves absorption by lowering levels of competing amino acids).

May be decreased in depression.

Observational Study: The ratio of tryptophan to the amino acids competing with it for brain entry was lower in depressed alcoholic pts. than in both non-depressed alcoholic pts. and normal controls (*Branchey L. et al. Relationship between changes in plasma amino acids and depression in alcoholic patients. Am. J. Psychiat. 141:1212-1215, 1984*).

Observational Study: Compared to normal volunteers, 50 hospitalized females with primary unipolar depression were found to have significantly decreased free plasma tryptophan. Recovered depressives had significantly lower tryptophan levels than controls, and recovered pts. who were not on antidepressants significantly increased tryptophan levels (*Coppen A, Wood K. Tryptophan and depressive illness. Psychological Med. 8:49-57, 1978*).

Observational Study: In a study of 18 women with puerperal depression, those with the most severe depressions had the lowest tryptophan levels (*Stein G et al. Relationship between mood disturbances and free and total plasma tryptophan in postpartum women. Brit. Med. J. 2:457, 1976*).

Supplementation may be effective.

Review Article: 8 studies on the action of tryptophan in pts. who were unipolar or of uncertain polarity were reviewed. Although 5 reported improvement in the majority of pts., they lacked control measures; thus no therapeutic effect has yet been demonstrated when tryptophan is given alone. (*Chouinard G et al. Tryptophan in the treatment of depression and mania. Adv. Biol. Psychiat. 10:47-66, 1983*).

Review Article: Doses of 6 gm or slightly less seem most effective for unipolar depressives as negative studies have tended to use larger doses and positive studies have used doses in this range (*Walinder J. Combination of tryptophan with MAO inhibitors, tricyclic antidepressants and selective 5-HT reuptake inhibitors. Adv. Biol. Psychiat. 10:82-93, 1983*).

See Also:

Young SN et al. Tryptophan in the treatment of depression. Adv. Exp. Med. Biol. 133:727-37, 1981

- with a monamine oxidase inhibitor:

Data from 4 studies indicate that tryptophan will potentiate the action of a monamine-oxidase inhibitor (*Chouinard G - op cit*). However, toxic reactions have been reported (*Pope HG et al. Toxic reactions to the combination of monamine oxidase inhibitors and tryptophan. Am. J. Psychiat. 142(4):491-2, 1985*).

- with a <u>tricyclic antidepressant</u>:

> May be useful as a potentiating agent (*Walinder J. Combination of tryptophan with MAO inhibitors, tricyclic antidepressants and selective 5-HT reuptake inhibitors. <u>Adv. Biol. Psychiat.</u> 10:82-93, 1983*).

<u>L-Tyrosine</u>:   2 gms. 3 times daily (100 mg./kg.) (2 wk. trial)

> Give with carbohydrates, as insulin lowers peripheral levels of competing amino acids by 2/3 (*Wurtman RJ.- quoted in <u>Med.World News</u> January 26, 1984*).

Supplementation may be beneficial.

> **Experimental Double-blind Study:** 3/5 unipolar drug-free pts. had at least a 50% reduction in the Hamilton depression scale after 4 wks. of supplementation with tyrosine 100 mg/kg daily in 3 divided doses compared to 1/4 controls receiving placebo. 2 placebo pts. were withdrawn due to deterioration of their condition. The reduction in depression rating score was positively correlated with the increase in fasting plasma tyrosine (p less than 0.1), suggesting that an adequate tyrosine level was necessary for improvement. There were no side effects except for mild gastric upset when tyrosine was taken without food (*Gibson CJ, Gelenberg A. Tyrosine for the treatment of depression. <u>Adv. Biol. Psychiat.</u> 10:148-159, 1983*).

> **Experimental Double-blind Case Study:** 30 year-old female with unipolar depression received tyrosine 100 mg/kg (6 gms) in 3 divided doses daily. After 2 wks. depression had been alleviated but she rapidly deteriorated when crossed over to placebo. Depression was alleviated once again when switched back to tyrosine (*Gelenberg AJ et al. <u>Am. J. Psychiat.</u> 137:622-3, 1980*).

> **Experimental Study:** After 2 amphetamine-dependent depressed pts. who had failed to respond to tricyclics, MAO inhibitors and electoconvulsive therapy were given tyrosine, one was able to eliminate amphetamines completely, while the other was able to decrease the dosage by 2/3, suggesting that a noradrenaline deficiency was corrected (*Goldberg IK. L-tyrosine in depression. Letter to the Editor. <u>Lancet</u> 2:364, 1980*).

- -

COMBINED SUPPLEMENTATION:

<u>L-5-Hydroxytryptophan</u> plus
<u>L-Tyrosine</u>:

> **Review Article:** After many double-blind studies, the author has concluded that L-5-hydroxytryptophan 200 mg daily combined with carbidopa 150 mg daily (a peripheral decarboxylase inhibitor) or L-tyrosine is an effective treatment for depression because it enhances both 5HT and catecholamine metabolism. L-tryptophan 5 gm daily, which increased only 5HT metabolism, was no more effective than placebo. (*van Praag HM. Studies in the mechanism of action of serotonin precursors in depression. <u>Psychopharm. Bull.</u> 20(3):599-602, 1984*).

- -

OTHER FACTORS :

Rule out <u>food sensitivities</u>.

> Provocative testing with foods and food extracts has been reported to induce depression as well as other mental symptoms.

Review Article: Foods may cause mental and behavioral symptoms by a variety of mechanisms including cerebral allergy, food addiction, hypoglycemias, caffeinism, hypersensitivity to chemical food additives, reactions to vasoactive amines in foods, and reactions to neuropeptides formed from foods (*Rippere V. Some varieties of food intolerance in psychiatric patients: An overview. Nutr. Health 3(3):125-36, 1984*).

Negative Experimental Double-blind Study: 19 pts. with neurotic symptoms who believed their symptoms were due to food allergy were investigated with exclusion diets and open food reintroductions followed by double-blind provocation tests for foods reported to cause reactions. Testing failed to produce evidence that any of them was food-sensitive (*Pearson DJ et al. Food allergy: How much in the mind? An objective clinical and psychiatric study of suspected food hypersensitivity. Lancet 1:1259-61, 1983*).

Experimental Double-blind Study: 30 pts. complaining of psychological symptoms who were found to have elevated MMPI scores noted significantly greater cognitive-emotional symptoms when tested with foods and chemicals than when tested with placebo (*King DS. Can allergic exposure provoke psychological symptoms? a double-blind test. Biol. Psychiat. 16(1):3-19, 1981*).

Allergic disorders are more common among depressives.

Observational Study: The incidence of allergy was about 33% in a gp. of depressed pts. compared to only 2% of a control gp. of schizophrenics (*Nasr S et al. Concordance of atopic and affective disorders. J. Affect. Dis. 3:291, 1981*).

Observational Study: 85% of 109 depressed children and adults were found to be atopic (*Ossofsky HJ. Affective and atopic disorders and cyclic AMP. Compre. Psychiat. 17:335, 1976*).

Tricyclic antidepressants are potent anti-histamines and this property may help to explain their effectiveness (*Richelson E. Pharmacology of antidepressants in use in the United States. J. Clin. Psychiat. 43:4, 1982; Hoffer A. Allergy, depression and tricyclic antidepressants. J. Ortho. Psychiat. 9(3):164-70, 1980*).

Rule out hydrochloric acid deficiency.

Case Report: Pt. with 17 year history of endogenous depression and signs suggestive of vitamin deficiency showed a dramatic response to hydrochloric acid given before meals along with vitamin B complex (*Keuter EJW. Nutr. Abs. Rev. 29:273, 1959*).

DERMATITIS HERPETIFORMIS

See Also: CELIAC DISEASE

NUTRIENTS:

<u>Para Amino Benzoic Acid:</u>   200 mg. four to five times daily

Supplementation may be beneficial.

Experimental Study: PABA was a successful treatment, even in pts. who were not controlling their intake of gluten (*Zarafonetis CJD et al. Paraaminobenzoic acid in dermatitis herpetiformis.* <u>*Arch. Dermatol. Syph.*</u> *63:115-132, 1951*).

- -

<u>Selenium:</u>

May be deficient.

Observational Study: The glutathione peroxidase level of 72 pts. was significantly lower than that of controls (p less than 0.001) (*Juhlin L et al. Blood glutathione-peroxidase levels in skin diseases: Effect of selenium and vitamin E treatment.* <u>*Acta Dermatovener (Stockholm)*</u> *62:211-14, 1982*).

- -

OTHER FACTORS:

Rule out <u>food sensitivities</u>.

Reference (<u>hypoallergenic diet</u>):

van der Meer JB et al. Rapid improvement of dermatitis herpetiformis after elemental diet. <u>*Arch. Dermatol. Res.*</u> *271:455, 1981*

References (<u>gluten</u>):

Review Article: A gluten-free diet is the therapy of choice. IgG, IgA and IgM antibodies against gliadin (the principal protein in gluten-containing grains) have been identified in DH pts., along with elevated serum gluten levels (<u>*Int. Clin. Nutr. Rev.*</u> *4(2):100, 1984*).

Observational Study: In a study of 45 pts., morphological changes in the mucosa of the small intestine were associated with higher intakes of gluten, although gastric morphologic and functional changes also characteristic of DH (e.g. achlorhydric atrophic gastritis) did not appear to be associated with gluten intake (*Andersson H et al. Influence of the amount of dietary gluten on gastrointestinal morphology and function in dermatitis herpetiformis.* <u>*Human Nutr.: Clin. Nutr.*</u> *38C:279-85, 1984*).

Experimental Study: 12 pts. whose skin rashes had been effectively controlled for an average of over 7 yrs. without medication on a gluten-free diet were challenged with gluten. After an ave. of 12 wks., the rash returned in 11/12, suggesting that a life-long gluten-free diet is required (*Leonard J et al. Gluten challenge in dermatitis herpetiformis.* <u>*New Eng. J. Med.*</u> *308:816, 1983*).

See Also:

> *Fry L et al.   Long term follow-up of dermatitis herpetiformis with and without dietary wheat gluten withdrawal. Brit. J. Derm. 107:631-40, 1982*

> *Frodin T et al. Gluten free diet for dermatitis herpetiformis: The long term effect of cutaneous, immunological and jejunal manifestations. Acta Dermatovener 61:405, 1981*

References (milk):

Case Report: 74 year-old man with characteristic lesions, upper abdominal pain and loose stools for 10 years was treated with a milk-free diet which improved his dermatitis in less than a week but only slightly lessened his dyspepsia. Both the dermatitis and the dyspepsia were completely controlled with a gluten and milk-free diet, while reintroduction of milk and milk proteins caused recurrence of the dermatitis. After 4 mo. of a gluten-free diet, reintroduction of gluten no longer provoked recurrence of the dermatitis (*Engquist A, Pock-Steen OC. Dermatitis herpetiformis and milk-free diet. Lancet 2:438, 1971*).

Case Report: Pt. improved on a gluten and milk-free diet, although only milk provocation resulted in recurrence of the dermatitis (*Pock-Steen OC, Niordson AM. Milk sensitivity in dermatitis herpetiformis. Brit. J. Dermatol. 83:614-19, 1970*).

Rule out hydrochloric acid deficiency.

> *Note: While gastric anacidity had been reported in the past to be a relatively common condition which was associated with various dermatologic disorders and a number of other illnesses, the presence of achlorhydria is no longer accepted unless a potent parietal-cell stimulant (such as histamine) is employed in gastric analysis. More recent studies suggest that histamine-fast anacidity is uncommon before the fifth decade of life and, although it probably does not occur in a normal stomach, its presence is not necessarily associated with symptoms (Rappaport EM. Achlorhydria: Associated symptoms and response to hydrochloric acid. New Engl. J. Med. 252(19):802-5, 1955).*

Observational Study: 4 pts. underwent a fractional gastric analysis following a routine Ewald test meal. Hypoacidity was defined as values for total and free acids of 1/2 normal or less, while hyperacidity was defined as values 10-15 points above normal or values which were relatively high at the start of the test. 3/4 (75%) of the pts. were found to have hypoacidity, while 1/4 (25%) had hyperacidity. For 1 pt., the severity of the eruption correlated with both the presence of GI symptoms and abnormal gastric secretions while, for 2 pts., the severity of the eruption correlated with abnormal gastric secretions but there were no GI complaints (*Ayres S. Gastric secretion in psoriasis, eczema and dermatitis herpetiformis. Arch. Dermatol. Syph. 20:854-57, 1929*).

DIABETES MELLITUS

See Also: ATHEROSCLEROSIS
CATARACTS
NEURALGIA and NEUROPATHY
ULCERS (ISCHEMIC)

OVERVIEW:

1. Interventions which may <u>improve glucose tolerance</u>:

Many studies have shown that <u>high fiber, high complex carbohydrate diets</u> are beneficial. While <u>sugar</u> seems to have an adverse effect, recent studies comparing the glycemic response to both simple and complex carbohydrates have suggested that each food which is rich in carbohydrates needs to be separately evaluated.

In regard to specific nutrients, the evidence for manipulating them is considerably weaker. Increasing the intake of organic <u>chromium</u> either separately or by supplementing with high-chromium <u>brewer's yeast</u> is best documented. Limited controlled studies also suggest that <u>biotin</u> and <u>pyridoxine alpha-ketoglutarate</u> may be beneficial. Many other nutrients have been found to be beneficial, but the evidence is generally anecdotal.

Deficiencies of several minerals have been shown to have an adverse effect. Deficiencies of <u>chromium</u>, <u>copper</u>, <u>manganese</u> and <u>zinc</u> are associated with glucose intolerance, while deficiencies of <u>phosphorus</u> and <u>potassium</u> are associated with insulin resistance.

2. Interventions which may <u>reduce diabetic complications</u>:

A. Neuropathy:

Supplementation with several of the B complex vitamins has been reported to be beneficial. In uncontrolled studies, increasing <u>inositol</u> has been followed by improved sensory nerve function and evoked nerve action potential amplitudes, although there were no benefits in a double-blind study of inositol supplementation. <u>Pyridoxine</u> is lower in pts. with neuropathy, and pts. with B_6 deficiency noted pain relief following B_6 supplementation in an uncontrolled study. There is also very preliminary evidence that <u>niacin</u> and <u>vitamin B_{12}</u> may be beneficial.

B. Nephropathy:

The development of nephropathy was retarded in rats made diabetic with streptozotocin when they were supplemented with <u>nicotinamide</u>, but evidence is lacking that human diabetics would also benefit from supplementation.

C. Retinopathy:

<u>Magnesium</u> is particularly low in diabetics with proliferative retinopathy, but it is not known if supplementation would be beneficial.

D. Microangiopathy:

There is reason to believe that a marginal <u>vitamin C</u> deficiency may contribute to the development of microangiopathy. Similarly, a <u>phosphorus</u> deficiency may be detrimental, but studies demonstrating benefit from supplementation with these nutrients are lacking.

- -

> *KEY: A = may benefit microangiopathy*
> *G = may improve glucose tolerance*
> *K = may benefit nephropathy*
> *N = may benefit neuropathy*
> *R = may benefit retinopathy*

- -

BASIC DIET:

High <u>complex carbohydrate</u> diet.
(G)

Review Article: Diets that are proportionally high in carbohydrates have been shown to improve blood glucose control by enhancing insulin sensitivity, provided adequate insulin is present (*Chait A. Dietary management of diabetes mellitus. <u>Contemp. Nutr.</u> 9(2), February, 1984*).

Review Article: A diet high in complex carbohydrates is advisable for virtually all diabetics (*Special report: Principles of nutrition and dietary recommendations for individuals with diabetes mellitus: 1979. <u>Diabetes</u> 28:1027-30, 1979*).

High <u>fiber</u> diet.
(G)

Associated with improved glucose tolerance.

Review Article: With a high fiber diet, diabetics can eventually decrease their insulin or tablet medication (*Philipson H. Dietary fibre in the diabetic diet. <u>Acta Med. Scand.</u> (suppl.) 671:91-93, 1983*).

Experimental Study: 10 pts. were placed on a high-fiber diet using readily available, low-cost foodstuffs. Although only 3 pts. approached the projected dietary fiber intake, after 3 mo. significant correlations were found between the mean plasma glucose changes and the dietary fiber contents (p less than 0.05) and between the mean serum triglyceride changes and the dietary fiber increments (p less than 0.05) (*Rosman MS. The effect of long-term high-fibre diets in diabetic outpatients. <u>S. Afr. Med. J.</u> 63(9):310-13, 1983*).

Observational Study: Diabetes is rare in African villagers who eat large amounts of fiber but is common in Western countries where people eat fiber-depleted diets (*Trowell HC. Dietary-fiber hypothesis of the etiology of diabetes mellitus. <u>Diabetes</u> 24(8):762-65, 1975*).

See Also:

Kay RM et al. Diets rich in natural fibre improve carbohydrate tolerance in maturity-onset, non-insulin dependent diabetics. <u>Diabetologia</u> 20:12-23, 1981

Rivellese A et al. Effect of dietary fibre on glucose control and serum lipoproteins in diabetic patients. <u>Lancet</u> 2:447, 1980

Specific Fibers:

<u>Guar Gum:</u>

Experimental Study: Guar reduced both plasma glucose and insulin responses to an oral glucose load, and delayed gastric emptying. Glucose absorption was significantly reduced during perfusion of the jejunum with guar, but returned to control values during subsequent guar-free perfusions, suggesting that guar improves glucose tolerance predominantly by reducing glucose absorption in the small intestine, probably by inhibiting the effects of intestinal motility of fluid convection (*Blackburn NA et al. Mechanism of action of guar gum in improving glucose tolerance in man.* <u>Clin. Sci.</u> *66(3):329-36, 1984*).

<u>Legumes:</u>

Experimental Crossover Study: 18 non-insulin-dependent and 9 insulin-dependent diabetics were put on a high carbohydrate diet containing leguminous fiber (HL) for 6 wks. and a standard low carbohydrate diet (LC) for 6 wks. in random order. Preprandial and mean 2 hr. postprandial blood glucoses were significantly lower on the HL diet in both gps., as were several measures of diabetic control. In addition, total cholesterol was significantly reduced in both gps. and the HDL/LDL cholesterol ratio increased significantly in the NIDDM gp., suggesting that use of a LC diet is no longer justified (*Simpson HCR et al. A high-carbohydrate leguminous fiber diet improves all aspects of diabetic control.* <u>Lancet</u> *1:1-5, 1981*).

<u>Pectin:</u>

Experimental Study: Insulin-dependent diabetics were given a milk shake of skim milk, vanilla and 7 gms of apple pectin (equivalent to 2 apples) 10 minutes before a meal of meat, rice, cheese and bread. Following the meal 35% less insulin was required to return blood sugar levels to baseline (*Poynard T et al. Reduction of post-prandial insulin needs by pectin as assessed by the artificial pancreas in insulin-dependent diabetics.* <u>Diabete. & Metab.</u> *8(3):187-89, 1982*).

<u>Vegetarian</u> diet.
(G)

Benefits may be due to its high fiber and low fat content.

Associated with reduced risk of death from diabetes.

Observational Study: During 21 yrs. of follow-up, the risk of diabetes as an underlying cause of-death among 25,600 caucasian Seventh-day Adventists was 1/2 of the risk for all USA caucasians. Within this population, the male vegetarians (those who consumed fish rarely and meat/poultry less than once weekly) had a substantially lower risk than non-vegetarians of diabetes as an underlying or contributing cause of death. The prevalence of reported diabetes was lower for both vegetarian males and females compared to non-vegetarians. These associations were not due to differences in weight, other dietary factors or physical activity and were stronger in males than in females (*Snowdon DA, Phillips RL. Does a vegetarian diet reduce the occurrence of diabetes?* <u>Am. J. Public Health</u> *75(5):507-12, 1985*).

Restrict <u>sugar</u>.
(G,K,R)

Sucrose added to the diet of laboratory animals or increased in the diet of healthy volunteers has been shown to be associated with impaired glucose tolerance, retinopathy and nephropathy (*Cohen AM et al. Experimental models in diabetes, in <u>Sugars in Nutrition</u>. San Francisco, Academic Press, 1974, pp. 483-*

511), and reduced insulin sensitivity of the tissues (*Bruckdorfer KR et al. Insulin sensitivity of adipose tissue of rats fed with various carbohydrates. Proc. Nutr. Sci. 33:3A, 1974*).

Review Article: Sucrose alone may be a very important etiologic factor in diabetes in the 10% of the population which is carbohydrate sensitive. In the rest of the population, sucrose still must be considered an important risk factor due to its synergistic interaction with dietary cholesterol and triglycerides (*Reiser S, Szepesi B. SCOGS report on the health aspects of sucrose consumption. Letter to the Editor. Am. J. Clin. Nutr. 31:9-11, 1978*).

Like sucrose, fructose has been shown to have a hyperlipidemic effect in diabetics.

Experimental Controlled Study: 12 men with a hyperinsulinemic response to sucrose loading and suitable controls were each alternately fed a diet with either 15% fructose or starch. Fructose caused a general increase in both the total serum cholesterol and in the LDL cholesterol in most subjects in both groups, while triglycerides rose significantly only in the hyperinsulinemic group (*Hallfrisch J et al. The effects of fructose on blood lipid levels. Am. J. Clin. Nutr. 37:740-8, 1983*).

See Also:

Simko V. *Am. J. Clin. Nutr. 33:2217, 1980*

When served as part of a meal, sugar still adversely affects glucose tolerance compared to complex carbohydrates.

Experimental Study: 10 men & 8 women received diets in which 50% of calories were derived from carbohydrate or which either 35% was complex and 15% simple carbohydrates (low sugar diet) or 15% complex and 35% simple carbohydrates (high sugar diet). Summation of glucose responses 30-180 minutes following an oral GTT was significantly higher in men only after they consumed the high sugar diet. Corresponding insulin responses were significantly higher in men consuming the high-sugar compared to the low-sugar diet. Insulin binding was significantly lower during the baseline period and after the high-sugar diet compared to the low-sugar diet. Results indicate that sugars adversely affect indices of glucose tolerance when they replace complex carbohydrates even in a high-fiber, low-saturated fat diet (*Reiser S et al. Am. J. Clin. Nutr. 43:151-59, 1986*).

Negative Experimental Controlled Study: 22 pts. with either Type I or Type II diabetes were compared to 10 healthy controls. In both gps. meals containing sucrose did not produce a significantly higher rise in blood glucose compared to meals containing potato, wheat or glucose, nor was the urinary excretion of glucose greater in diabetic patients after consuming the sucrose containing meal. Peak serum insulin concentrations in controls and pts. with Type II diabetes were not significantly different in response to any one of the test carbohydrates (glucose, fructose, sucrose, potato starch and wheat starch) (*Bantle J et al. New Engl. J. Med. 309:7-12, 1983*).

Negative Experimental Controlled Study: 8 insulin-requiring diabetics and 8 normal controls were given 4 different snacks randomly on 4 different days containing high amounts of either fructose, glucose, sucrose or starch. There was no significant difference observed in the diabetics, and virtually no effect on blood sugar levels in general (*Steel JM et al. Human Nutrition: Applied Nutrition 37A:3-8, 1983*).

Sugar increases urinary chromium excretion, and glucose intolerance is a sign of chromium deficiency (*see "Chromium" below*).

Experimental Controlled Study: 37 pts. consumed sequentially for 6 wks. each a diet containing 35% of calories from complex carbohydrates and 15% from sucrose, and a diet containing 15% of calories from complex carbohydrates and 35% from sucrose. Chromium content of each diet was 16 mcg/1000 calories. 27/37 had an increase in urinary chromium excretion during the high sucrose diet compared to the low sucrose diet ranging from 10-300%, while 10/37 had no change. Absorption of chromium did not differ between the 2 diet periods (*Kozlovsky AS et al. Effects of diets high in simple sugars on urinary chromium losses. Metabolism 35:515, 1986*).

- -

COMBINED DIET:

High complex carbohydrate and plant fiber diet.
(G)

Diet is high in cereal grains, legumes and root vegetables and restricts simple sugar and fat. 70-75% of calories come from complex carbohydrates, 15-20% from protein and 5-10% from fat, with a total fiber content of almost 100 gm daily. (More information and dietary guidelines are available from: *HFC Diabetes Research Foundation, 1872 Blairmore Rd., Lexington, Ky. 40502*).

The HFC diet has led to discontinuation of insulin therapy in approx. 60% of NIDDM pts., and has significantly reduced doses in the other 40% (*Vahouny G, Kritchevsky D. Dietary Fiber in Health and Disease. New York, Plenum Press, 1982; Anderson JW, Ward K. High-carbohydrate, high-fiber diets for insulin-treated men with diabetes mellitus. Am. J. Clin. Nutr. 32:2312-21, 1979; Anderson JW. High polysaccharide diet studies in patients with diabetes and vascular disease. Cereal Foods World 22:12-22, 1977*).

- -

NUTRIENTS:

General:

Review Article: Available evidence suggests that micronutrient supplementation of antioxidants, yeast-chromium, magnesium, zinc, pyridoxine, gamma-linolenic acid, and carnitine, may aid glucose tolerance, stimulate immune defenses, and promote wound healing, while reducing the risk and severity of some of the secondary complications of diabetes (*McCarty MF, Rubin EJ. Rationales for micronutrient supplementation in diabetes. Med. Hypotheses 13(2):139-51, 1984*).

Biotin:
(G)

Works both synergistically with insulin and independently in lowering blood glucose levels.

Experimental Placebo-controlled Study: Pts. with insulin-dependent DM were removed from insulin therapy and treated with biotin 16 mg daily or placebo for 1 week. Fasting blood sugar levels fell significantly in pts. on biotin, while they rose as expected in pts. on placebo. Since biotin levels are typically elevated in diabetics, the authors speculate that it may be abnormally bound and/or biologically unavailable (*Coggeshall JC et al. Biotin status and plasma glucose in diabetics. Annals N.Y. Acad. Sci. 447:389-92, 1985*).

Myo-inositol:
(N)

Supplements have resulted in improvement in symptoms of neuropathy, perhaps because sorbitol accumulation (and the resulting adverse effects) may be a direct effect of inositol loss.

Negative Experimental Double-blind Study: 28 young diabetics received either inositol 6 gm daily or placebo. After 2 mo., there were no differences in vibratory perception threshold, motor and sensory conduction velocity or amplitude of nerve potential and muscle tissue inositol levels were unchanged (*Gregersen G et al. Oral supplementation of myoinositol: Effects on peripheral nerve function* *in human diabetics and on the concentration in plasma, erythrocytes, urine and muscle tissue in human diabetics and normals. Acta Neurol. Scand. 67:164-72, 1983).*

Experimental Study: 20 pts. with diabetic neuropathy demonstrated significant improvement in sensory nerve function after the total mean daily inositol intake was increased from 772 to 1648 mg (*Clements RS et al. Dietary myo-inositol intake and peripheral nerve function in diabetic neuropathy. Metabolism 28:477, 1979*).

Experimental Study: Diabetics supplemented with inositol 1 gm daily demonstrated substantial increases in the amplitude of evoked nerve action potentials (*Salway JG et al. Effect of myo-inositol on peripheral-nerve function in diabetes. Lancet 2:1282, 1978*).

>   *Note: Inositol content of foods is analyzed in: Clements RS, Darnell B. Myo-inositol content of common foods: Development of a high-myo-inositol diet. Am. J. Clin. Nutr. 33:1954-1967, 1980*

Niacin:
(G,K)

A component of glucose tolerance factor (GTF); thus a deficiency will interfere with GTF synthesis (*Mertz W. Effects and metabolism of glucose tolerance factor. Nutr. Rev. 33(5):129-35, 1975*).

Supplementation may retard the development of nephropathy.

Animal Experimental Study: Rats with streptozotocin-induced diabetes were supplemented with nicotinamide. Compared to controls, the development of diabetic nephropathy was retarded (*Wahlberg G et al. Protective effect of nicotinamide against nephropathy in diabetic rats. Diabetes Res. 2:307, 1985*).

Pyridoxine: 100 mg. daily
(N)

Shown to be low in diabetics, and especially low in diabetics with neuropathy.

Observational Study: Serum pyridoxal concentrations were measured in 50 pts. with diabetic neuropathy and found to be significantly lower compared with randomly selected diabetics matched for age and sex without clinical evidence of neuropathy (*McCann VJ, Davis RE. Serum pyridoxal concentrations in patients with diabetic neuropathy. Aust. N. Z. J. Med. 8:259-61, 1978*).

Supplementation may reduce symptoms of diabetic neuropathy.

Experimental Study: 10 insulin-dependent diabetics with neuropathy and signs of pyridoxine deficiency were supplemented with 50 mg pyridoxine 3 times daily. Most noted some initial relief of pain and paresthesias in about 10 days. Improvement continued throughout the experimental period with amelioration or resolution of symptoms. Each pt. noted that the eyes "felt better." After the experimental period 7/10 pts. requested to be maintained on the supplementation. Within 3 wks., those who stopped noted a recurrence of symptoms which abated when supplementation was resumed (*Jones CL, Gonzales V. Pyridoxine deficiency: A new factor in diabetic neuropathy. J. Am. Podiatry Assoc. 68(9):646-53, 1978*).

Supplementation may cure gestational diabetes.

Experimental and Observational Study: 13/14 pregnant women shown by the oral glucose tolerance test to have gestational diabetes had an increased urinary xanthurenic acid excretion after an oral tryptophan load, indicating a relative pyridoxine deficiency. All were treated with pyridoxine 100 mg daily for 14 days after which the deficiency was corrected and glucose tolerance improved considerably. Only 2/14 then had sufficiently impaired glucose tolerance to justify the diagnosis of gestational diabetes (*Coelingh Bennink HJT, Schreurs WHP. Improvement of oral glucose tolerance in gestational diabetes by pyridoxine. Brit. Med. J. 3:13-15, 1975*).

In normals, however, subclinical pyridoxine deficiency may be associated with <u>improved</u> glucose tolerance.

Observational Study: 16 clinically normal subjects with pyridoxine deficiency (diagnosed by RBC transaminase activity and the 6 hr. tryptophan loading test) were compared to 16 controls. The deficient subjects had fasting normoglycemia with hypoinsulinemia (p less than 0.01) and a normal postglucose increment to insulin, but peak blood glucose and incremental glucose were significantly lower than in the controls (p less than 0.01), suggesting enhanced sensitivity to the hypoglycemic action of insulin. Supplementation resulted in a tendency for insulin levels to rise (NS) and a significant increase in growth hormone levels. It is suggested that impairment in growth hormone reserve may be the basis for the increased insulin sensitivity (*Rao RH. Glucose tolerance in subclinical pyridoxine deficiency in man. Am. J. Clin. Nutr. 38(3):440-44, 1983*).

<u>Thiamine</u>:   100 mg. daily (2 week trial)
(N)

Required in glucose metabolism to form thiamine diphosphate which acts in the direct oxidative pathway.

Supplementation is said to decrease the symptoms of <u>sensory neuropathy</u>.

Clinical Observation: About 80% of pts. were found to improve (*Mirsky, Stanley, M.D., pres. of N.Y. affiliate of Am. Diabetes Assoc.& author of <u>Diabetes: Controlling It the Easy Way</u>, Random House, 1981.*)

<u>Vitamin B$_{12}$</u>:
(N)

Supplementation may benefit <u>neuropathy</u>.

Animal Experimental Study: 24 rats made diabetic showed muscle wasting and severe growth retardation and were found to have excessive urinary methylmalonic acid excretion but no abnormalities in the excretion of pyruvic or other ketoacids. The serum total cobalamin was almost double that of controls. Following an injection of methylcobalamin, an active form of B$_{12}$, the methylmalonic aciduria was abolished within 24 hours. Since it is known that impaired tissue availability or utilization of cobalamins may rapidly produce neurological disorders, results suggest that a disturbance in tissue cobalamin enzymes are an important factor in the development of diabetic neuropathy (*Bhatt HR et al. Can faulty vitamin B$_{12}$ (cobalamin) metabolism produce diabetic neuropathy? Letter to the Editor. Lancet 2:572, 1983*).

See Also:

> *Davidson S. The use of vitamin B$_{12}$ in the treatment of diabetic neuropathy. J. Florida Med. Assoc. 15:717-20, 1954*

> *Sancetta SM et al. The use of vitamin B$_{12}$ in the management of the neurological manifestations of diabetes mellitus, with notes on the administration of massive doses. Ann. Int. Med. 35:1028-48, 1951*

Vitamin C: 2 grams daily
(A,G)

Review Article: *Ginter EM, Chorvathova V.* Nutr. & Health *2:3-11, 1983*

Frequently low in the plasma (but not in the leukocytes) due to increased urinary excretion (*Zebrowski EJ, Bhatnagar PK. Urinary excretion pattern of ascorbic acid in streptozotocin diabetic and insulin treated rats.* Pharm. Res. Commun. *11(2):95-103, 1979*) and increased oxidation to dehydroascorbic acid (*Som S et al. Ascorbic acid metabolism in diabetes mellitus.* Metabolism *30(6):572-7, 1981*).

> *Note: Dehydroascorbic acid, whose structure is closely related to alloxan, causes diabetes mellitus in rats (Patterson JW. The diabetogenic effect of dehydroascorbic acid and dehydroisoascorbic acids.* J. Bio. Chem. *183:81, 1950). Large doses of ascorbic acid can cause a rise in DHAA level with associated elevation in blood sugar (Chatterjee IB et al. Synthesis and some major major functions of vitamin C in animals.* Ann. N.Y. Acad. Sci. *258:24, 1975). Diabetics have markedly elevated DHAA levels (Chattergee - ibid). It is possible that the addition of "capillary active" bioflavonoids such as rutin or quercetin will prevent any adverse effects of ascorbic acid supplementation (Clemetson AB. Ascorbic acid and diabetes mellitus.* Med. Hypotheses *2:193-4, 1976), although such adverse effects, and their prevention by bioflavonoids, have not been confirmed (See: "*Bioflavonoids*" and "*Glutathione*" below).*

A marginal vitamin C deficiency may contribute to the development of microangiopathy, since low insulin levels and hyperglycemia accelerate the cellular changes leading to atherosclerosis by impairing ascorbic acid uptake into the vascular epithelium, and studies have correlated experimental ascorbic acid deficiencies with atherogenic processes, presumably by altering glycosaminoglycan metabolism.

In vitro Experimental Study: In a study of the effect of glucose on uptake of L-[1-14C] ascorbic acid by fibroblasts, ascorbic acid intake was inhibited instantly by glucose in a concentration dependent fashion, suggesting that local ascorbic acid deficiency in tissues could be a natural consequence of hyperglycemia and that additional ascorbic acid might be helpful to individuals averting deleterious effects of hyperglycemia on tissue ascorbic acid supply (*Padh H et al. Glucose inhibits cellular ascorbic acid uptake by fibroblasts in vitro.* Cell Biol. Int. Rep. *9(6):531-38, 1985*).

Animal Experimental Study: The absence of insulin or the presence of higher glucose concentrations significantly inhibited ascorbic acid uptake in heart endothelial cells. This inhibition could be overcome by doubling the ascorbic acid concentration (*Kapeghian JC, Verlangieri AJ. The effects of glucose on ascorbic acid uptake in heart endothelial cells: Possible pathogenesis of diabetic angiopathies.* Life Sci. *34(6):577-84, 1984*).

See Also:

> *Verlangieri AJ, Sestito J. Effect of insulin on ascorbic acid uptake by heart endothelial cells: Possible relationship to retinal atherogenesis.* Life Sciences. *29(1):5-9, 1981*

> *Mann GV. Hypothesis: The role of vitamin C in diabetic angiopathy.* Perspect. Biol. Med. *17:210-17, 1974*

Supplementation lowers cholesterol and triglycerides in maturity-onset diabetics.

Experimental Study: 60% of maturity-onset diabetic pts. with hypercholesterolemia given 500 mg ascorbic acid daily for 1 year experienced at least a 40% reduction in cholesterol levels along with a moderate decline of triglyceridemia. Since significantly lower vitamin C concentrations have been found in the blood and particularly in the leukocytes of these pts., these results suggest that the long-term administration removed the tissue ascorbate deficiency and improved the liver's ability to compensate for the increased endogenous synthesis of cholesterol by enhanced transformation to bile acids (*Ginter E et al. Hypocholesterolemic effect of ascorbic acid in maturity-onset diabetes mellitus. Int. J. Vit. & Nutr. Res. 48(4):368-73, 1978*).

Supplementation may improve <u>glucose tolerance</u>.

(WARNING: ascorbic acid may skew the results of urine tests for glucose)

Experimental Study: Pts. were given 500 mg vitamin C twice daily. After 10 days, glucose tolerance was improved in all pts. (*Sandhya P, Das UN. Vitamin C therapy for maturity onset diabetes mellitus: Relevance to prostaglandin involvement. IRCS Med. Sci. 9/7 (618), 1981*).

<u>Vitamin E:</u>
(G)

WARNING: As Vitamin E may reduce the insulin requirement, diabetics on insulin should be started on 100 I.U. or less daily and the dosage raised slowly with adjustment of the insulin dose (*Vogelsang A. Vitamin E in the treatment of diabetes mellitus. Ann. N.Y. Acad. Sci. 52:406, 1949*).

Diabetics appear to have an increased requirement for vitamin E (*Lubin B, Machlin L. Biological aspects of vitamin E. Ann. N.Y. Acad. Sci. 1982, p. 393*).

Deficiency may promote cellular damage due to free radical oxidation (*Galli C, Socin A. Biological actions and possible uses of vitamin E. Acta Vitaminol. Enzymol. 4:245-52, 1984*).

Supplementation may be beneficial.

Animal Experimental Study: Microvascular complications are believed to be due to platelet hyper-aggregability resulting from an imbalance of PGI_2 and TXA_2 production. Vitamin E supplementation at 10 and 100 times the normal requirement enhanced PGI_2 production and suppressed TXA_2 synthesis in streptozotocin-diabetic rats, restoring their ratio to that of normal controls (*Gilbert VA et al. Differential effects of megavitamin E on prostacyclin and thromboxane synthesis in streptozotocin-induced diabetic rats. Horm. Metabol. Res. 15:320-25, 1983*).

Case Report (<u>necrobiosis lipoidica diabeticorum</u>): "Moderately good success" following 400 I.U. daily (*Ayres S Jr., Mihan R. Vitamin E and dermatology. Cutis 16:1017-1021, 1975*).

Case Reports (<u>necrobiosis lipoidica diabeticorum</u>): A woman with a large, yellow ulcerating lesion on the right leg received 150 mg. of vitamin E twice weekly plus 100 mg. orally 3 times daily after meals. After 2 weeks, the ulcers closed and normal skin formation began. Another woman with 3 lesions which had been present for a year received the same treatment with clearing of the lesions in 3 weeks (*Block MT. Vitamin E in the treatment of diseases of the skin. Clin. Med. 60:31, 1953*).

Case Reports (<u>gangrene of the toes</u>): 3/3 patients had excellent results from treatment with 100-150 mg. of vitamin E orally 3 times daily and 150 mg. I.M. 2-3 times weekly. Strongly recommended by the author (in conjunction with antibiotics) even in advanced cases to prevent debridement and amputation (*Block - ibid*).

- -

<u>Calcium:</u>

Diabetes appears to enhance the deposition of calcium in arterial walls which may contribute to the development of hypertension and atherosclerosis.

Animal Experimental Study: Rat aortic smooth muscle exhibited a progressive increase in both membrane and intracellular calcium content from the 1st to the 8th week after the animals were made diabetic (*Turlapaty PD et al. Ca^{2+} uptake and distribution in alloxan-diabetic rat arterial and venous smooth muscle. Experientia 36(11):1298-99, 1980*).

Observational Study: Several types of blood vessels obtained from pts. were found to contain an increased calcium content (*Neubauer B. A quantitative study of peripheral arterial calcification and glucose tolerance in elderly diabetics and non-diabetics. Diabetologia 7:409-13, 1971*).

Chromium:
(G)

A necessary component of glucose tolerance factor (GTF), a substance present in brewer's yeast known to improve glucose tolerance in laboratory animals by potentiating the effect of insulin on carbohydrate metabolism (*Haylock SJ et al. Separation of biologically active chromium-containing complexes from yeast extracts and other sources of glucose tolerance factor (GTF) activity. J. Inorg. Biochem. 18(3):195-211, 1983; Mertz W, Schwarz K. Chromium (III) and the glucose tolerance factor. Arch. Biochem. Biophys. 85:292-5, 1959*).

Glucose intolerance is one of the signs of chromium deficiency (*Freund H et al. Chromium deficiency during total parenteral nutrition. JAMA 241(5):496-8, 1979*).

Serum chromium levels are positively correlated with serum insulin levels.

Observational Study: In a gp. of 20 normal college students, fasting serum chromium levels correlated with fasting serum insulin levels (p less than 0.05), with the percentage of ideal body weight (p less than 0.01), and with triceps skinfold thickness (p less than 0.02). The relative chromium response at insulin peak was inversely correlated with the total insulin (p less than 0.05) as well as with the ratio of total insulin to total glucose (p less than 0.02). The 10 low insulin (LI) secretors had a significantly higher relative chromium response than the high insulin (HI) secretors (p less than 0.005), and the ratio of total insulin to total glucose was significantly lower in LI than HI (p less than 0.001) (*Liu VJ, Abernathy RP. Chromium and insulin in young subjects with normal glucose tolerance. Am. J. Clin. Nutr. 25(4):661-67, 1982*).

Supplementation (in its trivalent form) has been shown to improve glucose tolerance in some human studies.

Experimental Double-blind Study: 85 elderly women (ages 59-82), 62% of whom were on medications that could affect glucose metabolism, were divided into "high risk" and "low risk" categories on the basis of a 2 hr. GTT and received either chromium (CrCl$_3$ 200 mcg) or placebo. After 10 wks. there were no significant differences between experimental subjects and controls except for a small but significant improvement after a GTT in the high risk, non-medicated group. This sub-group was found to have a significantly lower median chromium intake compared to the experimental low risk non-medicated group, suggesting that suboptimal chromium status may account for the difference. Because it appears that medications may have obscured this effect in the medicated subjects, the researchers suggest that future studies omit medicated subjects (*Martinez OB et al. Dietary chromium and effect of chromium supplementation on glucose tolerance of elderly Canadian women. Nutr. Res. 5:609-20, 1985*).

Negative Experimental Double-blind Study: Two gps. of diabetic and non-diabetic subjects received either 68 mcg chromium daily in the form of brewer's yeast or tortula yeast placebo. While hair chromium increased about 25% for both gps. supplemented with chromium, the decrease in fasting blood sugar among chromium-supplemented diabetics (from 204 to 194 mg/dl) was not significant compared to placebo (*Hunt AE et al. Effect of chromium supplementation on hair chromium concentration and diabetic status. Nutr. Res. 5:131-140, 1985*).

Experimental Study: 5 elderly pts. received 200 mcg daily of chromium chloride for 12 weeks. Glucose tolerance improved from 60-120 minutes after glucose challenge, although the difference was significant only at 60 minutes. Plasma insulin levels were unchanged; however glucose utilization and beta-cell sensitivity to glucose increased significantly (*Potter JF et al. Glucose metabolism in glucose-intolerant older people during chromium supplementation.* Metabolism *34:199-204, 1985*).

Negative Experimental Double-blind Crossover Study: 10 non-insulin-dependent diabetics received trivalent chromium 200 mcg daily. After 6 wks., 24 hr. urinary chromium showed a 9-fold increase indicating a positive chromium balance. There was no significant difference between chromium and placebo in glucose tolerance and fasting or 2 hr. postglucose serum insulin levels, but the 1 hr. postglucose insulin level was slightly lower on chromium (p less than 0.01). Serum total cholesterol, triglycerides, and the HDL, LDL and VLDL subfractions were unchanged (*Uusitupa MIJ et al. Effect of inorganic chromium supplementation on glucose tolerance,insulin response, and serum lipids in noninsulin dependent diabetics.* Am. J. Clin. Nutr. *38:404, 1983*).

See Also:

> *Saner G et al. Alterations of chromium metabolism and effect of chromium supplementation in Turner's syndrome patients.* Am. J. Clin. Nutr. *38(4):574-78, 1983*

> *Riales RR, Albrink MJ. Effect of chromium chloride supplementation on glucose tolerance and serum lipids including high-density lipoprotein of adult men.* Am. J. Clin. Nutr. *34:2670-8, 1981*

Copper:
(G)

Copper deficiency is associated with glucose intolerance (*Klevay LM et al. Diminished glucose tolerance in two men due to a diet low in copper.* Am. J. Clin. Nutr. *37:717, 1983*).

See Also:

> *Fields M et al. Effect of copper deficiency and experimental diabetes on glucose metabolism.* Fed. Proc. *42:528, 1983*

Magnesium:
(R)

Frequently low in diabetics, especially those with proliferative retinopathy (*Ceriello A et al. Hypomagnesemia in relation to diabetic retinopathy.* Diabetes Care *5:558-9, 1982*).

Observational Study: Magnesium levels were examined in the plasma, red blood cells and urine of 109 diabetics and 33 normal controls. Diabetics had considerably lower magnesium levels, especially those with proliferative retinopathy, suggesting that derangement of magnesium metabolism may have some relationship to the onset and/or development of the disease (Magnesium Bulletin *Vol. 1, 1983*).

See Also:

> *Mather HM et a. Hypomagnesemia in diabetes.* Clin. Chem. Acta *95:235-42, 1979*

> *McNair P et al. Hypomagnesemia, a risk factor in diabetic retinopathy.* Diabetes *27:1075-77, 1978*

Magnesium is an important cofactor in glycolysis (*Wimsurst JM, Manchester KL. Comparison of ability of Mg and Mn to activate the key enzymes of glycolysis.* FEBS Letters *27:321-6, 1972*).

Reductions in the magnesium content of aortas are associated with elevations in their calcium content (which may lead to atherosclerosis and hypertension), while elevations of magnesium produce lower calcium content (*Altura BM, Altura BT.   Magnesium ions and contraction of vascular smooth muscles: Relationship to some vascular diseases. Fed. Proc. 40(12):2672-9, 1981*).

Magnesium supplementation helps to prevent calcification of blood vessels and atherosclerosis (*Seelig MS, Heggtveit HA.   Magnesium interrelationships in ischemic heart disease: A review. Am. J. Clin. Nutr. 27(1):59-79, 1974*).

Manganese:
(G)

Levels in diabetics are 1/2 those of normals (*Kosenko LG. Klin. Med. 42:113, 1964*).

An important cofactor in the key enzymes of glycolysis (*Wimhurst JM, Manchester KL.   Comparison of ability of Mg and Mn to activate the key enzymes of glycolysis. FEBS Letters 27:321-6, 1972*).

Deficiency can lead to glucose intolerance which can be reversed by supplementation.

Animal Experimental Study: Manganese-deficient guinea pigs developed hyperglycemia and their offspring were found to have pancreatic abnormalities (*Editorial: Manganese and glucose tolerance. Nutr. Rev. 26:207-10, 1968*).

Case Report: A 21 year-old insulin-dependent diabetic received oral manganese chloride 3-5 mg daily which resulted in a consistent fall in blood glucose, often to severely hypoglycemic levels, with modification of the GTT. On the other hand, oral manganese failed to affect the blood sugar level in 3 middle-aged diabetics, 3 juvenile diabetics and 1 case of diabetes resulting from chronic pancreatitis (*Rubenstein AH et al. Hypoglycemia induced by manganese. Nature 194:188-9, 1962*).

See Also:

Everson GJ, Schrader RE.   Abnormal glucose tolerance in manganese-deficient guinea pigs. J. Nutr. 94:89-94, 1968

Manganese and glucose tolerance. Nutr. Rev. 26(7):207-9, 1968

Phosphorus:
(A,G)

Deficiency causes an impaired response to insulin (*DeFronzo RA, Lang R. New Engl. J. Med. November 27, 1980*).

Insulin-dependent diabetics appear to have a fluctuating disorder in the oxygen-releasing capacity of their erythrocytes which is believed to play a role in the pathogenesis of diabetic <u>angiopathy</u>. The position of the oxyhemoglobin dissociation curve is positively correlated with levels of RBC 2,3-diphosphoglycerate (2,3-DPG) which, in turn, varies in response to the plasma concentration of inorganic phosphate (*Ditzel J. Oxygen transport impairment in diabetes. Diabetes 25:832-8,1976*).

Supplementation with inorganic phosphate salts may thus improve RBC oxygen-releasing capacity (and thereby help to prevent the development of <u>angiopathy</u>) by preventing the inhibitory effect of a low concentration of inorganic phosphorus on red cell oxygen delivery.

Experimental Study: After 2 yrs. of supplementation with dibasic calcium phosphate 2 gm 3 times daily with meals, pts. felt less tired and diabetic control was improved. They showed no evidence of adverse effects including soft tissue calcification, urinary calculus formation, hyper- or hypocalcemia (*Ditzel - ibid*).

Potassium:
(G)

Potassium deficiency during a protein-modified fast causes a decrease in peripheral insulin levels and insulin resistence at the postreceptor sites.

Experimental Study: Caloric deprivation in 20 obese non-diabetic subjects (15 mmol K in a protein-modified fast) was followed by a negative potassium balance, decreased serum potassium, decreased peripheral insulin levels, increased insulin receptors and a striking reduction of peripheral glucose utilization. The addition of oral potassium chloride supplementation (64 mmol daily) was associated with significantly higher peripheral insulin levels and improvement of peripheral glucose utilization (*Norbiato G et al. Effects of potassium supplementation on insulin binding and insulin action in human obesity: Protein-modified fast and refeeding. Europ. J. Clin. Invest. 44:414-9, 1984*).

Zinc:
(G)

Deficiency may adversely affect carbohydrate and fat metabolism even though serum levels are normal.

Experimental Study: 6 non-diabetic young men were alternately fed diets containing either 16.5 or 5.5 mg zinc. While serum zinc was unchanged, the low zinc diet was associated with a significant increase in fasting blood glucose and a significant increase in the percent of total fatty acids as arachidonic acid. Results suggest that a low zinc intake mildly alters carbohydrate and fat metabolism before a change in serum zinc is evident (*Solomon SJ, King JC. Effect of low zinc intake on carbohydate and fat metabolism in men. Fed. Proc. 42:391, 1983*).

Diabetics tend to hyperexcrete zinc.

Observational Study: 60 adult insulin-treated diabetics with normal serum creatinine and absence of proteinuria had significantly increased zinc excretion rates compared to normals which correlated positively with the degree of glycosuria but gave no evidence of a state of zinc depletion, suggesting that there is compensatory hyperabsorption and/or increased zinc in the diet (*McNair P et al. Hyperzincuria in insulin treated diabetes mellitus: Its relation to glucose homeostasis and insulin administration. Clin. Chim. Acta 112:343-48, 1981*).

See Also:

> Tarui S. *Studies of zinc metabolism: III. Effect of the diabetic state on zinc metabolism: A clinical aspect. Endocrinol. Japan 10:9-15, 1963*

- -

Bioflavonoids: 1 gram daily
(A,G,N,R)

Strengthens capillary basement membranes *(see "VASCULAR FRAGILITY")*.

Supplementation with certain "capillary active" bioflavonoids such as rutin or quercetin will prevent vitamin C from being oxidized in the jejunum to dehydroascorbic acid which is damaging to capillary endothelial cells *(see "Vitamin C" above)* (*Clemetson AB. Ascorbic acid and diabetes mellitus. Med. Hypotheses 2:193-4, 1976; Clemetson AB, Anderson L. Plant polyphenols as antioxidants for ascorbic acid. Ann. N.Y. Acad. Sci. 136:339, 1966*).

May stimulate insulin secretion (*Middleton E, Drzewieki G. Naturally occurring flavonoids and human basophil histamine release. Arch. Allergy Applied Immunol. 77:155-7, 1985*).

- Quercetin:

A naturally occurring flavonoid which inhibits aldose reductase, an enzyme involved in the synthesis of sorbitol from glucose. Sorbitol is not easily transported in or out of cells and thus accumulates intracellularly, drawing water in by osmosis while low molecular weight compounds are lost in an attempt to maintain osmotic equilibrium. Diabetic animals have been shown to be unusually prone to accumulate sorbitol leading, possibly, to the development of cataracts, retinopathy, neuropathy and other complications (*Cogan DG et al. Aldose reductase and complications of diabetes. Ann. Int. Med. 101:82-91, 1984*).

Experimental Placebo-controlled Study: Sorbinil, a drug known to be a potent aldose reductase inhibitor, was given to 11 diabetics with neuropathy unresponsive to numerous drugs; 8 were also given a placebo. 8/11 supplemented pts. noted moderate to marked relief, usually starting the 3rd or 4th day. Each of the 4 who also had amyotrophy had improvement in pain and mild to moderate improvement in muscle strength which was confirmed by tests of autonomic nerve function and nerve conduction velocity (*Jaspan J et al. Treatment of severely painful diabetic neuropathy with an aldose reductase inhibitor: Relief of pain and improved somatic and automatic nerve function. Lancet 2:758-62, 1983*).

Animal Experimental Study: Oral quercitin given to diabetic rodents resulted in a significant decrease in sorbitol accumulation in lens tissue and, when given continuously, in a delay in the onset of cataracts (*Varma SD et al. Diabetic cataracts and flavonoids. Science 195:205, 1977*).

Coenzyme Q:
(G)

May be deficient.

Observational Study: 8.3% of pts. were deficient in CoQ_{10} compared to 1.9% of controls. Around 20% of pts. receiving oral hypoglycemic drugs were deficient (*Kishi T et al. Bioenergetics in clinical medicine. XI. Studies on coenzyme Q and diabetes mellitus. J. Med. 7:307, 1976*).

Supplementation may be beneficial.

Experimental Study: 39 stable diabetics received CoQ_7 (interchangeable in the body for CoQ_{10}) for 2-18 weeks. Fasting blood sugar was reduced by at least 20% in 12/39 pts (36%) and by at least 30% in 12/39 pts. (31%), while ketone bodies fell by at least 30% in 13/22 pts. (59%) (*Shigeta Y et al. Effect of coenzyme Q_7 treatment on blood sugar and ketone bodies of diabetics. J. Vitaminol. 12:293, 1966*).

Glutathione: (found in brewer's yeast)

A tripeptide composed of the amino acids cysteine, glutamic acid and glycine.

Reduces dehydroascorbic acid to vitamin C in red blood cells. Frequently low in diabetics which may be a cause of increased levels of dehydroascorbic acid (*Banerjee S. Physiological role of dehydroascorbic acid. Indian J. Physiol. Pharmacol. 21(2):85-93, 1977*) which is thought to have destructive effects (*See "Vitamin C" above*).

Omega-3 Fatty Acids:
(G)

Supplementation may decrease insulin resistance.

Experimental Study: Non-insulin dependent pts. who were supplemented with omega-3 fatty acids became more insulin-sensitive (*Abstracts. The Netherlands Soc. for the Study of Diabetes, March 17 and 23, 1984, Utrecht. Netherlands J. Med. 29(2):65-70, 1986*).

Omega-6 Fatty Acids:
(A,G)

$$\text{linoleic acid} \rightarrow \text{gammalinolenic acid} \rightarrow \text{DGLA} \rightarrow \text{PGE}_1$$

High linoleic acid diet is associated with decreased progression of microangiopathy and cardiac ischemia.

Experimental Controlled Study: Half of a gp. of 102 newly diagnosed diabetics were placed on a normal Western diet while the rest were placed on a linoleic acid enriched diet. After 5 yrs., 3 males in the normal diet gp. but none in the linoleic acid gp. had died of MI. Of the survivors, 6% of males and 4% of females in the linoleic acid gp. had cardiac ischemia vs. 22% of males and 16% of females in the control group. The incidence of microangiopathy was also significantly lower in the linoleic acid gp. (27% of males and 32% of females vs. 62% of males and 55% of females) (*Houtsmuller AJ et al. Favourable influences of linoleic acid on the progression of diabetic micro and macroangiopathy. Nutr. Metab. 24 (Supp. 1):105-18, 1980*).

Prostaglandin E_1 (PGE$_1$), which is derived from linoleic acid, has insulin-like actions and potentiates insulin effects (*Haessler HA, Crawford JD. Insulin-like inhibition of lipolysis and stimulation of lipo-genesis by prostaglandin E$_1$. J. Clin. Invest. 46:1065-70, 1967*).

The first step in the conversion of linoleic acid to PGE$_1$ requires delta-6-desaturase, an enzyme whose activity may be inhibited in diabetes, as suggested by animal models (*Mercuri O et al. Depression of microsomal desaturation of linoleic to gamma-linolenic acid in the alloxan-diabetic rat. Biochim. Biophys. Acta 116:409-11, 1966*).

Evening primrose oil, which is high in the PGE$_1$ precursor gamma linolenic acid (the compound formed by the action of delta-6-desaturase on linoleic acid), may benefit diabetic neuropathy.

Experimental Double-blind Study: 22 diabetics whose neuropathy was demonstrated both clinically and by nerve function tests received either evening primrose oil 4 gm daily or placebo. After 6 mo., all 8 variables tested improved in the EPO gp. but worsened in the placebo group (*Jamal GA et al. Gamma-linolenic acid in diabetic neuropathy. Lancet 1:1098, 1986*).

Pyridoxine Alpha-ketoglutarate (PAK):
(G)

Supplementation may be beneficial.

Experimental Double-blind Study: A gp. of 30 insulin-treated type I diabetics and a gp. of 30 phenformin-treated type II diabetics were each randomly divided into 2 sub-groups. Half of each gp. received PAK 600 mg 3 times daily, while half received placebo. After 4 wks., both gps. receiving PAK showed significant decreases in fasting glucose, glycosylated hemoglobin, lactate and pyruvate compared to pre-treatment levels. All values returned to pre-treatment levels within 3 wks. of discontinuing PAK. There were no side-effects or abnormalities in CBC, liver enzymes or BUN. Results suggested that PAK "potentiated the effects of insulin and phenformin" (*Passariello N et al. Effects of pyridoxine alpha-ketoglutarate on blood glucose and lactate in type I and type II diabetics. Int. J. Clin. Pharmacol. Ther. Toxicol. 21:252-56, 1983*).

— —

<u>Brewer's Yeast</u>:
(G)

The richest known source of glucose tolerance factor (GTF) *(Mertz W. Effects and metabolism of glucose tolerance factor. <u>Nutr. Rev.</u> 33(5):129-35, 1975).*

Chromium-enriched brewer's yeast may improve glucose tolerance and lipid metabolism.

Experimental Single-blind Study: 24 elderly subjects (including 8 non-insulin-dependent diabetics) randomly received either chromium-rich brewers' yeast 9 gm daily or chromium-poor tortula yeast. After 8 wks., glucose tolerance, insulin sensitivity and total lipids improved only in the gp. receiving brewers' yeast *(Offenbacher E, Stunyer F. Beneficial effect of chromium-rich yeast on glucose tolerance and blood lipids in elderly patients. <u>Diabetes</u> 29:919-25, 1980).*

See Also:

Freiberg SM et al. Effects of brewer's yeast on glucose tolerance. <u>Diabetes</u> 24 (Suppl. 2):433, 1975 (Abstract)

Chromium may not be essential to glucose tolerance factor.

In vitro Experimental Study: Fractions of extracts of brewer's yeast were purified. Although addition of chromium to the growth medium increased the yield of glucose tolerance factor, the purified substance contained no chromium and GTF activity was isolated in cationic and anionic small amino-acid or peptide-like molecules *(Davies DM et al. The isolation of glucose tolerance factors from brewer's yeast and their relationship to chromium. <u>Biochem. Med.</u> 33(3):297-311, 1985).*

In vitro Experimental Study: An insulin-enhancing factor was isolated from brewer's yeast grown on a chromium-containing medium. The active fraction was found to have little more than a background level of chromium, while the major chromium-containing fraction was found not to have insulin-enhancing activity *(Held DD et al. Isolation of a non-chromium insulin-enhancing factor from brewer's yeast. <u>Fed. Proc.</u> 43:472, 1984).*

<u>Sardine Oil</u>:

Rich in eicosapentaenoic acid (omega-3 fatty acid) and vitamin E.

Supplementation may increase RBC membrane fluidity, thus potentially reducing symptoms due to impaired red cell deformability (such as <u>intermittent claudication</u>).

Experimental Study: Dietary sardine oil 2.7 gm daily was given to diabetic and control subjects. Compared to controls, RBC membrane fluidity was lower in the diabetics prior to supplementation. After 4 wks., membrane fluidity was increased in both diabetics and controls, and remained elevated for the entire 8 wk. study, with disappearance of the difference in RBC membrane fluidity between diabetics and controls *(Kamada T et al. Dietary sardine oil increases erythrocyte membrane fluidity in diabetic patients. <u>Diabetes</u> 35:604, 1986).*

- -

OTHER FACTORS:

Rule out <u>hydrochloric acid deficiency</u>.

> *Note: While gastric anacidity had been reported in the past to be a relatively common condition which was associated with a number of illnesses, the presence of achlorhydria is no longer accepted unless a potent parietal-cell stimulant (such as histamine) is employed in gastric analysis. More recent studies suggest that histamine-fast anacidity is uncommon before the fifth decade of life and, although it probably does not occur in a normal stomach, its presence is not necessarily associated with symptoms (Rappaport EM. Achlorhydria: Associated symptoms and response to hydrochloric acid. <u>New Engl. J. Med.</u> 252(19):802-5, 1955).*

Experimental Controlled Study: Vagal response to feeding was evaluated in 17 insulin-dependent diabetics, 24 post-vagotomy pts. and 10 normals. Compared to normals, diabetics both with and without neuropathy had a decreased acid secretion and delayed gastric emptying following sham feeding similar to vagotomized patients. This was not due to hyperglycemia, since 3 pts. given IV insulin during sham feeding showed the same abnormality. (*Richardson CT et al. Diabetics have reduced acid secretion and delayed digestion. <u>Am. Family Physician</u> June, 1978, p. 143*).

Observational Study: 50 pts. under age 40 and 50 pts. ages 40 and older were randomly selected from a gp. in whom gastric analysis had been performed. 18% of the younger gp. and 64% of the older gp. were achlorhydric, an incidence considerably higher than that reported for normals. Of the 41/100 with achlorhydria, 11 (27%) were anemic compared to 3 (5.1%) of the 59 non-achlorhydric patients. Similarly, 7/41 with achlorhydria (17%) had neuritis vs. 2/59 (3%) of the non-achlorhydric patients. These differences suggest a causal association (*Rabinowich IM. Achlorhydria and its clinical significance in diabetes mellitus. <u>Am J. Dig. Dis.</u> 16:322-32, 1949*).

Review Article: Based on a review of 8 studies, the average incidence of achlorhydria in DM was 32.8% (*Joslin EP et al. <u>The Treatment of Diabetes Mellitus</u>, 8th Edition. Lea & Febiger, 1946*).

See Also:

> *Hosking DJ et al. Vagal impairment of gastric secretion in diabetic autonomic neuropathy. <u>Brit. Med. J.</u> June 14, 1975, pp. 588-90*

If deficient, supplementation may benefit <u>neuritis</u> due to inadequate thiamine absorption.

> **Case Reports:** 3 pts. with severe neuritis are described whose diabetes was under good control and who had failed to benefit from thiamine supplementation. After receiving HCl supplementation, all showed marked improvement. An additional large gp. of cases showed similar results (*Rabinowich - op cit*).

Avoid <u>obesity</u>.

The exaggerated serum insulin levels observed after administration of glucose to maturity-onset diabetic patients correlate with the degree of obesity and do not differ quantitatively from the hyperresponse of insulin to glucose in obesity (*Karam JH et al. The relationship of obesity and growth hormone to serum insulin levels. <u>Ann. N.Y. Acad. Sci.</u> 131(1):374-87, 1965; Karam JH et al. Excessive insulin response to glucose in obese subjects as measured by immunochemical assay. <u>Diabetes</u> 12(3):197-204, 1963*).

DUMPING SYNDROME

BASIC DIET:

High fiber diet.

    - <u>Guar Gum</u>:   5 grams per meal

        Experimental Double-blind Study: Prevented dumping syndrome and increased tolerance to foods not previously tolerated in 9/11 pts. (*Harju E, Larmi TKI. Efficacy of guar gum in preventing the dumping syndrome. <u>J. Parenteral & Enteral Nutr.</u> 7(5): 470-2, 1983*).

    - <u>Pectin</u>:

        Experimental Study: 12 pts. recovering from abdominal surgery developed characteristic G.I. distress and hypoglycemia after drinking a glucose solution. When 1/3 oz. pectin was added to the solution, gastric emptying time was prolonged to near normal in 6 pts., while in 5 the emptying time was slowed but not normalized. In all 11, blood glucose levels were more stable and symptoms were minimized (*Leeds AR et al. Pectin in the dumping syndrome: Reduction of symptoms and plasma volume changes. <u>Lancet</u> 1:1075-8, 1981*).

NUTRIENT:

<u>Folic Acid</u>:

Supplementation may be beneficial in post-gastrectomy syndrome.

    Case Report: 51 year-old male post-partial gastrectomy for pyloric stenosis resulting from duodenal ulcer presented with severe diarrhea and abdominal pain which failed to respond to standard treatments. X-rays showed that the stoma was functioning perfectly, although precipitately. Folic acid 5 mg orally twice daily was given. By the next day his stools were reduced from 8-14 daily to 4 and since the second day stools have been reduced to 2 formed stools daily although all medication has been discontinued (*Young C. Folic acid in dumping syndrome. Letter to the Editor. <u>Can. Med. Ass. J.</u> 65:72, 1951*).

DYSMENORRHEA

NUTRIENTS:

Niacin:

Supplementation may be beneficial.

Experimental Study: 80 pts. received niacin 100 mg twice daily and every 2-3 hours during cramps and were followed for up to 3 years. About 90% were relieved. The effectiveness of niacin seemed to be enhanced by the addition of rutin 60 mg and ascorbic acid 300 mg daily. Supplementation had to start at least 7-10 days prior to menses to be effective, and its benefits often remained for several months after discontinuation. A preliminary trial suggests that niacinaminde may be as effective (*Hudgins AP. Vitamins P, C and niacin for dysmenorrhea therapy. West. J. Surg. & Gyn. 62:610-11, 1954*).

Pyridoxine and
Magnesium:

Supplementation may be beneficial.

Experimental Study: Pts. received aminoacid-chelated Mg and pyridoxine 100 mg of each every 2 hours as needed during menses and 4 times daily throughout the cycle until RBC magnesium returned to normal. There was a progressive decrease in intensity and duration of menstrual cramps over 4-6 months (*Abraham GE. Primary dysmenorrhea. Clin. Obstet. Gynecol. 21(1):139-45, 1978*).

Vitamin E:

Supplementation may be beneficial.

Experimental Placebo-controlled Study: 100 young women (ages 18-21) with spasmotic dysmenorrhea received either alpha-tocopherol tablets 50 mg 3 times daily or placebo for 10 days premenstrually and for the next 4 days. After 2 cycles, 34/50 (68%) in the experimental gp. improved compared to 9/50 (18%) of the controls (*Butler EB, McKnight E. Vitamin E in the treatment of primary dysmenorrhoea. Lancet 1:844-47, 1955*).

- -

Iron:

Supplementation may be beneficial.

Experimental Study: 12 pts. with primary dysmenorrhea, most of whom had iron-deficiency anemia, reported dimunution or complete disappearance of menstrual pain following iron supplementation (*Shafer N. Iron in the treatment of dysmenorrhea: A preliminary report. Curr. Ther. Res. 7:365-66, 1965*).

Essential fatty acids:

Evening Primrose oil is a rich source of gamma-linolenic acid, precursor of prostaglandin E_1.

MaxEPA is a refined source of eicosapentaenoic acid, precursor of prostaglandin E_3.

The E series prostaglandins are said to produce myometrial relaxation (*Abraham GE - op cit*) although the results of clinical trials have not been reported.

ECZEMA
(ATOPIC DERMATITIS)

NUTRIENTS:

Vitamin A:

Supplementation may be beneficial.

WARNING: High doses may be toxic and thus must be given under close medical supervision.

Experimental Study: 10 children are described with chronic eczema who received oral vitamin A palmitate 25-200,00 IU daily for 3-21 months. 3/9 who tolerated it showed some improvement and 6 had marked improvement with a decrease in skin dryness. There was no evidence of vitamin A toxicity (*Strosser AV, Nelson LS. Synthetic vitamin A in the treatment of eczema in children. Ann. Allergy 10:703-4, 1952*).

- -

Selenium:

May be deficient.

Observational Study: The glutathione peroxidase level of 40 pts. with atopic dermatitis was significantly lower than that of controls (p less than 0.01). Similarly the level of 68 pts. with eczema was also significantly lower (p less than 0.001) (*Juhlin L et al. Blood glutathione-peroxidase levels in skin diseases: Effect of selenium and vitamin E treatment. Acta Dermatovener (Stockholm) 62:211-14, 1982*).

- -

Omega-6 Fatty Acids:

$$\text{linoleic acid} \rightarrow \text{GLA} \rightarrow \text{DGLA} \rightarrow \text{prostaglandin E}_1$$

Evening primrose oil is rich in GLA, the conversion of which from linoleic acid may be reduced in atopic eczema. Suggested adult dosage: 2 gm twice daily.

Experimental Double-blind and Observational Study: 50 young adult pts. had variable but higher levels of linoleic acid and lower levels of LA metabolites than did healthy controls. During supplementation with EPO, they showed no significant change in LA, a slight elevation in GLA, significant increases in DGLA and PGE_1 in the higher dose groups, and a significant increase in arachidonic acid when all gps. were considered together (*Manku MS et al. Reduced levels of prostaglandin precursors in the blood of atopic patients: Defective delta-6-desaturase function as a biochemical basis for atopy. Prostaglandins Leukotrienes Med. 9(6):615-28, 1982*).

Supplementation may be beneficial.

Experimental Double-blind Crossover Study: 60 adults and 39 children received primrose oil and placebo for 12 weeks in random order at various random doses (1-3 gm daily for adults and 1-2 gm daily for children). Itching improved significantly with both low and high doses. Overall severity improved by 30% in the low-dose gps. and by 43% in the high-dose groups (*Wright S, Burton JL. Oral evening-primrose-seed oil improves atopic eczema. Lancet November 20, 1982, pp. 1120-22*).

See Also:

Experimental Double-blind Crossover Study: *Wright S. Atopic dermatitis and essential fatty acids: A biochemical basis for atopy? Acta Derm. Venereol. (Stockholm) Suppl. 114:143-45, 1985*

- -

OTHER FACTORS:

Rule out food sensitivities.

Observational Study: 35.7% of 56 adult pts. had serum antibodies against wheat gliadin and/or milk using ELISA, compared with 9.2% of the controls (p less than 0.0005), and 30.4% had IgG antibodies reactive with gliadin compared with 6.5% of the controls (p less than 0.0005), suggesting that antigen absorption from the gut may play a role in the pathogenesis of the disease (*Finn RA et al. Serum IgG antibodies to gliadin and other dietary antigens in adults with atopic eczema. Clin. Exp. Dermatol. 10(3):222-28, 1985*).

Experimental Double-blind Study: 18/30 unselected pts. who had moderate to severe chronic eczema and required daily medication showed substantial improvement when placed on an elemental diet for 3-12 days. These responders were then challenged with various foods; challenge with certain foods caused immediate or delayed flaring of eczema or such other reactions as rhinitis, diarrhea and angioedema. Egg, soy, peanut, chocolate, milk and potato were among the worst offenders. Once a safe rotary diet was established, pts. received either 4-800 mg oral cromolyn or placebo. While pts. on placebo were unchanged, those on cromolyn showed a 19-26% further reduction in eczema (*Kniker WT. Paper presented at the 5th International Food Allergy Symposium, American College of Allergists, 1984*).

Experimental Double-blind Study: 33 afflicted children underwent a 10 day elimination of allergic foods followed by food challenges. 35 challenges elicited symptoms, 31 of which involved the skin, 17 the gastrointestinal tract, 8 the nasal passages and 6 the respiratory tract within 10 - 90 minutes. All 60 placebo challenges were negative (*Sampson HA, Jolie PL. Increased plasma histamine concentrations after food challenges in children with atopic dermatitis. New Eng. J. of Med. 311:371-6, 1984*).

Experimental Double-blind Study: Over 50% of 26 afflicted children with high serum IgE levels developed cutaneous signs after food challenges (*Sampson HA. Role of immediate food sensitivity in the pathogenesis of atopic dermatitis. J. Allergy Clin. Immuno. 71:473-80, 1983*).

Experimental Study: 228/319 (71.5%) of children with chronic eczema refractory to treatment placed on elimination diets and subsequently challenged with various foods were judged to be allergic to specific foods due to the response of their eczema to dietary manipulations (*K-i U. The role of food allergy in the management of chronic eczema in childhood. Abstract. Acta Paedia. Jpn. Japanese ed. 82(2), 1982. 24:395, 1982*).

Observational Study: Polyethylene glycol was used as a probe molecule to measure GI absorption which was found to be greater in pts. with known food allergy and/or eczema than in normals, suggesting either that abnormal food absorption precedes and causes eczema or that eczema also affects the GI tract causing increased absorption secondarily (*Jackson P et al. Intestinal permeability in patients with eczema and food allergy. Lancet 1:1285, 1981*).

Experimental Double-blind Crossover Study: 20/36 afflicted children completed a 12 week double blind, crossover trial of an egg and cow's milk exclusion diet. 14 responded more favorably to the antigen-avoidance diet versus only 1 to the control diet. There was no correlation between positive prick test to egg and cows' milk antigen and response to the trial diet (*Atherton DJ et al. A double-blind cross-over trial of an antigen-avoidance diet in atopic eczema.* *Lancet* *February 25, 1978 pp.401-3*).

Rule out <u>hydrochloric acid deficiency</u>.

> *Note: While gastric anacidity had been reported in the past to be a relatively common condition which was associated with a number of illnesses, the presence of achlorhydria is no longer accepted unless a potent parietal-cell stimulant (such as histamine) is employed in gastric analysis. More recent studies suggest that histamine-fast anacidity is uncommon before the fifth decade of life and, although it probably does not occur in a normal stomach, its presence is not necessarily associated with symptoms (Rappaport EM. Achlorhydria: Associated symptoms and response to hydrochloric acid. <u>New Engl. J. Med.</u> 252(19):802-5, 1955).*

Experimental and Observational Study: Of 106 cases of subacute or chronic eczema which had resisted all forms of local treatment, 26 (25%) had no HCl and only 27 (26%) had normal HCl levels. The severity of the condition seemed to correlate with the extent of the HCl deficiency and also seemed to be associated with signs of B complex deficiency. Supplementation of HCl and vitamin B complex was followed by improvement in the HCl deficient patients (*Allison JR. The relation of deficiency of hydrochloric acid and vitamin B complex in certain skin diseases. <u>Southern Med. J.</u> 38:235-241, 1945*).

Observational Study: 11 pts. underwent a fractional gastric analysis following a routine Ewald test meal. Hypoacidity was defined as values for total and free acids of 1/2 normal or less, while hyperacidity was defined as values 10-15 points above normal or values which were relatively high at the start of the test. 8/11 (72%) of the pts. were found to have hypoacidity, while 2/11 (18%) had normal acid and 1/11 (9%) had hyperacidity. For 7/11 (63%) of the pts., the severity of the eruption correlated with both the presence of GI symptoms and abnormal gastric acid levels (*Ayers S. Gastric secretion in psoriasis, eczema and dermatitis herpetiformis. <u>Arch. Dermatol. Syph.</u> 20:854-57, 1929*).

Case Report: A 52 year-old pt. with a 46 yr. history of eczema as well as a history of gas in the stomach and bowels for at least the past year presented with a red, lichenified face and a less severe eruption on the hand and thigh. The pt. was found to be deficient in hydrochloric acid and was treated with dilute HCl. For nearly 1 yr. the patient's skin condition has been practically normal (*Ayers S. Gastric secretion in psoriasis, eczema and dermatitis herpetiformis. <u>Arch. Dermatol. Syph.</u> 20:854-57, 1929*).

EPILEPSY

BASIC DIET:

For the rare child whose seizures cannot be controlled by drugs, a <u>low carbohydrate, high fat</u> diet may be beneficial. While <u>ketogenic</u> diets may be effective (*Bower BD et al. The use of ketogenic diets in the treatment of epilepsy, in Wharton B, Ed. <u>Topics in perinatal medicine</u>. London, Pitman, 1982*), they are unhealthy for growing children. In general, epileptic pts. should have normal, well-balanced meals at regular intervals, and children should not be allowed to take very large meals as these may predispose them to seizures (*Passmore R, Eastwood MA. <u>Davidson and Passmore: Human Nutrition and Dietetics</u>. Edinburgh, Churchill Livingstone, 1986, p. 471*).

- -

NUTRIENTS:

Folic Acid:

Low blood and cerebrospinal fluid levels are frequently caused by certain anti-convulsants such as phenytoin, primidone and phenobarbital, and total brain folate apparently is depleted following experimentally induced seizures, suggesting that folic acid metabolism is intimately involved in the epileptogenic process (*Smith DB, Obbens EAMT. Antifolate-antiepileptic relationships, in Botez MI, Reynolds EH, Eds. <u>Folic Acid in Neurology, Psychiatry, and Internal Medicine</u>. New York, Raven Press, 1979*).

Supplementation may be beneficial.

> WARNING: Administration of folic acid supplements to pts. on anti-convulsants can result in a marked fall in serum vitamin B_{12} levels (*Hunter R et al. Effect of folic-acid supplement on serum-vitamin-B_{12} levels in patients on anticonvulsants. <u>Lancet</u> September 27, 1969*).

> WARNING: A number of uncontrolled studies suggest that folate supplementation may have an epileptogenic effect. Several controlled studies, however, have failed to confirm this observation, suggesting that such an effect is very rare (*Smith DB, Obbens EAMT - op cit*).

Experimental Double-blind Study: Pts. on phenytoin supplemented with oral folate for a minimum of 1 year had a significant improvement in seizure frequency, while those given placebo also showed some improvement, suggesting that the improvement on folic acid was not only due to the effect of folate (*Givverd FB et al. The influence of folic acid on the frequency of epileptic attacks. <u>Europ. J. Clin. Pharm.</u> 19(1):57-60, 1981*).

Negative Experimental Study: Correction of folate deficiencies in epileptics on anti-convulsants failed to significantly alter seizure frequency or severity or psychological test performance. Serum folate concentrations rose (and both anti-convulsant and barbiturate levels fell) but cerebrospinal fluid folate levels failed to rise, suggesting that anti-convulsants may interfere with the conversion of folic acid to the form which can pass the blood-brain barrier (*Mattson R et al. Folate therapy in epilepsy. <u>Arch. Neurol.</u> 29:78, 1973*).

189

Pyridoxine:

Supplementation may be beneficial.

Case Reports: 3 infants with symptomatic and cryptogenic seizures with hypsarrhythmia received a total dose of 0.2 - 0.4 g/kg pyridoxine. The seizures stopped within 3-6 days (*Blennow G, Starck L. High dose B6 treatment in infantile spasms. Hippokrates Verlag GmbH. 17(1):7-10, 1986*).

Experimental Study: 17/19 infants and children (ages 3 mo. - 13 yrs.) with uncontrollable infantile spasms or their sequelae improved in 2-14 days on oral pyridoxal phosphate 20-50 mg/kg in 2-3 divided doses. 3 had complete relief, 6 showed transient relief and 8 showed marked reduction of seizures and improvement in the EEG. 6 developed elevated transaminases, 2 developed nausea and vomiting, and 1 developed lethargy (*Nakazawa M. High-dose vitamin B6 therapy in infantile spasms - The effect and adverse reactions. Brain & Development 5(2):193, 1983*).

Case Report: An 8 month-old boy with seizures which were unresponsive to anti-convulsants received 50 mg B6 IV. The seizure stopped within minutes and he remained seizure-free for 6 days. When seizure activity recurred, it was promptly stopped again with IV B6. For the next 22 months he received 25 mg oral B6 daily and had no further seizures. B6 was stopped and seizures recurred until B6 was restarted (*Bachman DS. Annals Neurol. December, 1983*).

– –

Magnesium:

May suppress epileptic bursts.

Animal Experimental Study: Parenteral magnesium sulfate was able to directly suppress neuronal burst firing and interictal EEG spike generation at serum levels below those producing paralysis, corroborating the clinical observation that magnesium can produce an anticonvulsant effect in pts. apart from neuromuscular blockade and suggesting that it may have clinical applicability in treating a wider range of acute convulsions (*Gorges LF, G:ucer G. Effect of magnesium on epileptic foci. Epilepsia 19(1):81-91, 1978*).

Blood levels may be deficient, while CSF levels may be elevated.

Observational Study: Compared to controls, epileptic children had a significantly decreased concentration of plasma magnesium and a positive correlation was found between the severity of the epilepsy and hypomagnesemia. A significant increase in CSF magnesium was also found (*Benga I et al. Plasma and cerebrospinal fluid concentrations of magnesium in epileptic children. J. Neurol. Sci. 67(1):29-34, 1985*).

Observational Study: Compared to non-neurologic controls, mean serum Mg in 225 epileptic children was significantly lower (p less than 0.001). There was no relationship between serum Mg levels and serum concentrations of anti-epileptic drugs (*Shoji Y. Serum magnesium and zinc in epileptic children. Brain & Development 5(2):200, 1983*).

If blood levels are deficient, supplementation may be beneficial.

Experimental and Observational Study: 75% of 21 children (age 9 - 14) were deficient and most of these improved after administration of magnesium chloride solution (5 mg./kg. daily) (*Pediatria Romania 31(4):343-347, 1982*).

Case Report: Immediately following 4 hrs. of continuous exercise in heat, a 23-year-old man displayed epileptic-type convulsions while, 1 wk. earlier, he completed an identical exercise program without convulsions at normal room temperature. Upon assessment, the only abnormality found was that, during the exercise in heat, an abnormally low serum magnesium prevailed for most of the test. Treatment with phenobarb and magnesium chloride enteric tablets reversed the biochemical abnormality. He subsequently heat acclimatized and repeated similar exercise tests as before without any ill effects (*Jooste PL et al. Epileptic-type convulsions and magnesium deficiency. Aviat. Space Environ. Med. 50(7):734-35, 1979*).

Manganese:

May be deficient.

Observational Study: Blood Mn levels of 197 pts. (maximum age: 22) were compared to 120 ambulatory pts. without neurologic disease. Levels were found to be lower, with the difference being highly significant (*Dupont CL, Tanaka Y. Blood manganese levels in children with convulsive disorder. Biochem. Med. 33(2):246-55, 1985*).

Observational Study: Epileptics were found to have significantly lower hair and blood manganese levels than normals. Although tissue manganese levels were not consistently lower, most subjects with frequent seizures had levels falling below the lowest control level (*Papavasiliou PS et al. Seizure disorders and trace metals: Manganese tissue levels in treated epileptics. Neurology 29:1466, 1979*).

Observational Study: Blood Mn levels were significantly lower in pts. than in controls (p less than 0.005) (*Sohler A, Pfeiffer CC. A direct method for the determination of manganese in whole blood: Patients with seizure activity have low blood levels. J. Orthomol. Psychiat. 8(4):275-80, 1979*).

If deficient, supplementation may be beneficial.

Clinical Observation: Helpful in controlling both major and minor motor seizures (*Pfeiffer CC, LaMola S. Zinc and manganese in the schizophrenias. J. Orthomol. Psychiat. 12:215-234, 1983*).

Experimental and Observational Study: 1/3 of a gp. of epileptic children were found to have lower blood manganese levels than normal children. A boy with seizures which were unresponsive to medications was found to have a blood manganese level which was half the normal value; when supplemented, he had fewer seizures and improvement in gait, speech and learning. (*Tanaka Y. Low manganese level may trigger epilepsy. JAMA 238:1805, 1977*).

Zinc:

May be deficient.

Observational Study: Compared to normal controls, mean serum zinc in 225 epileptic children was significantly lower (p less than 0.01). Serum zinc levels were especially low in children with West or Lennox syndromes. There was no relationship between serum zinc levels and serum concentrations of anti-epileptic drugs (*Shoji Y. Serum magnesium and zinc in epileptic children. Brain & Development 5(2):200, 1983*).

Anticonvulsants may cause zinc deficiency either by reducing zinc absorption in the gut by chelation or by causing diarrhea. In that case, supplementation may be beneficial.

Experimental and Observational Study: 2 pts. presented with diarrhea and brownish-red scaly eruptions which followed substitution of high dose sodium valproate for phenytoin. Serum zinc concentrations were abnormally low and the pts. responded to zinc supplementation while the anticonvulsant was continued (*Lewis-Jones MS et al. Cutaneous manifestations of zinc deficiency during treatment with anticonvulsants. Brit. Med. J. 290:603-4, 1985*).

Since serum zinc is low and copper high in epileptics, seizures are theorized to occur when the zinc/copper ratio falls suddenly in the absence of adequate taurine (*Barbeau A, Donaldson J. Zinc, taurine and epilepsy. Arch. Neurol. 30:52-58, 1974*).

- -

Choline: Start with 4 gms. daily
            Increase to 12 - 16 gms. by third month

Supplementation may be beneficial.

Experimental Study: 4 pts. with complex partial seizures who failed to respond to drugs had shorter seizure duration and less post-seizure fatigue but a slight increase in seizure frequency following supplementation. Pts. considered themselves much improved (*McNamara JO. Neurology December, 1980*).

Dimethyl Glycine: 100 mg. twice daily

DMG is formed in the metabolism of homocysteine to methionine and is a precursor of glycine, a neuroinhibitory amino acid.

Supplementation may be beneficial.

Case Report: A 22 year-old man with long-standing mental retardation and mixed complex, partial and grand mal seizures had been having 16-18 generalized seizures per week despite phenobarbitol and carbamazepine for the previous 6 months. Within 1 wk. of starting DMG 90 mg twice daily, his seizure frequency dropped to 3 per week. Two attempts to withdraw the DMG caused dramatic increases in seizure frequency (*Roach ES, Carlin L. N,N-dimethylglycine for epilepsy. Letter to the Editor. N. Engl. J. Med. 307:1081-82, 1982*).

See Also:

Freed WJ. N,N-dimethylglycine, betaine, and seizures. Letter to the Editor. Arch. Neurol. 41(11):1129-30, 1984

Roach ES, Gibson P. Failure of N,N-dimethylglycine in epilepsy. Letter to the Editor. Ann. Neurol. 14(3):347, 1983

Taurine: 500 mg 3 times daily

Taurine is a neuroinhibitory amino acid.

Low brain taurine concentrations have been found at the site of maximal seizure activity.

Observational Study: Low concentrations of taurine and glutamic acid along with high concentrations of glycine seem to characterize the site of maximum seizure activity (*Sturman J. Taurine in nutrition. Comprehen. Therapy 3:64, 1977*).

Supplementation may be beneficial.

Animal Experimental Study (rats): Administration of taurine affected the control of experimentally-induced seizures (*Mantovani J et al. Effects of taurine on seizures and growth hormone release in epileptic patients. Arch. Neuro. 35:672, 1979*).

Animal Experimental Study (rats): Taurine was found to have a potent, selective and long-lasting anti-convulsant action (*Huxtable R, Laird H. The prolonged anticonvulsant action of taurine on genetically determined seizure-susceptibility. Canadian J. Neurol. Sci. 5:220, 1978*).

See Also:

> *Maurizi C. Could supplementary dietary tryptophan and taurine prevent epileptic seizures? Med. Hypotheses 18:411-15, 1985*

> *Van Gelder NM. Antagonism by taurine of cobalt induced epilepsy in cat and mouse. Brain Res. 47:157, 1972*

- -

OTHER FACTORS:

Rule out food sensitivities.

Double-blind Case Report: Epilepsy was precipitated by ingestion of specific foods and carefully controlled, double-blind confirmation of the food-epilepsy relationship was demonstrated (*Crayton JW et al. Epilepsy precipitated by food sensitivity: Report of a case with double-blind placebo-controlled assessment. Clin. Electroencephalo. 12(4):192-8, 1981*).

Double-blind Case Report: 29 year-old male had a 4 year history of syncope and grand mal epilepsy as well as double vision, tachycardia, dizziness, edema, and spontaneous bruising. EEG was entirely normal. Phenytoin and other anti-convulsants only partly controlled his seizures. Following a 6 1/2 day fast, his symptoms cleared. Challenge with foods and chemicals precipitated seizures. A double-blind challenge with peanuts using a Levine tube confirmed that he was reacting to the food (*Rea WJ, Suits CW. Cardiovascular disease triggered by foods and chemicals, in Gerrard JW. Food Allergy: New Perspectives. Springfield, Illinois, Charles C. Thomas, 1980*).

Case Report: A 3 1/2 year old male with tuberous sclerosis, mental retardation and uncontrolled seizures was studied. Using a reversal design, the Feingold (salicylate and food additive elimination) diet was presented and withdrawn 3 times, and each presentation resulted in substantial reductions in seizure frequency. During a 21-week follow-up, seizure frequency remained low despite the phasing out of 1 drug, and seizures were reportedly eliminated 1 yr. later, while hyperactive behavior was unchanged (*Haavik S et al. Effects of the Feingold diet on seizures and hyperactivity: A single-subject analysis. J. Behav. Med. 2(4):365-74, 1979*).

See Also:

> **Review Article:** *Campbell MB. Allergy and epilepsy, in Speer, F., Editor. Allergy of the Nervous System. Springfield, Illinois, Charles C. Thomas, 1970, pp. 59-78*

FIBROCYSTIC BREAST DISEASE

See Also: CANCER
PREMENSTRUAL SYNDROME

BASIC DIET:

Avoid <u>methylxanthines</u> (found in <u>coffee</u>, <u>tea</u>, <u>chocolate</u>, <u>cola</u>).

Note: The studies suggest that total abstention is necessary to obtain clinical benefits.

Negative Experimental Study: In a controlled study of 192 women, women who reduced methylxanthine consumption at least 50% failed to benefit from the dietary change (*Parazzini F et al. Methylxanthine, alcohol-free diet and fibrocystic breast disease: A factorial clinical trial.* <u>Surgery</u> *99:576, 1986*).

Negative Observational Study: In a study of 2300 women, no association was found between fibrocystic breast disease and intake of caffeine-containing beverages (*Lubin F et al. A case-control study of caffeine and methylxanthines in benign breast disease.* <u>JAMA</u> *253(16):2388-92, 1985*).

Observational Study: In a study of 634 women with fibrocystic breast disease and 1066 controls, the occurrence of disease was positively associated with the ave. daily consumption of caffeine. Women who consumed 31-250 mg of caffeine/day had a 1.5-fold increase in odds of disease, while those who drank over 500 mg/day had a 2.3-fold increase. The association was particularly high among women with atypical lobular hyperplasia and sclerosing adenosis with concomitant papillomatosis or papillary hyperplasia, both of which have been associated with an increased breast cancer risk. There was no association with fibroadenoma or other forms of benign breast disease (*Boyle CA et al. Caffeine consumption and fibrocystic breast disease: A case-control epidemiologic study.* <u>JCNI</u> *72(5):1015-19, 1984*).

Experimental Controlled Study: 158 women with fibrocystic breast disease were randomly assigned to a methylxanthine-free diet or received no dietary advice. 4 months later there was a statistically significant reduction in clinically palpable breast findings in the abstaining gp. compared to controls, with the greatest improvement in the most severe cases. The absolute change was minor, however, and may be of little clinical significance. Comparison of mammograms before and after the diet failed to demonstrate major differences. Many women in the abstaining group were found to have substantial levels of caffeine in their breast fluid, suggesting that they were still consuming caffeine (*Ernster VL et al. Effects of a caffeine-free diet on benign breast disease: a randomized trial.* <u>Surgery</u> *91(3):263-67, 1982*).

Experimental Controlled Study: 37/45 women with fibrocystic breast disease who stopped all methylxanthines had resolution, 7 were improved and 1 was unchanged. 28 decreased consumption. Of these, 7 had resolution, 14 improved and 7 were unchanged. 12 made no changes: 2 had resolution, 1 improved and 9 were unchanged. Women with the disease were more likely than controls to have a famly history of breast cancer or fibrocystic breast disease and their breast tissue was more sensitive to adenylate cyclase than was normal tissue (*Minton JP et al. Clinical and biochemical studies on methylxanthine-related fibrocystic breast disease.* <u>Surgery</u> *90:299-304, 1981*).

Experimental Controlled Study: 47 women with benign breast lumps were asked to eliminate methylxanthines. Of the 20 who complied, the lumps completely disappeared in 13. Of the 27 who failed to comply, the lumps disappeared in only 1 (*Minton JP.* <u>JAMA</u> *March 23, 1979*).

See Also:

Minton JP. Caffeine and benign breast disease. Letter to the Editor. JAMA 254(17):2408-9, 1985

Minton JP et al. Caffeine, cyclic nucleotides, and breast disease. Surgery 86:105-09, 1979

- -

NUTRIENTS:

Vitamin A:

Supplementation may be beneficial.

WARNING: High doses of vitamin A can be toxic and should only be given under close medical supervision.

Experimental Study: 10/12 women with moderate to severe breast pain which had not responded to mild painkillers or caffeine withdrawal reported reduction in breast pain following supplementation with 150,000 IU vitamin A daily. In 5 pts. breast masses decreased at least 50% Two pts. had to stop supplementation due to severe headaches and 3 had mild reactions, while five had no side effects. Pts. who responded showed continued benefit at follow-up 8 months later, and side effects were rapidly reversed (*Band PR et al. Treatment of benign breast disease with vitamin A. Prev. Med. 13:549-54, 1984*).

Vitamin E: 400 - 600 I.U. daily (3 month trial)

Supplementation may be beneficial.

Negative Experimental Double-blind Study: In a randomized trial, 128 women with confirmed mammary dysplasia received placebo or 150, 300 or 600 IU daily of an alcohol form of vitamin E. Just over half reported benefits from placebo and from the highest dose of vitamin E. Vitamin E had no significant effects on any of the hormones measured (*London RS et al.   Obstet. & Gyn. 65:104-6, 1985*).

Experimental Controlled Study: 22/26 responded to 600 I.U. of D,L alpha-tocopheryl acetate in 8 weeks following an initial placebo trial. Cystic lesions and tenderness disappeared in 10, and 12 had a decrease in the number and size of the lesions with or without pain relief (*London RS et al. Nutr. Res. 2:243-247, 1982*).

Experimental Double-blind Study: 17 pts. with mammary dysplasia and 6 controls received placebo for 1 menstrual cycle followed by alpha-tocopheryl acetate 600 IU daily for 2 cycles. 15 pts. (88%) showed a clinical response and the ratio of progesterone to estradiol, which is abnormal in mammary dysplasia pts., rose from 30 to 53 in pts. and was unchanged in controls, suggesting that vitamin E may reduce future risk for malignant breast disease (*London RS et al. Endocrine parameters and alpha-tocopherol therapy of patients with mammary dysplasia. Cancer Res. 41:3811-13*).

Experimental Study: 17 women with mammary dysplasia and 6 age-matched controls received DL-alpha-tocopheryl acetate 600 IU daily. After 4 months, 15 (88%) showed objective and subjective remission. Elevated levels of LH and FSH were decreased to normal levels, suggesting that vitamin E may also normalize abnormal hormone levels (*Sundaram GS et al. Serum hormones and lipoproteins in benign breast disease. Cancer Res. 41:3814-6, 1981*).

Experimental Study: 29 women with chronic fibrocystic breast disease which was aggravated premenstrually took 300 or 600 I.U. daily for 3 months. 16 had moderate to complete symptom relief; the remaining 13 had palpable breast softening, with reduction of cyst size or complete elimination of cysts (*Abrams AA. Use of vitamin E in chronic cystic mastitis. New Engl. J. Med. 272:1080-1081, 1965*).

See Also:

> *London RS et al. The effect of alpha-tocopherol on premenstrual symptomatology: A double-blind study. II. Endocrine correlates. J. Am. Col. Nutr. 3:351-56, 1984*

- -

Iodine: 1 - 10 drops daily (prescription source)
example: SSKI (30 mg. = 1 drop)

If deficient, supplementation may be beneficial.

Animal Experimental Study: Iodine deficient rats developed lesions which resembled histologically human fibrocystic breast disease. This finding was more notable on older rats (*Krouse TB et al. Age-related changes resembling fibrocystic disease in iodine-blocked rat breasts. Arch. Pathol. Lab. Med. 103:631-4, 1979*).

Animal Experimental Study: Estrogen given to iodine-deficient rats resulted in lesions which resembled histologically human fibrocystic breast disease (*Eskin BA et al. Mammary gland dysplasia in iodine deficiency. JAMA 200:115-19, 1967*).

- -

Omega-6 Fatty Acids:

Example: Evening primrose oil 1500 mg twice daily.

Supplementation may be beneficial in mastalgia.

Experimental Study: In a gp. of 291 pts. with severe persistent breast pain in whom breast cancer had been excluded, 45% of those with cyclical mastalgia had good or useful responses to evening primrose oil, compared to 27% of those with non-cyclical mastalgia (*Pye JK et al. Clinical experience of drug treatments for mastalgia. Lancet 2:373-77, 1985*).

Experimental Double-blind Study: 41 pts. with cyclical breast symptoms were treated with evening primrose oil. After 2 mo., significant improvement was observed in patients' assessment of breast tenderness and nodularity, general wellbeing and irritability, and in physicians' assessment of breast nodularity and tenderness. There were no substantial side-effects and responses were sustained for up to 18 mo. with continued supplementation (*Pashby NL et al - 1984*).

- -

Ginseng:

WARNING: May be harmful.

Review Article: Several recent studies have linked ginseng to breast pain and tenderness, as well as to vaginal bleeding, probably because it contains small amounts of estrone, estradiol and estriol (*Porrath, Saar - quoted in Am. Med. News January 27, 1984*).

GALLBLADDER DISEASE
(CHOLECYSTITIS AND CHOLELITHIASIS)

BASIC DIET:

Increase <u>dietary fiber</u> and avoid <u>refined carbohydrates</u>.

Observational Study: Gallstone formation in young people was correlated with an increased sugar intake (soft drinks and sweets) as well as an increased energy or fat intake, suggesting that sugar may increase cholesterol synthesis by stimulating insulin secretion (*Report: How sugar can get you stoned.* <u>New Scientist</u> *vol. 14, March 21, 1985*).

Observational Study: Dietary habits were reviewed for 267 hospitalized pts. with newly diagnosed gallstones and compared to 214 matched controls in the community and 359 hospital patient controls. Refined sugar intake in drinks and sweets was a risk factor independent of obesity (*Scragg RKR et al.* <u>Brit. Med. J.</u> *288:1113, 1984*).

Experimental Controlled Study: 13 pts. with radiolucent gallstones ate refined or unrefined carbohydrate diets for 6 wks. each, in random order. While the unrefined carbohydrate diet averaged 27 gms of fiber daily, the refined carbohydrate diet averaged only 13 gms of fiber daily The bile saturation index was higher in 12/13 during the refined carbohydrate period (*Thornton JR et al. Diet and gallstones: Effects of refined carbohydrates on bile cholesterol saturation and bile acid metabolism.* <u>Gut</u> *24:2-6, 1983*).

Experimental Study: 11 healthy individuals added 30 grams of wheat bran to their diet for 2 months. There was a decrease in bile saturation index in all 5 subjects whose initial index was 1 or higher but no change in those whose initial index was less than 1 (*Watts JM et al. The effect of added bran to the diet on the saturation of bile in people without gallstones.* <u>Am. J. Surg.</u> *135:321, 1978*).

Experimental Study: 9 pts. added 50 gms. of wheat bran to their regular diet. After 4 wks., they demonstrated a significant decrease in bile cholesterol, bile saturation index, and proportion of deoxycholic acid in the total bile acid pool. 3 pts. who remained on the diet for at least 6 months demonstrated a significant increase in HDL cholesterol (*McDougall RM et al. Effect of wheat bran on serum lipoproteins and biliary lipids.* <u>Can. J. Surg.</u> *21:433, 1978*).

<u>Vegetarian diet</u>.

Observational Study: In a study of over 700 women ages 40-69 over several years, omnivorous women (#632) had about twice the incidence of gallstones as vegetarian women (#130), perhaps because they eat more fat and less fiber (*Pixley F et al. Effect of vegetarianism on development of gall stones in women.* <u>Brit. Med. J.</u> *291:11-12, 1985*).

Animal Experimental Study (hamster): Substitution of soy for casein (milk protein) significantly inhibited gallstone formation, and had a solubilizing effect when gallstones were preestablished (*Kritchevsky D, Klurfeld DM. Influence of vegetable protein on gallstone formation in hamsters.* <u>Am. J. Clin. Nutr.</u> *32:2174, 1979*).

Eat a regular <u>breakfast</u>.

Observational Study: Women who skipped breakfast or had only coffee experienced a much greater incidence of gallstones than those who ate a morning meal (*Capron JP et al. Meal frequency and duration of overnight fast: A role in gall-stone formation? <u>Brit. Med. J.</u> 283:1435, 1981*).

Avoid <u>obesity</u> and high <u>fat</u> intake.

Observational Study: 267 hospital pts. with newly-diagnosed gallstones were compared to 241 matched controls from the community and 359 hospital controls. High fat intake in the young and obesity in women under 50 years of age were found to be risk factors (*Scragg RKR et al. <u>Brit. Med. J.</u> 288:1113, 1984*).

Negative Experimental Study: The response of the gallbladder to meals containing differing amounts of fat was independent of the meal's fat content for 6 male and 9 female pts. with gallstones (*Mogadam M. <u>Am. J. Gastroenterol.</u> October, 1984*).

Case Report: 41 year old woman with a large gallstone who was also 55 pounds overweight went on a 1000 calorie diet. Ater 15 months, she had lost 42 pounds and her gallstone had disappeared. After 19 months, she was down to her ideal weight and her gallbladder was functioning normally (*Thornton JR. <u>Lancet</u> September 1, 1979*).

Observational Study: The authors found that a hypocaloric diet associated with a low fat intake and protein mostly of vegetable origin was negatively associated with cholelithisis (for calorie intakes below 3000 Kcal.) in the period following the second world war in southeast France when starvation was common. This correlation no longer held in the 1970's, however, suggesting that very low caloric intake is protective against cholesterol stones (*Sarles H et al. Diet and cholesterol gallstones: A multicenter study & Diet and cholesterol gallstones: A further study. <u>Digestion</u> 17:121-134, 1978*).

Note: Fatty meals <u>do not</u> provoke biliary colic.

Experimental Controlled Study: 15 pts. were randomly given either a breakfast with over 30 gm. of fat, less than 15 gm. of fat, or no fat, or an infusion of cholecystokinin (the primary stimulant of the gallbladder). Each person ultimately was placed into each of the 4 conditions over 4 days. No predictable pattern of response to any meal was noted, suggesting that the gallbladder dynamics in response to various meals are independent of a meal's fat content. Since the passage of gallstones into the cystic or common duct is a random event, fat-restricted diets offer no significant therapeutic advantage to pts. with asymptomatic gallstones (*Mogadam M et al. Gallbladder dynamics in response to various meals: Is dietary fat restriction necessary in the management of gallstones? <u>Am. J. Gastroenterol.</u> 79(11):745-47, 1984*).

Note: The incidence of gallstones is <u>higher</u> when fats come from polyunsaturates rather than from saturated fats and cholesterol.

Observational Study: The incidence of gallstones found at autopsy of 424 male pts. who had been on the standard American diet was compared to that of 422 male pts. who had been on a diet high in polyunsaturates and low in saturated fats and cholesterol. 14% of those on the standard diet had gallstones versus 34% of the others (*Sturdevant RA et al. Increased prevalence of cholelithiasis in men ingesting a serum-cholesterol-lowering diet. <u>N. Engl. J. Med.</u> 288(1):24-27, 1973*).

NUTRIENTS:

Vitamin C:

Deficiency may be associated with cholesterol gallstones.

Animal Experimental Study (guinea pig): All of 14 hypovitaminotic C animals on a high cholesterol diet developed gallstones compared to none of the controls on the identical high cholesterol diet. Compared to the controls, there was a lower bile acid/cholesterol ratio in their bile (*Jenkins SA. Vitamin C and gallstone formation: A preliminary report.* _Experientia_ *33:1616-17, 1977*).

Animal Experimental Study (guinea pig): 26 animals were given a scorbutic diet for 14 days followed by a maintenance dose of 0.5 mg. of ascorbic acid every 24 hours, while a control group of 26 animals was given a normal diet and 10 mg. of ascorbic acid. After 3 months the animals were given an injection of cholesterol and sacrificed. The C-deficient animals were found to have decreased levels of bile acids (making gallstone formation more likely), increased levels of cholesterol in their livers and twice as much cholesterol in their blood (*Ginter E.* _Science_ *February 16, 1973*).

Vitamin E:

Deficiency may be associated with cholesterol gallstones.

Animal Experimental Study (hamster): All of a group of animals on a vitamin E-deficient diet developed cholesterol stones even on a fat-free, cholesterol-free diet, while none of another group on a regular diet developed them (*Dam H et al.* _Acta Physiol. Scand._ *36:329, 1956*).

Animal Experimental Study: Animals given large amounts of cholesterol, saturated fat, or unsaturated fat failed to develop cholesterol stones so long as vitamin E intake was adequate (*Christensen F et al.* _Acta Physiol. Scand._ *27:315, 1952*).

Animal Experimental Study: Cholesterol stones which developed in animals given a vitamin E deficient diet dissolved when vitamin E was given (*Dam H et al.* _Acta Path. Microbiol. Scand._ *30:256, 1952*).

Essential Fatty Acids:

Supplementation may be beneficial.

Experimental Study: 23 pts. took "Rowachol," an essential fatty acid preparation, for 6-12 months. 3 pts. had complete and 4 had partial dissolution of gallstones (*Bell GD, Doran J. Gall stone dissolution in man using an essential oil preparation.* _Brit. Med. J._ *1:24, January 6, 1979*).

Lecithin: 100 mg. three times daily

Lecithin is known to increase the capacity of the bile to solubilize cholesterol (*Duff GL et al.* _Am. J. Med._ *11:92, 1951*).

Supplementation may normalize the abnormally low phospholipid to cholesterol ratio associated with cholesterol gallstones.

Experimental Study: 8 pts. with gallstones were treated for 18-34 months and demonstrated significant increases in bile phospholipid content and cholate/cholesterol ratio as well as a significant decrease in bile cholesterol (*Tuzhilin SA et al. The treatment of patients with gallstones by lecithin. Am. J. Gastroenterol. 65:231, 1976*).

Experimental Study: Pts. with gallstones have an abnormally low phospholipid-cholesterol ratio in their bile (2:1 in pts. vs. 6:1 in normals).   6 of these pts. were given 10 gm lecithin daily which resulted in a doubling of the bile concentration of phospholipids (*Tompkins RK et al. Relationship of biliary phospholipid and cholesterol concentrations to the occurrence and dissolution of human gallstones. Ann. Surg. 172(6):936-45, 1970*).

Supplementation may reduce the size of cholesterol gallstones.

Experimental Study: 1/8 pts. with gallstones treated for 18-34 months demonstrated a decrease in size of the stones as well as a change in their shape (*Tuzhilin - op cit*).

- with Cholic Acid: cholic acid: 750 mg. daily
                      lecithin: 2250 mg. daily

Experimental Study: 7 pts. with radiolucent gallstones and 2 pts. with radiolucent biliary tree stones were treated for 6 months.   In 2 pts. the stones disappeared and in 1 the stones decreased in size (*Tooli J et al. Gallstone dissolution in man using cholic acid and lecithin. Lancet 2:1124, 1975*).

Experimental Study: 5/5 pts. with radiolucent gallstones or biliary tree stones demonstrated a decreased bile lithogenic index following 6 months of treatment (*Tooli - ibid*).

Taurine:

Supplementation may be beneficial.

Animal Experimental Study: Mice were fed a cholesterol-free diet, a lithogenic diet containing cholesterol and sodium cholate, or a lithogenic diet supplemented with 5% taurine. Gallstone formation was only observed in the mice fed the lithogenic diet without taurine for more than 3 weeks, and the cholesterol mass in the liver decreased after the 3rd week in the taurine-supplemented mice, suggesting that the inhibitory effect of dietary taurine on cholesterol gallstone formation may be related to a decrease in the cholesterol content of the liver (*Yamanaka Y et al. Effect of dietary taurine on cholesterol gallstone formation and tissue cholesterol contents in mice. J. Nutr. Sci. Vitaminol. 31(2):226-32, 1985*).

OTHER FACTORS:

Rule out food sensitivities.

Experimental Study: 69 pts. with gallstones or post-cholecystectomy syndrome were placed on an elimination diet consisting of beef, rye, soy, rice, cherry, peach, apricot, beet, and spinach. After 1 week, additional foods were added systematically and each symptom-provoking food was retested several times. All pts. were relieved of their symptoms, with improvements usually occurring in 3-5 days. Egg was by far the most frequent offender (93%), followed by pork (64%) and onion (52%) (*Breneman JC. Allergy elimination diet as the most effective gallbladder diet. Ann. Allergy 26:83, 1968*).

Experimental Study: Ingestion of offending foods caused disturbances in emptying of the gallbladder, as evidenced by measurements of its size. Some differences between control and experimental measurements were seen at 1 hour, but the major differences were usually seen at the end of 2 hours and were associated with typical symptoms of a gallbladder attack along with such allergic symptoms as shortness of breath, sneezing, headaches and hives (*Necheles H et al. Allergy of the gallbladder: A study using the Graham-Cole test and the leukopenic index. Am. J. Dig. Dis. 7:238, 1940*).

Experimental Study: Pts. with bronchial asthma developed gall bladder distress after ingesting wheat which ceased after wheat elimination (*Graham EA et al. Diseases of the Gall Bladder and Bile Ducts. Philadelphia, Lea & Febiger, 1928*).

See Also:

Ficari A, De Muro P. *Experimental studies on allergic cholecystitis. Gastroenterol. 6:302-14, 1946*

Rule out hydrochloric acid deficiency.

Experimental Study: 26/50 pts. with cholelithiasis showed evidence of gastric hyposecretion with the augmented histamine test, and 16/18 showed persistent reflux of duodenal reflux by the pyloric regurgitation test. Results suggest that, when gallstones form, duodenal reflux may be an associated factor that produces dysfunction and destruction of oxyntic cells. These changes may cause hyposecretion, while the presence of bile and pancreatic juices in the stomach may cause flatulent dyspepsia (*Capper WM et al. Gallstones, gastric secretion, and flatulent dyspepsia. Lancet 1:413-15, February 25, 1967*).

See Also:

Fravel RC. *The occurrence of hypochlorhydria in gallbladder disease. Am. J. Med. Sci. 159:512-17, 1920*

GLAUCOMA

NUTRIENTS:

<u>Thiamine:</u>

May be deficient.

Observational Study: Pts. usually have lower blood levels than normals despite equal dietary intake (*Asregadoo ER. <u>Ann. Ophthalmol.,</u> July 1979*).

<u>Vitamin C:</u>

Low intake may be associated with higher intraocular pressures.

Observational Study: Average intraocular pressure of 31 subjects (ages 26-74) with a mean daily intake of 75 mg vitamin C was significantly higher (p less than 0.001) than that of a matched gp. with a mean daily intake of 1200 mg (*Lane BC. Evaluation of intraocular presure with daily, sustained closework stimulus to accommodation to lowered tissue chromium and dietary deficiency of ascorbic acid (vitamin C). Ph.D. dissertation, 1980, New York University*).

Supplementation may be beneficial.

Negative Experimental Study: 6 pts. with open angle glaucoma failed to benefit from the addition of 1.5 gm ascorbic acid 3 times daily for 3-12 weeks to their usual medications (*Fishbein SL, Goldstein S. The pressure lowering effect of ascorbic acid. <u>Ann. Ophthalmol.</u> 4:498-91, 1972*).

Experimental Controlled Study: 25 subjects (ave. age 63 yrs.) with moderate ocular hypertension received 0.5 gm ascorbic acid orally 4 times daily. After 6 days intraocular pressure fell significantly (*Linner E. The pressure lowering effect of ascorbic acid in ocular hypertension. <u>Acta. Ophthalmol.(Copen.)</u> 47:685-9, 1969*).

Experimental Study: A single dose of 500 mg/kg ascorbic acid reduced intraocular pressure in 39/39 pts. by an average of 16 mm Hg but usually caused GI symptoms. Ascorbic acid 100-150 mg/kg 3-5 times daily resulted in almost normal intraocular pressures in 15/16 pts. by 45 days, some of whom were uncontrollable with acetazolamide and 2% pilocarpine, with only 3-4 days of GI symptoms (*Virno M et al. Oral treatment of glaucoma with vitamin C. <u>Eye, Ear, Nose, Throat Monthly</u> 46:1502-8, 1967*).

Experimental Controlled Study: 22 normal subjects received 500 mg ascorbic acid orally twice daily. After 1 wk., intraocular pressure was significantly lower and returned to baseline by 1 wk. after ascorbic acid was discontinued (*Linner E. Intraocular pressure regulation and ascorbic acid. <u>Acta Soc. Med. Upsal.</u> 69:225-32, 1964*).

See Also:

Bietti G. Further contributions on the value of osmotic substances as means to reduce intraocular pressure. <u>Trans. Ophthamol. Soc. U.K.</u> 86:247-54, 1966

Topical application may be beneficial.

Experimental Controlled Study: 10% aqueous solution of ascorbic acid was applied topically in one eye of 19 subjects (ave. age 63 yrs.) 3 times daily for 3 days resulting in a significant drop in mean intraocular pressure in the treated eye only (*Linner - op cit*).

Rutin: 20 mg. three times daily

Supplementation may be beneficial.

Experimental Study: 17/26 eyes with uncomplicated primary glaucoma improved (demonstrated a 15% or greater reduction in intraocular pressure) and responded better to miotics after at least 4 weeks of supplementation (*Stocker FW. New ways of influencing the intraocular pressure. NY State J. Med. 49:58-63, 1949*).

- -

OTHER FACTORS:

Rule out <u>food sensitivities</u>.

Experimental Study: 113 pts. with chronic simple glaucoma demonstrated an immediate rise in intraocular pressure of up to 20 mm upon challenge with food or other allergens (*Raymond LF. Allergy and chronic simple glaucoma. Ann. Allergy 22:146-50, 1964*).

Experimental Study: In 3 cases of simple glaucoma, treatment with miotics and attempted desensitization with autogenous bacterial antigens was supplemented by the removal of food antigens (as determined from the pulse testing method of Coca) from their diets. In 1 case, ocular tension was brought under control only after the institution of an allergen-free diet. In the other 2 cases, surgery and medical treatment controlled the tension but failed to check the progressive visual field loss which showed marked improvement after the institution of an allergen-free diet (*Berens C et al. Allergy in glaucoma. Manifestations of allergy in three glaucoma patients as determined by the pulse-diet method of Coca. Ann. Allergy 5:526-35, 1947*).

GOUT

BASIC DIET:

Low <u>purine</u> diet (avoid meats, esp. organ meats, seafood, lentils, beans and peas).

May decrease uric acid by up to 1 milligram.

Restrict <u>alcohol</u>, especially <u>beer</u> (which has a higher purine content than wine or spirits).

Increases lactate production which competes with uric acid for renal clearance (*Emmerson BT. Therapeutics of hyperuricaemia and gout.* <u>*Med. J. Aust.*</u> *141:31-6, 1984*).

Increases purine nucleotide degradation in the liver increasing oxypurine and thus uric acid production (*Emmerson BT - ibid*).

Experimental Controlled Study: the major dietary difference of men with gout versus controls was that 41% (25/41) of the afflicted men drank more than seven 12 ounce cans of beer daily compared to 17% of the healthy men which was associated with a significantly higher intake of purine nitrogen, half of which was derived from beer (*Gibson T et al. A controlled study of diet in patients with gout.* <u>*Ann. Rheum. Dis.*</u> *42(2):123-27, 1983*).

Avoid <u>fructose</u>.

Increases urate production (*Emmerson BT. Effect of oral fructose on urate production.* <u>*Ann. Rheum. Dis.*</u> *33:276, 1974; Perheentupa J, Raivio K. Fructose-induced hyperuricaemia.* <u>*Lancet*</u> *2:528, 1967*).

- -

NUTRIENTS:

<u>Folic Acid:</u>   10 - 75 mg daily

>   WARNINGS: Monitor serum B_{12} level.
>   Watch for signs of toxicity, esp. restlessness.

Inhibits xanthine oxidase which is required for uric acid production (*Kalckar HM, Klenow H. Milk xanthopterin oxidase and pteroylglutamic acid.* <u>*J.Biol.Chem.*</u> *172:349-350, 1948*).

Said to reduce uric acid with greater safety than drugs (*Oster KA. Evaluation of serum cholesterol reduction and xanthine oxidase inhibition in the treatment of atherosclerosis, in* <u>*Recent Advances in Studies on Cardiac Structure*</u> *3:73-80, 1973*).

See Also:

Negative Experimental Study: *Boss GR et al. Failure of folic acid (pteroylglutamic acid) to affect hyperuricemia.* <u>*J. Lab. Clin. Med.*</u> *96:783, 1980*

Niacin:

WARNING: Supplementation may be harmful.

May precipitate an attack of gout as nicotinic acid competes with uric acid for renal excretion (*Pfeiffer CC. Mental and Elemental Nutrients. New Canaan, Conn. Keats Publishing, 1975, p. 121*).

Vitamin A:

WARNING: Supplementation may be harmful.

Review Article: Elevated retinol levels may play an important role in the development of some attacks of gouty arthritis (*Marson AR. Letter to the Editor. Lancet 1:1181, 1984*).

Vitamin C:

May lower serum uric acid by increasing renal excretion.

Experimental Study: Supplementation with 4 gms or more vitamin C daily increased renal excretion of uric acid. While supplementation with less than 8 gms vitamin C daily did not affect serum uric acid levels, 8 gms daily decreased serum uric acid levels by 1.2 to 3.1 mg percent (*Stein HB et al. Ascorbic acid-induced uricosuria: A consequence of megavitamin therapy. Ann. Int. Med. 84(4):385-8, 1976*).

HEADACHE

See Also: PAIN

BASIC DIET:

Avoid <u>caffeine</u>:

Caffeine intake is correlated with headache prevalence.

Observational Study: In a cross-sectional study of 4558 Australians, the proportion of subjects reporting headache increased significantly with mean caffeine intake. A multiple logistic regression model showed that the association between headache prevalence and usual daily caffeine consumption remained significant in both males and females after controlling for age, adiposity, smoking, alcohol intake and occupation. The relative risk of headache for people consuming 240 mg of caffeine (4-5 cups of coffee or tea) daily is 1.3 for males and 1.2 for females. Coffee consumption had no significant effect over and above that attributable to its caffeine content (*Shirlow MJ, Mathers CD. A study of caffeine consumption and symptoms: Indigestion, palpitations, tremor, headache and insomnia.* <u>Int. J. Epidemiol.</u> *14(2):239-48, 1985*).

Discontinuation of regular intake may cause a withdrawal headache.

Review Article: Caffeine withdrawal headache begins with a feeling of "cerebral fullness" about 18 hours after caffeine ingestion and quickly develops into a diffuse, throbbing, painful headache that is exacerbated by exercise. Discomfort peaks from 3-6 hours after onset (*Greden JF et al. Caffeine-withdrawal headache: A Clinical Profile.* <u>Psychosomatics</u> *21:411-18, 1980*).

- -

NUTRIENTS:

<u>Copper</u>:

Dietary copper may trigger migraine headaches.

Review Article: The migraine-inducing effect of Cu is associated with its role in the metabolism of vasoneuroactive amines, such as serotonin, tyramine, and catecholamines which makes foods which contain high amounts of copper (such as chocolate) or which increase the intestinal absorption of copper (such as citrus) potential headache triggering agents, especially when Cu metabolism is abnormal (*Harrison DP. Copper as a factor in the dietary precipitation of migraine.* <u>Headache</u> *26(5):248-50, 1986*).

- -

<u>Choline</u>:

RBC choline levels may be deficient in pts. with <u>cluster headache</u>.

Experimental and Observational Study (cluster headache): Compared to age-related controls, erythrocyte choline concentrations were low in patients both during and between cluster periods.

206

During lithium treatment, choline levels rose 78 times (*de Belleroche J et al. Erythrocyte choline concentrations and cluster headache. Brit. Med. J. 288:268-70, 1984*).

Omega-3 Fatty Acids:

Example: "MaxEPA" - a fish oil concentrate.

May change the balance of prostaglandins and leukotrienes - powerful mediators of inflammation and immune responses.

Supplementation may be beneficial.

Experimental Study (<u>migraine headache</u>): 15 pts. received supplements of omega-3 fatty acids. 8/15 had fewer headaches and less pain; 3 were unchanged, and 4 became worse (*Hitzemann RJ, associate professor of psychiatry and behavioral sciences, State U. of N.Y. at Stony Brook - 1986*).

Experimental Placebo-controlled Study (<u>migraine headache</u>): 8 pts. with severe and frequent migraines received vegetable oil capsules in divided doses with meals for 6 weeks, followed by substitution of 15 gm. EPA for 6 weeks. Compared to the vegetable oil placebo, EPA supplementation cut the incidence of severe headaches by more than half, and gave people twice as many headache-free hours, possibly by reducing platelet aggregation and platelet serotonin release (*Glueck Charles, U. of Cincinnati College of Medicine - 1986*).

Experimental Double-blind Study (<u>migraine headache</u>): 6 chronic sufferers were given 20 gm. fish oil daily. Significant headache relief was found in 5 of the 6 patients (*Mc Carren T et al. Am. J. Clin. Nutr. 41:874a, 1985*).

- -

Feverfew:

WARNING: Take with meals for no longer than 14 days at a time.

An inhibitor of platelet aggregation which prevents the release of excessive levels of arachidonic acid (*Heptinstall S et al. Extracts of feverfew inhibit granule secretion in blood platelets and polymorphonuclear leucocytes. Lancet 1:8437, 1985; Collier HO et al. Extract of feverfew inhibits prostaglandin biosynthesis. Lancet 2:1054, 1981*).

Said to have similar analgesic properties as the non-steroidal anti-inflammatory drugs.

Experimental Double-blind Study: 17 <u>migraine</u> pts. who ate fresh leaves of feverfew daily as prophylaxis (ave. of 2.44 leaves or 60 mg) received either feverfew 50 mg in capsules or placebo. The pts. in the 2 gps. did not differ in the amt. of feverfew usually consumed or in the duration of consumption. The mean frequency of attacks in pts. receiving placebo increased from 1.22 monthly prior to the study to 3.43 attacks during the final 3 mo. of the 6 mo. study, while pts. taking feverfew showed no change. In addition, those taking feverfew reported a far lower incidence of nausea and vomiting during episodes than those taking placebo. There was one report each of transient palpitations, colicky abdominal pain and heavier menstruation. Pts. in the placebo gp. reported symptoms of nervousness, tension and insomnia which are believed to be due to withdrawal effects (*Johnson ES et al. Efficacy of feverfew as prophylactic treatment of migraine. Brit. Med. J. 291:569-73, 1985*).

Observational Study: A survey of 270 pts. who had taken feverfew for prolonged periods suggested that the herb decreased the frequency and severity of migraine attacks with only minor side-effects (*Mahaja AN, Bailey JM. A platelet phospholipase inhibitor from the medicinal herb feverfew (tanacetum parthenium). Prostaglandins, Leukotrienes & Med. 8:653-60, 1982*).

- -

OTHER FACTORS:

Rule out <u>food sensitivities</u>.

General:

Experimental Double-blind Study (<u>migraine headache</u>): 6/43 adults with recurrent migraines became headache-free following an elimination diet and 13/43 experienced 66% or greater headache reduction. 11/16 skin test-positive pts. responded to the diet, while only 2/27 skin test-negatives did. Double-blind challenges provoked migraines in 5/7, while placebo challenges failed to provoke them (*Mansfield LE et al. Food allergy and adult migraine: Double-blind and mediator confirmation of an allergic etiology. <u>Ann. Allergy</u> 55:126, 1985*).

Experimental Study (<u>migraine headache</u>): A nutritionally supported fast week followed by food sensitivity management achieved major improvement for 80% of a group of 19 migraineurs (*Hughes EC et al. Migraine: A diagnostic test for etiology of food sensitivity by a nutritionally supported fast and confirmed by long-term report. <u>Annals of Allergy</u> 55:28-32, 1985*).

Experimental Double-blind Study (<u>migraine headache</u>): Foods which provoked migraine in 9 pts. with severe migraine refractory to medications were identified. The pts. were then given either sodium cromoglycate or placebo in a double-blind manner along with provoking foods. Sodium cromoglycate exerted a protective effect on the symptoms and immune complexes were not produced in the protected patients (*Monro J et al. Migraine is a food-allergic disease. <u>Lancet</u> September 29, 1984, pp. 719-21*).

Experimental Double-blind Study (<u>migraine headache</u>): 93% of 88 children with severe frequent migraine recovered on oligoantigenic diets; the causative foods were identified by sequential reintroduction, and the role of the foods provoking mgraine was established by a double-blind controlled trial in 40 of the children (*Egger J et al. Is migraine food allergy?: A double-blind controlled trial of oligoantigenic diet treatment. <u>Lancet</u> October 15, 1983, pp.865-9*).

Case Report (<u>tension headache</u>): Chronic tension headaches in a middle-aged woman were treated over a period of a year with alternating dietary and stress manangement approaches. While the dietary approach was effective, stress management training was not (*O'Banion DR et al. Dietary & stress management in tension headache treatment. <u>Clin. Ecology</u> 1:75-83, Fall-Winter 1982-3*).

Experimental Study (<u>migraine headache</u>): Certain flavonoid phenolic compounds in foods and alcoholic beverages inhibit phenolsulfotransterase P (PST-P), an important enzyme which deactivates phenols. Pts. with a history of diet-induced migraine have lower platelet levels of PST-P, while both healthy controls and migraine pts. whose headaches are not food-induced have normal levels. Many red wines cause 100% inhibition of PST-P, while white wines, whiskey and brandy cause less inhibition, and vodka and gin least of all (<u>*APA Psychiatric News*</u> *June 7, 1985; Littlewood J et al. Platelet phenolsulfotransterase deficiency in dietary migraine. <u>Lancet</u> 1:983-6, 1982*).

Review Article: At least 25 syndromes have been described in which foods or food and drug combinations cause head and neck pain, including coloring and flavoring agents, alcoholic products, chocolate, coffee and tea, foods containing tyramine, vitamins, minerals, pesticides, and several others (*Seltzer S. Foods, and food and drug combinations, responsible for head and neck pain. <u>Cephalalgia</u> 2(2):111-24, 1982*).

Experimental Study: (<u>migraine, tension and mixed headache</u>): 5 women were treated by controlling dietary factors. Baseline and treatment phases were repeated to indicate replicability and longitudinal trends. Dietary changes during treatment phases resulted in complete elimination of headache pain in 4 of the 5 subjects (*O'Banion DR. Dietary control of headache pain: Five case studies. <u>J. Holistic Med.</u> 3:140-151, 1981*).

Experimental Study (migraine headache): 24 migraineurs were placed on a diet containing tyramine, excluding tyramine, or unregulated. In evaluating headaches occurring within 12 hrs. after ingestion, there were no significant differences in migraine severity in any group, although some headaches were time-locked to alcohol, chocolate and fasting, suggesting that these substances may either have produced headaches or may merely have triggered impending attacks (*Medina JL, Diamond S. The role of diet in migraine. Headache 31-4, 1978*).

Chocolate:

Reactions have been blamed on its phenylethylamine content (at least 3 mg/2 oz bar).

Experimental Controlled Study (migraine headache): 36 pts. who attributed their migraines to chocolate received either phenylethylamine or placebo (lactose). 18/18 reported attacks 12 hrs. following phenylethylamine ingestion vs. 6/18 reported attacks following placebo (*Schweitzer JW et al. Chocolate, beta-phenylethylamine and migraine re-examined. Nature 257:256, 1975*).

Experimental Double-blind Study (migraine headache): 13/80 pts. developed attacks after chocolate but in only 2 could these reactions be reproduced with consistency (*Moffett AM et al. Effect of chocolate in migraine: A double-blind study. J. Neurol. Neurosurg. Psychiat. 37:445, 1974*).

Negative Double-blind Study (migraine headache): 100 pts. showed no evidence of an increase in frequency of headaches following ingestion of tyramine, phenylethylamine or chocolate, despite their conviction that chocolate would cause them to develop headaches (*Moffett AM et al. Migraine and diet. Letter to the Editor. Lancet 2:7885, 1974*).

HEARTBURN
(REFLUX ESOPHAGITIS)

BASIC DIET:

Avoid <u>foods which affect lower esophageal sphincter function</u>.

General References:

Castell DO. Diet and the lower esophageal sphincter. <u>Am. J.Clin. Nutr.</u> November, 1975, pp. 1296-8

Castell DO. The lower esophageal sphincter. <u>Ann. Int. Med.</u> 83:390, 1975

Alcohol:

Has been shown to relax the lower esophageal sphincter and to decrease the peristaltic force (*Hogan WJ et al. Ethanol induced acute esophageal sphincter motor dysfunction. <u>J. Appl. Physiol.</u> 32:755, 1972*).

Chocolate:

Has been shown to relax the lower esophageal sphincter (*Babka JC, Castell DO. On the genesis of heartburn. <u>Am. J. Dig. Dis.</u> 18:391, 1973*).

Effect on the LES may be due to its methylxanthine content, as chocolate syrup with a low fat content (1%) still lowers LES pressure (*Castell DO. Diet and the lower esophageal sphincter. <u>Am. J. Clin. Nutr.</u> 28:1296-98, 1975*).

Coffee:

Has been shown to both relax the lower esophageal sphincter and stimulate gastric acid secretion (<u>*JAMA*</u> *July 17, 1981*).

> **Experimental Study:** Caffeine slightly relaxed the LES even in the dose range commonly encountered in 1-2 cups of coffee during the first 30-45 minutes after ingestion, at the same time that it produced maximal stimulation of gastric acid (*Dennish GW, Castell DO. Caffeine and the lower esophageal sphincter. <u>Am. J. Digest. Dis.</u> 17:993-96, 1972*).

Fat:

Has been shown to relax the lower esophageal sphincter, even in normal subjects (*Nebel OT, Castell DO. Kinetics of fat inhibition of the lower esophageal sphincter. <u>J. Appl. Physiol.</u> 35:6, 1973*).

High <u>fiber</u> diet.

> **Review Article:** Epidemiological studies indicate that hiatus hernia is a "Western" disease. It is postulated that the unnaturally raised intra-abdominal pressures that are necessitated to evacuate the firm stools resulting from consumption of low-residue diets are an important etiological factor (*Burkitt DP, James PA. Low-residue diets and hiatus hernia. <u>Lancet</u> 2:128-30, 1973*).

HEPATITIS

BASIC DIET:

Low <u>sugar</u> diet.

> **Experimenal Study:** 21 normal subjects received a typical American diet containing 25-30% sucrose for 18 days, and a "calorically diluted" diet containing less than 10% sucrose for 12 days. Serum GOT and GPT levels rose significantly when subjects consumed the high sucrose diet and returned to baseline levels on the low sucrose diet, with the rise apparently due both to surplus calories and excess sucrose consumption. In 2 subjects, the rise in enzyme levels on the high sucrose diet was so great that they had to be withdrawn from the study. Serum triglycerides were also significantly greater on the high sucrose diet. (*Porikos KP, van Itallie TB. Diet-induced changes in serum transaminase and triglyceride levels in healthy adult men. Role of sucrose and excess calories. <u>Am. J. Med.</u> 75:624, 1983*).

- -

NUTRIENTS:

<u>Vitamin B12</u>:

Supplementation by injection may be beneficial in <u>viral</u> hepatitis.

> **Experimental Controlled Study:** 13/26 pts. with viral hepatitis selected alternately received B12 100 mcg IV daily in addition to standard treatment. While liver function tests were unmodified, the experimental gp. had less anorexia and jaundice and the mean duration of illness was 34.8 days compared to 45.8 days in the controls (*Jain ASC, Mukerji DP. Observations on the therapeutic value of intravenous B12 in infective hepatitis. <u>J. Indian Med. Assoc.</u> 35:502-5, 1960*).

> **Experimental Controlled Study:** IV B12 brought about rapid return of appetite and liver size to normal in pts. with viral hepatitis. In addition, the serum bilirubin returned to normal earlier (in 10 wks. compared to 18 wks. in the control gp.) and the mean duration of illness was reduced brom 54 to 48 days (*Campbell RE, Pruitt FW. Vitamin B12 in the treatment of viral hepatitis. <u>Am. J. Med. Sci.</u> 224:252, 1952*).

<u>Vitamin B12</u> and
<u>Folic Acid</u>:

Supplementation may be beneficial in <u>viral</u> hepatitis.

> **Experimental Study:** Supplementation was associated with feeling better sooner and shorter duration of illness (50 vs. 60 days) (*Campbell RE, Pruitt FW. The effect of vitamin B12 and folic acid in the treatment of viral hepatitis. <u>Am. J. Med. Sci.</u> 229:8, 1955*).

<u>Vitamin C</u>:

Supplementation may hasten recovery.

> **Clinical Observation (<u>viral</u>):** 40 - 100 gms. orally or IV. Said to be "one of the easiest diseases for ascorbic acid to cure" with paradoxical cessation of diarrhea despite oral supplementation within 1

to 2 days. Stools and urine return to normal color within 2-3 days in acute cases and patients feel fairly well in 2-4 days with clearing of jaundice in about 6 days (*Cathcart, RF III. The method of determining proper doses of vitamin C for the treatment of disease by titrating to bowel tolerance. J. Orthomol. Psychiat. 10:125-32, 1981*).

Negative Experimental Controlled Study: *Knodell RG et al. Vitamin C prophylaxis for posttransfusion hepatitis: Lack of an effect in a controlled trial. Am. J. Clin. Nutr. 34:20 1981*

> *Note: This study has been criticized by Linus Pauling who claims that the data demonstrate a reduction in the incidence of illness with vitamin C. Also pts. receiving vitamin C had more transfusions than the control group; thus if the ratio of cases of post-transfusion hepatitis per transfusion is calculated, there is a 40-50% reduction in those who received 3.2 gm. vitamin C daily (Am. J. Clin. Nutr. 34:1978, 1981).*

Clinical Observation: Pts. treated with 400-600 mg/kg were well and back to work in 3-7 days (*Klenner FR. Observations on the dose of administration of ascorbic acid when employed beyond the range of a vitamin in human pathology. J. Applied Nutr. 23(3 & 4):61-88, Winter, 1971*).

Experimental Study: 245 infected children received 10 gm. ascorbic acid daily with rapid recovery (*Baetgen D. Results of the treatment of epidemic hepatitis in children with high doses of ascorbic acid in the years 1957 - 1958. Medizinische Monatschrift 15:30-36, 1961*).

Experimental Controlled Study: 10 gms. ascorbic acid was infused on several different occasions and compared with results of the previous year in patients who were not given the infusions. The infusions were associated with about a 50% reduction in the duration of the illness (*Baur H, Staub H. Treatment of hepatitis with infusions of ascorbic acid: Comparison with other therapies. JAMA 156(5):565, 1954 [abstract]*).

May prevent serum hepatitis in surgical patients.

Experimental Controlled Study: None of 1095 surgical patients given 2 gm. or more vitamin C daily developed serum hepatitis, while 7% (11/150) patients given less than 1.5 gm. vitamin C developed the disease (*Murata A. Virucidal activity of vitamin C: Vitamin C for prevention and treatment of viral diseases, in Hasegawa T, Editor. Proc. First Intersectional Cong. Int. Assoc. Microbiol. Soc., Volume 3. Tokyo U. Press, 1975, pp. 432-42*).

See Also:

> *Morishige F, Murata A. Vitamin C for prophylaxis of viral hepatitis B in transfused patients. J. Int. Acad. Prev. Med. 5(1):54, 1978*

- -

Catechin:

Supplementation may be beneficial.

Experimental Double-blind Study: 338 pts. with HBe-Ag-positive chronic hepatitis received either cianidanol (catechin) 1.5 gm daily for 2 wks. followed by 2.25 gm daily for 14 wks. or placebo. The HBeAg titer decreased by at least 50% in 44/144 (31%) of treated pts. compared to 21/140 (15%) of controls (p less than 0.01). Liver function tests also tended to improve in those whose antibody titers fell. The only side effect was a transient febrile reaction in 13 pts. (*Suzuki H et al. Cianidanol therapy for HBe-antigen-positive chronic hepatitis: A multicentre, double-blind study. Liver 6:35, 1986*).

HERPES SIMPLEX

NUTRIENTS:

<u>Vitamin C</u> and   200 mg. of each 3 times daily with meals at start of discomfort
<u>Bioflavonoids</u>:

Supplementation may be beneficial.

Experimental Double-blind Study: 14/38 with herpes labialis on vitamins developed blisters versus 10/10 on placebo. Compared to placebo, the duration of the illness decreased from 9 to 4.5 days (*Terezhalmy GT et al. The use of water soluble bioflavonoid-ascorbic acid complex in the treatment of recurrent herpes labialis. <u>Oral Surgery, Oral Medicine, Oral Pathology</u> 45:56-62, 1978*).

- -

<u>Zinc</u>:

Supplementation may be beneficial.

In vitro Experimental Study: Zinc sulphate 0.1 mM inhibited the synthesis of herpes simplex virus progeny, while 0.2 mM resulted in almost complete inhibition of replication (*Gordon YJ et al. <u>Antimicrobial Agents & Chemotherapy</u> 8:337, 1975*).

- with Vitamin C:

Supplementation may be beneficial.

Experimental Study: Following an eruption, pts. with recurrent herpes simplex type I received zinc sulphate 100 mg and vitamin C 250 mg twice daily for 6 weeks. There was either (1) complete suppression of the eruption for an indefinite period; (2) a local tingling sensation but without an eruption or with local swelling and a very limited area of vesiculation which receded within 24 hrs.; or (3) a violent eruption which was not followed by any further eruption providing supplementation was continued (*Fitzherbert J. Genital herpes and zinc. Letter to the Editor. <u>Med. J. Aust.</u> 1:399, 1979*).

- -

<u>L-Lysine</u>:   1 - 6 gm. daily between meals until healed (take with carbohydrate) then 500 mg. daily to prevent recurrence.

WARNING: follow cholesterol levels as lysine may stimulate the liver to increase its manufacture (*Schmeisser DD et al. Effect of excess dietary lysine on plasma lipids of the chick. <u>J.Nutrition</u> 113(9):1777-83, 1983*).

Supplementation, along with arginine restriction, may be beneficial.

lysine/arginine ratios of foods

good	bad
meat	chocolate (1:2)
potatoes	peanuts (1:3)
milk	other nuts
brewer's yeast	seeds
fish	cereal grains
chicken	
beans	
eggs	

Experimental Study: 41 pts. taking an average daily dose of 1248 mg of lysine hydrochloride showed evidence of decreasing recurrence rate of attacks and decreasing symptom severity of recurrences. A dose of 624 mg daily, however, was ineffective (*McCune et al. Cutis 34:366, 1984*).

Negative Experimental Double-blind Study: 21 pts. with recurring infections randomly received oral lysine HCl 400 mg 3 times daily or placebo at the start of an episode and were told to continue it for 4-5 months. In addition, all pts. avoided excessive ingestion of seeds, nuts or chocolate. Measures of episode frequency, duration and severity failed to detect substantial benefits from lysine either as prophylaxis or as treatment for episodes in progress (*DiGiovanna J, Blank H. Failure of lysine in frequently recurrent herpes simplex infection. Arch. Derm. 120:48-51, 1984*).

Experimental Double-blind Crossover Study: 65 pts. with recurrent herpes simplex labialis received either L-lysine monohydrochloride daily or placebo. After 12 wks., the gps. were crossed-over. On the whole, lysine prophylaxis had no effect on recurrence rates; however, significantly more pts. were recurrence-free during lysine than during placebo, suggesting that certain pts. may benefit (*Milman N et al. Lysine prophylaxis in recurrent herpes simplex labialis: A double-blind crossover study. Acta Dermatovener 60:85-87, 1980*

Experimental Study: Supplementation with lysine 800-1000 mg daily during overt infection and 312-500 mg daily for maintenance was followed by complete symptom suppression in 42/45 patients followed 2 months to 2 years with marked reduction of recurrences. Pain disappeared overnight and the initial lesion did not spread to multiple sites. Frequently, however, infection returned 1-4 wks. after stopping lysine (*Griffith RS et al. A multicentered study of lysine therapy in herpes simplex infection. Dermatologica 156:257-267, 1978*).

- -

TOPICAL APPLICATIONS:

<u>Vitamin E:</u>   Squeeze capsule onto cotton roll

Topical application may be beneficial.

    Experimental Study: Application brought immediate relief of gingivostomatitis followed by recession of lesions (*Strasoler S, Haber G. N.Y.S. Dental J. 11/78 pp. 382-383*).

- -

<u>Lithium Succinate Ointment:</u>

Topical application may be beneficial.

Experimental Double-blind Study: 7/10 patients with cold sores improved and the lesions regressed faster than expected compared to improvement in 3/10 patients given placebo (*Skinner GR. Lithium ointment for genital herpes. Letter to the Editor.* Lancet *2:288, 1983*).

<u>Zinc Sulfate Ointment (0.05%):</u>

Topical application may be beneficial.

Experimental Study: 200 pts. with Type I or Type II herpes applied 0.25% zinc sulphate in a saturated solution of camphor water 8-10 times daily starting within 24 hrs. of the appearance of lesions. The lesions usually cleared within 3-6 days. With applications every 30-60 min., the itching, burning, stinging and pain usually disappeared within 2-3 hours. Similarly, a 0.25% zinc sulphate solution had excellent results when used as a douche for women with vaginal herpes (*Finnerty EF. Topical zinc in the treatment of herpes simplex.* Cutis *February 1986, p.130*).

Review Article: Long-term topical application appears to greatly reduce or eliminate recurrences of orolabial and genital herpetic infections (*Eby G.   Use of topical zinc to prevent recurrent herpes simplex infection: Review of literature and suggested protocols.* Med. Hypotheses *17:157-65, 1985*).

See Also:

> **Experimental Study:** *Brody I. Topical treatment of recurrent herpes simplex and post-herpetic erythema multiforme with low concentrations of zinc sulphate solution.* Brit. J. Dermatol. *104:191, 1981*

<u>Lithium Succinate (8%), Zinc Sulfate (0.05%) and D,L Alpha Tocopherol (0.1%) Ointment:</u>

Topical application may be beneficial.

Experimental Double-blind Study: 73 patients with recurrent genital herpes treated within 48 hours of lesion onset with ointment applied 4 times daily for 1 week or placebo. Ointment significantly reduced pain duration from 7 to 4 days (*Skinner GRB. Lithium ointment for genital herpes.* Lancet *2:288, 1983*).

- -

OTHER FACTORS:

<u>Lactobacillus Acidophilus:</u>

May be beneficial.

Experimental Study: 38/40 patients given tablets reported relief within 48 hours (*Rapoport L, Levine WI. Treatment of oral ulceration with lactobacillus tablets. Report of forty cases.* Oral Surg. *20(5):591-93, 1965*).

See Also:

> *Gertenrich RL, Hart RW. Treatment of oral ulcerations with Bacid (Lactobacillus acidophilus).* Oral Surg. *30(2):196-200, 1970*

HERPES ZOSTER

NUTRIENTS:

Vitamin B₁₂: 500 micrograms I.M. daily

Supplementation by injection may be beneficial.

> **Experimental Study:** 21 patients showed "dramatic response ... as judged by relief of pain and the speed of disappearance of vesicles" with improvement starting the second or third day of treatment. None developed post-herpetic neuralgia (*Gupta AK, Mital HS. Indian Practitioner July, 1967*).

Vitamin C: 10 grams daily (1 gm./hr.) until lesions dry up

Supplementation may be beneficial.

> **Experimental Study:** 327 pts. were all cured following 3 days of IV vitamin C injections (*Zureick M. Treatment of shingles and herpes with vitamin C intravenously. J. des Praticiens 64:586, 1950*).

> **Experimental Study:** 8 pts. received injections of vitamin C. 7 reported cessation of pain within 2 hours after the first injection. 7 also showed drying of the blisters within 1 day and complete clearing in 3 days (*Klenner F. The treatment of poliomyelitis and other virus diseases with vitamin C. South. Med. & Surg. 111:209-14, 1949*).

Vitamin E: 1200 - 1600 I.U. daily (6 months trial) (for <u>post-herpetic neuralgia</u>)

Supplementation may be beneficial.

> **Experimental Study:** 9/13 pts. with postherpetic neuralgia reported complete or almost complete pain relief - including one who had had the pain for 19 years and one who had had the pain for 13 years. Of the other 4, 2 were moderately improved and 2 were slightly improved (*Mihan R, Ayres S. Post-herpes zoster neuralgia: Response to vitamin E therapy. Arch. Derm. 12/73*).

> **Negative Experimental Study:** 6 female (ages 56-72) and 2 male (ages 60-64) pts. were given D-alpha tocopheryl acetate 400 IU daily before meals. After 2 wks. the dose was increased to 800 IU daily for 2 wks. and then to 1600 IU daily for 6 weeks. In addition, 2 women used vitamin E cream (50 IU/gm) topically. After 10 wks., 7/8 pts. noted no change in either severity or frequency of the neuralgia (*Cochrane T. Post-herpes zoster neuralgia: Response to vitamin E therapy. Letter to the Editor. Arch. Derm. 111:396, 1975*).

> *Note: Ayres and Mihan have emphasized that 1200-1600 IU of D-alpha tocopheryl acetate or succinate for at least 6 mo. is necessary as well as avoiding any medication or foods (including mixed vitamins containing inorganic iron, white flour, vitamin-enriched cereals, and conjugated estrogens) which may inactivate vitamin E (Ayres S, Mihan R. Letter to the Editor. Arch. Derm. 111:396, 1975).*

"HYPERESTROGENISM"
(IMPAIRED ESTROGEN METABOLISM)

See Also: CANCER
FIBROCYSTIC BREAST DISEASE
MENORRHAGIA
PREMENSTRUAL SYNDROME

Through hydroxylation in the liver, estrogen is metabolized as follows:

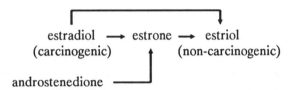

Estradiol is secreted by the ovary. Estrone is converted from estradiol or from androstenedione which is secreted by the adrenal cortex. Except for a small amount from the ovary, estriol is converted in the liver from estrone as well as from estradiol by a circuitous route.

Estradiol and estrone are extremely active stimulants of breast and uterine tissue, while estriol is less stimulating and may even be anticarcinogenic (*Follingstad AH. Commentary: Estriol, the forgotten estrogen? JAMA 239(1):29-30, 1978; Cole P, MacMahon B. Oestrogen fractions during early reproductive life in the aetiology of breast cancer. Lancet 1:604-6, 1969*).

> **Observational Study:** Urine was collected from women in their reproductive years in areas of the world of high and low breast cancer risk. Results were strikingly consistent with the hypothesis that women who metabolize a high proportion of their estrogens to estriol are at low risk for breast cancer (*MacMahon B et al. Urine oestrogen profiles of Asian and North American women. Int. J. Cancer 14:161-67, 1974; Dickinson LE et al. Estrogen profiles of Oriental and Caucasian women in Hawaii. N. Engl. J. Med. 291:1211-13, 1974*).

In the presence of sub-optimal liver function and/or nutritional deficiencies, the conversion of estradiol and estrone to estriol is blocked, causing <u>PMT-A</u>, one of the types of <u>premenstrual syndrome</u>. PMT-A is associated with symptoms of anxiety, irritability and nervous tension, occurring as early as the mid cycle, becoming progressively worse during the luteal phase and sometimes followed by mild to moderate depression and improvement with menses. Pts. have elevated blood estrogens (which are CNS stimulants) and decreased progesterone (a CNS depressant) during the luteal phase (*Abraham GE. Premenstrual tension syndromes: A nutritional approach. Anabolism 5(2):5-6, 1986*).

Also associated with increased estrogen levels is <u>prolonged menses</u> (over 4 days versus 3 days), <u>heavy bleeding</u> and an increased risk of <u>uterine fibroids</u>, <u>endometriosis</u> and <u>fibrocystic breast disease</u>.

> **Observational Study:** Women with periods of menstrual flow greater or equal to 1 wk as well as cycles of 27 days or less had more than double the risk for endometriosis compared to women with shorter flow and longer cycles. Women with greater menstrual pain were also at higher risk for endometriosis, while both smoking and regular exercise, which lower endogenous estrogen levels, were associated with decreased risk (*Cramer DW et al. JAMA April 11, 1986*).

The metabolism of estrogen can be evaluated by calculating the <u>estrogen quotient</u>. A 24 hour urine is obtained for fractionated estrogens. If the sum of the estrone and the estradiol is greater than the estriol, women may be at greater risk for illnesses related to estrogen excess.

High Risk: below 0.7
Low Risk: above 1.0

Observational Study: The presence of breast cancer was negatively correlated with the estrogen quotient (*Lemon HM et al. Reduced estriol excretion in patients with breast cancer prior to endocrine therapy. JAMA June 27, 1966, p. 112*).

- -

BASIC DIET:

High <u>protein</u> (about 1/2 gm protein/ lb. of body weight) diet.

Increases the cytochrome P-450-dependent hydroxylation of estradiol.

Experimental Study: 4 normal males (ages 20-35) were fed a high protein diet with 44% of calories as protein, 35% as carbohydrate and 21% as fat for 2 wks. and then a high carbohydrate diet (10% protein, 70% carbohydrate and 20% fat) for 2 wks. after a 3 wk. period in which they consumed their normal diets. The mean percentage oxidation of estradiol was substantially greater during consumption of the high protein diet than during the high carbohydrate diet (*Kappas A et al. Nutrition - endocrine interactions: Induction of reciprocal changes in the delta-4-5-alpha-reduction of testosterone and the cytochrome p-450-dependent oxidation of estradiol by dietary macronutrients in man. Proc. Natl. Acad. Sci. USA 80:7646-49, 1983*).

<u>Low fat, high fiber</u> diet.

Review Article: For Western women, dietary fiber may be important in the prevention of breast cancer, and both the early onset of menarche and a high fat diet are risk factors in breast cancer. Breast cancer may be estrogen-dependent and dietary fiber may increase the fecal excretion of estrogen. Perhaps high fat diets are necessarily low in fiber and low fiber intake rather than high fat intake is the reason why high dietary fat is a risk factor (*Hughes RE. Hypothesis: A new look at dietary fiber. Human Nutr.: Clin. Nutr. 40C:81-86, 1986*).

Dietary fat may influence estrogen metabolism due to:

1. the stimulation of animal fats upon the growth of colonic bacteria which are capable of synthesizing estrogen as well as of breaking the estrogen-glucuronide linkages (*Goldin BR, Gorbach SL. The relationship between diet and rat fecal bacterial enzymes implicated in colon cancer. J. Natl. Cancer Instit. 57:371-75, 1976*).

Observational Study: High fat diets were associated with metabolically very active anaerobic bacterial flora which were found to be able to produce estrone, estradiol and 17-methoxyestradiol from bacterial metabolites of cholesterol, suggesting that this is a mechanism by which dietary fat may influence estrogen patterns and breast cancer risk (*Hill MJ et al. Gut bacteria and aetiology of cancer of the breast. Lancet 2:472-73, 1971*).

2. increased arachidonic acid derived from animal fats. Arachidonic acid is the precursor of prostaglandin F_2 alpha which is luteolytic (*Dennefors BL et al. Progesterone and adenosine 3',5'-monophosphate formation by isolated human corpora lutea of different ages: Influence of human chorionic gonadotrophin and prostaglandins. J. Clin. Endocrino. & Metab. 3:227-34, 1943*) and thus could contribute to the increased estrogen/progesterone ratio seen in premenstrual syndrome (PMT-A).

<u>Vegetarian</u> diet.

Benefits may be due to its low fat and high fiber content.

Vegetarians excrete 2-3 times more estrogen in their feces and have 50% lower mean plasma levels of un-conjugated estrogens than do omnivores (*Goldin BR et al. Estrogen excretion patterns and plasma levels in vegetarian and omnivorous women.* <u>New Engl. J. Med.</u> *307:1542-47, 1982; Goldin BR et al. Effect of diet on excretion of estrogens in pre- and post-menopausal women.* <u>Cancer Res.</u> *41:3771-73, 1981*).

Restrict <u>sugar</u> intake to below 10% of calories.

May impair estrogen metabolism in the liver.

Experimental Study: 21 normal adult males received a typical Western diet containing 25-30% sucrose for 18 days and a "calorically diluted" diet containing less than 10% sucrose for 12 days. Serum GOT and GPT levels rose significantly on the high sucrose diet and returned to baseline levels on the low sucrose diet. The extent of the enzyme elevation was so great in 2 subjects that they had to be withdrawn from the study. Data analysis suggested that both surplus calories and ex-cess sucrose consumption contributed to the rise in enzyme levels which, the authors suggest, may be indicative of hepatic injury (*Porikos KP, van Itallie TB. Diet-induced changes in serum transaminase and triglyceride levels in healthy adult men. Role of sucrose and excess calories.* <u>Am. J. Med.</u> *75:624, 1983*).

- -

NUTRIENTS:

<u>Vitamin B Complex:</u>

If deficient, hepatic inactivation of estrogen may be impaired, and supplementation may be beneficial.

Experimental Study: In order to determine whether female pts. with signs and symptoms of nutri-tional deficiency also suffered from symptoms of estrogen excess, the nutritional status of pts. presenting with menorrhagia, metrorrhagia, cystic mastitis and/or premenstrual tension was inves-tigated. As a definite correlation was found, treatment of these conditions with vitamin B complex (containing thiamin 3-9 mg, riboflavin 4.5-9 mg and up to 60 mg of niacin and niacinamide along with the rest of the complex) was instituted with good results, suggesting that syndromes related to estrogen excess are caused by failure of the liver to inactivate estrogen because of deficiency of vitamin B complex (*Biskind MS. Nutritional deficiency in the etiology of menorrhagia, cystic mastitis and premenstrual tension, treatment with vitamin B complex.* <u>J. Clin. Endocrinol. Metabol.</u> *3:227-34, 1943*).

Animal Experimental Study: Estrone pellets were implanted in the spleens of adult castrate female rats so that the absorbed estrogen passed through the liver before reaching the systemic circulation. On a normal diet the animals remained anestrous, but when they were placed on a vitamin B com-plex-free diet, protracted estrus occurred. Addition of brewers yeast caused them to become anestrus, while subsequent dietary depletion again let to estrus, suggesting that the liver may have an important part in maintaining the body's estrogen level within the normal range and that a vitamin B deficiency may impair the hepatic estrogen-inactivating function (*Biskind MS, Biskind GR. Effect of vitamin B complex deficiency on inactivation of estrone in the liver.* <u>Endocrinology</u> *31:109-114, 1942*).

- Methionine:

Precursor of S-adenosylmethionine which has been shown to be beneficial in treating cholestasis due to estrogen excess (*Padova C et al. S-adenosyl-L-methionine antagonizes oral contraceptive-induced bile cholesterol supersaturation in healthy women: Preliminary report of a controlled randomized trial. Am. J. Gastroenterol. 79:941-44, 1984; Frezza M et al. Reversal of intrahepatic cholestasis of pregnancy in women after high dose S-adenosyl-L-methionine (SAMe) administration. Hepatology 4:274-78, 1984*).

- Pyridoxine: 300 mg. daily

If deficient, choline is unable to function properly as a lipotropic agent (*Engel RW. The relation of B-vitamins and dietary fat to the lipotropic action of choline. J. Biol. Chem 37:140, 1941*).

Deficiency lowers the hepatic clearance rate of estrogens resulting in hyperestrogenemia (*Abraham GE. Nutritional factors in the etiology of the premenstrual tension syndrome. J. Reproductive Med. 28(7):446-464, 1983*).

Vitamin E: 800 IU daily (mixed tocopherols)

An anti-oxidant which may be effective in the treatment of both premenstrual syndrome and fibrocystic breast disease, illnesses which may be due to impaired estrogen metabolism (*London RS et al. The effect of alpha-tocopherol on premenstrual symptomatology: A double-blind trial. J. Am. Coll. Nutr. 2:115-22, 1983; London RS et al. Nutr. Res. 2:243-47, 1982*).

– –

Selenium: 250 mcg. daily

An anti-oxidant required for the functioning of glutathione peroxidase, one of the peroxidases utilized in the liver to metabolize various substances.

– –

Bioflavonoids:

Examples: quercitin, apigenin

Inhibit human estrogen synthesis *in vitro* and may have a similar effect *in vivo* by competing with estrogen as a substrate (*Kellis Jr JT, Vickery LE. Inhibition of human estrogen synthetase (aromatase) by flavones. Science 255:1032-4, 1984*).

– –

OTHER FACTORS:

Lactobacillus Acidophilus:

Inhibits beta-glucuronidase, the fecal bacterial enzyme responsible for deconjugating liver-conjugated estrogen (*Goldin B, Gorsbach S. The effect of milk and lactobacillus feeding on human intestinal bacterial enzyme activity. Am. J. Clin. Nutr. 39:756-61, 1984*).

HYPERKINESIS

See Also: LEARNING DISABILTIES

BASIC DIET:

Limit <u>refined sugar</u>.

Negative Experimental Double-blind Crossover Study: 9 hospitalized behaviorally disturbed children (ages 9-13), 4 of whom met DSM III criteria for ADD with hyperactivity, were served breakfasts in which dietary protein, fat and complex carbohydrates were controlled while daily sucrose and total calories were varied. Aspartame was added to low-sucrose breakfasts to blind the children to that condition. They randomly received 12 high-sucrose and 12 low-sucrose breakfasts. The 4 ADD children received either methylphenidate or placebo under randomly generated double-blind conditions and were studied under 4 conditions of 6 days each: high sucrose-methylphenidate, low sucrose-methylphenidate, high sucrose-placebo and low sucrose-placebo. Subjects were rated by their teachers who were blind to the dietary condition using an abbreviated Conners scale for hyperactivity. While significant improvement in behavior was noted during methylphenidate treatment, no significant difference could be attributed to diet, and there was no significant Drug by Diet interaction (*Kaplan HK et al. Behavioral effects of dietary sucrose in disturbed children. Letter to the Editor.* <u>Am. J. Psychiat.</u> *143(7):944-45, 1986*).

Experimental Study: A moderate amount of sugar (about 1 ounce for a 40 lb child) eaten along with a meal balanced in fat, carbohydrate and protein improved classroom performance by speeding reaction time, decreasing errors and reducing activity levels. When eaten with a high-carbohydrate meal, however, sugar temporarily diminished classroom performance (*Wells, KC, Laboratory of Behavioral Medicine, Children's Hospital, Washington, D.C.- 1985*).

Negative Experimental Double-blind Study: 16 children said to become aggressive, overly active, loud and noncompliant when ingesting sugar were given a sugar-free home diet and openly challenged with a large dose (3 gm/kg) of sucrose. While there was no significant gp. behavioral change, 7/16 had a 15% increase from baseline in behavioral parameters. 5/7 were given a double-blind challenge test utilizing mint-flavored slushes of sucrose, honey, tapioca starch, or aspartame after a sucrose-free lunch. One reacted to both sucrose and honey, and on rechallenge reacted to honey again according to actometric readings, but this time not according the Stony Brook test, while he reacted to sugar only at the 70 minute Stony Brook. Another child who had reacted to sucrose reacted to placebo instead of sucrose when rechallenged. These results suggest that sugar is not related to abnormal behavior (*Mahan K et al. Sugar allergy and children's behavior. Abstract.* <u>Immunology and Allergy Practice</u>, *July, 1985, p. 81*).

Experimental Controlled Studies: (1) 12 children (ages 6-12) in a psychiatric hospital were given 50 gm of either sucrose or fructose; all showed increased classroom activity compared to controls, with no difference between sucrose and fructose. (2) A group of children who were under psychiatric care were followed for 6 months during which the sugar eaten at breakfast was adjusted to 1.25 gm/kg or switched to aspartame. Sugar added to protein or carbohydrates alone increased deviant behavior, but added to both together led to behavioral improvements. (3) In a study of 45 normal children, 1.75 gm/kg was compared to a breakfast of high protein, high carbohydrate, or no breakfast. Sugar in addition to a high carbohydrate breakfast increased deviant behavior, while sugar in addition to a high protein breakfast had no significant effect. These studies suggest that it is not sugar itself, but the absence of a well-balanced meal plus sugar that can lead to hyperactivity (*Conners CK - reported in* <u>Med. Tribune</u> *January 9, 1985*).

Negative Experimental Double-blind Study: Sucrose challenge studies revealed no changes in behavior or learning in 16 hyperactive boys when compared to aspartame placebo (*Wolraich M et al. Effects of sucrose ingestion on the behavior of hyperactive boys. J. Pediatrics 106(4):675-82, 1985*).

Negative Experimental Single-blind Study: 50 children whose mothers believed that they became hyperkinetic from sugar received either sucrose or saccharin in a lemon beverage; no consistent response to sucrose was observed, although some of the children could tell the difference between the taste of saccharin and sugar (*Gross MD. Effect of sucrose on hyperkinetic children. Pediatrics 74(5):876-7, 1984*).

Experimental Double-blind Study: Sugar consumption was tabulated for a group of hyperactive children and a control group and trained observers, blind to the purpose of the study, evaluated the children's behavior by categories viewing a videotape made through a one-way mirror. Sugar consumption was found to significantly correlate with observed restlessness and destructive-aggressive behavior (*Prinz RJ et al. J. Behavioral Ecology Vol.2,No.1, 1981*)

Observational Study: 28 hyperactive children were found to have higher sugar consumption than 28 normal controls (*Prinz RJ et al. Dietary correlates of hyperactive behavior in children. J. Consulting Clin. Psychol. 48:760-9, 1980*).

Observational Study: Glucose metabolism, blood chemistry and hematology were studied for 265 hyperkinetic children. Compared to published norms, glucose tolerance tests were abnormal in 76% (i.e. greater than 20 points above or below the median value). 50% had flat glucose curves, 15% had excessive peaks with rapid declines, and 11% had excessive peaks with slow recovery, suggesting that abnormal glucose metabolism may be a factor in the etiology of hyperkinesis (*Langseth L, Dowd J. Glucose tolerance and hyperkinesis. Fd. Cosmet. Toxicol. 16:129, 1978*).

- -

NUTRIENTS:

Vitamin B Complex:

Supplementation may be beneficial to selected individuals.

Experimental Single-blind Studies: 100 children were given megadoses of various B complex vitamins or placebo. 15% responded to pyridoxine, 8% to thiamine and several to niacinamide. Half of those who benefited from pyridoxine were worse on thiamine and visa versa (*Brenner A. The effects of megadoses of selected B complex viatmins on children with hyperkinesis: Controlled studies with long term followup. J. Learning Disabil. 15:258, 1982*).

- Niacin:

Supplementation may be beneficial.

Experimental Single-blind Study: 33 children under age 13 with disturbed and disturbing behavior were placed on nicotinamide (or rarely, if no response, on nicotinic acid) with doses increasing from 1.5 to 6 gm daily along with ascorbic acid 3 gm daily and, rarely, very small doses of tranquilizers or anti-depressants. Upon recovery (free of symptoms and signs, performing well in school, getting on well with their families and with the community), they were switched from niacin to placebo tablets while the ascorbic acid and other chemotherapy was unchanged. The mother and the author, but not the child, were aware of the switch. Only 1/33 children failed to respond to B3 therapy and all relapsed within 30 days after the placebo was substituted and recovered again when B3 was restarted. The author suggests a trial of niacin for children showing evidence of at least 3 of the following: hyperactivity, deteriorating school performance, perceptual changes and inability to acquire or maintain social relationships (*Hoffer A. Vitamin B3 dependent child. Schizophrenia 3:107-113, 1971*).

- <u>Niacin</u> and
<u>Pyridoxine</u>:

Supplementation may be beneficial.

Case Report: 14 year-old pt. received nicotinamide 3 gm daily and pyridoxine 0.5 gm daily. When seen for follow-up 2 mo. later he was markedly improved (*Hoffer A. Treatment of hyperkinetic children with nicotinamide and pyridoxine. Letter to the Editor.* <u>*Can. Med. Assoc. J.*</u> *107:111-12, 1972*).

- <u>Pyridoxine</u>:   20-30 mg/kg/day (500mg 2-3 times daily for 110 pound child)

May be effective <u>if</u> pts. have low blood serotonin levels.

Experimental Double-blind Study: 30 children with ADD had normal blood serotonin levels and failed to benefit from megavitamin therapy, including pyridoxine (*Haslam RH, Dalby JT.* <u>*New Engl. J. Med.*</u> *309:1328, 1983*).

Experimental Double-blind Crossover Study: For 6 children with low whole blood serotonin levels, B6 increased serotonin levels and was more effective than Ritalin in decreasing hyperkinesis and, in contrast to Ritalin, its benefit continued into the following placebo period (*Coleman M et al. A preliminary study of the effect of pyridoxine administration in a subgroup of hyperkinetic children: A double-blind crossover comparison with methylphenidate.* <u>*J. Biol. Psych.*</u> *14(5):741-51, 1979*).

Experimental Study: When pyridoxine was administered to hyperkinetic children with low serotonin, serotonin increased to normal and the hyperkinesis disappeared (*Bhagavan et al.* <u>*Pediatrics*</u> *vol. 55, 1975*).

- -

Calcium:

Supplementation may be beneficial if deficient.

Case Report: 9 year old boy diagnosed as hyperactive at age 4 had been on methylphenidate for 2 1/2 years. EEG revealed unusual electrical discharges in the rt. temporal region, and blood tests revealed a very low calcium level. Increasing milk intake resulted in marked behavioral improvement (*Walker S III. Drugging the American child: We're too cavalier about hyperactivity.* <u>*J. Learning Disabil.*</u> *8:354, 1975*).

- -

Essential Fatty Acids:

May be deficient.

Observational Study: A survey of a large number of hyperactive children revealed the following findings which support the hypothesis that many such children have a deficiency of essential fatty acids either because they cannot metabolize linoleic acid normally, or because they cannot absorb EFAs normally from the gut, or because the EFA requirements are higher than normal:
1. Most foods which cause symptoms in these children are weak inhibitors of the conversion of EFAs to prostaglandins (PGs).
2. Males (who have much higher EFA requirements than females) are more commonly affected.
3. Excessive thirst, a cardinal sign of EFA deficiency, is found in a high proportion.
4. Many have eczema, allergies and asthma which reports suggest can be alleviated by EFAs.

5. Many are zinc deficient which is required for the conversion of EFAs to PGs.

6. Some are badly affected by wheat and milk which give rise to exorphins in the gut which can block the conversion of EFAs to PGE₁.

(*Colquhoun I, Bunday S. A lack of essential fatty acids as a possible cause of hyperactivity in children. Med. Hypotheses 7:673-9, 1981*).

Supplementation may be beneficial.

Experimental Study: 5 hyperactive children received evening primrose oil 1-1.5 gm twice daily with good results (*Colquhoun - ibid*).

- -

COMBINED TREATMENT:

Negative Experimental Double-blind Study: 41 ADD children and 75 controls participated. Serum ascorbic acid and pyridoxine levels were not significantly different between groups. The ADD gp. received 13 wks. of supplementation as recommended by Cott (*Cott A. The Orthomolecular Approach to Learning Disabilities. Academic Therapy Pub., San Rafael, Calif., 1977, pp. 26-9*) consisting of initial doses of ascorbic acid 1 gm, niacinamide 1 gm and pyridoxine 200 mg with increments every 2 wks. until the final doses were 3 times the initial ones. 12/38 ADD children completing the trial showed improvement and were placed in a double-blind, repeated crossover trial with 4 consecutive 6 wk. treatment periods. Teacher assessment saw no difference in hyperactivity between treatments and parents as well as classroom observers rated the children as worse during the megavitamin treatment periods. There was also a significant rise in aspartate transaminase after megavitamin therapy (attributed to niacinamide), suggesting that such therapy may be potentially dangerous (*Haslam RHA et al. Effects of megavitamin therapy on children with attention deficit disorders. Pediatrics 74:103-111, 1984*).

Negative Experimental Double-blind Study: 31 children with minimal brain dysfunction randomly received either niacin 1 gm, ascorbic acid 1 gm, pyridoxine 100 mg, pantothenate calcium 200 mg and glutamic acid 500 mg, each twice daily, or placebo. After 2 wks., only 2 children, both in the placebo gp., improved sufficiently so as to be able to discontinue stimulants. Change scores as rated blindly by teachers and parents failed to show a significant difference between supplementation and placebo groups (*Arnold LE et al. Megavitamins for minimal brain dysfunction: A placebo-controlled study. JAMA 240:2642, 1978*).

- -

OTHER FACTORS:

Rule out food sensitivities.

Experimental Double-blind Controlled Study: 86/140 (61%) children with behavior disorders experienced significant improvement with a modified elimination and challenge protocol, 75% (64/86) of whom reacted to double-blind challenge with salicylates but not to placebo (*Swain A et al. Salicylates, oligoantigenic diets, and behavior. Letter to the Editor. Lancet, July 6, 1985, pp. 41-2*).

Experimental Double-blind Crossover Study: 62/76 (82%) overactive children treated with an oligoantigenic diet improved, and 21 of them achieved a normal range of behavior. 28 of the improved children completed a double-blind, crossover, placebo-controlled trial in which suspicious foods were reintroduced. Symptoms returned or worsened much more often when pts. were on these foods compared to placebo. Of the 48 foods incriminated, artificial colors and preservatives were the commonest provoking substances (*Egger J et al. Controlled trial of oligoantigenic treatment in the hyperkinetic syndrome. Lancet 1:540-5, 1985*).

Observational Study: 25 children with "tension fatigue syndrome" and their parents were studied. 100% were found to have allergic pallor and sleep disturbance, 92% catarrhal symptoms, 84% abnormal EEG,

80% urinary problems, 72% night sweats, 72% alimentary problems and 60% respiratory problems. All the subjects had an unusually high preference for refined carbohydrate food and chemical additives ("junk and fast foods") compared to siblings, and the majority had drug sensitivities. 100% of parents had similar problems with food and chemical sensitivities, tension fatigue syndrome, obesity, anxiety/tension symptoms, depressive-phobic symptoms or hallucinatory symptoms (*Menzies IC. Disturbed children: The role of food and chemical sensitivities. Nutrition and Health 3:39-54, 1984*).

Experimental Double-blind Study: 13 hyperkinetic children and 13 controls were challenged with 20 different food and inhalant allergenic extracts, 20 phenolic food components and traditional antigens, and observed for behavioral changes consistent with hyperactivity. Acetyl salicylate was the phenolic compound provoking the greatest frequency of responses (80%), while the greatest responses from foods were from sugar, corn, beef and egg (25-30%). Cat hair and house dust provoked positive responses in 25% (*McGovern J et al. Int. J. Biosocial Res. 4:40-2, 1983*).

Experimental Study: A gp. of children with attention deficit disorder with hyperactivity (ADD/HA) were placed on a week-long fast supported with a chemically defined diet. Pre- and post-tests included several standard objective psychological tests and 3 neurological tests. The concordance among tests was high and results divided the children into 2 groups: 7 were judged as ill primarily due to food hypersensitivity, and 3 had an etiology which was only partly due to food hypersensitivity (*Hughes EC et al. Food sensitivity in attention deficit disorder with hyperactivity (ADD/HA): A procedure for differential diagnosis. Ann. Allergy 49:276-80, 1982*).

NIH Consensus Panel Report: Decreases in hyperactivity in children on special diets (when properly documented) were inconsistent as were reports of behavioral changes by observers (*Consensus Conference - NIAID and NICHHD. Defined diets and childhood hyperactivity. JAMA 248:290, 1982; NIH Consensus Development Conference. Defined diets and childhood hyperactivity. Clin. Ped. 21:627, 1982*).

NIH Consensus Panel Report: There is no clear proof that the Feingold (salicylate and food additive elimination) diet reduces hyperkinetic behavior, although there are enough individual instances of improvement to warrant a trial of the diet for 1-2 months "after thorough and appropriate evaluation of the child and family - including consideration of other possible therapies" (*NIH panel finds Finegold diet unproved but OKs trying it briefly. Med. World News February 15, 1982, pp. 19-20*).

Experimental Double-blind Study: 14 children who met the clinical criteria of hyperkinetic syndrome were tested for reactions to foods, food colors and inhalent antigens by provocative testing methods and a mixture of neutralizing doses and placebo was given for 3 wks. each in random order. The allergy extract could be differentiated from placebo on the basis of improved activity and behavior patterns by 11/14 (78%) parents and 7/13 (54%) teachers (*O'Shea JA, Porter SF. Double-blind study of children with hyperkinetic syndrome treated with multi-allergen extract sublingually. J. Learning Disabilities 14(4):189-191&237, 1981*).

Negative Experimental Double-blind Crossover Study: In a randomized design, 11 children maintained on the Feingold (salicylate and food additive elimination) diet were challenged with food coloring and placebo (one each wk.). Evaluations by parents, teachers, and psychiatrists and psychological testing failed to provide evidence of an effect from food coloring (*Mattes JA, Gittelman R. Effects of artificial food colorings in children with hyperactive symptoms. Arch. Gen. Psychiat. 38:714-8, 1981*).

Observational Study: In a gp. of 90 hyperactive children, food allergy on the basis of RAST results was significantly associated with hyperactivity only in those who also had learning disability and minimal brain dysfunction (*Tryphonas H, Trites R. Food allergy in children with hyperactivity, learning disabilities and/or minimal brain dysfunction. Ann. Allergy 42:22-7, 1979*).

Rule out <u>aluminum</u> toxicity.

Observational Study: 28 children suffering from hyperactivity or learning disorders were found to have elevated serum aluminum levels (17 $\pm$ 6.9 mcg while normal is below 10 mcg) (*Howard JMH. Clinical import of small increases in serum aluminum. <u>Clin. Chem.</u> 30(10):1722-3, 1984*).

Rule out <u>lead</u> toxicity.

Observational Study: While middle class hyperactive children did not have significantly higher chelated urine lead levels than normals, there was a trend for a greater proportion of hyperactive children than normals to have toxic lead levels, and hyperactive children had significantly higher lead levels than their own siblings (p less than 0.02), suggesting that lead levels are weakly associated with hyperactivity in middle class children (*Gittelman R, Eskenazi B. Lead and hyperactivity revisited. An investigation of nondisadvantaged children. <u>Arch. Gen. Psychiat</u> 40:827-33, 1983*).

Observational Study: Black, inner-city hyperactive children had higher chelated urine lead levels than nonhyperactive children from the same area (62% vs. 29%) (*David O et al. Lead and hyperactivity. <u>Lancet</u> 2:900-3, 1972*).

See Also:

Negative Observational Study: *Hole K et al. Lead intoxication as an etiologic factor in hyperkinetic behavior in children: A negative report. <u>Acta Paediatr. Scand</u> 68:759, 1979*

HYPERTENSION

See Also: PREGNANCY AND NUTRITION

OVERVIEW:

Nutritional manipulation been proven to be an effective treatment method. A <u>high fiber, low fat</u> (with a high percentage of polyunsaturates), <u>low salt</u> diet is suggested.

The intake and metabolism of 4 minerals (<u>calcium</u>, <u>magnesium</u>, <u>potassium</u> and <u>sodium</u>) are of major importance in blood pressure regulation. Relatively higher intakes of calcium, magnesium and potassium, and a relatively lower intake of sodium, appear to be beneficial.

In addition, early studies suggest that supplementation with <u>omega-3 fatty acids</u> in fish oils or <u>coenzyme Q_{10}</u> may be beneficial.

Elevated blood <u>cadmium</u> levels appear to be related to hypertension, and <u>zinc</u> may counteract these effects. Blood <u>lead</u> levels are also positively correlated with BP.

General Reference: *Borgman RF. Dietary factors in essential hypertension. <u>Prog. Food Nutr. Sci.</u> 9:109-47, 1985*

- -

BASIC DIET:

<u>High fiber</u> diet.

> **Experimental Study:** 300 health food shop customers received an increased cereal fiber intake of 100 gm/wk which was followed by a reduction in systolic and diastolic BP of 4 and 3 mm Hg respectively (*Burr ML et al. Dietary fibre, blood pressure and plasma cholesterol. <u>Nutr. Res.</u> 5:465-72, 1985*).

> **Experimental Study:** 12 diabetic men were placed on a 2 wk. diet containing more than 3 times the dietary fiber and fat of the control diet along with a 50% increase in sodium and potassium. Ave. B.P. dropped 10%. In subjects who had had normal B.P.,systolic pressures were 8% lower and diastolic pressures were 10% lower. In hypertensive subjects, systolic pressures dropped 11% and diastolic pressures 10% (*Anderson JW. <u>Annals Int. Med.</u> May, 1983*).

> See Also:

> > *Silman AJ. Dietary fibre and blood pressure. <u>Brit. Med. J.</u> January 26, 1980, p. 250*

> > *Wright A et al. Dietary fibre and blood pressure. <u>Proc. Nutr. Soc.</u> 39:3A, 1980*

> > *Wright A et al. Dietary fibre and blood pressure. <u>Brit. Med. J.</u> 2:1541, 1979*

<u>Vegetarian</u> diet.

> Benefits may be due to its high content of fiber, polyunsaturates, vegetable protein, potassium and/or magnesium (*Rouse IL et al. Blood pressure lowering effects of a vegetarian diet: Controlled trial in normotensive subjects. <u>Lancet</u> 1:5-9, 1983*).

Associated with lower systolic and diastolic BP.

Observational and Experimental Study: Systolic BP of 97 Seventh-day Adventist vegetarians was almost 5 mm Hg lower than that of 113 Morman omnivores and the diastolic BP was 4-5 mm Hg lower when adjusted for age, height and weight despite similar strengths of religious affiliations, consumption of alcohol, tea and coffee and use of alcohol. In a controlled intervention study, mean systolic and diastolic BP and serum cholesterol fell significantly during feeding with a vegetarian diet. Dietary analysis indicated that a vegetarian diet provided more polyunsaturated fat, fiber, vitamin C, vitamin E, magnesium, calcium and potassium and significantly less total fat, saturated fat and cholesterol than an omnivore diet (*Rouse IL et al. Vegetarian diet, blood pressure and cardiovascular risk. Aust. N.Z. J. Med. 14(4):439-43, 1984*).

Experimental Controlled Study: 59 healthy omnivorous subjects were randomly assigned to a control gp. or to one of two experimental gps. whose members ate an omnivorous diet for the first 2 wks. and a lacto-ovo-vegetarian diet for one of two 6-wk. experimental periods. Mean systolic and diastolic B.P. changed significantly only in the experimental gps., dropping during the vegetarian diet in both gps. and rising in the experimental gp. which reverted to the omnivorous diet. Diet-related changes were some 5-6 mm. Hg systolic and 2-3 mm. Hg diastolic and did not appear to be mediated by changes in sodium or potassium intake but could be mediated by changes in dietary fat, since the vegetarian diet is lower in total fat and has a higher P/S ratio (*Rouse IL et al. Blood pressure lowering effects of a vegetarian diet: Controlled trial in normotensive subjects. Lancet 1:5-9, 1983*).

Observational Study: 98 vegetarians were compared to a matched gp. of nonvegetarians. The ave. BP was 126/77 for the vegetarians and 147/88 for the control gp., a significant difference. Only 2% of the vegetarians had hypertension (BP above 160/95) compared to 26% of the non-vegetarians. Both gps. had a similar sodium intake and excreted the same amounts of sodium, while potassium intake and excretion was significantly higher in the vegetarians; thus it appears that the high potassium intake of vegetarians could account for the diet's anti-hypertensive effect (*Ophir O et al. Am. J. Clin. Nutr. 37:755-762, 1983*).

Low fat diet (with high percentage of polyunsaturates).

Polyunsaturates may lower B.P. because they are metabolized into prostaglandins which are vasodilators and enhance sodium and water excretion (*Iacono JM et al. Reduction of blood pressure associated with dietary polyunsaturated fat. Hypertension 4(Supp. III):III-34, 1982*).

See also: "*Omega-3 Fatty Acids*" and "*Omega-6 Fatty Acids*" below.

Experimental Controlled Study: 84 middle-aged Finns were randomly allocated into 2 groups. In both gps., the proportion of energy from fats was reduced from 38-24%. In gp. I, the polyunsaturated/saturated fat ratio was increased from 0.2 to 0.9 while, in gp.II, it was only increased to 0.4. After 12 wks., mean systolic BP decreased 4 mm Hg in gp. I (p less than 0.01) and 3 mm Hg in gp. II (p less than 0.01). Mean diastolic BP decreased 5 mm Hg in Gp. I (p less than 0.001) and 4 mm Hg in gp. II (p less than 0.01). These reductions were reversed during a subsequent switch-back period. Results show no significant further BP reduction with more than a moderately increased P/S ratio when the saturated fat intake is markedly reduced (*Puska P et al. Dietary fat and blood pressure: An intervention study on the effects of a low-fat diet with two levels of polyunsaturated fat. Prev. Med. 14(5):573-84, 1985*).

Experimental Study: Finns, who consume more saturated and less polyunsaturated fats compared to Italians and Americans, have a higher incidence of hypertension. When 30 Finnish couples aged 40-50 were placed for 6 wks. on a low-fat diet high in polyunsaturates and low in saturated fats with no change in sodium intake, systolic BP dropped 7.5 mm Hg and diastolic BP dropped 2.8 mm Hg. Six wks. after normal diets were resumed, systolic and diastolic BP increased by 7.7 and 6.3 mm Hg, respectively (*Iacono JM et al.   Effect of dietary fat on blood pressure in a rural Finnish population. Am . J. Clin. Nutr. 38(6):860-69, 1983*).

Experimental Controlled Study: 57 healthy Finnish couples ages 30-50 were studied. Those following a diet low in fat and high in polyunsaturates for 6 wks. experienced a significant drop in systolic BP from 139 mm. Hg to 129 mm. Hg, and in diastolic BP from 89 mm. Hg to 81 mm. Hg. Slightly hypertensive subjects had a greater drop than normotensives. BP rose to baseline when the low fat diet was discontinued. These drops did not occur in other subjects who either continued their regular diet or reduced salt intake from 192 mmol. to 77 mmol., suggesting that reducing dietary fat may be more effective than reducing salt (*Puska P et al.   Controlled, randomised trial of the effect of dietary fat on blood pressure. Lancet 1:1-5, 1983*).

See Also:

> *Smith-Barbaro PA, Pucak GJ.   Dietary fat and blood pressure. Ann. Int. Med. 98:828-31, 1983*

> *Rao R et al.   Effect of polyunsaturated vegetable oils on blood pressure in essential hypertension. Clin. Exp. Hypertension 3:27-38, 1981*

Low sugar diet.

Experimental Study: The BP of 20 healthy normotensive men was examined after they had ingested various sugar solutions following an overnight fast. Ingestion of water, lactose or galactose produced no change in BP, while systolic BP 1 hr. after glucose ingestion rose significantly (10 mg Hg) for 2 hours and ingestion of sucrose produced a significant increase (9 mm Hg) that lasted for 1 hour (*Rebello T et al. Short-term effects of various sugars on antinatriuresis and blood pressure changes on normotensive young men. Am. J. Clin. Nutr. 38(1):84-94, 1983*).

Animal Experimental Study: Rats fed a diet similar to the common American diet (40% fat, 45% carbohydrates, 15% proteins) with 10-20% of total calories from sucrose (and the other 25-35% of total calories from starch) had significantly increased blood pressures compared to rats fed starch as their sole carbohydrate (*Ahems RA et al.   Moderate sucrose ingestion and blood pressure in the rat. J. Nutr. 110:725-31, 1980*).

Experimental Controlled Study: Average diastolic blood pressures of normal subjects fed 200 gms sucrose daily over 5 weeks were significantly higher than those who avoided sucrose (78 mm Hg compared to 73 mm Hg) (*Ahems RA. Fed. Proc. vol. 34, 1975*).

See Also:

> **Review Article:** *Hodges R, Rebello T.   Carbohydrates and blood pressure. Ann. Int. Med. 98:838-41, 1983*

Increase consumption of raw foods.

Experimental Study: For an mean duration of 6.7 mo., 32 pts. ingested an ave. of 62% of their calories in the form of uncooked food. Mean diastolic BP was significantly reduced by 17.8 mm Hg. In addition, there was a significant mean weight loss of 3.8 kg and 80% of those who smoked or drank alcohol abstained spontaneously (*Douglass J et al.   Effects of a raw food diet on hypertension and obesity. South. Med. J. 78(7):841, 1985*).

Restrict alcohol.

Review Article: Excessive alcohol intake is associated in many studies with proportionally higher arterial pressures and an increased prevalence of hypertension; thus hypertensive pts. should consume less than 2 oz. ethanol daily (*Nonpharmacological approaches to the control of high blood pressure. Final report of the subcommittee on nonpharmacological therapy of the 1984 Joint National Committee on Detection, Evaluation, and Treatment of High Blood Pressure. Hypertension 8(5):444-67, 1986*).

Experimental Controlled Study: 16 hypertensive men who were moderate (80 gm./ day) alcohol consumers were studied for 1 week. Medications were stopped and 8 consumed moderate amts. of beer for 4 days and then stopped, whereupon both systolic and diastolic B.P. dropped significantly. The other 8 were abstinent for 4 days and then consumed moderate amts. of beer which was followed in 2 days by a significant rise in both systolic and diastolic B.P. (*Potter JF, Beevers DG. Lancet 1:119-122, 1984*).

Observational Study: Alcohol consumption was studied in relation to BP for 883 men and 959 women aged 20-74 who were not on antihypertensive drugs. After the data were controlled for smoking, exercise and medication use, the amount of alcohol consumption was directly correlated with both systolic and diastolic BP for both men and non-estrogen-using women over 50 (*Fortmann, SP et al. The association of blood pressure and dietary alcohol: Differences by age, sex, and estrogen use. Am. J. Epidemiol. 118(4):497-507, 1983*).

Avoid caffeine.

Research regarding the long-term effects of caffeine intake upon blood pressure is inconclusive (*Borgman RF. Dietary factors in essential hypertension. Prog. Food Nutr. Sci. 9(1-2):109-47, 1985*).

Review Article: Drinking coffee results in increased BP after an interval of caffeine abstinence but, during chronic caffeine intake, this pressor response disappears and adaptation to the circulatory effects of caffeine develops (*Smits P et al. Circulatory effects of coffee in relation to the pharmacokinetics of caffeine. Am. J. Cardiol. 56(15):958-63, 1985*).

Experimental Double-blind Study: 9/18 borderline pts. received placebo during the first 3 days of the study, caffeine 250 mg with meals 3 times daily during the next 7 days, and placebo during the final 4 days, while the rest received placebo throughout the study. Systolic BP was immediately increased (9.2 +/- 3.4 mm Hg) after the first dose of caffeine. On the first day of caffeine, systolic BP was increased by a mean of 7.3 +/- 4.0 mm Hg, but this was no longer significant afterwards. Diastolic BP showed a trend toward increasing, but never reached significance. It is concluded that prolonged administration of caffeine is not associated with significant elevation in blood pressure in borderline hypertensives (*Robertson D et al. Caffeine and hypertension. Am. J. Med. 77(1):54-60, 1984*).

- -

NUTRIENTS:

Vitamin A:

Lower intake associated with hypertension.

Observational Study: The intake of 17 nutrients was surveyed in over 10,000 adult Americans who denied a history of hypertension. A significant decrease in vitamin A intake was 1 of the 4 nutritional factors that distinguished hypertensive from normotensive subjects (*McCarron DA et al. Blood pressure and nutrient intake in the United States. Science 224(4656):1392-98, 1984*).

Vitamin B Complex:

Supplementation may be beneficial.

Experimental Study: 45 pts. with coronary heart disease and hypertension received daily supplementation with thiamine diphosphate 50 mg, riboflavin 40 mg, calcium pantothenate 200 mg, nicotinic acid 200 mg and lipoic acid 50 mg. After 10 days, the content of unsaturated (linoleic and arachidonic) fatty acids increased while that of saturated (stearic and palmitic) fatty acids decreased (*Vodoevich VP, Buko VU. [Effect of the B-group vitamin complex on the blood content of saturated and unsaturated fatty acids in patients with ischemic heart disease and hypertension.] Vopr. Pitan. (2):9-11, 1986*).

Vitamin C:

Lower intake associated with hypertension.

Observational Study: The intake of 17 nutrients was surveyed in over 10,000 adult Americans who denied a history of hypertension. A significant decrease in vitamin C intake was 1 of the 4 nutritional factors that distinguished hypertensive from normotensive subjects (*McCarron DA et al. Blood pressure and nutrient intake in the United States. Science 224(4656):1392-98, 1984*).

Supplementation may be beneficial.

Observational Study: Blood pressures and serum vitamin C levels of healthy Japanese men (aged 30-39) were examined. Compared to men with high vitamin C levels, men with low vitamin C levels had 7.4 times the prevalence of hypertension, and men with intermediate levels had 4.6 times the prevalence. Results suggest why some populations with high vitamin C intake have a low mortality rate from heart disease and atherosclerosis (*Yoshioka M et al. Inverse association of serum ascorbic acid level and blood pressure or rate of hypertension in male adults aged 30-39 years. Int. J. Vitam. Nutr. Res. 54:343-7, 1984*).

Vitamin D:

Supplementation may be beneficial.

Observational Study: Women between the ages of 20 and 35 who consumed at least 400 IU daily in their diets had significantly lower systolic BP (*Sowers MF et al. The association of intakes of vitamin D and calcium with blood pressure among women. Am. J. Clin. Nutr. 42:135-42, 1985*).

— —

Calcium: 1000 - 2000 mg. daily   (2 month trial)

Alterations in calcium metabolism may be a primary factor in the development of hypertension.

Review Article: It appears that there are parallel deviations in plasma renin activity, circulating ionized calcium, and calcium-regulating hormones, which suggest a calcium deficiency in some hypertensives, and a calcium excess in others (*Resnick LM. Alterations of dietary calcium intake as a therapeutic modality in essential hypertension. Can. J. Physiol. Pharmacol. 64(6):803-7, 1986*).

Review Article: Abnormalities in calcium homeostasis may be a primary factor in the pathogenesis of hypertension. The effects of sodium or chloride or both on BP may represent, in selected situations, secondary influences mediated through induced changes in calcium homeostasis. Reduced dietary calcium is the most consistent nutritional correlate of hypertension in the U.S., and there is increasing data relating disordered calcium metabolism to altered vascular smooth muscle function and increased peripheral vascular resistance (*McCarron DA. Is calcium more important than sodium in the pathogenesis of essential hypertension? Hypertension 7(4):607-27, 1985*).

Review Article: While certain studies suggest that increased calcium availability may be associated with increased BP, others suggest that a calcium deficiency may contribute to the pathogenesis of hypertensive disease. Calcium metabolic indices may predict and even determine dietary sodium sensitivity in hypertension, as well as the BP responsiveness to antihypertensive drug therapy.

Moreover, oral calcium supplementation may posesss antihypertensive actions in specifically targeted renin subgroups of essential hypertensive subjects. It may ultimately be the calcium-regulating hormones, rather than circulating calcium levels, that mediate BP and possibly even the renin deviations observed among differing hypertensives (*Resnick LM et al. Calcium metabolism and the renin-aldosterone system in essential hypertension. J. Cardiovasc. Pharmacol. 7 Suppl. 6:S187-93, 1985*).

Review Article: Epidemiological surveys, animal experiments, and clinical trials support an inverse relationship between calcium and BP. Current basic research "suggests that when adequate levels of available calcium are present in cells, calcium acts as a calcium channel blocker, controlling its own influx across the cell membrane" (*Henry HJ et al. Increasing calcium lowers blood pressure: The literature reviewed. J. Am. Diet. Assoc. 85:182-5, 1985*).

See Also:

Review Article: *Hypertension: Is there a place for calcium? Lancet February 15, 1986, pp. 359-61*

Dietary calcium is negatively correlated with blood pressure.

Observational Study: The correlation between low calcium intake and hypertension appears to be stronger than either high sodium or low potassium intakes and hypertension (*Harlan WK et al. Blood pressure and nutrition in adults. The National Health and Nutrition Examination Survey. Am. J. Epidemiol. 120:17-27, 1984*).

Observational Study: Of 17 nutrients examined in the large Health and Nutrition Examination Survey (HANES I) of 10,372 adults who denied a history of hypertension and intentional dietary modification, dietary calcium was the only one which had a significant, consistent and independent association with BP among previously undiagnosed hypertensives (*McCarron DA et al. Blood pressure and nutrient intake in the United States. Science 224(4656):1392-98, 1984*).

Observational Study: Compared to 44 normal controls, 46 pts. reported significantly less daily calcium ingestion. The intake of other nutrients, including sodium and potassium, was very similar in the 2 groups, and the hypertensives differed from the controls primarily in nonfluid dairy products (*McCarron DA et al. Dietary calcium in human hypertension. Science 217(4556):267-69, 1982*).

Calcium excretion is positively correlated with blood pressure.

Observational Study: In a study of 194 young males and 174 young females (ages 19-35), males with elevated BP had greater calcium excretion than normotensives despite adequate calcium status and an equivalent calcium intake (*Medeiros DM et al. Blood pressure in young adults as influenced by diet, anthropometrics, calcium status and serum lipids. Nutr. Res. 6:359-68, 1986*).

Supplementation may be beneficial to pts. with low serum ionized calcium.

Review Article: "Calcium has enhanced anti-hypertensive effects in low renin subjects, having lower ionized calcium and higher endogenous 1,25-dihydroxyvitamin D values, and in subjects on higher dietary salt intake" (*Resnick LM. Alerations of dietary calcium intake as a therapeutic modality in essential hypertenion. Can. J. Physiol. Pharmacol. 64(6):803-7, 1986*).

See Also:

Resnick LM, Laragh JH. Renin, calcium metabolism and the pathophysiologic basis of antihypertensive therapy. Am. J. Cardiol. 56(16):68H-74H, 1985

Calcium supplementation may lower elevated blood pressure, perhaps by reducing the concentration of circulating parathyroid hormone which, in turn, may lower intracellular calcium by slowing calcium transport into arterial cells (*Belizan JM et al. The mediating role of the parathyroid gland in the effect of low calcium intake on blood pressure in the rat. Arch. Latinoam. Nutr. 34(4):666-75, 1984*).

Experimental Double-blind Study: 90 pts. (ages 16-29) with mild primary hypertension and elevated PTH or serum calcium randomly received either calcium as calcium citrate 1 gm daily or placebo. Calcium supplementation did not affect systolic BP. After 6 wks., the calcium-treated gp. had a mean 3.1 mm Hg greater drop in diastolic BP than the controls (p = 0.04). After 12 wks., the difference was 2.4 mm Hg (p = 0.11). Calcium-treated pts. with a baseline plasma parathyroid hormone higher than the median showed a 6.1 mm Hg greater drop at 6 wks. (p = 0.01) and a 5.4 mm Hg greater drop at 12 wks. (p = 0.01). Calcium-treated pts. whose BP values were above the median had a 6.1 mm Hg greater drop at 6 wks. and a 5.4 mm Hg greater drop at 12 weeks. Similarly, calcium-treated pts. whose serum calciums were above the median had a 6.5 mm Hg greater drop at 6 wks. and a 4.8 mm Hg drop at 12 wks. (*Grobbee DE, Hofman A. Effect of calcium supplementation on diastolic blood pressure in young people with mild hypertension. Lancet 2:703-7, 1986*).

Experimental Double-blind Crossover Study: The diets of 48 borderline hypertensives and 32 normals were randomly supplemented with either 1 gm calcium daily or placebo. After 8 wks., there was little change in the BP of normotensives except for a small but significant fall in supine diastolic BP. 44% of the hypertensives, however, had at least a 10 mg reduction in BP. Overall, hypertensives on calcium had a 5.6 mm decrease in standing systolic BP, a 3.8 mm decrease in supine BP, and a 2.3 mm decrease in supine diastolic BP, while standing diastolic BP was unaffected. Effects began to be noted after 6 weeks (*McCarron DA, Morris CD. Blood pressure response to oral calcium in persons with mild to moderate hypertension: A randomized double-blind placebo-controlled crossover trial. Ann. Int. Med. 103:825-31, 1985*).

Experimental Controlled Study: Part of a gp. of 81 normotensive and 34 medicated hypertensive women (ages 35-65) supplemented their diets with 1.5 gm calcium daily. After 4 yrs., total calcium intake was found to be unrelated to BP in normotensives; however, there was a significant decrease in systolic BP (13 mm) in supplemented hypertensives and a significant increase in systolic BP (7 mm) in unsupplemented hypertensives (*Johnson NE et al. Am. J. Clin. Nutr. 42:12-17, 1985*).

Experimental Study: 26 pts. with essential hypertension, low serum ionized calcium levels and no history of calcium stones or hypercalcemia were given 2 gms. calcium carbonate daily. Within 3 months, 16 responders (systolic decline of at least 10 mm Hg) decreased BP from an ave. of 160/94 to 128/81 (*Laragh J, Resnick LM - quoted in Med. World News March 1985 pp. 13-14*).

Experimental Double-blind Study: 46 young normotensive adults randomly received either 1 gm. calcium daily or placebo for 2 wks. Compared to the placebo gp., the experimental gp. significantly reduced BP. In men, there was a maximal 9% reduction by 6 wks.; in women there was a maximal 5% reduction by 9 wks. (*Belizan JM et al. Reduction of blood pressure with calcium supplementation in young adults. JAMA 249:1161-1165, 1983*).

Calcium and Phosphorus:

Low dietary calcium to phosphorus ratios are associated with hypertension (*Parrot-Garcia M, McCarron DA. Nutr. Rev. 42:205-13, 1984; Nutr. Rev. 42:223-25, 1984*).

Calcium and Vitamin D:

Supplementation may be beneficial.

Observational Study: Women between the ages of 55 and 80 who consumed at least 800 mg calcium and 400 IU vitamin D daily had significantly lower systolic BP than those who failed to do so

(Sowers MF et al.   The association of intakes of vitamin D and calcium with blood pressure among women.   Am. J. Clin. Nutr. 42:135-42, 1985).

<u>Magnesium:</u>

Mg is a potent vasodilator because of its ability to displace calcium from the same smooth muscle cell surfaces as well as its interference with the metabolism of acetylcholine at the myoneural junction. With Mg deficiency there is an increased flow of calcium into vascular muscle cells which increases contractility and potentiates the constrictor effects of humoral pressor substances. Reversible hypertension is a clinical finding in hypomagnesemia and Mg depletion; 50% of Mg depleted pts. are hypertensive and their B.P. returns to normal with supplementation. Mg deficiency is also associated with loss of cellular K *(Anabolism 2(6):1, 1983; Altura BM, Altura BT. Interactions of Mg and K on blood vessels: Aspects in view of hypertension. Magnesium 3(4-6):175-94, 1984; Altura BM, Altura BT. Magnesium ions and contraction of vascular smooth muscles: Relationship to some vascular diseases. Fed. Proc. 40(12):2672-9, 1981).*

Observational Study: Erythrocyte free magnesium levels were consistently low in 11 untreated hypertensives as compared to 7 normotensives (p less than 0.001) and 8 treated hypertensives (p less than 0.005), and showed an inverse correlation with both systolic and diastolic BP (p less than 0.001). Significant relationships were also found between intracellular free magnesium and extracellular serum calcium ion levels (p less than 0.001) as well as serum concentrations of total magnesium (p less than 0.001). Results suggest that abnormalities of intracellular magnesium metabolism may contribute to the pathophysiology of essential hypertension *(Resnick LM et al. Intracellular free magnesium in erythrocytes of essential hypertension: Relationship to blood pressure and serum divalent cations. Proc. Natl. Acad. Sci. USA 81(2):6511-5, 1984).*

Animal Experimental Study: Compared to controls, rats maintained for 3 months on diets either moderately or severely deficient in Mg demonstrated significant elevations in BP as well as decreased microvascular circulation *(Altura B et al. Magnesium deficiency and hypertension: Correlation between magnesium-deficient diets and microcirculatory changes in situ. Science 223:1315-17, 1984).*

Observational Study: 1000 stable, treated essential hypertensives were studied. 4.5% had definite hypomagnesemia and, regardless of their potassium levels, required a greater number of anti-hypertensive drugs for the same degree of BP control as hypertensives with normal magnesium levels. Since normal serum Mg may still be associated with celluar Mg depletion, the prevalence of Mg depletion may have been greater *(Whang R et al. Hypomagnesemia and hypokalemia in 1,000 treated ambulatory hypertensive patients. J. Am. Col. Nutr. 1:317-322, 1982).*

Supplementation may be beneficial.

Negative Experimental Double-blind Study: 40 pts. on diuretics received either magnesium oxide 301 mg or placebo. After 6 mo., there was no significant difference in systolic or diastolic BP between the 2 groups *(Henderson DG et al. Effect of magnesium supplementation on blood pressure and electrolyte concentrations in hypertensive patients receiving long term diuretic treatment. Br. Med. J. 293:664, 1986).*

Negative Experimental Double-blind Crossover Study: 17 mild-moderate hypertensives randomly received either 15 mmol daily of magnesium or placebo. After 1 mo., neither gp. demonstrated significant changes in BP *(Cappuccio FP et al. Lack of effect of oral magnesium on high blood pressure: A double blind study. Brit. Med. J. 291:235-8, 1985)*

Note: As calcium supplementation may take at least 6 wks. to lower BP, this trial may have been too short for reductions to occur.

Experimental Double-blind Study: After 6 mo., magnesium supplementation (15 mmol daily as magnesium aspartate) lowered BP by 12/8 mm Hg in 19 of 20 subjects in the experimental gp. compared to 0/4 in the placebo gp. (*Dyckner T, Wester O. Effect of magnesium on blood pressure. Br. Med. J. 286:1847-9, 1983*).

Potassium:

Dietary potassium is negatively associated with hypertension.

Observational Study: The intake of 17 nutrients was surveyed in over 10,000 adult Americans who denied a history of hypertension. A significant decrease in potassium intake was 1 of the 4 nutritional factors that distinguished hypertensive from normotensive subjects, and higher intakes of potassium were associated with lower mean systolic BP and lower absolute risk of hypertension (*McCarron DA et al. Blood pressure and nutrient intake in the United States. Science 224(4656):1392-98, 1984*).

Observational Study: In a study of 685 men and women ages 20-79, dietary potassium as estimated on a dietary history was significantly and negatively correlated with age-adjusted systolic pressure in both men and women and with age-adjusted diastolic pressure in women (*Khaw KT, Barrett-Connor. Dietary potassium and blood pressure in a population. Am. J. Clin. Nutr. 39:963-8, 1984*).

Observational Study: 98 vegetarians were compared to a matched gp. of nonvegetarians. The ave. BP was 126/77 for the vegetarians and 147/88 for the control gp., a significant difference. Only 2% of the vegetarians had hypertension (BP above 160/95) compared to 26% of the non-vegetarians. Both gps. had a similar sodium intake and excreted the same amounts of sodium, while potassium intake and excretion was significantly higher in the vegetarians; thus it appears that the high potassium intake of vegetarians could account for the diet's anti-hypertensive effect (*Ophir O et al. Am. J. Clin. Nutr. 37:755-762, 1983*).

Supplementation may be beneficial.

Experimental Double-blind Crossover Study: 20 healthy young males received either increased oral potassium (64 mmol daily) or placebo while on a normal sodium unrestricted diet. A significantly greater proportion had lower systolic and diastolic blood pressures on potassium than on placebo and the mean diastolic BP was significantly lowered by 2.4 mm HG on potassium. Change in diastolic pressure correlated negatively with change in 24 hr. urinary potassium and positively with change in 24 hr. urinary sodium/potassium ratio in individual subjects (*Khaw KT, Thom S. Randomised double-blind cross-over trial of potassium on blood pressure in normal subjects. Lancet 2:1127-29, 1982*).

Sodium:

Moderate restriction may possibly delay or prevent the development of hypertension (*Kaplan NM. Nondrug treatment of hypertension. Ann. Int. Med. 102:359-73, 1985*) and may be associated with a 5-10 mm. Hg. decrease in the 1/3-1/2 of hypertensives who are salt-sensitive (*Kawasaki T et al. The effect of high-sodium and low-sodium intakes on blood pressure and other related variables in human subjects with idiopathic hypertension. Am. J. Med. 64:193-98, 1978*).

Review Article: Although long-term studies are sorely lacking, sodium restriction to 2 gm/day has been shown to be manageable and safe and probably will benefit those hypertensive patients who are sodium-sensitive (*Nonpharmacological approaches to the control of high blood pressure. Final report of the Subcommittee on Nonpharmacological Therapy of the 1984 Joint National Committee on Detection, Evaluation, and Treatment of High Blood Pressure. Hypertension 8(5):444-467, 1986*).

Review Article: Data from 13 randomized trials showed the hypotensive effect of sodium restriction to be small and restricted largely to systolic BP,which fell by an average of 3.6 mm Hg (range 0.5-10.0 mm Hg). The reduction increased with age and in those with higher BP. Results suggest that sodium restriction may be of limited use in young pts. with mild hypertension (*Grobbee DE, Hofman A. Does sodium restriction lower the blood pressure?* Br. Med. J. *293:27-9, 1986*).

Negative Observational Study: Because of apparently elevated rates of hypertension in Gila Bend Papago indians and a high sodium level (440 mg/L) in the water supply, 342 indians and 375 non-indians living in the area 25 yrs. of age or older were interviewed. No consistent associations were found between any of the sodium values (dietary sodium intake and urinary sodium) and systolic or diastolic BP. Mean BP for the Gila Bend whites were lower in most age gps. than in comparison US white populations, and the prevalence of hypertension was not significantly higher than national rates (*Welty TK et al. Effects of exposure to salty drinking water in an arizona community: Cardiovascular mortality, hypertension prevalence, and relationships between blood pressure and sodium intake.* JAMA *255(5):622, 1986*).

Review Article: Restricting sodium is more reasonable for lowering BP of hypertensives than preventing hypertension in normotensives. Strict salt restriction to less than 1 gm daily lowers BP in approx. 60% of hypertensives, and less stringent restriction to 2-5 gm daily is also beneficial to roughly 1/2 of patients. Since it is usually difficult to lower salt to below 4 gm/day, this degree of restriction seems realistic. If BP does not fall an ave. of 5 mm Hg over 2 mo., it is probably pointless to continue restriction, unless the pt. is motivated to attempt a 1-2 mo. trial of restricting sodium to below 1 gm daily (*Egan B. Nutritional and lifstyle approaches to the prevention and management of hypertension.* Comprehen. Therapy *11(8):15-20, 1985*).

Negative Observational Study: Among normotensive young adults, the less table salt reportedly consumed, the higher the systolic and diastolic BP measured (*Phillips K et al.* Am. J. Public Health *75:405-6, 1985*).

Review Article: While evidence linking salt and hypertension is growing stronger, there is still uncertainty. It appears that, in the middle range of sodium intake, another factor, linked perhaps to the renal handling of sodium, contributes to the prevalence of hypertension (*Simpson FO. Salt and hypertension: Current data, attitudes, and policies.* J. Cardiovasc. Pharmacol. *6 Suppl. 1:S4-9, 1984*).

Negative Observational Study: The intake of 17 nutrients was surveyed in over 10,000 adult Americans who denied a history of hypertension. Not only did a significant increase in sodium intake fail to distinguish hypertensive from normotensive subjects, but higher intakes of sodium were associated with lower mean systolic BP and lower absolute risk of hypertension (*McCarron DA et al. Blood pressure and nutrient intake in the United States.* Science *224(4656):1392-98, 1984*).

Negative Observational Study: BP and salt intake was measured in 3566 men and women who had never been diagnosed as hypertensive. No significant difference in BP was found between those with the lowest and highest 10% of salt use, suggesting that moderate reduction of salt consumption by the general population to prevent hypertension is unjustified (*Holden RA et al. Dietary salt intake and blood pressure.* JAMA *250:365-9, 1983*).

Experimental Controlled Study: 1500 men and women were randomly selected in 3 towns. In 2 of the towns, subjects cut salt intake 30%; in the third, no dietary change was made. Follow-up measurements found that BP was 6.4% lower among the subjects in the low-salt towns as compared to the control town (*Farquhar J., Stanford U. - reported in* Time *3/15/82*).

Experimental Double-blind Crossover Study: 19 pts. with mild to moderate essential hypertension (ave. untreated supine BP - 156/98 mg Hg) were advised not to add salt to food and to avoid sodium-laden foods. After 2 wks. they received either Slow Sodium (Ciba) or placebo. The mean supine BP was 7.1 mg Hg (6.1%) lower in the fourth week of placebo than that in the fourth week of Slow sodium (p less than 0.001) (*MacGregor GA et al. Double-blind randomised crossover trial of moderate sodium restriction in essential hypertension. Lancet 1:351-55, 1982*).

See Also:

> *Freis E. Salt, volume and the prevention of hypertension. Am. J. Cardiol. 38:768-81, 1976*

- with potassium supplementation:

> **Review Article:** "Although the addition of potassium may reduce the hypertensive effect of a high-sodium intake, the potential hazards and considerable cost of large amounts of potassium supplements make this practice unacceptable. A more sensible approach is to reduce the intake of high-sodium, low-potassium processed foods and increase the intake of low-sodium, high-potassium natural foods. In addition, potassium chloride should be partially substituted for sodium chloride in cooking and at the table" (*Kaplan NM. Non-drug treatment of hypertension. Ann. Int. Med. 102:359-73, 1985*).

> **Negative Experimental Study:** 12 pts. were randomly given 1 of 3 diets: control, 180 mmol sodium and 60 mmol potassium; sodium-restricted, 80 mmol sodium and 60 mmol potassium; or potassium-supplemented, the same as the control diet plus 140 mmol/d of potassium elixir. On the basis of intra-arterial BP after 4-6 wks. on each diet, neither of the altered diets was associated with significant overall falls in BP, although 7/12 pts. had some fall on the lower sodium diet (*Richards AM et al. Blood-pressure response to moderate sodium restriction and to potassium supplementation in mild essential hypertension. Lancet 1:757-61, 1984*).

> **Observational Study:** Dietary intakes of 1939 subjects suggest that the sodium/potassium ratio may be a major determinant in the etiology of hypertension and that a high potassium diet may help to counteract the deleterious effects of sodium on blood pressure (*Miller GD. Relationship between urinary sodium and potassium, and arterial blood pressure: An epidemiologic study. J. Nat. Med. Assoc. 76(1):47-52, 1984*).

> See Also:

> > *Parfrey PS et al. Blood pressure and hormonal changes following alteration in dietary sodium and potassium in mild essential hypertension. Lancet 1:59, 1981*

> > *Parfrey PS et al. Blood pressure and hormonal changes following alteration in dietary sodium and potassium in young men with and without a family predisposition to hypertension. Lancet 1:113, 1981*

Zinc:

May counteract the deleterious effects of cadmium on BP (*see "Cadmium" below*).

- -

Coenzyme Q: 60 mg daily
(BP reduction takes 4-12 weeks)

Often deficient in hypertensives.

> **Observational Study:** Enzymatic assays revealed that 39% of 59 pts. were deficient compared to 6% of 65 controls (*Yamagami T et al. Bioenergetics in clinical medicine. Studies on coenzyme Q10 and essential hypertension. Res. Commun. Chem. Pathol. Pharmacol. 11:273, 1975*).

Supplementation may be beneficial.

Experimental Study: 25 essential hypertensives received CoQ_{10} 60 mg daily. After 8 weeks, there was a highly significant decrease in mean BP and 54% had a mean BP reduction of greater than 10% (*Yamagami T et al. Correlation between serum coenzyme Q levels and succinate dehydrogenase coenzyme Q reductase activity in cardiovascular disease and the influence of coenzyme Q administration, in Folkers K, Yamamura Y, Eds., Biomed. & Clin. Aspects of Coenzyme Q. Amsterdam, Elsevier Science Publishers, 1984, pp. 253-62*).

See Also:

Folkers K et al. Bioenergetics in clinical medicine. XVI. Reduction of hypertension in patients with coenzyme Q_{10}. Res. Commun. Chem. Pathol. Pharmacol. 31:129, 1981

Yamagami T et al. Bioenergetics in clinical medicine. III. Administration of coenzyme Q_{10} to patients with essential hypertension. Res. Commun. Chem. Pathol. Pharmacol. 14:721, 1976

Omega-3 Fatty Acids:

("MaxEPA" is a fish oil concentration high in omega-3 fatty acids including eicosapentaenoic acid.)

Supplementation may be beneficial.

Experimental Double-blind Crossover Study: 16 hypertensives received MaxEPA 16.5 gm daily or placebo. Mean BP was significantly lower by about 5% after EPA but not after placebo, although the reduction in diastolic BP did not reach statistical significance (*Norris PG et al. Effect of dietary supplementation with fish oil on systolic blood pressure in mild essential hypertension. Br. Med. J. 293:104, 1986*).

Experimental Crossover Study: After 2 wks. on a mackerel diet (high in omega-3 fatty acids) or a control herring diet, 15 subjects had "markedly lower" systolic and diastolic BP as well as significant decreases in cholesterol and triglycerides after the mackerel but not the herring diet (*Singer P et al. Lipid and blood-pressure-lowering effect of mackerel diet in man. Atherosclerosis 49(1):99-108, 1983*).

Experimental Study: The addition of 3 tbsp. (40 ml) cod liver oil (containing 10 gm omega-3 fatty acids) daily to the diet of 8 volunteers for 25 days was associated with a significant BP reduction (p less than 0.05) (*Lorenz R et al. Platelet function, thromboxane formation and blood presure control during supplementation of the Western diet with cod liver oil. Circulation 67(3):504-11, 1983*).

Omega-6 Fatty Acids:

$$\text{linoleic acid} \rightarrow \text{GLA} \rightarrow \text{DGLA} \rightarrow \text{Prostaglandin E}_1$$

Evening primrose oil is a rich source of GLA.

Supplementation may be beneficial.

Animal Experimental Study: Spontaneously hypertensive rats from 4 to over 24 wks. of age fed a standard diet supplemented with 10% evening primrose oil experienced a lowering of BP in the first 19 wks. of life which did not occur to controls supplemented with 10% hydrogenated coconut oil, 10% safflower oil or fed just a standard diet (*Soma M et al. The effects of hydrogenated coconut oil, safflower oil and evening primrose oil on development of hypertension and sodium handling in spontaneously hypertensive rats. Can. J. Physiol. Pharmacol. 63:325-30, 1985*).

Animal Experimental Study: Rats treated daily with 1 ml. EPO showed a significant decline in the vasopressor response to renin and angiotension II (*Scholkens BA et al. Evening primrose oil, a dietary prostaglandin precursor, diminishes vascular reactivity to renin and angiotensin II in rats. Prost. Leuko. Med. 8:273, 1982*).

See Also:

> *Mills DE et al. Gamma-linolenic acid attenuates cardiovascular responses to stress in borderline hypertensive rats. Lipids 20(9):573-77, 1985*

- -

OTHER FACTORS:

Rule out <u>food sensitivities</u>.

Experimental Study: 15 migraineurs with diastolic BP of 100 mm Hg or greater followed a 5-day elimination diet consisting usually of lamb and pears. The exclusion diet and avoidance of other precipitants resulted in reduction of diastolic BP to 90 mm Hg or below in every patient. BP rose when foods causing reactions were tested and fell to normal when these foods were avoided (*Grant CG. Food allergies and migraine. Lancet May 5, 1979, pp. 966-69*).

Experimental Study: 6 cases of hypertension are described with "definite and positive" evidence of a relationship between familial non-reaginic food allergy and hypertension. Food eliminations produced excellent clinical results in 2, good results in 2 and unfavorable results in 2 (*Price AS. The role of food allergy in hypertension: An experimental study. Rev. Gastroenterol. 10:233-45, 1943*).

Rule out <u>cadmium</u> toxicity.

Observational Study: Untreated hypertensives showed blood cadmium levels 3 - 4 times those in matched normotensives (*Glauser SC et al. Blood cadmium levels in normotensive and untreated hypertensive humans. Lancet 1:717-18, 1976*).

See Also:

> *Ostergaard K. Cadmium and hypertension. Lancet March 26, 1977, pp. 677-78*

> *Perry H et al. Hypertension following chronic, very low dose cadmium feeding. Proc. Soc. Experiment. Biol. & Med. 156:173-76, 1977*

> *Thind GS et al. Trace elements in human arterial hypertension. Physiologist August, 1976, p. 388*

<u>Zinc</u> counteracts the negative effects of cadmium on BP.

Observational Study: Compared to 37 healthy controls, 39 pts. had a higher total blood cadmium level, (p less than 10^{-5}), a lower plasma zinc level (p less than 10^{-7}), and a higher total blood cadmium to plasma zinc ratio. A negative correlation was found between blood cadmium and plasma zinc, and between BP (systolic and diastolic) and plasma zinc. A positive correlation was found between BP and blood cadmium, and therefore the blood cadmium to plasma zinc ratio (*Bartolin R et al. [Blood cadmium and plasma zinc in hypertensive patients. Apropos of 76 cases.] Rev. Med. Interne. 6(3):280-84, 1985*).

Animal Experimental Study: Supplementation with a zinc chelate was able to reverse cadmium-induced experimental hypertension in rats (*Schroeder HA, Buckman J. Cadmium hypertension: Its reversal in rats by a zinc chelate. Arch. Environ. Health 14:693, 1967*).

Rule out <u>lead</u> toxicity.

Observational Study: Lead levels previously considered safe were found to be associated with increased B.P. (*Harlan WR et al. Blood lead and blood pressure. Relationship in the adolescent and adult US population. <u>JAMA</u> 253(4):530-34, 1985*).

Observational Study: The Second Annual Health and Nutrition Survey (NHANES II, 1976-1980) substantially supports the growing evidence from both animal and epidemiologic studies that a causal association exists between serum lead and hypertension (*Peirkle JL et al. The relationship between blood lead levels and blood pressure and its cardiovascular risk implications. <u>Am. J. Epid.</u> 121:246-58, 1985*).

See Also:

Weiss ST et al. The relationship of blood lead to blood pressure in a longitudinal study of working men. <u>Am. J. Epidemiol.</u> 123(5):800-08, 1986

Shaper AG, Pocock SJ. Blood lead and blood pressure [editorial]. <u>Br. Med. J. [Clin. Res.]</u> 291:1147-49, 1985

"HYPOGLYCEMIA" (FUNCTIONAL)

See Also: ALCOHOLISM
            TINNITUS

BASIC DIET:

High fiber diet.

> **Experimental Study:** Of the different fibers, apple pectin and oat bran have the most pronounced effects on the hypoglycemic index (the fall in blood glucose in the 90 min. before reaching the nadir divided by the value of the nadir) (*Langseth L et al. Fd. Cosmet. Toxicol. 16:129-38, 1978*).

> **Experimental Study:** Pts. ingesting high-methoxy pectin had a marked reduction in hyperinsulinemia (*Anthony D et al. Diabetes 22:664-7, 1973*).

High protein, low carbohydrate diet.

> Said to be beneficial as blood sugar response to protein ingestion in both normals and functional hypoglycemics is flatter than for glucose, suggesting that there may be a smaller subsequent hypoglycemic swing (*Conn JW. The glycemic response to isoglucogenic quantitites of protein and carbohydrate. J. Clin. Invest. 15:665-71, 1936; Conn JW, Newburgh LH. The advantage of a high protein diet in the treatment of spontaneous hypoglycemia. J. Clin. Invest. 15:673-78, 1936*).

> **Experimental Study:** Flat GTT curve pts. with hypoglycemic symptoms responded well to a high protein, low carbohydrate diet (*Shah S et al. Flat G.T.T.: The significance of the flat glucose tolerance test. J. Kansas Med. Soc. November, 1975, pp. 263-67*).

> **Negative Experimental Study:** 7 pts. with impaired glucose tolerance (3 with diabetes mellitus and 4 with post-prandial hypoglycemia) had a significant deterioration in glucose tolerance when they changed from a low protein, high carbohydrate diet to a high protein, low carbohydrate diet (*Anderson JW, Herman RH. Effects of carbohydrate restriction on glucose tolerance of normal men and reactive hypoglycemic patients. Am. J. Clin. Nutr. 28:748, 1975*).

> **Experimental Controlled Study:** As compared to high carbohydrate meals, high protein meals resulted in greater blood sugar stability with avoidance of hypoglycemic symptoms and higher metabolic rates (*Thorn GW et al. A comparison of the metabolic effects of isocaloric meals of varying compositions with special reference to the prevention of post-prandial hypoglycemic symptoms. Ann. Int. Med. 18(6):913-19, 1943*).

Avoid refined carbohydrates.

> **Experimental Study:** 8 pts. (ages 19-52) with glucose nadirs less than 55 mg/dl accompanied by symptoms of reactive hypoglycemia, peak plasma cortisol of more than 18 mcg/ml, and at least a 5 mcg/ml rise in plasma cortisol from its value at the glucose nadir were placed on a low refined carbohydrate diet. Mean daily consumption of refined carbohydrates decreased from 147 gm to 20 gm, mean total carbohydrate consumption decreased from 307 to 221 gm, mean daily protein consumption increased from 89 to 99 gm, and mean fat consumption decreased from 107 to 95 grams. 7/8 became asymptomatic and the other was substantially improved. When total grams of refined carbohydrate in-

creased, symptoms returned (*Sanders LR et al. Refined carbohydrate as a contributing factor in reactive hypoglycemia. Southern Med. J. 75:1072, 1982*).

Avoid <u>alcohol</u>.

The increase in gastric acidity which follows alcohol ingestion might cause excessive release of gut secretagogues which augment beta-cell responsiveness to glucose fluctuations, leading to excessive insulin release (*Freinkel N, Getzger BE. Oral glucose tolerance curve and hypoglycemias in the fed state. <u>New Engl. J. Med.</u> 280:820-8, 1969*).

See Also:

> O'Keefe SJD, Marks V. Lunchtime gin and tonic as a cause of reactive hypoglycemia. <u>Lancet</u> *1:1286, 1977*

> Arky RA. <u>The Biology of Alcoholism</u>. New York, Plenum Press, 1971

- -

NUTRIENTS:

<u>Niacinamide</u>: time release spansules 100 mg/kg in divided doses

Supplementation may be beneficial (*Shansky A. Vitamin B₃ in the alleviation of hypoglycemia. <u>Drug & Cosmetic Industry</u> 129(4):68, 1981*).

- -

<u>Chromium</u>:

Supplementation may be beneficial.

> **Experimental Double-blind Crossover Study:** 8 female pts. were supplemented with 200 mcg chromium (as chromic chloride) daily. By 3 months, hypoglycemic symptoms were alleviated and the glucose nadir following a glucose load was raised at 2 to 4 hours (*Anderson RA et al. Chromium supplementation of humans with hypoglycemia. <u>Fed. Proc.</u> 43:471, 1984*).

<u>Magnesium</u>: 340 mg. daily (6 week trial)

May reduce glucose-induced insulin secretion (*Curry DL et al. Magnesium modulation of glucose-induced insulin secretion by the perfused rat pancreas. <u>Endocrinology</u> 101:203, 1977*); thus deficiency may contribute to reactive hypoglycemia by enhancing glucose-induced insulin secretion.

Supplementation may be beneficial.

> **Experimental Controlled Study:** After Mg supplementation, blood glucose of hypoglycemics failed to drop below fasting levels during GTT. 57% felt better vs. 25% of subjects on placebo (*<u>Magnesium Bulletin</u> vol. 4, no. 2, 1982*).

- -

OTHER FACTORS:

Rule out <u>food sensitivities</u>.

> **Clinical Observation:** Said to cause 75% of functional hypoglycemia (*Breneman JC. <u>Basics of Food Allergy</u>. Springfield, Illinois, Charles C. Thomas, 1978*).

IMMUNODEPRESSION

See Also: INFECTION

GENERAL REVIEW ARTICLE: "The importance of diet in multiple aspects of the immune response is inescapable. Although only a few trials have attempted to apply knowledge derived from *in vitro* and animal data to humans, the ability to modulate or "reset" the immune response by manipulating dietary intake will surely continue to be studied in the future" (*Corman LC. Effects of specific nutrients on the immune response. Selected clinical applications. Med. Clin. North Am. 69(4):759-91, 1985*).

- -

BASIC DIET:

Adequate dietary <u>protein</u>.

> Deficiency is immunosuppressive (*Levy JA. Nutrition and the immune system, in Stites DP et al. <u>Basic and Clinical Immunology</u>. 4th Edition. Los Altos, Ca., Lange Medical Publications, 1982, pp. 297-305*).

Low <u>fat</u> diet.

> Excessive lipid intake (particularly of <u>cholesterol</u> and of <u>polyunsaturated fatty acids</u>) is associated with immunodepression (*Chandra RK. Nutrition and immunity - Basic considerations. Part 1. <u>Contemp. Nutr.</u> 11(11), 1986; Levy JA. Nutrition and the immune system, in Stites DP et al. <u>Basic and Clinical Immunology</u>. 4th Edition. Los Altos, Ca., Lange Medical Publications, 1982, pp. 297-305*).

Avoid <u>sugar</u>.

> May impair cell-mediated immunity.

>> **Experimental Study:** 7 healthy adults ingested 75 gm glucose. *In vitro* lymphocyte transformation in response to PHA at 30 and 60 minutes was significantly depressed to 79.4% and 83.3% of fasting levels, respectively. At 2 hrs., lymphocyte transformation had returned to fasting levels. Addition of physiologic doses of insulin decreased *in vitro* lymphocyte transformation by 40%. Results suggest that glucose ingestion may affect *in vitro* measures of cellular immunity by increasing serum insulin, which competes with mitogens for binding sites on lymphocytes. In addition, glucose may impair cell-mediated immunity *in vivo* (*Bernstein J et al. Depression of lymphocyte transformation following oral glucose ingestion. <u>Am. J. Clin. Nutr.</u> 30:613, 1977*).

> May impair humoral immunity.

>> **Experimental Animal Study (mice):** "As the nutritional quality of the diet is reduced by progressively diluting the diet with sucrose in 10 percent increments, the production of antibodies was decreased proportionately" (*Nalder BN et al. <u>J. Nutr.</u> April, 1972*).

> May impair phagocytosis.

>> **Experimental Study:** Healthy volunteers ingested 100 gm portions of carbohydrate from glucose, fructose, sucrose, honey or orange juice. Each significantly decreased the phagocytic index (the capacity of neutrophils to engulf bacteria). Starch ingestion did not have this effect. The maximal

decrease in phagocytic activity occurred between 1-2 hrs. after ingestion, but the values remained below control levels 5 hrs. after feeding (*Sanchez A et al. Role of sugars in human neutrophilic phagocytosis. Am. J. Clin. Nutr. 26:180, 1973*).

NUTRIENTS:

Beta-Carotene:

Modest doses stimulate immune responses (*Chandra RK. Nutrition and immunity - Basic considerations. Part 1. Contemp. Nutr. 11(11), 1986*).

Supplementation may increase the number of helper T cells.

Experimental Controlled Study: After 1 wk., beta-carotene 180 mg daily significantly increased the frequency of OKT4$^+$ cells (helper/inducer T cells) in normal volunteers; after 2 wks., it significantly increased the frequency of OKT3$^+$ cells (all T cells). The frequency of OKT8$^+$ cells (suppressor T cells) was unaffected compared to controls (*Alexander M et al. Oral beta-carotene can increase the number of OKT4$^+$ cells in human blood. Immunology Letters 9:221-24, 1985*).

Vitamin A:

Deficiency reduces the response of both T and B cells to mitogens and antigens, while modest doses stimulate immune responses (*Chandra RK. Nutrition and immunity - Basic considerations. Part 1. Contemp. Nutr. 11(11), 1986*).

Severe deficiency leads to atrophy of the thymus and spleen and a marked decrease in circulating leukocytes and lymphocytes (*Levy JA. Nutrition and the immune system, in Stites DP et al. Basic and Clinical Immunology. 4th Edition. Los Altos, Ca., Lange Medical Publications, 1982, pp. 297-305*).

While essentially nothing is known about the effects of high intakes of vitamin A on IgE production or immediate hypersensitivity, it can both increase and suppress cellular immune function depending upon the system tested and the concentration used (*Watson RR. Regulation of immunological resistance to cancer by beta carotene and retinoids, in Nutrition, Disease Resistance, and Immune Function. New York, Marcel Dekker, Inc., 1984, pp. 345-55*).

Supplementation may reverse post-operative immunosuppression.

Experimental Controlled Study: Lymphocytes were counted on the first and seventh days post-surgery. The experimental gp., which received 300,000-450,000 units of vitamin A acetate for 7 days, showed no change, while the lymphocyte counts fell in the control gp. (*Cohen B et al. Reversal of postoperative immunosuppresion in man by vitamin A. Surg. Gynecol. Obstet., 149:658-62, 1979*).

Supplementation may enhance responses to weak immunogens and reverse immunosuppression.

Animal Experimental Study: Lymphocytes from BCG-sensitized mice were stimulated specifically with purified protein derivative and nonspecifically with phytohemagglutinin. In the vitamin A-injected animals there was significant enhancement of the spleen lymphocyte transformation not only in the PPD-sensitive cells but also in the T cells at large. In addition, vitamin A was able to restore to normal the cellular and humoral forms of immunity in prednisolone and cyclophosphamide-treated animals (*Nuwayri-Salti N, Murad T. Immunologic and anti-immunosuppressive effects of vitamin A. Pharmacology 30(4):181-87, 1985*).

While modest increases in dietary vitamin A can enhance cell-mediated immunity, including natural killer cell activity, an excess of vitamin A depresses these immune responses (*Levy JA. Nutrition and the im-*

mune system, in Stites DP et al. Basic and Clinical Immunology. 4th Edition. Los Altos, Ca., Lange Medical Publications, 1982, pp. 297-305).

Vitamin B Complex:

Deficiencies are associated with decreased antibody responses and impaired cellular immunity (*Chandra RK. Nutrition and immunity - Basic considerations. Part 1. Contemp. Nutr. 11(11), 1986*).

- Folic Acid:

Deficiency is associated with impaired responses to mitogens *in vitro* and delayed hypersensitivity responses in both animals and man (*Levy JA. Nutrition and the immune system, in Stites DP et al. Basic and Clinical Immunology. 4th Edition. Los Altos, Ca., Lange Medical Publications, 1982, pp. 297-305; Beisel WR. Single nutrients and immunity. Am. J. Clin. Nutr. 35:417-68 [Suppl.], 1982*).

- Pantothenic Acid:

Deficiency depresses humoral antibody responses to various antigens in experimental animals and man (*Beisel WR. Single nutrients and immunity. Am. J. Clin. Nutr. 35:417-68 [Suppl.], 1982*).

- Pyridoxine:

Since pyridoxine is required for normal nucleic acid and protein synthesis and for cellular multiplication, isolated pyridoxine deficiencies cause more profound effects on immune system functions than deficiencies of any other B gp. vitamin. Also, unlike any other B vitamin, deficiencies appear to inhibit cell-mediated immune functions as well as humoral responsiveness to a variety of test antigens (*Axelrod AE, Traketellis AC. Relationship of pyridoxine to immunological phenomena. Vitam. Horm. 22:591-607, 1964*).

Deficiency is associated with a reduction in number and function of both T and B lymphocytes, reduced delayed hypersensitivity responses, greatly diminished response to antigenic challenge, decreased secretion of immunoglobulins, reduced thymic epithelial cell function and reduced phagocytic activity of neutrophils (*Levy JA. Nutrition and the immune system, in Stites DP et al. Basic and Clinical Immunology. 4th Edition. Los Altos, Ca., Lange Medical Publications, 1982, pp. 297-305*).

- Riboflavin:

Deficiency in animals is associated with a diminished ability to generate humoral antibodies in response to test antigens (*Beisel WR. Single nutrients and immunity. Am. J. Clin. Nutr. 35:417-68 [Suppl.], 1982*).

- Vitamin B_{12}:

Deficiency is associated with impaired lymphocyte response to mitogens and a modest reduction in the phagocytic and bacteriocidal capacity of polymorphonuclearleukocytes (*Levy JA. Nutrition and the immune system, in Stites DP et al. Basic and Clinical Immunology. 4th Edition. Los Altos, Ca., Lange Medical Publications, 1982, pp. 297-305*).

Vitamin C:

WARNING: In the presence of high levels of stress, large supplementary doses may impair the immune response.

Animal Study: Large daily doses of vitamin C resulted in severe lymphopenia in stressed mice. Since stress abruptly increases adrenal corticosteroids in plasma following the release of vitamin C by the adrenals, it is hypothesized that large doses of vitamin C may maintain high levels of plasma corticosteroids which, in turn, may reduce the organism's immune response when stress is present (*Richardson J. Vitamin C and immunosuppression. Med. Hypotheses 21(4):383-85, 1986*).

Extreme deficiency impairs phagocyte function and cellular immunity (*Chandra RK. Nutrition and immunity - Basic considerations. Part 1. Contemp. Nutr. 11(11), 1986*).

Deficiency is associated with a reduced delayed hypersensitivity response that appears to be due to an inability to develop a local inflammatory response rather than to an immunologic defect in lymphocytes (*Levy JA. Nutrition and the immune system, in Stites DP et al. Basic and Clinical Immunology. 4th Edition. Los Altos, Ca., Lange Medical Publications, 1982, pp. 297-305*).

Supplementation may increase immunoglobulin levels.

Experimental Controlled Study: Healthy students received vitamin C 1000 mg daily.   After 77 days, their serum IgA, IgM and C3 levels showed a statistically significant increase compared to controls (*Prinz W et al.   The effect of ascorbic acid supplementation on some parameters of the human immunological defense system. Int. J. Vitam. Nutr. Res. 47(3):248-57, 1977*).

See Also:

> *Vallance S.   Relationships between ascorbic acid and serum proteins of the immune system.   Brit. Med. J. 2:437-38, 1977*

Supplementation may improve immune competence in the elderly.

Experimental Placebo-controlled Study: After 1 mo., vitamin C 500 mg/day IM enhanced the proliferative response of T lymphocytes *in vitro*, and tuberculin skin hypersensitivity *in vivo* in elderly volunteers, but not in controls receiving placebo.   Serum immunoglobulins were unchanged as were the proportion of E-rosette-forming cells (*Kennes B et al.   Effect of vitamin C supplements on cell-mediated immunity in old people.   Gerontology 29(5):305-10, 1983*).

Massive supplementation may suppress the symptoms of acquired immune deficiency syndrome.

Case Reports: Preliminary clinical experience suggests that massive doses of ascorbate (50-200 gm daily) may suppress the symptoms of AIDS and reduce the risk of secondary infections despite continued helper T-cell suppression (*Cathcart R.   Vitamin C in the treatment of acquired immune deficiency syndrome.   Med. Hypotheses 14:423-33, 1984*).

Vitamin D:

Deficiency may depress immune responses.

Observational and Experimental Controlled Study: 30% of 63 elderly men and women failed to react to intracutaneous injections of 5 recall antigens; these same subjects were found to have significantly lower vitamin D levels than the subjects with normal immunoreactivity and most were deficient.   5 of the gp. with anergy who were vitamin D deficient were supplemented with oral vitamin D or exposed to ultraviolet radiation daily.   After 2-3 mo., both vitamin D levels and delayed hypersensitivity responses had normalized, while a control gp. of untreated subjects was unchanged (*Toss G, Symreng T.   Delayed hypersensitivity response and vitamin D deficiency.   Int. J. Vit. Nutr. Res. 53(1):27-31, 1983*).

See Also:

> *Gray TK, Cohen MS. Vitamin D, phagocyte differentiation and immune function.* <u>*Surv. Immunol. Res.*</u> *4(3):200-212, 1985*

Vitamin E:

WARNING: Megadoses may inhibit immune functions and impair the bactericidal function of polymorphonuclear leukocytes.

> **Experimental Study:** 18 healthy male volunteers received d,l-alpha-tocopheryl acetate 300 mg daily. After 21 days, there was diminished *in vitro* bactericidal activity of neutrophils and responsiveness of lymphocytes to PHA; however, when PHA was used for skin testing, DDH reactions were unchanged (*Prasad JS. Effect of vitamin E supplementation on leukocyte function.* <u>*Am. J. Clin. Nutr.*</u> *33:606-8, 1980*).

Deficiency depresses immunoglobulin response to antigens, lymphocytic proliferative responses to mitogens and antigens, delayed dermal hypersensitivity reactions, and general host resistance (*Beisel WR et al. Single-nutrient effects on immunologic functions.* <u>*JAMA*</u> *245(1):53-58, 1981*).

Supplementation may enhance immune responses (*Chandra RK. Nutrition and immunity - Basic considerations. Part 1.* <u>*Contemp. Nutr.*</u> *11(11), 1986*). In addition to probably increasing the number of antibody-forming cells, supplementation enhances cell-mediated responses, including the delayed hypersensitivity reaction, and the clearance function of reticuloendothelial cells (*Levy JA. Nutrition and the immune system, in Stites DP et al.* <u>*Basic and Clinical Immunology.*</u> *4th Edition. Los Altos, Ca., Lange Medical Publications, 1982, pp. 297-305*).

> **Animal Experimental Study:** High levels of vitamin E supplementation increased some immune functions in mice and altered the levels of corticosterone (*Lim TS et al. Effect of vitamin E on cell-mediated immune responses and serum corticosterone in young and maturing mice.* <u>*Immunology*</u> *44:289, 1981*).

See Also:

> *The effect of vitamin E on immune responses.* <u>*Nutr. Rev.*</u> *45(1):27-29, 1987*

The elderly may require a higher intake to maintain immune function.

> **Animal Experimental Study:** Vitamin E administered in high doses to aging animals caused several indices of immune function to be equal to those of younger animals, suggesting that they have higher vitamin E requirements than young animals in terms of immune system responsiveness (*Blumberg J. - reported in* <u>*Med. Tribune*</u> *January 8, 1986*).

- -

Copper:

Deficiency is associated with an increased incidence of infection and impairment of cell-mediated immunity. The function of the reticuloendothelial system is depressed and the microbicidal activity of granulocytes is reduced. Impaired antibody response to heterologous red blood cells and low levels of thymic hormone activity have been reported (*Chandra RK. Nutrition and immunity - Basic considerations. Part 1.* <u>*Contemp. Nutr.*</u> *11(11), 1986; Chandra RK. Trace element regulation of immunity and infection.* <u>*J. Am. Coll. Nutr.*</u> *4(1):5-16, 1985*).

Iodine:

Deficiency is associated with reduced microbicidal activity of polymorphonuclear leukocytes (*Chandra RK. Nutrition and immunity - Basic considerations. Part 1. Contemp. Nutr. 11(11), 1986*).

Iron:

Deficiency may result in impaired immunity due to impairment of bacteriocidal capacity of neutrophils and impairment of the lymphocyte proliferation response (*Chandra RK. Nutrition and immunity - Basic considerations. Part 1. Contemp. Nutr. 11(11), 1986; Chandra RK. Trace element regulation of immunity and infection. J. Am. Coll. Nutr. 4(1):5-16, 1985*).

Immunodepression can occur with as little as a 10% decrease in dietary iron (*Levy JA. Nutrition and the immune system, in Stites DP et al. Basic and Clinical Immunology. 4th Edition. Los Altos, Ca., Lange Medical Publications, 1982, pp. 297-305*).

Magnesium:

Magnesium-deficient animals have primarily a reduction in antibody-forming cells. Immunoglobulin levels are decreased, the humoral response to particular antigens is diminished, and thymic atrophy can take place (*Levy JA. Nutrition and the immune system, in Stites DP et al. Basic and Clinical Immunology. 4th Edition. Los Altos, Ca., Lange Medical Publications, 1982, pp. 297-305*).

Selenium:

Especially when associated with a vitamin E deficiency, cell-mediated immunity is impaired (*Chandra RK. Trace element regulation of immunity and infection. J. Am. Coll. Nutr. 4(1):5-16, 1985*). Phagocytosis is decreased, and T cells appear to be coated by factors that suppress their response to mitogens and antigens (*Levy JA. Nutrition and the immune system, in Stites DP et al. Basic and Clinical Immunology. 4th Edition. Los Altos, Ca., Lange Medical Publications, 1982, pp. 297-305*).

Deficiency may impair humoral immunity in laboratory animals.

> **Animal Experimental Study:** Mice were fed either a selenium-deficient (SD) or a control diet. Offspring were then fed the diet of the mother. While the first generation did not differ, the second generation SD gp. had reduced body and spleen weights and decreased lymphocytes per spleen compared to controls. In the first generation SD gp., a reduced IgG antibody response following exposure to sheep RBC was observed both *in vitro* and *in vivo*; in the second generation SP gp., both IgG and IgM antibody response was reduced (*Mulhern SA et al. Deficient levels of dietary selenium suppress the antibody response to first and second generation mice. Nutr. Res. 5:201-10, 1985*).

Zinc:

WARNING: Excessive intake may impair lymphocyte and neutrophil responses.

> **Experimental Study:** 11 healthy adult men ingested 150 mg of elemental zinc twice daily. After 6 wks., there was a reduction in lymphocyte stimulation response to phytohemagglutinin as well as chemotaxis and phagocytosis of bacteria by polymorphonuclear leukocytes (*Chandra RK. Excessive intake of zinc impairs immune responses. JAMA 252:1443-46, 1984*).

Deficiency is associated with depression of immune and other host defense mechanisms, including T cell response and chemotaxis of neutrophils. Thymic hormone activity is very low (*Chandra RK. Nutrition and immunity - Basic considerations. Part 1. Contemp. Nutr. 11(11), 1986; Chandra RK. Trace element regulation of immunity and infection. J. Am. Coll. Nutr. 4(1):5-16, 1985*).

Experimental Study: 6 young men consumed a semipurified diet providing 0.28 mg zinc and 0.8 kg protein daily. After 4-9 wks., there were significant decreases in plasma, whole blood, urinary, seminal and fecal zinc along with impairment of leukocyte chemotaxis and clinical signs indicative of decreased resistance to infection (*Baer MT et al. Nitrogen utilization, enzyme activity, glucose intolerance and leukocyte chemotaxis in human experimental zinc depletion.* Am. J. Clin. Nutr. *41(6):1220-35, 1985*).

May be deficient in pts. with <u>acquired immunodeficiency syndrome</u> (*Weiner RG. AIDS and zinc deficiency. Letter to the Editor.* JAMA *252(11):1409-10, 1984*).

If deficient, supplementation may be beneficial.

Experimental Study: Individuals over age 50 and most young Down's Syndrome children were found to have reduced concentrations of thymic hormone. This reduction could be completely prevented by the addition of zinc sulfate to plasma samples taken from these individuals and, in fact, induced concentrations of thymic hormone comparable to those of healthy young people (*Fabris N et al. Thymic hormone deficiency in normal ageing and Down's Syndrome. Is there a primary failure of the thymus?* Lancet *1:983-86, 1984*).

Experimental and Observational Study: 22% of 203 elderly men and women (ages 60-97) were anergic; the same subjects were those with the lowest zinc intakes and serum zinc levels. 5 of these anergic subjects were supplemented with 55 mg zinc daily. After 4 wks., their immune responses had normalized (*Wagner PA et al. Zinc nutriture and cell-mediated immunity in the aged.* Int. J. Vit. Nutr. Res. *53(1):94-101, 1983*).

Experimental Study: 83 normal volunteers received zinc sulfate 660 mg daily (150 mg elemental zinc). After 1 mo., the response of lymphocytes to mitogens *in vitro* was significantly improved. This effect was not correlated with initial serum zinc concentrations (*Duchateau J et al. Influence of oral zinc supplementation on the lymphocyte response to mitogens of normal subjects.* Am. J. Clin. Nutr. *34:88-93, 1981*).

Experimental Study: Following supplementation, T-lymphocytes of pts. with low zinc levels and poor immune function proliferated and persistent infections were cured (*Fed. Am. Soc. Experiment. Biol. Abst. April, 1979*).

- -

<u>L-Carnitine:</u>

Supplementation may be beneficial.

In vitro Experimental Study: L-carnitine increased the proliferative response of both murine and human lymphocytes following mitogenic stimulation, increased polymorphonuclear chemotaxis and, even at minimal concentrations, neutralized lipid-induced immunosuppression (*Se Simone C et al. Vitamins and immunity: Influence of L-carnitine on the immune system.* Acta Vitaminol. Enzymol. *4(1-2):135-40, 1982*).

<u>Dimethylglycine:</u>

Supplementation may enhance both humoral and cell-mediated immunity.

Experimental Double-blind Study: Compared to age-matched controls who received calcium gluconate 300 mg daily, 10 healthy volunteers receiving DMG 120 mg daily along with calcium gluconate 180 mg daily showed a fourfold increase in antibody response to pneumococcal vaccine after 10 wks. (p less than 0.01). While production of leukocyte inhibitory factor in response to concanavalin A was similar in the 2 gps., those taking DMG had a significantly higher mean response of leukocyte inhibition factor to streptokinase-streptodornase (p less than 0.01) and to pneumococcal antigens after immunization with vaccine (p less than 0.001) (*Graber CD et al. Immunomodulating properties of dimethylglycine in humans. J. Infectious Dis. 143(1):101-5, 1981*).

In vitro Experimental Study: The *in vitro* response of lymphocytes from diabetic pts. and those with sickle cell disease to phytohemagglutinin, concanavalin A, and pokeweed mitogen were increased almost threefold after addition of DMG (*Graber CD - ibid*).

Essential Amino Acids:

Deficiencies are known to be immunosuppressive (*Levy JA. Nutrition and the immune system, in Stites DP et al. Basic and Clinical Immunology. 4th Edition. Los Altos, Ca., Lange Medical Publications, 1982, pp. 297-305*).

Essential Fatty Acids:

Deficiency results in lymphoid atrophy and depressed immune responses (*Chandra RK. Nutrition and immunity - Basic considerations. Part 1. Contemp. Nutr. 11(11), 1986*).

Animal Experimental Study: Mice were fed a diet totally deficient in essential fatty acids. After 28 days, reduced antibody response was demonstrated against T-cell dependent and T-cell independent antigens, and in both primary and secondary responses, suggesting that essential fatty acids play a crucial role in maintaining the functional integrity of humoral immunity (*DeWille JW et al. Effects of essential fatty acid deficiency, and various levels of dietary polyunsaturated fatty acids, on humoral immunity in mice. J. Nutr. 109(6):1018-27, 1979*).

Excess (for example, of arachidonic or linoleic acids) induces atrophy of lymphoid tissue and diminishes T cell immune responsiveness to antigenic stimulation (*Chandra RK. Nutrition and immunity - Basic considerations. Part 1. Contemp. Nutr. 11(11), 1986*).

Glutamine:

Deficiency is immunosuppressive (*Kafkewitz D, Bendich A. Am. J. Clin. Nutr. 37:1025-30, 1983*).

Omega-6 Fatty Acids:

$$\text{linoleic acid} \rightarrow \text{GLA} \rightarrow \text{DGLA} \rightarrow \text{Prostaglandin E}_1$$

Supplementation may be beneficial.

Theoretical Discussion(AIDS): Repeated viral infections may disrupt the biosynthesis of prostaglandin E_1 (PGE$_1$) which plays an important role in the regulation of T lymphocyte function and thus may contribute to the risk of developing acquired immunodeficiency syndrome. In order to restore PGE$_1$ synthesis, the author suggests supplementation with gammalinolenic acid in addition to:
1. pyridoxine (assists in the conversion of GLA to DGLA)
2. ascorbic acid IV along with L-lysine (assists in the conversion of DGLA to PGE$_1$ and enhances interferon production and phagocytic activity)
3. Zinc (assists in the conversion of DGLA to PGE$_1$)
4. Eicosapentaenoic acid (inhibits the conversion of DGLA to arachidonic acid)
5. Niacin (assists in the synthesis of the anti-oxidant NADPH)
6. Riboflavin (assists in the synthesis of glutathione reductase).
(*Marcus S. Breakdown of PGE$_1$ synthesis is responsible for the acquired immunodeficiency syndrome. Med. Hypotheses 15:39-46, 1984*).

Theoretical Discussion: The evidence is reviewed that prostaglandin E$_1$ plays an important role in the regulation of T lymphocyte function, and that either a deficiency or an excess can have a deleterious effect. It is suggested that PGE$_1$ precursors such as cis-linoleic acid (cLA) and gammalinolenic acid (GLA) (in addition to pyridoxine, zinc and vitamin C) may be utilized to promote T cell activation, and that supplementation with evening primrose oil, which contains about 70% cLA and 10% GLA, may be beneficial (*Horrobin DF et al. The nutritional regulation of T lymphocyte function. Med. Hypotheses 5:969-85, 1979*).

Taurine:

Supplementation strengthens both the phagocytic and bactericidal capacities of rat neutrophils (*Masuda M et al. Influences of taurine on functions of rat neutrophils. Jap. J. Pharmacol. 34(1):116-18, 1984*).

- -

OTHER FACTORS:

Rule out cadmium toxicity.

Produces immunosuppression by reduction of lymphocyte formation of IgG and IgM in laboratory animals. Also reduces bactericidal activity of alveolar macrophages (*Halstead BW. Immune augmentation therapy. J. Int. Acad. Prevent. Med. 9(1):5-19, 1985*).

Rule out lead toxicity.

Causes immunosuppression similar to that of cadmium (see above) (*Halstead BW. Immune augmentation therapy. J. Int. Acad. Prevent. Med. 9(1):5-19, 1985*).

Rule out mercury toxicity.

In laboratory animals, inhibits the serological response to viral antigens and diminishes production of neutralizing antibodies (*Halstead BW. Immune augmentation therapy. J. Int. Acad. Prevent. Med. 9(1):5-19, 1985*).

INFECTION

See Also: IMMUNODEPRESSION

OVERVIEW:

1. A low fat, low cholesterol, low sugar diet may be beneficial.

2. Deficiencies of the following nutrients will increase susceptibility to infection and thus should be corrected: folic acid, pantothenic acid, pyridoxine, riboflavin, vitamin A, vitamin C, vitamin E, copper, iron, magnesium, zinc.

3. Excesses of the following nutrients will increase susceptibility to infection and thus should be corrected: vitamin A, copper, iron, zinc.

4. Appropriate levels of supplementation with the following nutrients may reduce susceptibility to infection: vitamin C, vitamin E, zinc, dimethylglycine, essential fatty acids, quercetin, garlic.

5. Cadmium and lead toxicity will increase susceptibility to infection.

6. Lactobacillus acidophilus has significant antibacterial activity _in vitro_. It may be beneficial intravaginally in bacterial vaginitis; whether it is effective orally in treating bacterial infections of the lower GI tract is uncertain.

- -

BASIC DIET:

Avoid protein-calorie malnutrition.

> **Review Article:** Protein-calorie malnutrition is associated with impaired immunocompetence and increased susceptibility to infection (_Chandra RK. Trace element regulation of immunity and infection. J. Am. Coll. Nutr. 4(1):5-16, 1985_).

Low fat, low cholesterol diet.

> Decreases susceptibility to infection (_Beisel WR. Single nutrients and immunity. Am. J. Clin. Nutr. 35:417-68 (suppl.), 1982_).

Avoid sugar.

> Impairs cell-mediated immunity.

> > **Experimental Study:** Lymphocyte transformation (response to phytohemagglutinin) was significantly depressed at 30 and 60 minutes in 7 subjects following a 75 gram glucose load but returned to fasting levels at 2 hours (_Bernstein J, Alpert S, Nauss KM et al. Depression of lymphocyte transformation following oral glucose ingestion. Am. J. Clin. Nutr. 30:613, 1977_).

> > **Experimental Study:** Ingestion of 100 grams of carbohydrate from glucose, fructose, sucrose, honey or orange juice but not starch significantly decreased the phagocytic index as measured by the

capacity of neutrophils to engulf bacteria. Values were still below control values 5 hours after inges-tion (*Sanchez A et al. Role of sugars in human neutrophilic phagocytosis. Am. J. Clin. Nutr. 26:180, 1973*).

See Also:

> *Cheraskin E. Sucrose, neutrophilic phagocytosis and resistance to disease. Dental Survey 52(12):46-48, 1976*

- -

NUTRIENTS:

Folic Acid:

> If deficient, host resistance is reduced and lymphocytic functions are impaired (*Beisel WR. Single nutrients and immunity. Am. J. Clin. Nutr. 35:417-68 (suppl.), 1982*).

Pantothenic Acid:

> If deficient, depresses humoral antibodiy responsiveness to various antigens, but has not been shown to impair cell-mediated immunity (*Beisel WR. Single nutrients and immunity. Am. J. Clin. Nutr. 35:417-68 (suppl.), 1982*).

Pyridoxine:

> If deficient, inhibits cell-mediated immune functions as well as humoral responsiveness to a variety of test antigens (*Axelrod AE, Trakatellis AC. Relationship of pyridoxine to immunological phenomena. Vitam. Horm. 22:591-607, 1964*).

Riboflavin:

> If deficient, humoral immunity is impaired (*Beisel WR. Single nutrients and immunity. Am. J. Clin. Nutr. 35:417-68 (suppl.), 1982*).

Vitamin A: 10,000 - 20,000 I.U. daily

> Severe deficiency causes increased susceptibility to infection yet, although an increased supply of vitamin A may intensify antibody production, a definitely positive effect on the course of infections has not been established (*Hof H. [Vitamin A, the "anti-infective" vitamin?] MMW 118(46):1485-88, 1976*).

Deficiency impairs leukocytic and reticulo-endothelial system function.

> **Animal Experimental Study:** Following injections with E. coli, vitamin A-deficient rats demonstrated impaired leukocytic phagocytic activity and a reduction in the functional integrity of the reticulo-endothelial system (*Ongsakul M et al. Impaired blood clearance of bacteria and phagocytic activity in vitamin A deficient rats. Proc. Soc. Exp. Biol. Med. 178(2):204-8, 1985*).

> **Negative Animal Experimental Study:** Vitamin A-deprived mice with markedly reduced liver vitamin A content which were either immunized with sheep erythrocytes or infected with L. monocytogenes responded the same as controls, suggesting that neither the immune system nor the phagocytic system was impaired (*Hof H, Wirsing CH. Anti-infective properties of vitamin A. Z. Ernah-rungswiss 18(4):221-32, 1979*).

Deficiency is associated with decreased cellular immune response to antigens.

Observational Study: In 100 healthy people over age 60, those with higher plasma concentrations of vitamin A exhibited delayed hypersensitivity reactions to significantly more antigens than people with lower concentrations (p less than 0.01) *(Chavance M et al. Nutritional support improves antibody response to influenza virus in the elderly. Letter to the Editor.* <u>Br. Med. J.</u> *November 9, 1985, pp. 1348-49).*

Supplementation causing vitamin A excess enhances lymphocytic response to antigens and antibody responses, and may diminish host susceptibility to infection *(Beisel WR. Single nutrients and immunity.* <u>Am. J. Clin. Nutr.</u> *35:417-68 (suppl.), 1982).*

Experimental Controlled Study: 147 preschool-age children with a history of frequent respiratory illness randomly received either vitamin A 450 mcg/day or placebo. After 11 mo., supplemented children experienced 19% fewer episodes of respiratory symptomatology (p less than 0.05) compared to controls, even though their plasma retinol levels did not change. Children with prior histories of lower respiratory illness or of allergy benefited most *(Pinnock CB et al. Vitamin A status in children who are prone to respiratory tract infections.* <u>Aust. Paediatr. J.</u> *22(2):95-99, 1986).*

Observational Study: In 100 healthy people over age 60, those with higher plasma concentrations of vitamin A reported less infections over the past 3 yrs., but the difference was not quite significant (p less than 0.07) *(Chavance M et al. Nutritional support improves antibody response to influenza virus in the elderly. Letter to the Editor.* <u>Br. Med. J.</u> *November 9, 1985, pp. 1348-49).*

Animal Experimental Study: Mice treated with a high dose of vitamin A showed increased antibody production against infection with L. monocytogenes, suggesting a stimulatory effect on the immune system and the mononuclear phagocytic system *(Hof H, Wirsing CH. Anti-infective properties of vitamin A.* <u>Z. Ernahrungswiss</u> *18(4):221-32, 1979).*

<u>Vitamin B$_{12}$:</u>

In untreated primary pernicious anemia:

1. neutrophil phagocytosis is impaired *(Kaplan SS, Basford RE. Effect of vitamin B$_{12}$ and folic acid deficiencies on neutrophil function.* <u>Blood</u> *47:801-5, 1976).*

2. lymphocyte function is impaired *(Das KC, Herbert V. The lymphocyte as a marker of past nutritional status: Persistence of abnormal lymphocyte deoxyuridine (uD) suppression test and chromosomes in patients with past deficiency of folate and vitamin B$_{12}$.* <u>Br. J. Haematol.</u> *38:219-33, 1978).*

<u>Vitamin C:</u>

Bacterial infections can reduce cellular uptake.

In vitro Experimental Study: Bacterial endotoxin instantly inhibited ascorbic acid uptake by fibroblasts in a dose dependent manner *(Aleo JJ, Padh H. Inhibition of ascorbic acid uptake by endotoxin: Evidence of mediation by serum factor(s).* <u>Proc. Soc. Exp. Biol. Med.</u> *179(1):128-31, 1985).*

Leukocyte and plasma concentrations of ascorbate are significantly decreased in the common cold *(Wilson CWM. Clinical pharmacological aspects of ascorbic acid.* <u>Ann. N.Y. Acad. Sci.</u> *258:355-76, 1975; Hume R, Weyers E. Changes in leucocyte ascorbic acid during the common cold.* <u>Scot. Med. J.</u> *18:3-7, 1973),* possibly due to increased degradation and excretion due to the greatly enhanced rates of oxidation of ascorbate in inflammation due to activated neutrophils *(Roberts P et al. Vitamin C and inflammation.* <u>Med. Biol.</u> *62:88, 1984).*

If deficient, phagocytic cell functions are impaired *(Beisel WR. Single nutrients and immunity.* <u>Am. J. Clin. Nutr.</u> *35:417-68 (suppl.), 1982).*

Supplementation may reduce the severity and duration (and possibly the incidence) of certain bacterial and viral infections including the common cold, although the evidence remains inconclusive.

Review Article: "It is now fairly clear that for preventing common colds, vitamin C has no worthwhile effect....There is ... a little more evidence for a small therapeutic effect ..., but it is not clear which symptom it relieves or how" (*Truswell AS. Ascorbic acid. N. Engl. J. Med. 315(11):709, 1986*).

Review Article: "The present consensus of scientific opinion fails to support the view that ascorbic acid supplementation using 1 to 2 g/day doses is effective in reducing susceptibility to common colds. At best, such doses may lessen the severity and/or duration of symptoms" (*Beisel WR. Single nutrients and immunity. Am. J. Clin. Nutr. 35:417-68 (suppl.), 1982*).

Observational Study: Plasma ascorbic acid levels were studied for 18 submarine crewmen before, during and after a 68-day patrol. While there were no significant health differences between those with the highest and those with the lowest levels, twice as many of those with the lowest developed upper respiratory infections (*J. Applied Nutr. vol. 34, no. 1, 1982*).

Experimental Double-blind Study: One twin from each of 95 pairs of identical twins ingested 1 gram of ascorbic acid per day for 100 days while the other received a placebo. Vitamin C cut the duration of cold symptoms by 19% but did not prevent the occurrence of colds (*Carr AB et al. Vitamin C and the common cold: Using identical twins as controls. Med. J. Aust. 2:411-12, 1981*).

Experimental Controlled Study: 353 healthy young volunteers received either natural orange juice with 80 mg ascorbic acid, synthetic orange juice with 80 mg ascorbic acid, or synthetic orange juice alone for 72 days. Vitamin C supplementation significantly increased the number of cold-free subjects and led to a 14-21% reduction in total number of cold symptoms (p less than 0.05) (*Baird IM et al. The effects of ascorbic acid and flavonoids on the occurence of symptoms normally associated with the common cold. Am. J. Clin. Nutr. 32:1686-90, 1979*).

Experimental Double-blind Study: 674 marines randomly received ascorbic acid 2 gms daily or placebo for 8 weeks. Compared to controls, there were no differences in the incidence of colds. The gp. taking ascorbic acid rated cold symptoms as less severe, although they did not have fewer sick calls, training days lost or different symptom complexes than controls (*Pitt HA, Costrini AM. Vitamin C prophylaxis in marine recruits. JAMA 241:908-11, March 2, 1979*).

Experimental Double-blind Study: 3 different dosages of vitamin C dependent upon body weight were administered to 44 school-aged monozygotic twins using a co-twin control study design. Paired comparisons after 5 months showed no significant overall treatment effect on cold symptoms, although treated girls in the youngest 2 gps. had significantly shorter and less severe illness episodes, and an effect on severity was also observed in the youngest gp. of boys (*Miller JZ et al. Therapeutic effect of vitamin C. A co-twin control study. JAMA 237(3):248-51, 1977*).

In vitro Experimental Study: Human cell cultures were incubated with ascorbic acid (equivalent to 6-10 gm daily) for 2 days when rhinovirus was added. 2 days later the amount of virus collected from the vitamin C-treated cultures was 1/40 that from untreated control cultures (*Schwerdt PR, Schwerdt CE. Effect of ascorbic acid on rhinovirus replication in WI-38 cells. Proc. Soc. Biol. Med. 148:1237, 1975*).

See Also:

Ludvigsson J et al. Vitamin C as a preventive medicine against common colds in children. Scand. J. Infect. Dis. 9(2):91-98, 1977

Tyrrell DA et al. A trial of ascorbic acid in the treatment of the common cold. Brit. J. Prev. Soc. Med. 31(3):189-91, 1977

Destro RL, Sharma V. An appraisal of vitamin C in adjunct therapy of bacterial and "viral" meningitis. Clin. Ped. 16:936, 1977

Coulehan JL et al. Vitamin C and acute illness in Navajo school children. New Engl. J. Med. 295(18):973-77, 1976

Geber WF, Lefkowitz SS, Hung CY. Effect of ascorbic acid, sodium salicylate and caffeine on the serum interferon level in response to viral infection. Pharmacology 13:228, 1975

Vitamin E:

Deficiency associated with increased infections due to diminished membrane-related chemotaxis and ingestion (*Baehner RL, Boxer LA. Role of membrane vitamin E and cytoplasmic glutathione in the regulation of phagocytic functions of neutrophils and monocytes. Am. J. Pediatr. Hematol. Oncol. 1(1):71-76, 1979*).

Observational Study: In 100 healthy people over age 60, the plasma alpha tocopherol concentration was negatively correlated (p less than 0.001) with the number of infections in the past 3 years (*Chavance M et al. Nutritional support improves antibody response to influenza virus in the elderly. Letter to the Editor. Br. Med. J. November 9, 1985, pp. 1348-49*).

Supplementation may enhance immune response and resistence to infectious agents.

Negative Experimental Study: 18 healthy subjects received D,L alpha-tocopheryl acetate 300 ml/day. After 21 days, diminished *in vitro* bactericidal activity of neutophils and responsiveness of lymphocytes to a mitogen were noted (*Prasad JS. Effect of vitamin E supplementation on leukocyte function. Am. J. Clin. Nutr. 33:606-8, 1980*).

Animal Experimental Studies: Mice, chicks, guinea pigs, turkeys and sheep receiving supplementation showed significantly increased immune responses and resistence to a variety of infectious agents (*Nockels CF. Protective effects of supplemental vitamin E against infection. Fed. Proc. 38:2134-8, 1979*).

- -

Copper:

WARNING: Excess copper may increase susceptibility to infection (*Beisel WR. Single nutrients and immunity. Am. J. Clin. Nutr. 35:417-68 (suppl.), 1982*).

Deficiency may be associated with increased susceptibility to infection due to impairment of cell-mediated immunity (*Chandra RK. Trace element regulation of immunity and infection. J. Am. Coll. Nutr. 4(1):5-16, 1985*).

Observational Study: 28 children (ages 10 mo. - 10 yrs.) with undue susceptibility to middle ear and respiratory infections were found to have significantly lower serum ceruloplasmin than 13 controls (*Acta Paediatr. Scand. 74:515-20, 1985*).

Review Article: In animal studies, copper deficiency has resulted in a lowered resistance to infection either through an impaired immune response or faulty leukocyte function (*Miller ER. Mineral X disease interactions. J. Anim. Sci. 60(6):1500-7, 1985*).

<u>Iron:</u>

WARNING: Excess supplementation can increase bacterial growth and replication and the release of certain exotoxins (*Beisel WR. Single nutrients and immunity. Am. J. Clin. Nutr. 35:417-68 (suppl.), 1982*).

In response to infection, iron is abruptly redistributed from serum into cellular storage sites to restrain bacterial growth by decreasing iron availability within bodily fluids.

Deficiency may be associated with increased susceptibility to infection (*Beisel WR. Single nutrients and immunity. Am. J. Clin. Nutr. 35:417-68 (suppl.), 1982*) as there is a slight decrease in the number of rosette-forming T cells and a significant impairment of lymphocyte response to mitogens and antigens. Polymorphonuclear leukocytes are unable to kill ingested bacteria and fungi in an efficient manner (*Chandra RK. Trace element regulation of immunity and infection. J. Am. Coll. Nutr. 4(1):5-16, 1985*).

Experimental Controlled Study: 28 children (ages 10 mo. - 10 yrs.) with undue susceptibility to middle ear and respiratory infections were found to have significantly lower serum iron (p less than 0.05) than 13 controls. Serum zinc was also significantly lower, but copper, magnesium, transferrin and ceruloplasmin did not differ between gps. (*Bondestam M et al. Subclinical trace element deficiency in children with undue susceptibility to infections. Acta Paediatr. Scand. 74(4):515-20, 1985*).

<u>Magnesium:</u>

While magnesium deficiency has not been shown to cause deficient immune responses in humans, deficient immune responses have been found in mice and rats fed diets moderately deficient in magnesium for extended periods (*Beisel WR. Single nutrients and immunity. Am. J. Clin. Nutr. 35:417-68 (suppl.), 1982*).

The ability of animals to cope with infection may be influenced by magnesium nutriture (*Miller ER. Mineral X disease interactions. J. Anim. Sci. 60(6):1500-7, 1985*).

<u>Phosphorus:</u>

The ability of animals to cope with infection may be influenced by phosphorus nutriture (*Miller ER. Mineral X disease interactions. J. Anim. Sci. 60(6):1500-7, 1985*).

<u>Selenium:</u>

The ability of animals to cope with infection may be influenced by selenium nutriture. The role of selenium in bactericidal action of the phagocytes is associated with oxidative functions believed important for killing phagocytized bacteria (*Miller ER. Mineral X disease interactions. J. Anim. Sci. 60(6):1500-7, 1985*).

<u>Zinc:</u>

WARNING: Excessive zinc intake <u>impairs</u> immune responses.

Experimental Study: 11 healthy adult men ingested 150 mg of elemental zinc twice daily. After 6 wks., there was a reduction in lymphocyte stimulation response to phytohemagglutinin as well as chemotaxis and phagocytosis of bacteria by polymorphonuclear leukocytes (*Chandra RK. Excessive intake of zinc impairs immune responses. JAMA 252(11):1443-46, 1984*).

Deficiency may be associated with impaired humoral and cellular immune responses (*Chandra RK. Trace element regulation of immunity and infection. J. Am. Coll. Nutr. 4(1):5-16, 1985; Pekarek RS et al. Humoral and cellular immune responses in zinc deficient rats. Nutr. Reports Int. 16(3):267-76, 1977; Gol-*

den MHN et al. Effect of zinc on thymus of recently malnourished children. Lancet November 19, 1977, pp. 1057-59).

Experimental Controlled Study: 28 children (ages 10 mo. - 10 yrs.) with undue susceptibility to middle ear and respiratory infections were found to have significantly lower serum zinc (p less than 0.001) than 13 controls. Serum iron was also significantly lower, but copper, magnesium, transferrin and ceruloplasmin did not differ between gps. (*Bondestam M et al. Subclinical trace element deficiency in children with undue susceptibility to infections. Acta Paediatr. Scand. 74(4):515-20, 1985*).

Animal Experimental Study: When mice which normally show adequate lymphokine release and resistance to infection were placed on a low zinc diet, they became more susceptible to candida albicans infection and their capacity to release migration inhibitory factor (MIF) decreased markedly (*Salvin SB, Rabin BS. Resistance and susceptibility to infection in inbred murine strains. IV. Effects of dietary zinc. Cellular Immunol. 87(2):546-52, 1984*).

Supplementation may improve immunoregulation even when not deficient.

Animal Experimental Study: When mice inbred to exhibit decreased cell-mediated immunity were fed diets that were high in zinc, their resistence to infection with candida albicans as well as their release of migration inhibitory factor (MIF) increased dramatically (*Salvin SB, Rabin BS. Resistance and susceptibility to infection in inbred murine strains. IV. Effects of dietary zinc. Cellular Immunol. 87(2):546-52, 1984*).

Experimental Study: 83 normal men & women received 150 mg of elemental zinc daily as zinc sulfate. After 4 wks., there was a significant improvement in T-cell function. The authors argue that the absence of a significant linear correlation between initial zinc levels and the degree of improvement in mitogen response suggests that the effect of zinc supplementation was not due to a pre-existing, latent zinc deficiency (*Duchateau J et al. Influence of oral zinc supplementation on the lymphocyte response to mitogens of normal subjects. Am. J. Clin. Nutr. 34:88-93, 1981*).

Note: The proposition that the immunoregulation of cell-mediated immunity is a pharmacological or medicinal effect of zinc is unsettled (Oral zinc and immunoregulation: A nutritional or pharmacological effect of zinc supplementation? Nutr. Rev. 40(3):72-4, 1982).

Supplementation may be effective for <u>trichomonal</u> infections even when metronidazole is ineffective.

Case Report: Pt. with vaginal trichomoniasis and low plasma zinc responded to metronidazole only after zinc supplementation raised her plasma zinc level into the normal range (*Willmott F et al. Lancet 1:1053, 1983*).

See Also:

Krieger JN, Rein MF. Zinc sensitivity of Trichomonas vaginalis: In vitro studies and clinical implications. J. Infec. Dis. 146:341, 1982

Supplementation may be effective for the <u>common cold</u>.

Experimental Double-blind Study: 146 volunteers were given a 7 day supply of zinc gluconate tablets 180 mg (each containing 23 mg elemental zinc) or placebo tablets. Adults and youngsters at least 60 lbs. were told to to suck on 2 tablets for at least 10 minutes at the outset of a cold, followed by 1 tablet every 2 waking hours up to a maximum of 12 daily for adults and 9 daily for youngsters. Smaller children were limited to a maximum of 6 daily. Treatment was to stop 6 hrs. after symptoms ceased, and no other treatments were permitted. While cold sufferers receiving zinc completely recovered in an ave. of 3.9 days, those receiving placebo took 10.8 days to become symptom-free. The treatment was equally effective for both mild and severe infections, and was beneficial even if supplementation was delayed. Many subjects became asymptomatic within hours and 1/5 of the zinc-treated group fully recuperated within one day (*Eby GA, Davis DR, Halcomb WW. Antimicrobial Agents & Chemotherapy 25:20-24, January, 1984*).

- -

Dimethylglycine: 50 mg. t.i.d.

Supplementation may be beneficial.

Experimental Double-blind Study: 20 subjects showed a fourfold increase in antibody response to pneumococcal vaccine compared to controls (p less than 0.01) as well as a significantly higher response of leukocyte inhibitory factor to streptokinase-streptodornase (p less than 0.01) and to pneumococcal antigens after immunization with vaccine (p less than 0.001). The *in vitro* responses to lymphocytes from pts. with diabetes and sickle cell disease to mitogens were increased almost three fold after addition of DMG. These results suggest that DMG enhances both humoral and cell-mediated immune reponses (*Graber CD et al. Immunomodulating properties of dimethylglycine in humans. J. Infect. Dis. 143(1):101-5, 1981*).

Essential Fatty Acids:

Review Article: The oils of evening primrose, fish and linseed are rich in linoleic, linolenic and eicosapen-taenoic acid, essential fatty acids which have anti-bacterial, anti-fungal and anti-viral actions (*Das UN. Antibiotic-like action of essential fatty acids. Can. Med. Assoc. J. 132:1350, 1985*).

Lactic Acid:

The predominant acid in normal vaginal fluid as lactate producers (lactobacillus and streptococcus species) are the predominant organisms (*Spiegel CA et al. Anaerobic bacteria in nonspecific vaginitis. N. Engl. J. Med. 303(11):601-7, 1980*).

Decrease is associated with Gardnerella vaginitis as organisms which produce other acids predominate (*Spiegel - ibid*).

Supplementation may be beneficial in Gardnerella vaginitis.

Experimental Controlled and Observational Study: Anaerobes dominated the flora in 62 bacterial vaginosis pts., while lactobacilli were the predominant organisms in 42 controls. Lactate-gel (pH 3.5, 5 ml) inserted into the vagina daily for 7 days was as effective as oral metronidazole 500 mg twice daily for 7 days. The women in both gps. became symptom-free and objectively improved. Anaerobes were significantly reduced (p less than 0.0001) in both gps. after treatment but Gardnerella was not significantly reduced. Results suggest that lactate-gel is an ideal treatment (*Andersch B et al. Treatment of bacterial vaginosis with an acid cream: A comparison between the effect of lactate-gel and metronidazole. Gynecol. Obstet. Invest. 21(1):19-25, 1986*).

Quercetin:

Inhibits the infectiousness and/or replication of both RNA and DNA viruses.

In vitro Experimental Study: Quercetin was effective against herpes simplex type 1, polio virus type 1, parainfluenzal virus type 3, and respiratory syncytial virus (*Kaul TN et al. Antiviral effect of flavonoids on human viruses. J. Med. Virol. 15:71-79, 1985*).

- -

Garlic:

Supplementation may be beneficial.

In vitro Experimental Study: Garlic demonstrated a broad spectrum of activity against 17 strains of fungi and was more effective than nystatin against pathogenic yeasts (*Adetumbi MA, Lau BH. Allium sativum (garlic): A natural antibiotic. Med. Hypotheses 12(3):227-37, 1983*).

See Also:

Prasad G, Sharma VD. *Efficacy of garlic (Allium sativum) treatment against experimental Candidiasis in chicks.* Brit. Vet. J. 136:448, 1980

Anonymous. *Garlic in Cryptococcal meningitis: A preliminary report of 21 cases.* Chinese Med. J. 93:123, 1980

Amer M, Taha M, Tosson Z. *The effect of aqueous garlic extract on the growth of dermatophytes.* Int. J. Dermatol. 19:285, 1980

- -

OTHER FACTORS:

Rule out cadmium toxicity.

Has adverse effects on host resistance to bacterial and viral infections (*Gainer JH. Effects of heavy metals and of deficiency of zinc on mortality rates in mice infected with encephalomyocarditis virus. Am. J. Vet. Res. 38:869-72, 1977; Cook JA et al. Influence of lead and cadmium on the susceptibility of rats to bacterial challenge. Proc. Soc. Exp. Biol. Med. 150:741-47, 1975*).

Rule out hydrochloric acid deficiency.

Review Article: The available data support the concept that gastric hypochlorhydria or achlorhydria increases both susceptibility to and severity of bacterial and perhaps also of certain parasitic enteric infections (*Giannella RA et al. Influence of gastric acidity on bacterial and parasitic enteric infections. Ann. Int. Med. 78:271-76, 1973*).

Lactobacillus Acidophilus:

Has significant anti-bacterial action.

In vitro Experimental Study: Acidophyllin, the antibacterial component of acidophilus, caused a 50% inhibition in growth of 27 different types of bacteria in lactic-acid-free preparations, 10 of which were common pathogens (*Shahani KM et al. Cultured Dairy Products Journal 12:8-11, 1977*).

See Also:

Review Article: Shahani KM, Ayebo AD. *Role of dietary lactobacilli in gastrointestinal microecology.* Am. J. Clin. Nutr. 33:2448-2457, 1980

Decrease (along with a decrease in lactate acid) is associated with Garnerella-associated ("non-specific") vaginitis.

Observational Study: 12 pts. believed to have Gardnerella-associated vaginitis on the basis of symptoms, vaginal pH above 4.5, a positive amine test and/or clue cells on wet smear (at least 3 out of the above 4 criteria) were examined on 52 different occasions, including 27 occasions during which they were asymptomatic. Lactobacilli were significantly more often present when they were symptom-free (p less than 0.05) and gardnerella was a common isolate whether or not the pt. was symptomatic, suggesting that its presence indicates a disturbed ecologic situation within the vagina, resulting in loss of predominance of lactobacilli and hence liability to develop symptoms (*Fredricsson B et al. Gardnerella-associated vaginitis and anerobic bacteria. Gynecol. Obstet. Invest. 17(5):236-41, 1984*).

Observational Study: Samples of vaginal fluid from 60 women of whom 25 had evidence of bacterial vaginosis were examined. An inverse relationship between the quantity of Lactobacillus morphotype (large gram-positive rods) and of the Gardnerella morphotype (small gram-variable rods) was noted on gram stain (p less than 0.001). Gram stains were consistent with BV in 25/25 women with the clinical diagnosis and in 0/35 controls, suggesting that a microscopically detectable changes in vaginial microflora from the Lactobacillus morphotype with or without the Gardnerella morphotype (normal), to a mixed flora with few or no Lactobacillus morphotypes (BV) can be used in the diagnosis of BV (*Spiegel CA et al. Diagnosis of bacterial vaginosis by direct gram stain of vaginal fluid. J. Clin. Microbiol. 18(1):170-77, 1983*).

Observational Study: Vaginal fluid from 53 women with nonspecific vaginitis and normal controls was analyzed. In normal vaginal fluid, lactate was the predominant acid, and the predominant organisms were lactobacillus and streptococcus species (lactate producers). In nonspecific vaginitis, lactate was decreased, whereas succinate, acetate, butyrate and propionate were increased, the predominant flora included Gardnerella (Haemophilus) vaginalis (acetate producer) and anaerobes, which included bacteroides species (succinate producers) and peptococcus (butyrate and acetate producers). After metronidazole therapy, symptoms and signs of nonspecific vaginitis disappeared, and lactate and lactate-producing organisms became predominant (*Spiegel CA et al. Anaerobic bacteria in nonspecific vaginitis. N. Engl. J. Med. 303(11):601-7, 1980*).

Supplementation may be beneficial in vaginitis.

Experimental Study: 94 pts. with non-specific vaginitis were treated with a vaginal lactobacillus preparation (Solco Trichovac/Gynatren),a vaccine containing at least $7x10^9$ inactivated microorganisms of various LA strains in each 0.5 ml dose. Concurrent with a decrease in pathogens, the growth of a normal lactobacilli flora was observed, and the degree of vaginal purity and vaginal pH returned to normal. A cure or at least a marked improvement of symptoms was documented in about 80% of patients. Since, in contrast to conventional therapy, this regimen protects against reinfection, it has a decisive advantage (*Karkut G. [Effect of lactobacillus immunotherapy on genital infections in women (SolcoTrichovac/Gynatren).] Geburtshilfe Fraunheilkd 44(5):311-14, 1984*).

Experimental Study: 444 women with trichomoniasis vaginalis were treated with lactobacillus acidophilis (SolcoTrichovac/Gynatren). One year after the first vaccination, 427 (96.2%) were followed up, and 92.5% of them were found to be cured of clinical symptoms, while the remaining 7.5% had either a positive slide or culture (*Litschgi MS et al. [Effectiveness of a lactobacillus vaccine on trichomonas infections in women. Preliminary results.] Fortschr. Med. 98(41):1624-27, 1980*).

Clinical Report: 20 pts. reported that they cured their candidia vulvovaginitis with preparations containing viable LA cultures (*Will TE. Lactobacillus overgrowth for treatment of moniliary vulvovaginitis. Letter to the Editor. Lancet 2:482, 1979*).

Experimental Study: Pts. with vaginal discharge were treated with yogurt. The results for those with nonspecific vaginitis were encouraging, while the treatment was ineffective in reducing Trichomonas vaginalis infestations (*Gunston KD, Fairbrother PF. Treatment of vaginal discharge with yoghurt. S. Afr. Med. J. 49(16):675-76, 1975*).

See Also:

Friedlander A et al. Lactobacillus acidophillus and vitamin B complex in the treatment of vaginal infection. Panminerva Med. 28(1):51-3, 1986

Karkut G. Effect of lactobacillus immunotherapy (Gynatren/SolcoTrichovac) on vaginal microflora when used for the prophylaxis and treatment of vaginitis. Gynakol Rundsch 24 Suppl. 3:17-24, 1984

Rule out <u>lead</u> toxicity.

Subtoxic oral doses have been shown to reduce host resistence to bacterial and viral infections in mice and rats (*Gainer JH. Effects of heavy metals and of deficiency of zinc on mortality rates in mice infected with encephalomyocarditis virus. Am. J. Vet. Res. 38:869-72, 1977; Cook JA et al. Influence of lead and cadmium on the susceptibility of rats to bacterial challenge. Proc. Soc. Exp. Biol. Med. 150:741-47, 1975*).

INFERTILITY

NUTRIENTS:

Pyridoxine:

Supplementation may be beneficial to infertile women.

Experimental Study: 12/14 women (ages 23-31) with premenstrual syndrome who had been infertile from 18 mo. - 7 yrs. were able to conceive following pyridoxine supplementation 100 - 800 mg daily depending upon the dosage needed to relieve PMS for at least 6 months. Of the 13 pregnancies (1 woman conceived twice), 11 occurred within the first 6 mo. of therapy, 1 occurred in the seventh mo. and the last occurred following 11 mo. of supplementation. In 5/7 women studied, there was a significant increase in progesterone levels with B6 supplementation (*Abraham GE, Hargrove JT - reported in* Med. World News *March 19, 1979*).

Vitamin C:

Supplementation may be beneficial to infertile men.

Experimental Controlled Study: 368 men complaining of an infertile marriage randomly received either vitamin C or mesterolone. After 9 mo., there was no significant difference in the wife's pregnancy rate between the 2 groups (*Hargreave TB et al. Randomised trial of mesterolone versus vitamin C for male infertility.* Brit. J. Urol. *56(6):740-44, 1984*).

Experimental Study: 35 men who could not impregnate their wives due to non-specific sperm agglutination affecting over 20% of their sperm were found to have ave. serum ascorbic acid concentrations of 0.2 mg/dL which is classified as borderline by the U.S. National Nutrition Research Council. They were supplemented with ascorbic acid 500 mg every 12 hours. After 3 wks., mean serum ascorbic acid in the 10 men who returned for evaluation had risen to 2.5 mg/dL and the ave. number of sperm that agglutinated had dropped to 11% (*Dawson EB et al - reported in Gonzalez ER. Sperm swim singly after vitamin C therapy. Medical News.* JAMA *A249(20):2747, 2751, May 27, 1983*).

Experimental Controlled Study: 179 men complaining of an infertile marriage randomly received either vitamin C or clomiphene citrate. After 6 mo., there was no significant difference in the wives' pregnancy rates between the 2 gps., suggesting that vitamin C may be preferable as an alternative treatment for male infertility (*Abel BJ et al. Randomised trial of clomiphene citrate treatment and vitamin C for male infertility.* Brit. J. Urol. *54(6):780-84, 1982*).

See Also:

Briggs MH. Vitamin C and infertility. Lancet *2:677-78, 1973*

Vaishwanar PS, Deshkar BV. Ascorbic acid content and quality of human semen. Am. J. Obstet. Gynecol. *95(8):1080-82, 1966*

- -

Zinc:

Level in seminal plasma is directly correlated with motility of spermatozoa.

Observational Study: Zinc levels in seminal plasma of normals were compared to those of oligospermic, asthenospermic and azoospermic subjects. A linear direct relationship was found between zinc levels and motility of spermatozoans (*Skandhan KP et al. Semen electrolytes in normal and infertile subjects. II. Zinc. Experientia 34(11):1476-77, 1978*).

Supplementation may be beneficial to infertile men.

Experimental Study: 37 males with infertility of over 5 yrs. duration whose sperm counts were less than 25 million (and, if over 15 million, whose sperm motility was under 30%) who had no other known cause of infertility received zinc sulfate 120 mg twice daily (60 mg elemental zinc daily) for 40-50 days. In pts. with initially low plasma testosterone (#22), mean sperm count increased significantly from 8-20 million. Testosterone also increased significantly and 9/22 wives became pregnant. In the 15/37 with initially normal plasma testosterone, sperm count increased, though not significantly, plasma testosterone did not change, and no pregnancies occurred (*Netter A et al. Effect of zinc administration on plasma testosterone, dehydrotestosterone and sperm count. Arch. Androl. 7:69, 1981*).

See Also:

Hartoma TR et al. Zinc, plasma androgens and male sterility. Letter to the Editor. Lancet 3:1125-26, 1977

- -

L-Arginine:

Supplementation may be beneficial to infertile men.

Review Article: The changes in arginine, ornithine and total amino acid concentrations of the seminal plasma in various types of pathospermia are discussed, and a procedure which detects the arginine-deficient type of pathospermia is introduced (*Papp G et al. The role of basic amino acids of the seminal plasma in fertility. Int. Urol. Nephrol. 15(2):195-203, 1983*).

Experimental Study: 178 men with mild to severe problems with sperm count and motility received L-arginine 4 gm daily. 111 had a marked improvement, 21 had a moderate improvement and 46 (25%) had no improvement (*Schachter A et al. Treatment of oligospermia with the amino acid arginine. J. Urology 110(3):311-13, 1973*).

INFLAMMATION

See Also: ALLERGY

NUTRIENTS:

Vitamin C:

A. Shown to have fibrinolytic activity (*Bordia A et al. Atherosclerosis 30:351-54, 1978*).

B. Shown to have anti-histaminic effects (*Nandi BK et al. Effect of ascorbic acid on detoxification of histamine under stress conditions. Biochem. Pharm. 23:643-47, 1974; Zuskin E et al. Inhibition of histamine-induced airway constriction by ascorbic acid. J. Allergy Clin. Immunol. 51(4):218-26, 1973*).

C. Stabilizes cell membranes due to its reducing properties (*Dolbreare FA, Martlage KA. Proc. Soc. Exp. Biol. Med. 139:540-43, 1972*).

D. Required for the hydroxylation of steroids (*Shahied II. Biochemistry of Food and the Biocatalysts. New York, Vantage Press, 1977, pp. 171-80; 251-59*).

E. Inflammation enhances excretion and thus may predispose to deficiency.

> **In vitro Experimental Study:** While resting human neutrophils did not oxidize ascorbic acid, the vitamin was effectively oxidized when added to suspensions of activated human neutrophils. Since oxidation favors degradation and excretion, inflammatory reactions could cause significantly accelerated losses of the vitamin (*Roberts P et al. Vitamin C and inflammation. Med. Biol. 62:88, 1984*).

Supplementation may be beneficial.

> **Animal Experimental Study:** Vitamin C (20 mg/kg) was as effective as phenylbutazone (50 mg/kg) and twice as effective as ASA (100 mg/kg) in inhibiting induced peritonitis-polyarthritis swelling in rats. It was also 60% as effective as phenylbutazone and 300% as effective as ASA in inhibiting adjuvant arthritis at the same dose (*Dolbreare - op cit*).

Vitamin E:

Supplementation may be beneficial.

> **Review Article:** Animal studies suggest that vitamin E has an anti-inflammatory action due to its strong action to protect lysosome and other membranes which may inhibit histamine liberation from granules of mast cells and serotonin liberation from inside the tissue cells. Supporting this theory is that fact that vitamin E acts slowly, protects enlargement of inflammation, shortens its prognosis, and has lesser effects in suppressing inflammation already existing (*Kamimura M. Antiinflammatory effect of vitamin E. J. Vitaminol. 18:204-09, 1972*).

- -

Zinc:

Important in the inflammatory response.

> **Review Article:** Zinc in physiological concentrations can cause approx. a 40% inhibition of im-
> munologically induced histamine and leukotriene release from both basophils and mast cells. In ad-
> dition, zinc modulates serotonin release from platelets, macrophage and neutrophil phagocytosis,
> lymphocyte proliferation, and immune hemolysis (*Marone G et al. Physiological concentrations of
> zinc inhibit the release of histamine from human basophils and lung mast cells. Agents Actions 18:103-
> 106, 1986*).

- -

Amino Acids:

- Creatine:

Supplementation may be beneficial.

> **Animal Experimental Study (rats):** Oral supplementation was as effective as phenylbutazone
> in suppressing acute and chronic inflammatory responses and did not produce GI ulceration at
> effective doses. It exhibited analgesic activity (*Khanna NK, Madan BR. Studies on the anti-in-
> flammatory activity of creatine. Arch. Int. Pharmacodyn. Ther. 231(2):340-50, 1978*).

- D-Phenylalanine:

Supplementation may be beneficial.

> **Theoretical Discussion:** D-phenylalanine and possibly other enkephalinase inhibitors may
> protect peripheral enkephalin or other endorphins generated from the adrenal medulla where
> high concentrations of precursors are present and may also inhibit enkephalinases in joints.
> Both of these actions would result in accumulaton of endorphins in synovial fluid, counteracting
> the effects of prostaglandin-mediated inflammation (*Millinger GS. Neutral amino acid therapy
> for the management of chronic pain. Cranio 4(2):156-63, 1986*).

> **Animal Experimental Study:** Locally injected endorphins antagonized the inflammatory effects
> of carrageenin injected into the rat paw (*Ferreira S, Nakamura M. Prostaglandin hyperalgesia:
> The opioid antagonists. Prostaglandins 18:191-200, 1979*).

- L-Tryptophan or
 DL-Tryptophan:

Supplementation may be beneficial.

> **Animal Experimental Study (rats):** Oral supplementation was as effective as phenylbutazone
> in suppressing acute and chronic inflammatory responses, but not by exerting a counter-irritant
> effect as do almost all anti-inflammatory drugs (*Madan BR, Khanna NK. Anti-inflammatory ac-
> tivity of L-tryptophan and DL-tryptophan. Indian J. Med. Res. 68:708-13, 1978*).

- DL-Valine:

Supplementation may be beneficial.

Animal Experimental Study (rats): Oral supplementation was effective in suppressing acute and chronic inflammatory responses, although it had no analgesic activity. Its effect was not via counter-irritation (*Khanna NK, Madan BR. Anti-inflammatory activity of DL-valine. Indian J. Exp. Biol. 16:834-36, 1978*).

Bioflavonoids:

- Quercetin:

Inhibits the lipoxygenase pathway of arachidonic acid metabolism (which produces some of the most potent inflammatory mediators) while exerting a lesser inhibitory effect on the cyclooxygenase pathway which, in addition to producing less potent activators of inflammation, also produces anti-inflammatory prostaglandins (*Bauman J et al. Prostaglandins 20(4):627-37, 1980*).

Inhibits histamine release from basophils and mast cells (*Middleton E, Drzewieki G. Naturally occurring flavonoids and human basophil histamine release. Arch. Allergy Appl. Immunol. 77:155-57, 1985; Amella M et al. Inhibition of mast cell histamine release by flavonoids and bioflavonoids. Planta Medica 51:16-20, 1985*).

Decreases neutrophil lysosomal enzyme secretion to stabilize cell membranes and decrease lipid peroxidation, leukotriene release, and collagen breakdown by hyaluronidase (*Busse WW et al. Flavonoid modulation of human neutrophil function. J. Allergy Clin. Immuno. 73:801-9, 1984*).

Omega-3 Fatty Acids:

("MaxEPA" is a refined source with 18% eicosapentaenoic acid.)

Supplementation may reduce inflammation by changing the balance of prostaglandins and leukotrienes (which are powerful mediators of inflammation) (*Moncada S et al. Leucocytes and tissue injury: The use of eicosapentaenoic acid in the control of white cell activation. Wien. Klin. Wochenschr. 98(4):104-6, 1986*).

Animal Experimental Study: Supplementation of a standard rat diet with 240 mg/kg/day EPA for 4wks. significantly decreased the concentration of PGE_2 and TXE_2 in inflammatory exudate derived from implantation of carrageenin impregnated sponges. In addition, edema induced by injection of carrageenin into rat paws was significantly reduced in animals fed an EPA-rich diet. Results suggest that supplementation with EPA could, mainly by reducing prostaglandin synthesis, offer a novel and non-toxic approach to the modulation of an inflammatory response (*Terano T et al. Eicosapentaenoic acid as a modulator of inflammation. Biochem. Pharmacol. 35(5):779-85, 1986*).

Experimental Study: The diets of 7 normal subjects were supplemented with 3.2 gm EPA or 1.8 gm MaxEPA daily for 6 weeks. EPA in neutrophils was increased 7 fold without any increase in arachidonic acid. When the neutrophils were activated, there was a 37% reduction in the release of arachidonic acid and a 48% reduction in the inflammatory products of this pathway. In addition, the adherence of neutrophils to bovine epithelial cells as monolayers treated with leukotriene B-4 was completely inhibited. The results suggest that diets enriched with fish oil-derived fatty acids have anti-inflammatory effects by inhibiting the 5-lipoxygenase pathway, thus causing a reduction in the release of leukotrienes along with a reduction in the release of superoxide from neutrophils (*Lee TH et al. Effect of dietary enrichment with eicosapentaenoic acid and docosahexaenoic acids on in vitro neutrophil and monocyte leukotriene generation and neutrophil function. New Engl. J. Med. 312:1217-23, 1985*).

Omega-6 Fatty Acids:

$$\text{linoleic acid} \rightarrow \text{GLA} \rightarrow \text{DGLA} \rightarrow \text{prostaglandin E}_1$$

Evening primrose oil is a rich source of GLA.

Supplementation may be beneficial in reducing acute inflammatory reactions.

In vitro Experimental Study: Rats were given EPO 0.75 ml daily in addition to their regular diets. After 2 wks., their neutrophils demonstrated a greater than 60% reduction in chemotaxis compared to controls, suggesting that EPO influences the responsiveness of inflammatory cells involved in acute immune reactions (*Kunkel SL et al. Suppression of chronic inflammation by evening primrose oil. Prog. Lipid Res. 20(1-4):885-88, 1981*).

Supplementation may be beneficial in reducing chronic inflammatory reactions.

Animal Experimental Study: Rats whose diets were supplemented with EPO 0.75 ml daily 2 wks. before adjuvant challenge demonstrated both a delay in the onset and suppression of the polyarthritis response (*Kunkel SL et al. Suppression of chronic inflammation by evening primrose oil. Prog. Lipid Res. 20(1-4):885-88, 1981*).

Proteolytic Enzymes:

Supplementation may speed healing of injuries.

Experimental Double-blind Study: 64 college football players randomly received 10 pills daily containing either a concentrated proteolytic enzyme mixture or placebo. The experimental gp. sustained fewer time-loss injuries and were able to return to performance sooner than the control group. The number of minor time-loss injuries sustained in the control gp. greatly exceeded the number sustained by the experimental gp., while the number of major injuries sustained in each gp. was of equal number (*Cichoke AJ, Marty L. The use of proteolytic enzymes with soft tissue athletic injuires. Am. Chiropractor, October 1981, p. 32*).

See Also:

Simonet H et al. Therapeutic use of enzymes as anti-inflammatory agents. Ed. Med. et Hyg., Geneve 1:108, 1961

- Bromelain: 1 gm. twice daily between meals

The proteolytic enzyme isolated from the pineapple plant.

Supplementation may be effective (*Cirelli MG. Five years of clinical experience with bromelains in therapy of edema and inflammation in postoperative tissue reaction, skin infections and trauma. Clin. Med. 74(6):55-59, 1967*).

A. Promotes fibrinolysis by activating the production of plasmin from plasminogen (*Ako H et al. Arch. Int. Pharmacodyn. 254:157-67, 1981; Felton GE. Fibrinolytic and antithrombotic action of bromelain may eliminate thrombosis in heart patients. Med. Hypotheses 6:1123-33, 1980; Tausig SJ. The mechanism of the physiological action of bromelain. Med. Hypotheses 6:99-104, 1980*).

B. Selectively stimulates the production of anti-inflammatory prostaglandin E$_1$, possibly due to the formation of active peptides formed from fibrinolysis (*Tausig - op cit*) or due to factor XII activation of low levels of thrombin (*Felton - op cit*).

C. Reduces edema.

Animal Experimental Study (rats): Oral bromelain reduced post-traumatic swelling in the hindlegs (*Uhlig G, Seifert J. Efficacy of proteolytic enzymes traumanase (Bromelain) on post traumatic edema. Forsch. Med. 99(15):554-56, 1981*).

Animal Experimental Study (rabbits): Bromelain's anti-inflammatory properties were equal or superior to those of indomethacin and salicylates following certain chemical assaults (ex. carrageenan), although it showed little anti-inflammatory activity with other chemicals where salicylates are effective (ex. mustard), suggesting that its mode of act on is through increasing vascular permeability to reduce edema and facilitate WBC mobility (*Ito C et al. Anti-inflammatory actions of proteases, bromelain, trypsin and their mixed preparations. Folia Pharmachol. Japan 75:227-37, 1979*).

Animal Experimental Studies: Bromelain reduced paw edema induced by egg white, carrageenin, dextran, serotonin, bradykinin, and yeast as well as reducing the increased permeability induced by histamine, bradykinin and serotonin (*Pirotta F, De Giuli-Morghen C. Drugs Exptl. Clin. Res. 4(1):1-20, 1978; Hiramatso Y. Chem. Abstracts 72:11264b, 1970*).

- Chymotrypsin:

Animal Experimental Study (rats): Following experimentally-induced pleural effusions, injections of chymotrypsin increased the rate of lymphatic flow from the pleural space without increasing capillary permeability (*Gabler WL, Fosdick LS. Proc. Soc. Exp. Biol. Med. 120:160-63, 1965*).

Note: Oral doses have been shown to raise plasma levels.

Experimental Study: Plasma chymotrypsin levels significantly increased in 27 pts. receiving oral supplementation (*Avakian S. J. Clin. Pharm. Therapeut. 5:712-15, 1964*).

- Trypsin:

Reduces edema.

Animal Experimental Study: Suppressed experimentally induced egg white edema in rats (*Martin GJ et al. Proc. Soc. Exp. Biol. Med. 86:636-38, 1954*).

Supplementation may be beneficial.

Experimental Study: In a study of 538 pts., 428 of whom had acute thrombophlebitis, there was "a dramatic subsidence of all signs and symptoms of acute inflammation in 99.3% when trypsin was administered IV" (*Innerfield I et al. Proc. Soc. Exp. Biol. Med. 112:189-90, 1963*).

- -

Feverfew:

WARNINGS: should not be taken without food or longer than 14 consecutive days.

A medicinal herb whose active component (parthenolide) inhibits the secretory action of polymorphonuclear leukocytes involved in the production of cytotoxic and chemotaxic compounds and appears to inhibit the synthesis of prostaglandins PGE2, thromboxane, and leukotrienes that are involved in the inflammatory and pain process (*Heptinstall S et al. Extracts of fevewfew inhibit granule secretion in blood platelets and polymorphonuclear leucocytes. Lancet 1:1071-74, 1985*).

See Also:

Berry MI. Feverfew faces the future. Pharm. J. 611-14, May, 1984

Makheja AN, Bailey JM. A platelet phospholipase inhibitor from the medicinal herb feverfew. Prostaglandins, Leukotrienes & Med. 8:653-60, 1982

Makheja AN, Bailey JM. The active principle in feverfew. Lancet 2:1054, 1981

Collier HO et al. Extract of feverfew inhibits prostaglandin biosynthesis. Lancet 2:1054, 1981

- -

COMBINED SUPPLEMENTATION:

Proteolytic Enzymes and
Flavonoids and
Vitamin C:

May be at least as effective as non-steroidal anti-inflammatory drugs.

Animal Experimental Study (rats): When compared against the action of 7 non-steroidal anti-inflammatory drugs by 4 tests (histamine-induced wheal, dextran and carrageenin induced edemas, and permeability to Evans blue in the peritoneal cavity), a combination of oral proteolytic enzymes (chymotrypsin & trypsin), flavonoids (hesperidin-methyl-chalcone & methyl-4-esculetol sodium monoethanoate) and ascorbic acid showed a "more complete spectrum of action than the non-steroid anti-inflammatory substances against the initial symptoms of inflammation" as only the combination was effective in decreasing the effects of histamine and dextran (*Taraye JP, Lauressergues H. Advantages of a combination of proteolytic enzymes, flavonoids and ascorbic acid in comparison with non-steroid inflammatory drugs. Arzneim.-Forsch. 27(1):1144-49, 1977*).

INSOMNIA

BASIC DIET:

Low <u>alcohol</u> consumption may be beneficial.

Experimental Study: 6 healthy young adults received either 0.16, 0.32 or 0.64 g/kg alcohol. The lowest dosage increased total sleep time and reduced awake activity, and both the lowest and medium dosages improved the sleep efficiency index. However, all 3 dosages reduced slow wave sleep in the latter part of the night, REM sleep was delayed and the REM/NREM reduced. In addition, results suggested that, at the highest dosage, disturbances in REM sleep were likely (*Stone BM. Sleep and low doses of alcohol. Electroencephalogr. Clin. Neurophysiol. 48(6):706-9, 1980*).

Avoid <u>caffeine</u>.

Observational Study: In a cross-sectional study of 4558 Australians, the proportion of subjects reporting insomnia increased significantly with mean caffeine intake. A multiple logistic regression model showed that the association between the prevalence of these symptoms and usual daily caffeine consumption remained significant in both males and females after controlling for age, adiposity, smoking, alcohol intake and occupation. The relative risk of insomnia for people consuming 240 mg of caffeine (4-5 cups of coffee or tea) daily is 1.4 for both males and females. Coffee consumption had no significant effect over and above that attributable to its caffeine content (*Shirlow MJ, Mathers CD. A study of caffeine consumption and symptoms: Indigestion, palpitations, tremor, headache and insomnia. Int. J. Epidemiol. 14(2):239-48, 1985*).

Experimental Study: Compared to controls, 6 subjects with caffeine-induced wakefulness had a longer plasma t 1/2 (mean 7.4 vs. 4.2 hr.) and slower plasma clearance of caffeine. Plasma caffeine concentration at midnight, 8 hrs. after afternoon coffee, was also higher (*Levy M, Zylber-Katz E. Caffeine metabolism and coffee-attributed sleep disturbances. Clin. Pharmacol. Ther. 33(6):770-75, 1983*).

Experimental Study: Following caffeine intake, normal subjects demonstrated an increase in longer episodes of intervening wakefulness plus drowsiness, but no significant change in the episode duration of any of the sleep stages; thus caffeine insomnia seems characterized by increased stability of wakefulness (*Brezinova V et al. Two types of insomnia: Too much waking or not enough sleep. Brit. J. Psychiat. 126:439-45, 1975*).

- -

NUTRIENTS:

<u>Myo-inositol</u>:   500 mg. daily

May have a calming effect (*Pfeiffer, Carl. Mental and Elemental Nutrients. New Canaan, Conn., Keats Publishing Company, 1975*).

Clinical Observation: The effect of myo-inositol supplementation on the EEG was found to resemble that of chlordiazepoxide and meprobamate (*Pfeiffer - ibid*).

<u>Niacinamide</u>:   1 gram at bedtime

Said to be particularly helpful for those who fall asleep readily but can't return to sleep after awakening during the night.

Animal Experimental Study: Found to have anti-conflict, anti-aggressive, muscle relaxant and hypnotic actions with effectiveness similar to that of minor tranquilizers (*M:ohler H et al. Nicotinamide is a brain constituent with benzodiazepine-like actions.* <u>Nature</u> *278:563-65, 1979*).

- -

<u>L-Tryptophan</u>:   1 gram 30-45 minutes before bedtime (higher doses may be needed in people over 40).
Avoid protein for 90 min. before and afterward.
Take with sugar.

Nutritional precursor of serotonin, a neurotransmitter which plays an important role in the induction and maintenance of sleep.

Review Article: Controlled studies have found that:
1. 1 gm at bedtime resulted in a 50% reduction in sleep latency (time between lights out and stage 2 sleep) in normal subjects.
2. Lower doses were less effective and higher doses produced very little improvement.
3. Sleep stages were not distorted unless 10-15 gm were ingested.
4. While mild insomniacs also benefited from a 1 gm dose, severe insomniacs usually responded to higher doses.
5. Chronic insomniacs, some of whom were psychiatric pts., did not respond to tryptophan in initial trials.
6. While serious insomniacs did not respond to low doses during the first week, sleep latencies did improve during the second week compared to those on placebo, suggesting that there could be a cumulative effect.
7. Experience with over 400 pts. showed a low to negligible level of side effects at doses below 15 grams.
(*Hartmann EL speaking at a symposium sponsored by the AMA - quoted in* <u>Clin. Psychiat. News</u>, *March, 1985*).

Experimental Study: 3/10 (30%) elderly pts. with persistent insomnia had "dramatic and sustained relief" from 1 - 4 gm at bedtime for 3 weeks (*Fitten LJ et al. L-tryptophan as a hypnotic in special patients.* <u>J. Am. Geriat. Soc.</u> *33:294, 1985*).

Experimental Controlled Study: 20 newborns weighing 6.5-7.5 lbs received a bottle feeding that contained either tryptophan (equivalent to 420 mg for a 150 lb man) or valine, and sleep was compared to that following a Similac feeding on another day. Infants receiving tryptophan entered quiet sleep 20 min earlier than when they received Similac, while the valine gp. entered quiet sleep 39 minutes later after valine than after Similac. While the total sleep of the tryptophan gp. was 14.4 min. longer on tryptophan than on Similac, the total sleep of the valine gp. was 36.2 minutes shorter (*Yogman M, Zeisel S. Diet and sleep patterns in newborn infants.* <u>New Engl. J. Med.</u> *309(19):1147, 1983*).

See Also:

Experimental Double-blind Study: *Hartmann E et al. Effect of amino acids on quantified sleepiness.* <u>Nutr. Behav.</u> *1:179-183, 1983*

Experimental Double-blind Study: *Spinweber C et al. L-tryptophan: Effects on daytime sleep latency and the waking EEG.* <u>Electroencephalo. Clin. Neurophysiol.</u> *55:652-61, 1983*

Review of Scientific Studies (including Animal and Placebo-Controlled Studies): *Hartmann E. Am. J. Psychiat. 134:366-370, 1977*

- -

OTHER FACTORS:

Rule Out <u>Food Sensitivities</u>:

Experimental Study: 8 infants with sleeplessness had extensive medical and psychological testing without the establishment of a causative diagnosis. Allergy evaluation showed *in vivo* and *in vitro* evidence of cow's milk allergy. Sleeplessness was eliminated with the removal of cow's milk protein from the diet and reproduced by its reintroduction (*Kah A et al. Insomnia and cow's milk allergy in infants. Pediatrics 76(6):880-84, 1985*).

IRRITABLE BOWEL SYNDROME

BASIC DIET:

Increase <u>dietary fiber</u>:

Example: Unprocessed <u>wheat bran</u>: 8 -10 tsp. daily

Experimental Placebo-controlled Study: 40 pts. received wheat bran 15 gm daily. A significant reduction in symptoms was noted after 12 wks., but not after 16 weeks, suggesting that wheat bran may benefit some pts., but is not an ideal treatment (*Kruis W et al. Comparison of the therapeutic effect of wheat bran, mebeverine and placebo in patients with irritable bowel syndrome.* <u>Digestion</u> *34:196, 1986*).

Experimental Double-blind Crossover Study: 38 pts. received either wheat bran 10-30 gm daily or placebo. Both bran and placebo significantly reduced the severity of most of the symptoms except for constipation which only improved significantly with bran. Pain and urgency were significantly more frequent with bran than with placebo (*Cann P et al. What is the benefit of coarse wheat bran in patients with irritable bowel syndrome?* <u>Gut</u> *25:168-73, 1984*).

Experimental Controlled Study: A diet composed of 30 gm fruit and vegetable fiber and 10 gm cereal fiber was compared to one with the opposite ratio. Both resulted in similar significant improvement in abdominal pain, bowel habits and state of well being (*Fielding J, Kehoe M. Different dietary fibre formulations and the irritable bowel syndrome.* <u>Irish J. Med. Sci.</u> *153:178-80, 1984*).

Experimental Controlled Study: 14 pts. on bran 20 gm daily showed a significant reduction in abdominal pain and "improvement in bowel habit" on bran compared to controls who excluded wholegrain cereal products (*Manning AP et al. Wheat fibre and irritable bowel syndrome: A controlled trial.* <u>Lancet</u> *2:417, 1977*

Negative Experimental Double-blind Study: The effect of biscuits containing bran (30 gm daily) was compared to biscuits without bran in a mixed gp. of pts. including pts. with diverticular disease and pts. taking laxatives. Results failed to support the use of bran (*Soltoft J et al. A double-blind trial of the effect of wheat bran on symptoms of irritable bowel syndrome.* <u>Lancet</u> *1:270-2, 1976*).

See Also:

Painter NS. Bran and the irritable bowel. Letter to the Editor. <u>Lancet</u> *1:540, 1976*

Harvey RF et al. Effects of increased dietary fibre on intestinal transit. <u>Lancet</u> *1:1278-80, 1973*

Avoid <u>sugar</u>.

Review Article: A diet high in refined carbohydrate is implicated in the etiology of irritable bowel syndrome and certain other diseases of the colon. It is suggested that spasm of the smooth muscle is the common pathogenetic mechanism, and the strength of the spasm producing increased pressure in the colonic lumen or wall and the length of time for which the colon has been affected are believed to determine the type of disease resulting. A diet high in refined carbohydrate allows the intense muscle spasm to occur because the physical buffering effect of fecal bulk is considerably reduced (*Grimes DS. Refined carbohydrate, smooth-muscle spasm and disease of the colon. Lancet 1:395-97, 1976*).

- -

NUTRIENTS:

Folic Acid:

Supplementation may be beneficial for chronic diarrhea.

> **Experimental Study:** 8 pts. with chronic diarrhea from diverse etiologies were treated with folic acid 40-60 mg daily with restoration of normal or almost normal stools in 2-5 days which reversed when folate was discontinued, suggesting that long-standing diarrhea is associated with the development of folate deficiency (*Carruthers LB. Chronic diarrhea treated with folic acid. Lancet 1:849, 1946*).

- -

Peppermint Oil: 3-6 capsules (0.2 ml/cap) daily
(capsules must be enteric coated to prevent premature oil release)

Inhibits GI smooth muscle action.

> **Experimental Study:** Pts. who took 3-6 capsules (0.2 ml per capsule) of peppermint oil daily were relieved of their symptoms, while the number of daily bowel movements was unaffected (*Dew MJ et al. Brit. J. Clin. Prac. 38:394-8, 1984*).

> **Experimental Double-blind Study:** Capsules of peppermint oil were effective in relieving symptoms (*Rees WRW et al. Treating irritable bowel syndrome with peppermint oil. Brit. Med. J. October 6, 1979, p. 835*).

> See Also:

> > *Somerville K et al. Delayed release peppermint oil capsules (Colpermin) for the spastic colon syndrome: A pharmacokinetic study. Brit. J. Clin. Pharmacol. 18:638-40, 1984*

- -

OTHER FACTORS:

Rule out food sensitivities.

> **Experimental Study:** 28 pts. with predominant diarrhea received skin prick testing for foods and received oral disodium cromoglycate 1500 mg daily for 8 weeks. 19 pts. with positive skin prick tests responded while only 1 of the remaining 9 pts. improved, suggesting that IBS with predominant diarrhea may be related to atopic food allergy (*Stefananini GF et al. Efficacy of oral disodium cromoglycate in patients with irritable bowel syndrome and positive skin prick tests to foods. Letter to the Editor. Lancet 1:207-8, 1986*).

> **Experimental Single-blind Study:**   17 pts. who had failed to respond to standard therapy were placed on a strict diet eliminating foods commonly associated with hypersensitivity. After 1 mo., 9/17 (53%) were free of symptoms. Foods were individually re-introduced and 7/17 (41%) identified reactions to specific foods which they continued to avoid. These pts. remained well for the following year when nasogastric tubes were inserted, and they were fed either known safe or test (excluded) foods. They correctly identified test foods on 10/12 occasions and safe foods on 10/12 occasions, a significant result (p less than 0.01). The test foods also caused an elevation of rectal prostaglandin E_2 levels. In a separate study, 17/28 pts. (60%) were found to be atopic compared to 6/26 (23%) matched controls (*Finn R et al. Expanding horizons of allergy and the total allergy syndrome. Clinical Ecology 3(3):129-131, 1985*).

Experimental Study: 11/28 pts. who had failed to respond to standard treatments were placed on a strict elimination diet of lamb, fresh white fish, cabbage, carrots, peas, 'Ryvita', milk-free margarine, and weak black tea. At 1 wk., 2 showed major improvement. The other 17 were put on the diet for 2 wks. and 9 improved significantly. Improvement was most likely in those with dominant diarrhea. Foods were then reintroduced at 2-day intervals in the 9 responders to identify provoking foods. At 1 yr., 7/9 of these pts. were still well so long as they avoided the foods to which they were intolerant. 17 out of the pts. (60%) were atopic on the basis of prick tests to standard inhalent antigens compared to 6/26 (23%) controls. This difference was significant (p less than 0.05) (*Smith MA et al. Food intolerance, atopy, and irritable bowel syndrome.* Lancet 2:1064, November 9, 1985).

Experimental Study: 122/188 (65%) of pts. who were placed on a diet eliminating frequently incriminated foods for 2 weeks benefited and were able to identify offending foods upon their re-introduction. Wheat, found to provoke symptoms in 65%, was by far the most common offender (*Alun Jones V, Hunter JO. Food intolerance in irritable bowel syndrome.* Clin. Ecology 3(1):35-8, 1985).

Experimental Blinded Study: 12/24 pts. were found to be atopic (positive skin tests, positive IgE RAST, positive histories) and 9/12 had elevated total serum IgE levels. All 24 pts. were placed on an exclusion diet and blind challenged 1-2 wks. later with 18 different foods and 6 food additives. 17 improved on the diet and 14/17 exacerbated during challenges. Of the 6 additives tested, sodium benzoate, sodium nitrite, erythrosine and carminic acid were symptom-producing. All pts. with elevated IgE were food-sensitive. In only 10 cases did the IgE RAST correlate with the results of provocation. Six months after starting an exclusion diet based on test results, 10 of 14 pts. with positive provocative test results were asymptomatic, while the other 4 had only mild symptoms. The presence of yeast in the stools (Candida albicans and Geotrichum candidum) appeared to be related to their food sensitivities as treatment with nystatin was followed by improvement in most of the affected patients (*Petitpierre M et al. Irritable bowel syndrome and hypersensitivity to food.* Ann. Allergy 54:538-40, 1985).

Observational Study: Endoscopy of pts. revealed patchy erythema with loss of visible vascularity and very occasional, mild, superficial ulceration. Histology revealed an excess of both mucosal eosinophils and IgE-containing cells, compatible with an IgE-mediated process. The main foods implicated were milk, soy and beef (*Jenkins HR et al. Food allergy: The major cause of infantile colitis.* Ann. Allergy vol. 53, October, 1984).

Negative Experimental Double-blind Study: Foods believed to provoke symptoms were first eliminated as were skin-test positive foods (i.e. foods such as wheat were not usually eliminated). About half the subjects reacted to an open trial of the remaining foods who were then subjected to double blind challenges. Reactions to the "placebo" capsules (which contained lactose, food coloring and beef- or pork-derived gelatin) were as frequent as reactions to the actual foods, suggesting that skin testing is unreliable as a method of identifying provoking foods (*Alun-Jones VA et al. Food intolerance and the irritable bowel.* Lancet 2:633, 1983).

Note: Subjects sensitive to milk, food coloring, beef or pork could have reacted to the "placebo" capsules, thus throwing the results into question.

Experimental Double-blind Study: 14/21 were found to be provoked by specific food challenges following 1 week on a single meat, a single fruit, and distilled or spring water. These reactions were confirmed in the 6 who were challenged double-blind. 9 reacted to wheat, 5 to corn, 4 to dairy products, 4 to coffee, 3 to tea and 2 to citrus. Rectal prostaglandin E_2 was significantly increased after positive challenges and sometimes remained elevated for more than 24 hours (*Alun-Jones VA et al. Food intolerance: A major factor in the pathogenesis of irritable bowel syndrome.* Lancet 2:1115-7, 1982).

Experimental Study: Based on a symptom survey listing atopic allergic symptoms, 17/22 (77%) pts. were judged to be possibly allergic. In addition, over 50 pts. with inflammatory bowel disease (including irritable bowel syndrome) treated with inhalent allergy hyposensitization and dietary changes consisting of rotation and diversification of allergic foods were considerably improved in both their respiratory and abdominal symptoms, suggesting an allergic diathesis (*Siegel J. Inflammatory bowel disease: Another possible facet of the allergic diathesis. Ann. Allergy 47:92-94, 1981*).

See Also:

Halpin TC et al. Colitis, persistent diarrhea, and soy protein intolerance. J. Pediat. 21:404, 1977

Rule out <u>hydrochloric acid deficiency.</u>

Experimental Study: HCl suplementation was effective in "gastrogenous" (i.e. achlorhydric) chronic diarrhea (*Bulletin Gen. de Therapeutique, Paris - abstracted in JAMA 39:55, 1902*).

<u>Lactobacillus Acidophilus:</u>

Supplementation may be beneficial.

Experimental Controlled Study: The effects of yogurt and Neomycin-kaopectate as treatment of infantile diarrhea were compared using 45 infants aged 1-27 months. Those treated with yogurt recovered more rapidly (*Niv M et al. Yogurt in the treatment of infantile diarrhea. Clin. Ped. 2:407-11, 1963*).

Experimental Studies (compilation of previous studies):
    15/21 cases of "constipation and diarrhea" responded
    46/50 cases of "functional diarrhea" responded
    32/39 cases of irritable colon and diverticulosis responded
    (*Lancet General Advertiser September 21, 1957*)

KIDNEY STONES (CALCIUM OXALATE)

See Also: OSTEOPOROSIS

OVERVIEW:

1. All patients:

    A. Avoid sugar.
    B. Vegetarian diet.
    C. Increase fiber.
    D. Supplement with magnesium 300 mg daily

2. Pts. with hypercalciuria:

    A. Limit calcium intake.
    B. Limit sodium intake.
    C. Avoid caffeine.

3. Pts. with hyperoxaluria:

    A. Limit oxalic acid intake.
    B. Supplement with pyridoxine 150 mg daily

3. Pts. with hypocitraturia or hyperuricosuria.

    Supplement with potassium citrate 60 meq daily.

4. Rule out cadmium toxicity.

- -

BASIC DIET:

Drink enough water throughout the day and night to produce 2-3 quarts of urine daily.

Limit calcium intake in the 30-50% of idiopathic stoneformers with hypercalciuria (including boiling water for 10 minutes to lower calcium content by precipitating calcium carbonate).

> **Case Report:** A pt. with recurrent kidney stones was found to have 7 mg/kg/day urinary calcium excretion when drinking unboiled water compared to 3 mg/kg/day when drinking boiled water. After switching to boiled water he remained free of symptoms for 3 years of follow-up (*Popovtzer MM et al. Letter to the Editor. N. Engl. J. Med. 310(11):721, 1984*).

> *Note: Lowering dietary calcium is <u>not</u> beneficial to pts. without hypercalciuria as the lower the calcium intake, the higher the urinary oxalate excretion (Brockis JG et al. The effects of vegetable and animal protein diets on calcium, urate and oxalate excretion. Brit. J. Urol. 54(6):590-93, 1982).*

Limit <u>sodium</u> intake in <u>hypercalciuria</u>.

Experimental Study: 4 pts. had hypercalciuria which was dependent on a high sodium intake. Moderate sodium restriction corrected the hypercalciuria (*Silver J et al. Sodium-dependent idiopathic hypercalciuria in renal-stone formers. <u>Lancet</u> 2:484-86, 1983*).

Remove <u>high oxalate foods</u>:

Foods with 25 mg/100 gm oxalate (highest concentration):

Beans, Cocoa, Instant Coffee, Parsley, Rhubarb, Spinach, Tea

Other frequently eaten foods relatively high in oxalates:

Beet tops, Carrot, Celery, Chocolate, Cucumber, Grapefruit, Kale, Peanut, Pepper, Sweet Potato

Dietary oxalate contributes to urinary oxalate excretion, although the increase in excretion between a low and high oxalate diet is relatively small.

Experimental Controlled Study: Oral loads of 400 mg sodium oxalate daily significantly increased urinary oxalate excretion in both 14 normals and 22 stone formers; however, 130 mg daily failed to produce significant increases and the degree of oxaluria did not differ at either dosage between normals and stone formers (*Butz M et al. Dietary influence on serum and urinary oxalate in healthy subjects and oxalate stone formers. <u>Urol. Int.</u> 35:309-15, 1980*).

Experimental Controlled Study: The effects of 6 days of low oxalate intake followed by 6 days of high oxalate intake on urinary oxalate excretion in 4 normals and 6 stone formers was compared. In the normals, the average 24-hour oxalate excretion increased from 19.3 mg to 30.3 mg, only 3.4% of the increase in dietary intake. In the stone formers, excretion increased from 14.5 mg to 24.4 mg (10.3% of the increase in dietary intake), suggesting that stone formers have a greater tendency to absorb oxalate and to excrete it in the urine (*Zarembski PM, Hodgkinson. Some factors increasing the urinary excretion of oxalate in man. <u>Clin. Chim. Acta</u> 25:1-10, 1969*).

In normals, about 40% of urinary oxalate is believed to be derived from glycine (*Crawhall JC et al. Conversion of glycine to oxalate in a normal subject. <u>Lancet</u> 2:810, 1959*) and 40% from ingested ascorbic acid (*Atkins GL et al. Quantitative aspects of ascorbic acid metabolism in man. <u>J. Biol. Chem.</u> 239:2975-80, 1964*), with only 20% coming from dietary oxalate.

Hyperoxaluria does not necessarily cause kidney stones.

Case Report: A healthy man ingested 490 mg oxalate as beetroot extract for 5 yrs and was found to have both hyperoxaluria and oxalate crystalluria but no evidence of kidney stones (*Butz - op cit*).

Most stone formers do not have hyperoxaluria.

Observational Study: 16.3% of 392 stone formers were found to have hyperoxaluria (*Rao RN et al. Dietary management of urinary risk factors in renal stone formers. <u>Brit. J. Urol.</u> 54:578-83, 1982*).

Avoid <u>sugar</u>.

Sugar ingestion is associated with increased urinary calcium concentration, especially in stone-formers (*Lennon EJ et al. A possible mechanism for diminished renal tubular calcium and magnesium reabsorption after glucose ingestion. <u>Clin. Res., Nat. Mtg. Abstr.</u> 16:388, 1968*).

Experimental Controlled Study: 18 healthy males were fed diets which were low, normal or high in refined carbohydrates (sucrose) for 1 month. Results suggested that normal dietary supplements of refined carbohydrate will significantly increase the number and magnitude of peaks of urinary calcium concentration at the time when oxalate excretion is also maximal; thus significant amounts of sugar or sugar products in the diet will increase the risk of the formation product of calcium oxalate being exceeded (*Thom JA et al. The influence of refined carbohydrate on urinary calcium excretion. Brit. J. Urology 50:459-464, 1978*).

Experimental Controlled Study: Ingestion of refined sugar significantly increased urinary calcium excretion and concentration in normals, stone-formers and relatives of stone-formers. The effect of sugar on the latter 2 gps. was far greater than on the normal subjects (*Lemann J et al. Possible role of carbohydrate induced calciuria in calcium oxalate kidney stone formation. New Engl. J. Med. 280:232-7, 1969*).

Sugar (sucrose or glucose) provokes an excessive insulin response in stone-formers.

Experimental Study: 59% of 39 pts. with idiopathic urolithiasis had an excessive insulin response to an oral sugar load (*Rao PN et al. Are stone formers maladapted to refined carbohydrates? Brit. J. Urol. 54(6):575-77, 1982*).

Insulin increases renal calcium output; thus sugar may increase calcium output in stone formers because of its effect upon insulin (*DeFronzo RA et al. The effect of insulin on renal handling of sodium, potassium, calcium and phosphate in man. J. Clin. Inves. 55:845-55, 1975*).

Sugar increases the urinary output of n-acetyl-glucosaminidase (NAG) which is only present in pts. with renal disease (*Dance N et al. The excretion of N-acetyl-beta-glucosaminidase and B-galactosidase by patients with renal disease. Clin. Chem. Acta 27:87-92, 1970*), suggesting that high sugar intake may cause renal damage which would contribute to the nephrocalcific foci believed necessary for the initiation of crystallization of supersaturated solutes from the urine (*Anderson CK. Renal histological changes in stone formers and non-stone formers, in Hodgkinson A, Nordin BEC, Eds., Proceed. Renal Stone Res. Sympos.. London, Churchill, 1969, pp. 133-6*).

Experimental Study: 14 young normal males who were found to normally ingest 115 gm sugar daily were given a high sugar diet of 260 gm daily (the ave. intake in England is about 125 gm daily). After 3 wks., the activity of NAG had significantly risen. 2 wks. after returning to their normal diet, the fall in NAG had not reached significance (*Yudkin J et al. Effects of high dietary sugar. Brit. Med. J. 281:1396, 1980*)

Avoid caffeine.

Increases urinary calcium excretion.

Experimental Study: 31 women ingested decaffeinated coffee at different times to which caffeine had been added. 3 hours afterwards, urinary calcium excretion increased significantly, but only in women taking estrogen, suggesting that caffeine ingestion may offset the beneficial effect of estrogen on calcium metabolism (*Hollingbery PW et al. Effect of dietary caffeine and aspirin on urinary calcium and hydroxyproline excretion in pre- and postmenopausal women. Fed. Proc. 44:1149, 1985*).

Experimental Study: 15 males drank decaffeinated coffee to which 0, 150 or 300 mg caffeine had been added. Total urinary 3 hr. excretion of calcium, magnesium, sodium and chloride increased significantly after caffeine intake, while zinc, phosphorus, potassium, creatinine and volume were unchanged (*Massey LK, Berg TA. The effect of dietary caffeine on urinary excretion of calcium, magnesium, phosphorus, sodium, potassium, chloride and zinc in healthy males. Nutr. Res. 5:1281-84, 1985*).

Observational Study: The caffeine intake of 168 women (ages 36-45) was studied over the long term. Subjects averaged about 2 cups of regular coffee daily and suffered from a net calcium loss of 22 mg daily. The addition of only 1 cup of regular coffee resulted in an additional 6 mg of daily calcium loss. In addition, women who consumed a high amount of caffeine also consumed fewer calcium-rich foods. The authors note that a negative calcium balance of only 40 mg daily is quite sufficient to explain the 1-1.5% loss in skeletal mass annually in postmenopausal women (*Heaney RP, Recker RR. Effects of nitrogen, phosphorus, and caffeine on calcium balance in women. J. Lab. & Clin. Med. 99:46-55, 1982*).

<u>Vegetarian</u> diet.

Meat intake is correlated with calcium oxalate stone formation as well as urinary output of calcium.

Observational Study: 30 meat eaters were compared to 30 vegetarians matched for age and sex. Intake of animal protein was found to be associated with increased calcium excretion. Urinary oxalate increased with the vegetable protein content of the diet but animal protein did not affect oxalate excretion (*Brockis JG et al. Brit. J. Urol. 54(6):590-93, 1982*).

Observational Study: Vegetarians have a 50-60% decreased risk of stones (*Robertson WG, Peacock M, Marshall DH. The prevalence of urinary stone disease in vegetarians. Eur. Urol. 8:334, 1982*).

Observational Study: Dietary analysis revealed that pts. with a history of recurrent nephrolithiasis have higher dietary intakes of animal protein than do single stone formers, and non-stone formers consume less animal protein than single stone formers. Stone formers were found to excrete more calcium, oxalate and uric acid than non-stone formers, while vegetarians excreted least of all (*Robertson WG et al. Should recurrent calcium oxalate stone formers become vegetarian? Brit. J. Urol. 51:427-31, 1979*).

Experimental Study: In normal subjects, high animal protein intake increased their urinary excretion of calcium oxalate and uric acid, while reducing the consumption of animal protein reduced their excretion (*Robertson, 1979 - ibid*).

Increase <u>dietary fiber</u>.

Observational Study: Fiber intake was lower in stone formers than in controls (*Griffith HM et al. A control study of dietary factors in renal stone formation. Brit. J. Urol. 53:416, 1981*).

Experimental Study: 24 grams of bran daily lowered calcium excretion by 20-25% in 73% of stone formers (*Shah PJR. Unprocessed bran and its effect on urinary calcium excretion in idiopathic hypercalciuria. Brit. Med. J. August 9, 1980, p. 426*).

- -

COMBINED DIETARY CHANGES:

While the dietary habits of 392 stone formers did not differ significantly from controls, dietary advice to <u>increase fiber</u> and <u>reduce sugar</u>, <u>refined carbohydrates</u> and <u>animal protein</u> produced a significant reduction in the urinary excretion of calcium, oxalate and uric acid, suggesting that this is the first line of management of idiopathic stone formers (*Rao PN et al. Dietary management of urinary risk factors in renal stone formers. Br. J. Urology 54(6):578-83, 1982*).

- -

NUTRIENTS:

Pyridoxine:

Essential for the normal metabolism of oxalic acid. Deficiency is associated with metabolic block in its degradation resulting in increased urinary oxalic acid and stone precipitation; thus supplementation may benefit at least certain hyperoxaluric patients.

Experimental Study: 12 pts. who had had an average of at least 1 stone annually for the past few years were supplemented with 10 mg. pyridoxine for 6 months. Urine oxalate decreased significantly and the results were better and faster than those from prescribing thiazides (*Murthy MSR et al. Effect of pyridoxine supplementation on recurrent stone formers. Int. J. Clin. Pharm., Therapy & Toxicol. 1982*).

Experimental Controlled Study: 24 stone formers experienced a reduction in the rate of recurrence of urolithiasis related to decreased oxaluria following supplementation with 60 mg, but not with 20 mg, pyridoxine daily (*Revusova V et al. The significance of oxaluria reduction by pyridoxine in prevention of calcium oxalate nephrolithiasis. Cas. Lek. Ces. 121(6):163-6, 1982*).

Experimental Study: 2 pts. with primary oxalosis were supplemented with pyridoxine hydrochloride 1 gm daily. 24 hr. urinary oxalate excretion decreased by 60% and 70%, respectively, with corresponding clinical benefit. In the 1 pt. with renal failure, serum creatinine decreased from 243 to 146 mumol/l after 15 mo. of treatment (*Will EJ, Bijvoet OL. Primary oxalosis: Clinical and biochemical response to high-dose pyridoxine therapy. Metabolism 28(5):542-48, 1979*).

Experimental Controlled Study: 4 stone formers with primary hyperoxaluria in whom tryptophan load studies failed to suggest pyridoxine deficiency were supplemented with 75 - 600 mg daily. Doses of 150 mg were found to cause a sustained maximal reduction in urinary oxalate excretion in 2/4 pts. at levels intermediate between normal and their pre-treatment baseline (*Gibbs DA, Watts RWE. The action of pyridoxine in primary hyperoxaluria. Clin. Sci. 38:277086, 1970*).

Experimental Controlled Study: Following loading with 10 mg. DL tryptophan for 2 days, 18 stone formers excreted more xanthurenic acid than 12 normals, suggesting a marginal B_6 deficiency (*Gershoff SN, Prien EL. Excretion of urinary metabolites in calcium oxalate urolithiasis: Effect of tryptophan and vitamin B6 administration. Am. J. Clin. Nutr. 8:812, 1960*).

Vitamin A:

Deficiency may promote the formation of kidney stones.

Animal Experimental Study: Rats fed a vitamin A-deficient diet were found to have reduced uromucoid excretion (uromucoid excretion is also decreased in pts. with uric acid stones or renal tubular acidosis with staghorn calculi) with hypercalciuria and reduced phosphate levels (*Bichler KH et al. Influence of vitamin A deficiency on the excretion of uromucoid and other substances in the urine of rats. Clin. Nephrol. 20:32-39, 1983*)..

Animal Experimental Study: 74% of rats fed a vitamin A-deficient, lactose-rich diet developed urinary calculi and half developed renal pelvic calculi. In addition they develped hypercalciuria and hyperoxaluria. A lactose-rich diet without vitamin A deficiency did not lead to stone formation, suggesting that the vitamin A deficiency was responsible for the lithogenic effect of lactose due to increased calcium absorption with consequent hypercalciuria (*Gershoff SN, McGandy RB. The effects of vitamin A-deficient diets containing lactose in producing bladder cacluli and tumors in rats. Am. J. Clin. Nutr. 34:483, 1981*).

Negative Experimental Controlled Study: The rate of dark adaptation, the thresholds of the completely dark adapted eye and blood vitamin A levels were determined for 20 pts. and compared to normal controls. In addition, in 78 autopsy cases with urolithiasis, the respiratory and urinary tracts were examined for the epithelial metaplasia characteristic of vitamin A deficiency. None of these cases showed evidence of vitamin A deficiency, suggesting that urolithiasis in humans is not usually associated with vitamin A deficiency (*Jewett HJ et al. Does vitamin A deficiency exist in clinical urolithiasis?* JAMA *121:566-69, 1943*).

Vitamin C:

WARNING: Megadoses (over 6 gm daily) can be harmful.

Review Article: Urinary oxalate excretion generally does not increase significantly for both normal subjects and stone-formers with ascorbic acid supplementation unless doses exceed 6 gm daily; however, oxalate excretion even at those high doses is still usually in the range achievable by dietary influences alone. The exceptions derive from anecdotal reports of a small number of cases and from one poorly-controlled trial with unstated methodology and questionable assay techniques (*Piesse JW. Nutritional factors in calcium containing kidney stones with particular emphasis on vitamin C.* Int. Clin. Nutr. Rev. *5(3):110-129, 1985*).

- -

Magnesium: 200 mg. twice daily

The urine of stone formers has a lowered magnesium/calcium ratio (*Takahasi E. The magnesium:calcium ratio in the concentrated urines of patients with calcium oxalate calculi.* Invest. Urol. *10:147, 1972*).

Supplementation inhibits calcium oxalate stone formation.

Experimental Controlled Study: 55 pts. who had had an average of 0.8 stones annually (460 stones in 10 previous years) were placed on 200 mg. magnesium hydroxide daily. After 2-4 years, only 8/55 developed stones and the average rate of stone development decreased 90% to 0.08 stones per person per year. Over 4 years, a control group of 43 pts. averaged a much higher formation rate and, after 4 years, 59% of them had developed new stones (*Johansson G et al. Effects of magnesium hydroxide in renal stone disease.* J. Am. Col. Nutr. *vol. 1, no. 2, 1982*).

Experimental Controlled Study: 56 consecutive pts. with renal calcium stones received prophylatic treatment with magnesium hydroxide 200 mg twice daily. After most pts. had received supplementation for at least 2 yrs., 45 were free of recurrences or formations of new stones. The mean stone episode rate during treatment was 0.03 stones/yr. compared to 0.8 stones/yr. before treatment. Of 34 pts. who served as controls, 15 experienced recurrences after 2 years. The only side-effect was minor GI discomfort (*Johannson G et al. Biochemical and clinical effects of prophylactic treatment of renal calcium stones with magnesium hydroxide.* J. Urol. *124:770-4, 1980*).

See Also:

Hallson PG et al. Magnesium reduces calcium oxalate crystal formation in human whole urine. Clin. Sci. *62:17, 1982*

Johansson G. Magnesium and renal stone disease. Acta Med. Scand. *(suppl.) 661:13-18, 1982*

- with pyridoxine: 10 mg. daily

Supplementation inhibits calcium oxalate stone formation.

Experimental Study: 149 pts. who had had at least 1 stone annually for 5 years (total of 871 stones) were placed on magnesium oxide 300 mg and pyridoxine 10 mg daily. In the next 4 1/2 - 6 years, only 17/149 (11%) developed stones (total of 71 stones). The rate of stone production decreased from an ave. of 1.3 stones per patient per year to 0.10 stones per pt. per yr. during therapy (*Prien EL, Gershoff S. Magnesium oxide-pyridoxine therapy for recurring calcium oxalate urinary calculi. J. Urology 112:509-12, 1974*).

Experimental Study: After 1 year, stone formers (average 1.1 stones per year) receiving 300 mg. MgO and 10 mg. pyridoxine daily had over a 90% reduction in stone formation (less than 0.1 stones per year), an increased capacity to maintain calcium oxalate in solution, a raised citric acid level and a decreased xanthurenic acid level (*Gershoff S, Prien EL. Effect of daily MgO and vitamin B6 administration to patients with recurring calcium oxalate kidney stones. Am. J. Clin. Nutr. 20:393, 1967*).

– –

Glutamic acid:

Note: As oral supplemental glutamic acid is metabolized, it is not yet known how to effectively increase urinary glutamic acid levels.

Low or absent in the urine of many stone formers (*McGeown MG. The urinary excretion of amino acids in calculus patients. Clin. Sci. 18:185, 1959*).

Effective *in vitro* in retarding calcium oxalate precipitation in the urine of stone formers, although this effect may be superfluous when pyridoxine levels are adequate.

In vitro Experimental Study: Urine from stone formers containing no GOT activity was incubated with exogenous GOT which markedly reduced the rate of calcium oxalate precipitation to a level approximating normal (*Azoury R et al. May enzyme activity in urine play a role in kidney stone formation? Urol. Res. 10:185, 1982*).

In vitro Experimental Study: The effects of physiological amounts of L-glutamic acid, alanine and L-aspartic acid on stone formation was assessed using simulated urine as an assay material. Only glutamic acid retarded the rate of crystal formation (*Azoury R et al. Retardation of calcium oxalate precipitation by glutamic-oxaloacetic-transaminase activity. Urol. Res. 10:169, 1982*).

Lysine:

Dietary deficiency will increase urinary calcium.

Animal Experimental Study: *Wolinsky L, Fosmire GJ. Calcium metabolism in aged mice ingesting a lysine-deficient diet. Gerontol. 28:156, 1982*

Potassium citrate: 60 mEq. daily
                           (available by prescription)

Stone formers may have hypocitraturia.

Observational Study: 7/46 pts. had hypocitraturia (*Menon M, Mahle CJ. Urinary citrate excretion in patients with renal calculi. J. Urology 129(6), 1158-60, 1983*).

Observational Study: Stone formers excrete less citric acid than normals (*Gershoff SN. Excretion of urinary metabolites in calcium oxalate urolithiasis: Effect of tryptophan and vitamin B6 administration. Am. J. Clin. Nutr. 8:812, 1960*).

See Also:

Nicar MJ et al. Low urinary citrate excretion in nephrolithiasis. Urology *21:8-14, 1983*

Supplementation may benefit stone formers with hypocitraturia as citrate augments inhibitor activity against calcium oxalate crystallization (*Harvey JA et al. Calcium citrate: Reduced propensity for the crystallization of calcium oxalate in urine resulting from induced hypercalciuria of calcium supplementation.* J. Clin. Endocrinol. Metabol. *61(6):1223-25, 1985*).

Experimental Study: Potassium citrate prophylaxis in hypocitraturic pts. over a 2-year period resulted in an 86% reduction in stone formation rate (*Pak CYC, Fuller C. Idiopathic hypocitraturic calcium-oxalate nephrolithiasis successfully treated with potassium citrate.* Ann. Int. Med. *104:33-37, 1986*).

Experimental Study: During the 3 yrs. prior to treatment, 9 calcium stone-forming pts. with distal renal tubular acidosis formed an ave. of 39.3 stones each. Treatment with oral potassium citrate 60-80 meq daily over a 34 mo. period resulted in complete inhibition of new stone formation in all pts. (*Preminger GM et al. Prevention of recurrent calcium stone formation with potassium citrate therapy in patients with renal tubular acidosis.* J. Urology *134(1):20-23, 1985*).

Experimental Study: Treatment of 89 recurrent calcium stone-forming pts. with potassium citrate 20 mEq 3 times daily over 1-4 yrs. resulted in a decrease in individual stone formation in 97.8% of pts. and remission in 79.8% (*Pak CYC et al. Long term treatment of calcium nephrolithiasis with potassium citrate.* J. Urol. *134(1):11-19, 1985*).

See Also:

Pak CYC et al. Correction of hypocitraturia and prevention of stone formation by combined thiazide and potassium citrate therapy in thiazide-unresponsive hypercalciuria nephrolithiasis. Am. J. Med. *1986*

Editorial: Citrate for calcium nephrolithiasis. Lancet *1:955, 1986*

Supplementation may benefit patients with hyperuricosuria in addition to hypocitraturia.

Experimental Study: 19 hyperuricosuric pts. with recurrent calcium oxalate kidney stones were treated with potassium citrate 60-80 meq daily. Urinary citrate levels, which were initially below normal, increased into the normal range. Stone formation declined from a mean of 1.55 per pt. per yr. to 0.38 per pt. per yr. (mean reduction of about 75%) during a mean observation period of 2.35 years (*Pak CYC, Peterson R. Successful treatment of hyperuricosuric calcium oxalate nephrolithiasis with potassium citrate.* Arch Int. Med. *146:863, 1986*).

- -

OTHER FACTORS:

Rule out cadmium toxicity.

Cadmium exposure has been associated with increased prevalence of urolithiasis.

Observational Study: A gp. of coppersmiths who had been chronically exposed to cadmium was studied over 6 years. The prevalence of urinary tract stones was just under 40% compared to 3.5% in the general population (*Scott R et al. the importance of cadmium as a factor in calcified upper urinary tract stone disease - A prospective 7-year study.* Brit. J. Urol. *54:584, 1982*).

Cadmium causes renal tubular damage which can lead to calcific foci in the kidneys (*Axellson B, Piscator M. Renal change after prolonged exposure to cadmium. Arch. Envir. Health 12:360-72, 1969*).

Stone formers excrete significantly more cadmium than normals (*Elliot JS, Ribeiro ME. the urinary excretion of trace metals in patients with calcium oxalate urinary stone. Invest. Urol. 10:253-55, 1973*).

Cadmium may encourage oxalate crystallization (*Eusebio E, Elliot JS. Effect of trace metals on the crystallisation of calcium oxalate. Invest. Urol. 4:431, 1967*).

LEARNING DISABILITIES

See also: HYPERKINESIS

BASIC DIET:

Avoid <u>refined carbohydrates</u>.

Refined carbohydrates have a much lower zinc to cadmium ratio than whole grains since zinc is more concentrated in the germ and bran while cadmium is most concentrated in the endosperm (*Schoeder HA. Losses of vitamins and trace minerals resulting from processing and preservation of foods. Am. J. Clin. Nutr. 24:562-73, 1971*). Learning disabilities in children whose carbohydrates are mainly derived from refined sources may thus be related to a relatively depressed zinc/cadmium ratio. (*See also: "Heavy Metal Toxicity" below.*)

Observational Study: The relationship between hair cadmium and lead and the refined carbohydrate ratio was investigated in 150 school children. Lead was not significantly correlated with diet, but cadmium showed a strong positive correlation with the proportion of refined carbohydrates in the diet, suggesting that the consumption of refined low-nutrient foods increases the body cadmium burden. In addition, a significant negative relationship between refined low-nutrient food intake and intellectual ability was shown, independent of the effects of cadmium, age, race, sex and socioeconomic status (*Lester ML et al. Refined carbohydrate intake, hair cadmium levels and cognitive functioning in children. J. Nutr. & Behavior 1:3-13, 1982*).

See Also:

> *Von Hilsheimer G. Allergy, Toxins, and the Learning Disabled Child. San Rafael, California, Academic Therapy Publications, 1974*

- -

NUTRIENTS:

Iron:

Deficiency associated with decreased attentiveness, attention, persistence and voluntary activity (*Pollitt E, Leibel R. Iron deficiency anemia and scholastic achievement in young adolescents. J. Pediatrics 88:372-81, 1976; Webb T, Oski F. Iron deficiency anemia and scholastic achievement in young adolescents. J. Pediatrics 82:827-30, 1973*).

Supplementation may be beneficial in cases of iron-deficiency whether or not anemia is present.

Experimental Study: In comparison to controls, Guatemalan infants with iron deficiency with or without anemia tended to score lower on the Bayley Scale of Mental Development, and preschool iron-deficient children with or without anemia were less likely to pay attention to relevant cues in problem solving situations. Iron repletion therapy was likely to result in improvement (*Pollitt E et al. Iron deficiency and behavioral development in infants and preschool children. Am. J. Clin. Nutr. 43(4):555-65, 1986*).

Experimental Placebo-controlled Study: 78 Javan children (average age 10.8) with iron-deficiency anemia were found to have significantly lower scores on a standardized achievement test than matched nonanemic children. They received ferrous sulphate 10 mg/kg daily for 5 mo. or placebo. Only supplemented children significantly improved their scores on the achievement test. (*Pollitt E. Cognitive effects of iron deficiency anaemia. Letter to the Editor. Lancet 1:158, 1985*).

Experimental Placebo-controlled Study: 18/28 Egyptian children with iron-deficiency anemia received 50 mg ferrous sulphate daily for 4 months while the rest received placebos. Before and after treatment, all children took Form F of the Matching Familiar Figure Test to assess efficiency and impulsivity. The anemic children's speed and accuracy initially was lower than that of the non-anemic children but improved after treatment for those treated with iron but not for those treated with placebo (*Pollitt - ibid*).

Selenium:

Excessive intake may be harmful.

Observational Study: In a study of 120 children drawn from a general school population, increasing hair selenium correlated significantly with increased scores on the Walker Problem Behavior Identification Checklist (WPBIC) scales measuring acting out, withdrawal, and total scale score (*Marlowe M et al. Hair selenium levels and children's classroom behavior. J. Orthomol. Med. 1(2):91-96, 1986*).

Observational Study: In a study of 400 public school children, learning disabled children were found to have significantly higher hair selenium than normal controls, and learning disabled children in special classes had significantly higher hair selenium than learning disabled children who remained in the regular classroom (*Ely DL et al. Aerometric and hair trace metal content in learning disabled. Environ. Res. 25:325-39, 1981*).

Zinc:

(*See also "Heavy Metal Toxicity" below.*)

Deficiency may be associated with learning disabilities due to behavioral disturbances.

Review Article: Children with zinc deficiencies are irritable, tearful and sullen. They are not soothed by close body contact and resent disturbances. Photophobia is present and gaze aversion is common (*Moynahan EJ. Zinc deficiency and disturbances of mood and visual behavior. Lancet 1:91, 1976*).

Cadmium, which may be elevated in LD children, displaces zinc in biochemical reactions to slow or halt processes normally catalyzed by zinc (*Venugopal B, Luckey TD. Metal Toxicity in Mammals. Vol. 2. New York, Plenum Press, 1980*), thus adequate zinc nutriture may protect against the adverse effects of cadmium.

Observational Study: School children ages 5-16 were evaluated using measurements of cognition as well as measurements of the body burden of pollutants and nutrients. Hair was used to assess zinc nutrient status. Results suggested that the degree of negative correlation of cadmium to cognitive performance was dependent upon hair zinc concentration even after the relation of other significant independent variables (age, sex, race and socioeconomic status) were partialled out (*Lester ML et al. Protective effects of calcium and zinc against heavy metal impairment of cognitive function - summarized in Thatcher RW, Lester ML. Nutrition, environmental toxins and computerized EEG: A mini-max approach to learning disabilities. J. Learning Disabilities 18(5):287-97, 1985*).

COMBINED DIETARY INTERVENTIONS:

Experimental Controlled Study: 16 children with behavioral and learning problems were placed on a dietary program in which toxic metals, refined foods, sugars, fats and salt were reduced, relevant vitamins and minerals supplemented, and fiber, wholegrains, complex carbohydrates and unprocessed foods increased according to their individual needs. Significant improvements in intelligence, behavior and learning were found compared to 16 matched controls who received only a multivitamin capsule in addition to normal diets over the 22 week trial period. In addition, among the experimental gp., cadmium levels fell by 28% and lead by 49% (*Colgan M, Colgan L. Do nutrient supplements and dietary changes affect learning and emotional reactions of children with learning difficulties?: A controlled series of 16 cases. <u>Nutrition and Health</u> 3:69-77, 1984*).

Experimental Controlled Study: Children with learning problems were supplemented with vitamins and minerals and placed on a special diet which eliminated refined sugars and emphasized whole grains, unprocessed, chemically free foods, and fresh or frozen but not canned vegetables. Every child showed evidence of improved school behavior and performance and parents noted relief from sinus problems, asthma, indigestion,"nerves" and skin problems. Comparison of baseline vs. third-year data of the treatment and control gps. for the Dolch Word List, Peabody Picture Vocabulary Test and reading and math achievement scores suggested greater improvement for the experimental subjects than for the controls. While baseline hair analyses showed 25% to be in the medium high range for lead, by the end of the first yr. none showed such an elevation. 45% were initially in the middle or high cadmium range but, but the end of the yr., 30% were in the middle range and 70% were in the low range. 55% were in the middle range for arsenic at the start, while all were in the low range by the end of the year (*Oliver B. The children who should have been passing but didn't. <u>J. Orthomol. Psychiat.</u> 12(3):235-41, 1983*).

Experimental Controlled Study: 24/33 learning disabled children received vitamin C 3 gm, niacinamide 3 gm, pantothenic acid 250 mg, pyridoxine 250 mg and a high-protein, low carbohydrate diet while the rest served as controls with no supplementation or dietary changes. Standardized testing over 1.1 yrs. revealed that while the experimental gp. did not progress faster in reading or spelling, they did improve faster in the abilities measured by the Illinois Test of Psycholinguistic Ability (ITPA). They also showed a greater reduction in general symptoms and soft neurological signs than controls (*Thiessen I, Mills L. The use of megavitamin treatment in children with learning disabilities. <u>J. Orthomol. Psychiat</u> 4(4):288-96, 1975*).

Case Report: A girl diagnosed as having minimal brain dysfunction had learning problems and displayed antagonism, uncooperativeness, and unprovoked raging temper tantrums. At 13 she was placed on a high-protein, sugar-free diet with vitamin C, nicotinamide and pyridoxine. Tantrums ceased after a few days but recurred after candy. Because she was unusually alert and cooperative after eating oysters (which have a high zinc content), a trial of zinc supplementation was begun. After chelated zinc 80 mg in the morning and 200 mg in the afternoon was added, there was dramatic behavioral improvement within 24 hours. Discontinuation of zinc supplements was followed by tantrums (*Kronick D. A case history: Sugar, fried oysters, and zinc. <u>Academ. Therap.</u> 11:119, 1975*).

OTHER FACTORS:

Rule out <u>food and chemical sensitivities</u>.

Negative Observational Study: 2343 children were surveyed as to the known presence of "allergies" and learning disabilities. Allergic children were found to function similarly to their peers and LD subjects were not reported to have been diagnosed as allergic more often or to have more severe symptoms than non-LD subjects (*McLoughlin JA et al. Allergies and learning disabilities. <u>Learning Disability Quarterly</u> 8:255-60, 1985*).

Note: The criteria for "allergy" were not defined and no evaluation for masked food sensitivities was performed.

Review Article: Food allergens enter the circulation and travel to any body site where they probably attach themselves by means of specific antibodies that are acting as receptors. The resulting immunologic reactions produce symptoms that are characteristic of each body site. Such symptoms could be clues to the diagnosis of the child who is dull, listless, confused, or unable to grasp simple concepts, or the child who is hyperactive, irritable, aggressive, and hostile (*Mayron LW. Allergy, learning, and behavior problems. J. Learning Disabilities 12(1):32-41, 1979*).

Rule out heavy metal toxicity.

Observational Study: Hair mineral analysis of 26 learning disabled students and 24 controls was performed to investigate the relationship between learning disabilities and hair mineral levels. Lead was significantly higher in the learning disabled gp. and there were also significant differences in the levels of 10 other minerals. Discriminant function analysis revealed that by using lead, calcium, silicon, aluminum, vanadium, mercury and zinc, subjects could be classified as normal controls or learning disabled with 91.7% and 76.1% accuracy, respectively (*Marlowe M et al. Hair mineral content as a predictor of learning disabilities. J. Learning Disabilities 17(7):418-21, 1984*).

Review Article: The results of 10 studies of toxic mineral levels in the hair suggest a correlation between learning disabilities and elevated levels of cadmium, lead, copper, and manganese (*Rimland B. Hair mineral analysis and behavior: An analysis of 51 studies. J. Learning Disabil. 16(5):279-85, 1983*).

Observational Study: Hair samples from 31 3rd and 4th grade learning disabled and 22 normal children were analyzed for content of 14 elements. The learning disabled children showed significantly higher levels of cadmium, manganese and lead compared to controls and significantly lower levels of chromium and lithium. A discriminant function was completed using cadmium, cobalt, manganese and chromium which separated the gps. with 98% accuracy. (*Pihl RO, Parkes M. Hair element content in learning disabled children. Science 198:204-6, 1977*).

Evidence of aluminum toxicity:

Observational Study: 28 children suffering from learning disorders or hyperactivity were found to have elevated serum aluminum levels (*Howard JMH. Clinical import of small increases in serum aluminum. Clin. Chem. 30(10):1722-3, 1984*).

Evidence of cadmium and lead toxicity:

Observational Study: 150 school children were divided into 4 gps. based upon WISC-R and WRAT test scores into gifted, normal, low achievers and very low achievers. There were significant differences between gps. in hair lead concentration and there was a significant linear trend from the gifted gp. to the very low achievers (i.e. the worse their test performance, the higher the lead level). In addition, polynomial regression analysis of either hair lead or cadmium concentrations as the independent variables and WISC-R verbal and performance I.Q. as the dependent variables showed a continuous negative relationship between intelligence measures and both independent variables. Further analysis suggested that lead independently accounted for a significant amount of the performance but not verbal I.Q. variance, while the reverse was true for cadmium (*Thatcher RW, Lester ML. Nutrition, Environmental toxins and computerized EEG: A Mini-max approach to learning disabilities. J. Learning Disabilities 18(5):287-97, 1985*).

Negative Observational Study: Moderate blood lead levels showed no evidence of an adverse effect on cognitive measures, reading tests or teacher behavior ratings for 63 inner city children (*Ernhart CB, et al. Subclinical lead level and developmental deficit: Re-analysis of data. J. Learning Disabilities 18(8): 475-9, 1985*).

Note: Blood mineral levels reflect primarily current exposure while hair mineral levels reflect exposure over several months and thus the results may differ.

See Also:

Thatcher RW et al. Effects of low levels of cadmium and lead on cognitive functioning in children. Arch. Env. Health 37:159, 1982

Evidence of <u>manganese</u> toxicity:

Three separate studies have shown an association between high hair manganese and learning disabilities in children. It is possible that higher manganese levels cause decreased dopamine turnover leading to increased locomotor activity (<u>*Int. Clin. Nutr. Rev.*</u> *vol. 4, no. 2, April, 1984*).

Observational Study: 16 learning disabled children were found to have a significantly higher hair manganese level than 44 normal children. Since infant formulas contain 3 to 100 times the manganese content of breast milk, the authors postulate that these formulas may contribute to an overload of manganese (*Collipp PJ et al. Manganese in infant formulas and learning disability.* <u>*Ann. Nutr. Metab.*</u> *27:488-94, 1983*).

LUPUS

See Also: AUTO-IMMUNE DISORDERS (GENERAL)

BASIC DIET:

Low calorie, low fat diet.

Review Article: Studies of diet in the mouse model of SLE have established the beneficial effects of a low calorie, low fat diet in these animals and suggest that a similar diet would be of benefit to humans (*Corman LC. The role of diet in animal models of systemic lupus erythematosus: Possible implications for human lupus. Semin. Arthritis Rheum. 15(1):61-69, 1985*).

Limit beef and dairy products.

Review Article: Studies of diet in the mouse model of SLE have established the beneficial effects of limiting proteins with a high content of phenylalanine and tyrosine, such as beef and dairy products, and suggest that a similar diet would be of benefit to humans (*Corman LC. The role of diet in animal models of systemic lupus erythematosus: Possible implications for human lupus. Semin. Arthritis Rheum. 15(1):61-69, 1985*).

- -

NUTRIENTS:

Beta Carotene:

Supplementation may be beneficial (discoid lupus).

Case Reports: 3 pts. with treatment-resistent chronic discoid lupus are described whose lesions flared with sun exposure. Beta-carotene 50 mg 3 times daily resulted in clearing of all lesions starting in 1 week (*Newbold PCH. Beta-carotene in the treatment of discoid lupus erythematosus. Brit. J. Dermatol. 95:100-101, 1976*).

Pantothenic Acid: example: calcium pantothenate 6-10 gm daily initially followed by 2-4 gm daily for "some months"

Supplementation may be beneficial.

Negative Experimental Study: 35 pts. with subacute or chronic lupus were unchanged or worse following supplementation with 2-600 mg daily of calcium pantothenate for 2-14 wks., as were 9 pts. supplemented with panthenol 1-4 mg daily for 4-16 wks. No other treatment was given concomitantly (*Cochrane T, Leslie G. The treatment of lupus erythematosus with calcium pantothenate and panthenol. J. Invest. Dermat. 18:365-67, 1952*).

Experimental Study: 30/37 pts. with subacute or chronic discoid lupus improved with massive panthenol therapy (*Goldman L. Preliminary and short report: Intensive panthenol therapy for lupus erythematosus. J. Invest. Dermat. 15:291, 1950*).

Experimental Study: Pts. with subacute and chronic discoid lupus showed satisfactory improvement with massive calcium pantothenate therapy (*Goldman L. Treatment of subacute and chronic discoid lupus erythematosus with intensive calcium pantothenate therapy. J. Invest. Dermat. 11:95, 1948*).

Vitamin A:

WARNING: Excessive tissue levels may be harmful.

Theoretical Discussion: Several lines of indirect evidence suggest that SLE could reflect a toxicity reaction to excessive tissue levels of vitamin A and that the remission often associated with long-term hemodialysis in pts. with end-stage renal disease may be due to a gradual reduction in vitamin A levels at the sites of SLE activity (*Mawson AR. Systemic lupus erythematosus, renal disease, hemodialysis and vitamin A. Med. Hypotheses 18(4):387-98, 1985*).

Deficiency may accelerate the disease process.

Animal Experimental Study: Mice susceptible to a lupus-like disease were fed a vitamin-A deficient diet or a normal control diet. The vitamin-A deficient animals were found to manifest more severe hyper-gammaglobulinemia and an earlier onset of both NTA and IgM anti-erythrocyte antibodies (*Gershwin ME et al. Nutritional factors and autoimmunity. IV. Dietary vitamin A deprivation induces a selective increase in IgM autoantibodies and hypergammaglobulinemia in New Zealand Black mice. J. Immunology 133(1):222-26, 1984*).

Vitamin B$_{12}$: 1000 mcg. I.M. twice weekly

IM supplementation may be beneficial.

Experimental Study: After 6 wks. of IM supplementation with B$_{12}$, 3/3 patients with lupus erythematosus who had failed to respond to oral and I.M. vitamin E had complete clearing of the lesions (*Block MT. Vitamin E in the treatment of diseases of the skin. Clin. Med. January 1953, pp. 31-34*).

Vitamin E: 1200 - 1600 I.U. daily
         (may also be applied locally to skin lesions)
         (effect enhanced by 50 mcg. selenium daily)

Supplementation may be beneficial.

Experimental Study (discoid lupus): 4 pts. receiving vitamin E 900-1600 IU daily of vitamin E showed complete or almost complete clearing, while 2 pts. receiving 300 IU daily had no benefit (*Ayres S, Mihan R. Is vitamin E involved in the autoimmune mechanism? Cutis 21:321-25, 1978*).

Experimental Study (lupus erythematosus): 12 pts. were treated with 100-150 mg. orally 3 times daily after meals plus 150 mg. I.M. in an aqueous solution 2-3 times weekly. 8 had excellent results, 1 had good results and 3 had poor results (*Block MT. Vitamin E in the treatment of diseases of the skin. Clin. Med. January 1953, pp. 31-34*).

See Also:

Ayres S, Mihan R. Lupus erythematosus and vitamin E: An effective and non-toxic therapy. Cutis 23:49-54, 1979

Burgess JF, Pritchard JE. Tocopherol (vitamin E) treatment of lupus erythematosus: Preliminary report. Arch. Dermatol. Syphilol. 57:953, 1948

- and <u>Pantothenic Acid</u>:

Supplementation may be beneficial.

> **Experimental Study:** 67 pts. with biopsy-confirmed LE were treated with pantothenic acid (ex. calcium pantothenate) 10-15 gm daily and vitamin E 1-2000 mg daily. All pts. showed marked improvement. Pts. with chronic discoid lupus began to show objective improvement in 4-6 months. Pts. with disseminated discoid lupus improved in 2 mo., while pts. in the subacute disseminated gp. improved in 1 month. The 3 pts. in the acute disseminated gp. also received steroid hormones initially and subsequently were maintained on the supplements without relapse for 7-19 months. The only side effects were transient nausea and gastric distress from the pantothenate (*Welsh AL. Lupus erythematosus: Treatment by combined use of massive amounts of pantothenic acid and vitamin E. <u>Arch. Derm. Syph.</u> 70:181-98, 1954*).

- and <u>Selenium</u>:

Supplementation may be beneficial in <u>SLE</u>.

> **Experimental Study:** 1 pt. with SLE was found to have a low level of of glutathione peroxidase compared to normal controls, while 5 pts. with discoid lupus had levels similar to the controls. The SLE pt. was treated with tablets containing 10 mg tocopheryl succinate and 0.2 mg selenium as Na_2SeO_3. Glutathione peroxidase levels increased slowly within 6-8 wks. and the clinical effect was encouraging (*Juhlin L et al. Blood glutathione-peroxidase levels in skin diseases: Effect of selenium and vitamin E treatment. <u>Acta Derm. Venereal. (Stockh.)</u> 62(3):211-14, 1982*).

- -

Omega-3 Fatty Acids:

Supplementation may be beneficial.

> **Animal Experimental Study:** The effect of fish oil on autoimmune lupus in mice showed that the substance "had the most striking protective effect seen thus far in any animal model of inflammatory disease" (*Robinson DR - reported in <u>Med. World News</u> July 14, 1986; Robinson DR et al. The protective effect of dietary fish oil on murine lupus. <u>Prostaglandins</u> 30(1):51-75, 1985*).

> **Animal Experimental Study:** Dietary supplementation of fish oil suppressed autoimmune lupus in mice, both delaying the onset of renal disease and prolonging survival (*Kelley VE et al. A fish oil diet rich in eicosapentaenoic acid reduces cyclooxygenase metabolites, and suppresses lupus in MRL-lpr mice. <u>J. Immunol.</u> 134(3):1914-19, 1985*).

See Also:

> *Prickett JD et al. A diet enriched with eicosapentaenoic acid suppress autoimmune nephritis in female (NZB x NZW) F1 mice. <u>Trans. Assoc. Am. Physicians</u> 95:145-54, 1982*

> *Note: An <u>essential fatty acid-deficient</u> diet has also been found beneficial for NZB/NZW F1 mice (Hurd ER, Gilliam JN. Beneficial effect of an essential fatty deficient diet in NZB/NZW F1 mice. <u>J. Invest. Dermatol.</u> 77(5):381-84, 1981*).

Omega-6 Fatty Acids:

Precursors of prostaglandin E_1.

Supplementation may be beneficial.

Animal Experimental Study: PGE$_1$ was successfully used to control the auto-immune inflammatory disease, including kidney damage, which spontaneously develops in New Zealand black/white mice - believed to be an excellent model of human systemic lupus erythematosus (*Zurier RB et al. Prostaglandin E$_1$ treatment of NZB/W mice, I. Arth. Rheum. 20:723-8, 1977; Krakauer K et al. Prostaglandin E$_1$ treatment of NZB/W mice, III. Immunol. Immunopathol. 11:256, 1978*).

Note: An essential fatty acid-deficient diet has also been found beneficial for NZB/NZW F1 mice (Hurd ER, Gilliam JN. Beneficial effect of an essential fatty deficient diet in NZB/NZW F1 mice. J. Invest. Dermatol. 77(5):381-84, 1981).

L-Tryptophan:

WARNING: Supplementation may be harmful.

Patients are said to have decreased serotonin levels, perhaps due to deficient conversion of tryptophan to serotonin. The tryptophan breakdown products may lead to auto-antibody production (*McCormick JP et al. Characterization of a cell-lethal product from the photooxidation of tryptophan: Hydrogen peroxide. Science 191:468-9, 1976*).

Review Article: An abnormal tryptophan metabolism is present with high excretion particularly of kynurenines and xanthurenic acid (*Cardin de'Stefani E, Costa C. [Changes in the metabolism of tryptophan in erythematosus.] Boll. Soc. Ital. Biol. Sper. 60(8):1535-40, 1984*).

Animal Experimental Study: A tryptophan deficient diet increased survival of animals with lupus (*Dubois. Lupus Erythematosus 2nd. edition, p. 121*).

- -

Alfalfa:

WARNING: May produce a lupus-like syndrome or aggravate SLE.

Animal Experimental Study: Hematologic and serologic abnormalities similar to those observed in human systemic lupus erythematosus developed in monkeys fed alfalfa sprouts. L-canavanine sulfate, a constituent, was incorporated into the diet and reactivated the syndrome (*Malonow MR et al. Systemic lupus erythematosus-like syndrome in monkeys fed alfalfa sprouts: Role of a nonprotein amino acid. Science 216:415-17, 1982*).

See Also:

Case Report: *Roberts JL, Hayashi JA. Exacerbation of SLE associated with alfalfa ingestion. Letter to the Editor. New Engl. J. Med. 308(22):1361, 1983*

- -

OTHER FACTORS:

Rule out food and chemical sensitivities.

Food allergies and other allergies may be more common in lupus pts. than in normals (*Carr RI et al. Antibodies to bovine gamma globulin (BCG) and the occurrence of a BCG-like substance in systemic lupus erythematosus sera. J. Allergy Clin. Immunol. 50(1):18-30, 1972*).

Observational Study: The frequency of a history of clinical manifestations of urticaria, pharyngitis, conjunctivitis and food allergy was significantly increased in 63 SLE pts. compared to pts. with other autoimmune diseases and normals, and SLE pts. had the highest incidence of different types of clinical manifestations per individual (*Diumenjo MS et al. [Allergic manifestations of systemic lupus erythematosus.] Allergol. Immunopathol. (Madr.) 13(4):323-26, 1985*).

Food and chemical exposures may influence disease activity in sensitive patients.

Experimental Study: 4 pts. with SLE developed remissions following food eliminations and nutritional supplementation, while another 70 pts. with lupus and lupus-like syndromes showed a "similar trend" (*Cooke HM, Reading CM. Dietary intervention in systemic lupus erythematosus: 4 cases of clinical remission and reversal of abnormal pathology. Int. Clin. Nutr. Rev. 5(4):166-76, 1985*).

Case Report: 36 year-old female developed episodic vomiting at age 5 and migraine at age 11. At age 16 she developed a polyarthritis and a diagnosis of SLE was made. Her disease progressed over the years with further involvement of the GI, GU, respiratory and vascular symptoms. Spontaneous bruising and petechiae occurred, together with peripheral edema. Antinuclear antibodies and LE preparations were positive repeatedly and she was placed on cortisone and cytotoxic drugs. Following admission to an environmental control unit, all meds were stopped. Joint stiffness and swelling gradually disappeared and her sed rate fell from 63 to 15 mm in 1 week, the lowest value in years. Food and chemical challenges precipitated a return of her symptoms (*Rea WJ, Brown OD. Mechanisms of environmental vascular triggering. Clin. Ecology 3(3):122-8, 1985*).

Rule out <u>hydrochloric acid deficiency</u>.

If deficient, supplementation may be beneficial.

Experimental Study: Of 9 pts. with lupus erythematosus, none had normal HCl levels and 2 had no detectable HCl. Signs of vitamin B complex deficiency seemed to correlate to the extent of the HCl deficiency and improvement followed supplementation with HCl and vitamin B complex (*Allison JR. The relation of hydrochloric acid and vitamin B complex deficiency in certain skin diseases. Southern Med. J. 38:235-241, 1945*).

MENOPAUSAL SYMPTOMS

NUTRIENTS:

<u>Bioflavonoids:</u>

Supplementation may be effective.

Experimental Study: Bioflavonoids (hesperiden and hesperiden methyl chalcone - citrus-derived) were much more effective than sub-therapeutic doses of estrogen and 2 other treatments which have been suggested (*Smith CJ. Non-hormonal control of vaso-motor flushing in menopausal patients. Chicago Med. March 7, 1964*).

<u>Vitamin E:</u>   results in 2 wks. - 3 mo.

Supplementation may be effective.

Experimental Study: Vitamin E 100 mg 3 times daily cured menopausal symptoms in 3/35 pts. and ameliorated symptoms in 16/35 within 3 months (*Gozan HA. The use of vitamin E in treatment of the menopause. N.Y. State Med. J. May 15, 1952, pp. 1289-91*).

Experimental Study: In a preliminary study, 37/59 pts. with hot flashes and sweats, 16/28 with back-aches and muscle pains, and 16/34 with menorrhagia improved on 10-25 mg vitamin E (Ephynal Acetate) daily. 79 additional pts. received either 50 or 100 mg vitamin E daily. At least 75% of pts. with hot flashes and sweats improved and 47-86% were relieved of backaches, jointaches and headaches within 4 weeks. 11/12 pts. with dizziness, 9/11 with palpitations, and 3/4 with dyspnea were relieved within 2 weeks. 43-70% of pts. with fatigue and 41-67% of pts. with nervousness were relieved within 8 weeks (*Kavinoky NR. Vitamin E and the control of climacteric symptoms. Ann. West. Med. & Surg. 4(1):27-32, 1950*).

Experimental Single-blind Study: 66 pts. with vasomotor symptoms were given 20-100 mg (ave. 30 mg) vitamin E in divided doses daily for 10 days-7 mo (ave. 31 days). 31 had good to excellent results and 16/66 had fair results, with prompt recurrence of symptoms after discontinuation of the vitamin. Placebo was substituted in 17 pts. followed by recurrence of symptoms which remitted again when vitamin E was resumed (*Finkler RS. The effect of vitamin E in the menopause. J. Clin. Endocrin. Metabol. 9:89-94, 1949*).

Experimental Study: 25 women with intractable hot flashes and a history of cancer which made estrogen supplementation inappropriate received 10-30 mg daily for 1-6 weeks. All responded with either complete relief or marked improvement of hot flashes and they reported positive mood chan-ges. There were no untoward side effects (*Christy CJ. Vitamin E in menopause. Am. J. Obstet. & Gyn. 50:84, 1945*).

See Also:

Blatt MHG et al. Vitamin E and climacteric syndrome: Failure of effective control as measured by menopausal index. Arch. Int. Med. 91:792, 1953

- -

<u>L-Tryptophan</u>:

Deficiency may be associated with menopausal depression.

Observational Study: A positive correlation was found between low blood levels of tryptophan and estrogen in depressed women who had recently gone through menopause (*Editorial: Tryptophan and depression.* <u>Brit. Med. J.</u> *1:242-3, 1976*).

MENORRHAGIA

NUTRIENTS:

<u>Vitamin A</u>:   25,000 I.U. twice daily for 15 days

If deficient, supplementation may be beneficial.

> **Experimental and Observational Study:** 71 women with menorrhagia were found to have significantly lower serum vitamin A levels than healthy controls. 40 of these women were treated with vitamin A 25,000 IU twice daily for 15 days. Menstruation returned to normal in 57.5% and diminished in an additional 35% (*Lithgow DM, Politzer WM. Vitamin A in the treatment of menorrhagia.* <u>*S. Afr. Med. J.*</u> *51:191-3, 1977*).

<u>Bioflavonoids</u> plus
<u>Vitamin C</u>:   200 mg 3 times daily

Supplementation may be beneficial.

> **Experimental Study:** Supplementation reduced symptoms in 14/16 pts. Of the 2 failing to respond, 1 had endometriosis and the other had metrorrhagia (*Cohen JD, Rubin, HW. Functional menorrhagia: Treatment with bioflavonoids and vitamin C.* <u>*Curr. Ther. Res.*</u> *2:539, 1960*).

- -

<u>Iron</u>:   100 mg daily

Patients with menorrhagia may be iron-deficient despite the absence of iron-deficiency anemia.

> **Observational Study:** Serum ferritin of menorrhagic pts. was significantly lower than that of controls despite the lack of significant differences in hemoglobin concentration, mean corpuscular volume and mean corpuscular hemoglobin (*Lewis GJ. Do women with menorrhagia need iron?* <u>*Brit. Med. J.*</u> *284:1158, 1982*).

Chronic iron deficiency can cause menorrhagia.

> **Experimental Studies:**
> 1. 74/83 pts. (in whom organic pathology had been excluded) responded to iron supplementation.
> 2. Pts. who failed to respond to iron had a high rate of organic pathology (fibroids, polyps,adenomyosis, etc.).
> 3. 44/57 responding pts. had an associated rise in serum iron.
> 4. When initial iron levels were high, there was a decreased response to supplementation.
> 5. Menorrhagia correlated with depleted bone marrow iron stores irrespective of serum iron level.
> 6. In a double-blind study, 75% of those on iron improved compared to 32.5% on placebo, a significant difference.
> (*Taymor ML et al. The etiological role of chronic iron deficiency in production of menorrhagia.* <u>*JAMA*</u> *187:323-27, 1964*)

See Also:

Samuels AJ.   Studies in patients with functional menorrhagia: The antihemorrhagic effect of the adequate repletion of iron.   Israel J. Med. Sci. 1:851, 1965

Supplementation with iron 100 mg daily will prevent iron deficiency.

Experimental Study: 15 pts. received iron 100 mg daily in connection with the menstrual period. Mean menstrual blood loss was 117 ml (range 21-117 ml), corresponding to 53 mg of iron (range 21-117 mg).   The mean absorption was 81 mg (range 49-145 mg), with 14/15 absorbing more iron than was lost by menstrual bleeding (*Arvidsson B et al.   Iron prophylaxis in menorrhagia.   Acta Obstet. Gynecol. Scand. 60:157-60, 1981*).

MITRAL VALVE PROLAPSE

NUTRIENTS:

Magnesium:

May be deficient.

Observational Study: 40 pts. were investigated and hypomagnesemia was a statistically significant finding, suggesting that it has an important role in causing the rhythm and neuropsychic disturbances (*Zeana C et al. Considerations on the pathogenesis of mitral valve prolapse. Med. Interne 23(3):165-70, 1985*).

Observational Study: Compared to 36 matched controls, 42 MVP pts. had significantly lower mean RBC Mg (p less than 0.01), but there were no significant differences in serum Mg or serum ionized calcium (*Galland L. Magnesium deficiency in mitral valve prolapse, in Halpern and Durlach, Eds. Magnesium Deficiency. First European Congress on Magnesium. Karger, Basel, 1985*).

Observational Study: Out of a gp. of 170 pts. evaluated for the investigation of neuromuscular hyperexcitability, 26% of 143 pts. with latent tetany on the basis of Chvostek's sign, EEG or EMG findings were found to have MVP, compared to none of 27 pts. without latent tetany. Although there were no significant differences in plasma and RBC Mg levels between the non-tetanic nervous pts., the tetanic pts. and the MVP pts., these values were all significantly lower than normal reference values (p less than 0.001) (*Durlach J et al. Latent tetany and mitral valve prolapse due to chronic primary magnesium deficit, in Halpern and Durlach, Eds. Magnesium Deficiency. First European Congress on Magnesium. Karger, Basel, 1985*).

Observational Study: EMG in 64/75 MVP pts. showed changes suggestive of spasmophilia with symptoms typical of this condition. The specific clinical signs of spasmophilia were elicited with a positive Chvostek sign in 20/30 (73.3%). Radiological, echo-cardiographical and hemodynamic studies underlined the hyperkinetic state of the left ventricle. There was a high incidence of low RBC magnesium levels. It is noted that chest pain suggestive of angina pectoris, mitral valve prolapse and spasmophilia are frequently associated (*G:erard R et al. [Mitral valve prolapse and spasmophila in the adult.] Arch. Mal Coeur 72(7);715-20, 1979*).

See Also:

Cohen L et al. Idiopathic magnesium deficiency in mitral valve prolapse. Am. J. Cardiol. 57(6):486-87, 1986

Supplementation may be beneficial.

Experimental Study: 12 pts. with MVP, ventricular hyperkinesia (LVH) and latent tetany received magnesium salts (pyrrolidone carboxylate 4.5 gm/day, lactate 3 gm/day) either alone or with a beta-blocker for a mean of 36.5 mo. (range 12-72 mo.). Following treatment, MVP and LVH were still present in 50%. Mean RBC magnesium was below normal prior to therapy and normal after therapy but no relationship was found between the increase in RBC magnesium and the disappearance or persistence of MVP and LVH (*Frances Y et al. Long-term follow-up of mitral valve prolapse and latent tetany. Preliminary data. Magnesium 5(3-4):175-81, 1986*).

Review Article: To the list of signs of latent tetany due to magnesium deficit, MVP should be added as an irreversible neuromuscular sign. When MVP is found, it should be described as a common local sign of tetany which will help determine treatment in pts. with dyskinetic but normal, unthickened valves and not those associated with heart disease. Mg therapy is the essential specific element of treatment. Beta-blockers or phenytoin are suggested as first time treatment. The effects of Mg therapy on the symptoms of MVP are even more dramatic when the signs of latent tetany have been controlled. Early control of tetany-producing magnesium deficit ensures the prevention of MVP. After at least 1 yr. of Mg treatment, the symptoms may be partially or even totally reversed in about 1/3 of cases (*Durlach J et al. Latent tetany and mitral valve prolapse due to chronic primary magnesium deficit, in Halpern and Durlach, Eds. Magnesium Deficiency. First European Congress on Magnesium. Karger, Basel, 1985*).

Experimental Blinded Study: 35 pts. with symptomatic MVP and latent tetany attributed to a primary Mg deficit received magnesium lactate 3 gms daily. 24 received magnesium for 16 wks., while 11 received placebo for 8 wks. followed by magnesium for 8 wks. Symptoms which improved during magnesium supplementation included palpitations, atypical chest pain, peripheral vascular spasms, psychological symptoms and muscle cramps. Trousseau's sign disappeared in the 10 cases in whom it was positive. No improvement occurred during placebo administration, but improvement did occur when pts. on placebo were switched to magnesium. Of those treated for 16 wks. with magnesium, 29.2% became asymptomatic after 4-12 wks., 45.8% had persistence of only 1-2 psychic symptoms (e.g. anxiety, depressive tendency), and the remaining 25% showed improvement, but it was less marked. Auscultatory signs of MVP were unchanged. Serum Mg levels tended to rise during supplementation (*Fernandes JS et al. Therapeutic effect of a magnesium salt in patients suffering from mitral valvular prolapse and latent tetany. Magnesium 4:283, 1985*).

MULTIPLE SCLEROSIS

See Also: AUTO-IMMUNE DISORDERS (GENERAL)

BASIC DIET:

Low fat diet.

A high fat diet impairs the conversion of linoleic acid to prostaglandin E_1 (PGE$_1$) (*Brenner RR. The oxidative desaturation of unsaturated fatty acids in animals. Mol. Cell. Biochem. 3:41-52, 1974*). PGE$_1$ levels may have a relationship to disease activity (*see "Omega-6 Fatty Acids" below*).

Experimental Study: 146 pts. were placed on a low fat diet and followed up to an average of 17 years. The course of the disease was less rapidly progressive than in untreated cases. If treated before significant disability developed, a high percentage of cases remained unchanged for up to 20 years. When treated later, the disease was slowly progressive. Pts. consuming the least fat and the largest amount of fluid (mono- and polyunsaturated) oils deteriorated the least (*Swank RL. Multiple Sclerosis: Twenty years on low fat diet. Arch. Neurol. 23:460-74, 1970*).

See Also:

Swank RL. The Multiple Sclerosis Diet Book. New York, Doubleday, 1977

- -

NUTRIENTS:

Pyridoxine:

Deficiency may predispose to MS.

Theoretical Discussion: Carbon monoxide pollution of the air is the one environmental factor present only in the localities where MS is common. Of 21,000 non-fatal cases of CM poisoning, a number developed a demyelinating condition. Similarly, animals exposed to CM develop CNS degeneration. It has been shown that CM exposure increases the need for pyridoxine, suggesting that a relative B$_6$ deficiency may cause MS in susceptible persons (*Mitchell DA, Schandl EK. Am. J. Clin. Nutr. August, 1973*).

Thiamine:

Supplementation by injection may be beneficial.

Case Reports: Intraspinal injections led to dramatic, though transient, improvements (*Stern EI. The intraspinal injection of vitamin B$_1$ for the relief of intractable pain, and for inflammatory and degenerative diseases of the central nervous system. Am. J. Surg. 34:495, 1938*).

- with Niacin:

> **Case Reports:** Pts. benefited from IV injections containing nicotinic acid 100 mg and thiamine 60 mg in each 10 cc solution (*Moore MT. Treatment of multiple sclerosis with nicotinic acid and vitamin B_1. Arch. Int. Med. 65:18, 1940*).

Calcium and
Vitamin D:

Deficiency during puberty has been theorized to predispose to MS. If so, supplementation during puberty may be preventative.

> **Theoretical Discussion:** Based on epidemiologic, biochemical and genetic evidence, it is hypothesized that demyelination in MS results from a breakdown due to abnormal lipid composition and structure produced during the period of brain development. Altered lipid concentrations and fatty acid profiles result from genetic deficiencies in enzymes that govern myelin synthesis and membrane asssembly which may occur because of inadequate supplies of vitamin D and calcium at times of rapid myelination and growth, especially adolescence. If this theory is correct, it may be possible to suppress the disease by dietary supplementation with vitamin D and calcium during puberty (*Goldberg P. Multiple sclerosis: Vitamin D and calcium as environmental determinants of prevalence. Intern. J. Environ. Stud. 6:19-27 & 121-29, 1974*).

- -

Essential Fatty Acids:

Epidemiologic studies have shown a negative correlation between the prevalence of the disease and the intake of polyunsaturated fatty acids (*Alter M et al. Arch. Neurol. 31:267, 1970*).

Polyunsaturates may be deficient in the brain, serum and RBC of MS pts. (*Gul S et al. J. Neurol. Neurosurg. Psychiat 33:506, 1970; Baker RWR et al. J. Neurol. Neurosurg. Psychiat. 33:506, 1970; Gerstl B et al. Brain 84:310, 1961*).

- Omega-3 Fatty Acids:

> Example: "MaxEPA": 3 capsules three times daily

> **Experimental Study** (*study design only*): *French JM. MaxEPA in multiple sclerosis. Br. J. Clin. Pract. (Symp. Suppl.) 31:117-21, 1984*

- Omega-6 Fatty Acids:

$$\text{linoleic acid} \rightarrow \text{GLA} \rightarrow \text{DGLA} \rightarrow \text{PGE}_1$$

Linoleic acid, a polyunsaturate which is the main essential fatty acid in the diet, tends to be low in the blood of MS pts. and to fall further during relapses (*Mertin H, Meade CJ. Relevance of fatty acids in MS. Brit. Med. Bull. 33:67-71, 1977; Sanders H et al. Further studies on platelet adhesiveness and serum cholesteryl linoleate levels in MS. J. Neurol. Neurosurg. Psych. 31:321-5, 1968; Thompson RHS. Proc. Roy. Soc. Med. 59:269, 1966*).

> **Observational Study:** Analyses of the fatty acids isolated from the peripheral blood lymphocytes of pts. vs. controls showed a small but significant decrease (p less than 0.01) in the relative percentage of linoleic acid. Determination of ester-linked fatty acids in RBC lipids showed a significant decrease (p less than 0.001) in the relative percentage of linoleic acid and an increase (p less than 0.01) in palmitic plus palmitoleic acids compared to controls. The fatty acid composition of the plasma neutral lipids plus free fatty acids showed a very significant

decrease (p much less than 0.001) in the relative percentage of linoleic acid, a small decrease (p less than 0.05) in arachidonic acid and significant increases in palmitic (p less than 0.001) and oleic acids (p less than 0.001) in pts. vs. controls (*Cherayil GD. Sialic acid and fatty acid concentrations in lymphocytes, red blood cells and plasma from patients with multiple sclerosis. J. Neurol. Sci. 63(1):1-10, 1984*).

Negative Observational Study: Compared to 33 controls, 30 pts. showed no significant decrease in serum linoleic acid, suggesting that a disturbance in linoleic acid metabolism is not inevitably associated with this disease (*Wolfgram F et al. Neurology 25(8):786-88, 1975*).

Epidemiologic studies of the relationship between the prevalence of MS and diet are consistent with the hypothesis that linoleic acid intake is negatively associated with MS (*Alter M et al. Multiple sclerosis and nutrition. Arch. Neurol. 31:267-72, 1974; Agranoff BW, Goldberg D. Diet and geographical distribution of multiple sclerosis. Lancet 2:1061-66, 1974*).

Supplementation with linoleic acid may be beneficial.

Review Article: Data from 3 double-blind trials of linoleic acid in pts. with a remitting-relapsing course were reanalyzed to determine whether inconsistency in the results was due to a relationship between pt. characteristics and treatment response. The combined data consisted of neurologic assessments over 2 1/2-year trials for 87 treated pts. and 85 control patients. Treated pts. with minimal or no disability at entry had a smaller increase in disability than did controls (p less than 0.05). In addition, treatment reduced the severity and duration of relapses at all levels of disability and duration of illness at entry to the trials. The authors suggest that treatment benefits compared to controls may have failed to demonstrate the full extent of potential benefits as oleic acid, the placebo used, may itself ameliorate MS-like illnesses (*Dworkin RH et al. Linoleic acid and multiple sclerosis: A reanalysis of three double-blind trials. Neurology 34:1441-45, 1984; Dworkin RH. Linoleic acid and multiple sclerosis. Lancet 1:1153-4, 1981*).

Studies reviewed:

1. Experimental Double-blind Study: *Bates D et al. Polyunsaturated fatty acids in the treatment of acute remitting multiple sclerosis. Brit. Med. J. 2:1390-1, 1978*

2. Negative Experimental Double-blind Study: *Paty DW et al. Linoleic acid in multiple sclerosis: Failure to show any therapeutic benefit. Ann. Neuro. Scand. 58:53-8, 1978*

3. Experimental Double-blind Study: *Millar JHD et al. Double blind trial of linoleate supplementation of the diet in multiple sclerosis. Brit. Med. J. 2:765-8, 1973*

Note: David Horrobin has suggested that the results of these studies were not optimal due to inadequate dosages and the use of dyes which his gp. has shown to block the conversion of EFA's to prostaglandins (Horrobin D. Multiple sclerosis: The rational basis for treatment with colchicine and evening primrose oil. Med. Hypotheses 5:365-78, 1979).

Supplementation with safflower oil (high in linoleic acid) may be beneficial.

Experimental Double-blind Crossover Study: 20 pts. received daily doses of safflower oil (high in polyunsaturates) for 5 wks. and daily doses of olive oil (low in polyunsaturates) for 5 weeks. Only the safflower oil diet appeared to help some of the pts. (*Utermohlen, Virginia, nutrition scientist at Cornell University - reported in Science 9/4/82*).

In the event that there is a block in the conversion of linoleic acid to GLA, supplementation with evening primrose oil, which has a high concentration of GLA, may be beneficial.

Experimental and Observational Study: 16 pts. were found to have abnormal blood rheology (whole blood filterability) and were supplemented with primrose oil 4 gm daily. After 3 wks., both blood rheology and hand grip strength were improved, suggesting that there was improved capillary perfusion in muscles (*Simpson LO et al. Dietary supplementation with Efamol and multiple sclerosis.* New Zea. Med. J. *98(792):1053-54, 1985*).

Experimental Study: Electrophoretic mobility studies of red cells from MS pts. indicate that treatment with unsaturated fatty acids must continue for at least 2 yrs. before normal reactivity is restored. Assuming this also applies to myelin, clinical trials need to last longer than 2 yrs. if treatment is to be effective (*Field EJ, Joyce G. Multiple sclerosis: Effect of gamma-linolenate administration upon membranes and the need for extended clinical trials of unsaturated fatty acids.* Eur. Neurol. *22:78, 1983*).

Experimental Study: 8 seriously disabled pts. were assessed using the Kurtzke disability score, the B-M manual dexterity test and a dynamometer and were treated with undyed EPO in capsules. After 6 mo., 3 showed some improvement on the Kurtzke score. While there was no improvement in grip strength, there was a significant improvement in manual dexterity (*Horrobin DF. Multiple sclerosis: The rational basis for treatment with colchicine and evening primrose oil.* Med. Hypotheses *5:365-78, 1979*).

See Also:

> *Field EJ, Joyce G. Effect of prolonged ingestion of gamma-linolenate by multiple sclerosis patients.* Eur. Neurol. *17:67-76, 1978*

D-Phenylalanine:

Supplementation may be beneficial.

Experimental Double-blind Study: 12 men and 38 women were treated with DPA and TENS (transcutaneous electrical nerve stimulation). 49/50 improved. Improvements included better bladder control, greater mobility and less depression (*Winter A. New treatment for multiple sclerosis.* Neurol. & Orthoped. J. of Med. & Surg. *5:1, April, 1984*).

- -

COMBINED SUPPLEMENTATION:

Case Reports: Pts. improved following daily supplementation (much of it by injection) of massive doses of various B complex vitamins, vitamin C, vitamin E, choline, lecithin, magnesium, calcium gluconate and pantothenate, aminoacetic acid-glycine, adenosine-5-monophosphoric acid and crude liver (*Klenner FR. Response of peripheral and central nerve pathology to mega-doses of the vitamin B-complex and other metabolites.* J. Applied Nutr. *25:16-40, 1973*).

Experimental Study: 15 pts. received intraspinal B_1 & B_6 injections combined with mixed tocopherols and vitamin B complex orally. 4 of the 6 pts. with advanced disease improved, and 1 of them relapsed after stopping all vitamin therapy for 1 year. Arrest of the progress of the disease was noted in the other 9 cases with improvement in symptoms, recession of neurologic signs and diminution of reflex overactivity (*Stone S. Pyridoxine and thiamine therapy in disorders of the nervous system.* Dis. Nerv. Sys. *11:131-138, 1950*).

- -

OTHER TREATMENTS:

Rule out <u>environmental sensitivities</u>.

> **Observational Study:** In a survey of 2000 pts. with MS and related diseases, those with the most severe cases were food sensitive, those with moderate symptoms were sensitive to molds or fungi, and the least affected were strongly sensitive to pollens (*Jonez HD. <u>Calif. Med.</u> 79:376-80, November, 1953*).

See Also:

> Boines GJ. *The multiple sclerosis diet. <u>Delaware Med. J.</u> 40(2):34, February, 1968*

> Jonez HD. *<u>Postgrad. Med.</u> vol. 11, no. 5, May, 1952*

> Jonez HD. *<u>Annals of Allergy</u> 6:550, 1948; Jan.-Feb. 1950; March-April 1950*

Rule out <u>mercury amalgam toxicity</u>.

There is an epidemiological correlation between MS and dental caries.

> **Observational Study:** Death rates from MS were "linearly related to the numbers of decayed, missing and filled teeth in six Australian and 48 American states and in 45 Asian and European countries," suggesting that dental caries "may be a precursor of one form of MS" (*Craelius W. Comparative epidemiology of multiple sclerosis and dental caries. <u>J. Epidemiol. Comm. Health</u> 32:155-65, 1972*).

The correlation between MS and rates of dental caries may be due to the placement of mercury amalgams.

> **Theoretical Discussion:** When silver amalgam fillings are exposed to gingival action and oxidation, inorganic mercury in the fillings (especially class V fillings and root canals) may be converted to an organic form which may act as a neurotoxin (*Ingalls TH. Epidemiology, etiology and prevention of multiple sclerosis. <u>Am. J. Forensic Med. & Path.</u> 4:55-61, 1983*).

Case Report: The author, an MS pt., was found to have lead toxicity (lead line in his gums, positive blood and urine studies) 4 yrs. after symptom-onset. Extraction of a suspicious tooth showed it to be grossly blackened from its amalgam interior, and a biopsy section of the adjacent ginviva stained for heavy metal depositions. Recently he abruptly developed diplopia following the pulverising of 50-year-old amalgam fillings which, he is convinced, was due to released mercury vapor which reached the oculomotor nerves (probably via the mandibular branch of the trigeminal) (*Ingalls TH. Triggers for multiple sclerosis. Letter to the Editor. <u>Lancet</u> 2:160, 1986*).

MUSCLE CRAMPS

See Also: PREGNANCY AND NUTRITION

NUTRIENTS:

<u>Vitamin E:</u>   200 I.U. four times daily after meals
(50 I.U. four times daily for children with "growing pains" or if history of cardiovascular or renal disorder)
Minimum trial: 4 weeks
Dosage can usually be reduced after maximal results are achieved

Supplementation may be beneficial.

Experimental Study: 50/50 pts. with muscle cramps responded to 450 I.U. daily (*Lotzof L. Med. J. Australia June 11, 1977*).

Experimental Study: 103/125 pts. with nocturnal leg and foot cramps, over half of whom had suffered for over 5 yrs., reported complete or nearly complete relief, 20/125 had a moderate to good response and only 2 failed to respond. Half responded to 300 I.U. or less, while half required 400 I.U. or more. Many had to continue vitamin E to prevent cramps from recurring. Response was usually within 1 week. Similar success was obtained with nocturnal rectal cramps, abdominal muscle cramps and cramps following heavy exercise (*Ayres S, Mihan R. Nocturnal leg cramps (systremma): A progress report on response to vitamin E. South. Med. J. 67(11):1308-12, 1974*).

See Also:

Cathcart RF 3rd. Leg cramps and vitamin E. JAMA 219(2):216-17, 1972

Ayres S Jr., Mihan R. Leg cramps (systremma) and "restless legs" syndrome. Response to vitamin E (tocopherol). Calif. Med. 111(2):87-91, 1969

- -

<u>Calcium:</u>

May affect leg cramps during pregnancy.

Review Article: Leg cramps in the pregnant woman may reflect alterations in calcium metabolism (*Pitkin RM. Endocrine regulation of calcium homeostasis during pregnancy. Clin. Perinatol. 10(3):575-92, 1983*).

Supplementation (or reduction in <u>phosphorus</u>) may prevent or relieve leg cramps during pregnancy.

Review Article: Leg cramps in the pregnant woman may reflect alterations in calcium metabolism (*Pitkin RM. Endocrine regulation of calcium homeostasis during pregnancy. Clin. Perinatol. 10(3):575-92, 1983*).

Experimental and Observational Study: 42 pregnant women with leg cramps failed to demonstrate any differences in total serum or ionized calcium concentrations compared to pregnant women without leg cramps. 21 pts. were treated with calcium 1 gm orally twice daily for 2 weeks. Leg cramps ceased in 9/21 and improved in 11/21 while only 3/21 matched controls improved. Treatment increased total serum calcium concentration but did not alter ionized serum calcium (*Hammar M et al. Calcium treatment of leg cramps in pregnancy. Effect on clinical symptoms and total serum and ionized serum calcium concentrations. Acta Obstet. Gynecol. Scand. 60(4):345-47, 1981*).

Experimental Study: Calcium supplementation, reduction of milk intake or aluminum hydroxide (to decrease phosphorus absorption) was effective in relieving leg cramps in a gp. of pregnant women. Effective treatment was accompanied by a rise in ionizable calcium and a reduction in blood phosphorus (*Page EW, Page EP. Leg cramps in pregnancy: Etiology and treatment. Obstet. Gyn. 1(94):1953*).

Magnesium:

Deficiency may be associated with muscle cramps.

Observational Study: 5 pts. with Crohn's disease and recurrent low serum Mg levels had symptoms of muscle cramps, tetany and bone pain (*Russell RI. Magnesium requirements in patients with chronic inflammatory disease receiving intravenous nutrition. J. Am. Coll. Nutr. 4(5):553-58, 1985*).

If deficient, supplementation may be beneficial.

Case Report: Leg cramps in a pt. with severe cardiac decompensation and hypomagnesemia improved after the infusion of magnesium sulfate 25 mmol IV (*Johansson BW. Magnesium infusion in decompensated hypomagnesemic patients. Acta Pharmacol. Toxicol. (Copenh.) 54 (Suppl. 1):125-28, 1984*).

Calcium plus Magnesium:

Supplementation may be beneficial.

Experimental Study: 112 children with "growing pains" or who kicked and screamed at night were given either dicalcium phosphate or bone meal (which contains both calcium and magnesium) 20 gr daily along with vitamins A and D. Over a 2-year period, all 57 children on bone meal were completely relieved, while 22/56 of the children on dicalcium phosphate were relieved. When the remaining children were switched to bone meal, all of them were completely relieved (*Martin EM. Report on the clinical use of bone meal. Can. Med. Assoc. J. 50:562, 1944*).

MUSCULAR DYSTROPHY

See Also: AUTO-IMMUNE DISORDERS (GENERAL)

NUTRIENTS:

Vitamin E:

MD closely resembles the muscular dystrophy induced in animals by deprivation of tocopherol which is reversed by oral but not parenteral tocopherol (*Milhorat AT, Bartels WE. The defect in utilization of tocopherol in progressive muscular dystrophy. Science 101:93-4, 1945*).

Supplementation may be beneficial.

Experimental Study: Pts.were supplemented with up to 300 mg. tocopherols daily, mainly in the form of wheat germ oil. Symptoms were arrested in 5/25 with progressive muscular dystrophy and moderate to marked improvement occurred. 3/5 with menopausal muscular dystrophy showed "remarkable" improvement (*Rabinovitch R et al. Neuromuscular disorders amenable to wheat germ oil therapy. J. Neurol. Neurosurg. Psychiat. 14:95-100, 1951*).

- with inositol:

Supplementation may be beneficial.

Experimental Study: 7 pts. given tocopherol or inositol alone showed no reduction in creatinuria, but 5 of them responded with reduced creatinuria when both substances were given in equimolar amounts for 1 or 2 days. This suggests that there is an inherited deficiency in muscular dystrophy preventing the formation of a condensation product of the 2 substances in the G.I. tract (*Milhorat - op cit*).

- -

Selenium:

Serum selenium is reduced in myotonic dystrophy and all its major symptoms (muscle dystrophy, infertility, alopecia, cataract and myocardial degeneration) can be cured or prevented in animals by selenium supplementation (*Orndahl G et al. Selenium therapy of myotonic dystrophy. Acta. Med. Scand. 213:237, 1983*).

- with Vitamin E:

Experimental Study: Pt. treated with 228 mcg. selenium (as 0.5 mg. sodium selenite) and 10 mg. vitamin E daily which was increased over 2 years to 3 mg. sodium selenite and 125 mg. vitamin E daily. After 6 months, gradual improvements were observed with regression of all symptoms (muscular weakness, myopathic facies, bilateral ptosis and mental tiredness) except active myotonia. 3 more pts. had begun treatment and all were slightly improved after 9 months (*Orndahl - ibid*).

– –

<u>Phosphatidyl Choline</u>:

Supplementation may be beneficial.

Case Report: Pt. with progressive muscular dystrophy ingested 20 gm. soy lecithin daily. After day 15 the creatinuria dropped slowly. When lecithin was discontinued, the creatine output remained at a low level for 6 days and then slowly rose to its previous level (*Milhorat AT et al. Effect of wheat germ on creatinuria in dermatomyositis and progressive muscular dystrophy. Proc. Soc. Exp. Biol. Med. 58:40-1, 1945*).

NEURALGIA AND NEUROPATHY

See Also: **CARPAL TUNNEL SYNDROME**
                                  DIABETES MELLITUS

NUTRIENTS:

<u>Folic Acid</u>:

Deficiency may be associated with peripheral neuropathy.

Observational Study: 7/34 pts.(21%) with severe folate deficiency and megaloblastosis due to GI or dietary causes had clinical or electrophysiological evidence of peripheral neuropathy that was usually mild and predominantly sensory. The presence of neuropathy was unrelated to age, sex, hemoglobin, mean cell volume, serum or red cell folate, or serum vitamin B_{12}. It is concluded that the neuropathy is at least in part the result of folate deficiency, although a contributing role of other deficiencies cannot be excluded (*Shorvon SD, Reynolds EH. Folate deficiency and peripheral neuropathy, in Botez MI, Reynolds EH, Eds.* <u>Folic Acid in Neurology, Psychiatry, and Internal Medicine</u>. *New York, Raven Press, 1979*).

If deficient, supplementation may be beneficial.

Review Article: Several clinical clues may lead to the suspicion of a folate-responsive polyneuropathy in a pt. with a long-standing low serum folate level: (a) hematological abnormalities; however, their absence does not rule out folate deficiency as an etiological factor; (b) chronic GI dysfunction with evidence of an irritable colon for years, sometimes with atrophy of the jejunal mucosa; (c) chronic low-residue diet; (d) a neurological picture indicative of a mild and predominantly sensory demyelinating type of polyneuropathy, at times associated with signs of posteroloateral cord involvement (*Botez MI et al. Polyneuropathies responsive to folic acid therapy, in Botez MI, Reynolds EH.* <u>Folic Acid in Neurology, Psychiatry, and Internal Medicine</u>. *New York, Raven Press, 1979*).

Case Reports: 5 pts. with <u>polyneuropathy</u> (2 men and 3 women), 2 of whom had subacute combined degeneration of the spinal cord, had low serum folate levels compared to controls, long-standing GI disease, and deficient folate intake. The D-xylose absorption test gave low values in all pts., while none displayed the classical malabsorption syndrome. They had substantial improvement or recovered after periods ranging from 9-39 mo. of supplementation with oral folic acid 5-15 mg daily (*Botez MI et al. Polyneuropathy and folate deficiency.* <u>Arch. Neurol.</u> *35:581-84, 1978*).

Case Report: 26 year-old male complaining of left wrist and hand weakness and paresthesias in the forearm and dorsum of the hand due to a polyneuropathy was found to have a folate deficiency (in the absence of other vitamin deficiencies) and celiac disease. The discrete clinical signs and the relatively pronounced electrophysiologic signs did not improve after therapy with vitamin B complex but improved after folic acid 2.5 mg daily, suggesting that the polyneuropathy was due to the folate deficiency (*Fehling C et al. Folate deficiency and neurological disease: One case with a close association.* <u>Arch. Neurol.</u> *30:263-65, 1974*).

See Also:

Enk C et al. Reversible dementia and neuropathy associated with folate deficiency 16 years after partial gastrectomy. Scand. J. Haematol. 25:63, 1980

Manzoor M, Runcie J. Folate-responsive neuropathy: Report of 10 cases. Brit. Med. J. 1:1176, 1976

Niacin:

Supplementation may be beneficial.

Experimental Study: 74 consecutive Bell's palsy pts. were treated with nicotinic acid 100-250 mg with "excellent results" noted in all pts. within 2-4 weeks (*Kime CE. Bell's palsy: A new syndrome associated with treatment by nicotinic acid. Arch. Otolaryngol. 68:28-32, 1958*).

Experimental Study: 8 pts. with trigeminal neuralgia received nicotinic acid 1-200 mg IV daily. 4 were completely cured, 3 were partial cures and 1 was a treatment failure. In successful cases, a few injections were followed by complete pain relief lasting for months, and when an injection was given during an actual paroxysm, the relief was immediate (*Furtado D, Chicorro V. Rev. Clin. Espan., Madrid 5:416, 1942*).

Pyridoxine:

WARNING: Pyridoxine supplementation may <u>cause</u> a sensory neuropathy in doses as low as 200 mg daily over 3 years (usually 2-5 gm daily). The neurotoxicity is believed to be due to exceeding the liver's ability to phosphorylate pyridoxine to the active coenzyme, pyridoxal phosphate. The resulting high pyridoxine blood level could be directly neurotoxic or may compete for binding sites with pyridoxal phosphate resulting in a relative deficiency of the active metabolite (*Parry GJ. Sensory neuropathy with low-dose pyridoxine. Neurology 35:1466-68, 1985*). Supplementation in the form of pyridoxal phosphate should thus avoid this danger.

Deficiency may cause a pyridoxine-responsive neuropathy.

Experimental Study: Using electrodiagnostic criteria, pts. with carpal tunnel syndrome (CTS) were categorized into 4 groups of at least 7 subjects each: CTS, peripheral neuropathy (PN), CTS and PN, and normal. Based on RBC glutamine oxaloacetic acid transaminase (EGOT) activity with vs. without pyridoxal phosphate, a significant difference in pyridoxine metabolic activity (PMA) was found between gps. by both chi square (p less than 0.05) and analysis of variance (p less than 0.05) which was associated with the presence or absence of PN. There was no difference in PMA when gps. were separated on the basis of CTS, suggesting that a PMA abnormality is highly correlated, not with CTS, but with PN, and that pts. with CTS responding to pyridoxine may have an unrecognized PN (*Byers CM et al. Pyridoxine metabolism in carpal tunnel syndrome with and without peripheral neuropathy. Arch Phys. Med. Rehabil. 65(11):712-16, 1984*).

Case Report: 51 year-old non-alcoholic, non-diabetic female developed a sensorimotor peripheral neuropathy and pyridoxine deficiency associated with long-term phenelzine therapy (*Heller CA, Friedman PA. Pyridoxine deficiency and peripheral neuropathy associated with long-term phenelzine therapy. Am. J. Med. 75(5):887-88, 1983*).

Review Article: Isoniazid, which competitively inhibits the actions of the coenzymes derived from pyridoxine, can produce a peripheral neuropathy. The routine use of pyridoxine supplementation to prevent peripheral neuropathy in high risk populations receiving isoniazid is recommended (*Snider DE Jr. Pyridoxine supplementation during isoniazid therapy. Tubercle 61(4):191-96, 1980*).

Intraspinal injections may be effective in <u>sciatic neuritis</u> and <u>Korsakoff's polyneuritis</u>.

Experimental Study: 8/8 cases of sciatic neuritis without evidence of nerve root compression (most of whom had failed to improve after prolonged bed rest and local sciatic nerve infiltration) improved with intraspinal B_6 injections. 2/2 cases of Korsakoff's polyneuritis unresponsive to large doses of B complex orally and I.V. also responded rapidly to 2 intraspinal B_6 injections along with the addition of oral natural mixed tocopherols (*Stone S. Pyridoxine and thiamine therapy in disorders of the nervous system. Dis. Nerv. Sys. 11:131-8, 1950*).

<u>Thiamine:</u>

Deficiency known to cause a polyneuropathy (the essential feature of dry beriberi).

Supplementation may be beneficial for <u>trigeminal neuralgia</u>.

Experimental Study: 37/58 pts. with trigeminal neuralgia were "markedly improved" following treatment with thiamine chloride 10 mg daily IM or IV, liver extract by injection 3 times weekly (total of 22.5 USP units), and a high vitamin, low carbohydrate diet with 30 cc orally of an aqueous concentrate of rice polishings daily, providing 1500 IU B_1 as well as other components of the vitamin B complex. Treatment had to be continued for as long as 6 mo. before maximal benefits were obtained (*Borsook H et al. The relief of symptoms of major trigeminal neuralgia (tic douloureux) following the use of vitamin B_1 and concentrated liver extract. JAMA April 13, 1940, p. 1421*).

<u>Vitamin B_{12}</u>: 1000 micrograms IM as needed

Deficiency may cause a peripheral neuropathy, even in the absence of the classic findings of pernicious anemia, which responds to supplementation.

Placebo-controlled Case Reports: Vitamin B_{12} 15 gamma IM was rapidly effective in relieving pain in 3 pts. believed to have neuritis due to malnutrition but not in pts. with other painful illnesses, including 2 with brachial neuritis. It was also ineffective in reducing pain threshold in 2 normal controls, suggesting that it did not have an analgesic effect:
1. 43 year-old male alcoholic with 8 wk. history paresthesias of legs and feet with pain preventing ambulation. BP was 165/105 and his heart was slightly enlarged. Both feet were sweating excessively and were acutely painful spontaneously and to touch. Calves were tender and atrophic. Tendon reflexes were hypoactive, and there was decreased touch and vibratory sensation in the legs and feet. Gait was unsteady but the Romberg was negative. HGb was 10 gms and RBC count was 3.9 million. He failed to improve in 1 wk on a control vitamin B-poor diet and was then given 1 cc normal saline IM without effect. When given a similar injection containing 15 gamma vitamin B_{12}, all spontaneous pain vanished with 1/2 hour, he could walk normally and pain to touch was gone. With a good diet and vitamin B supplementation, the neuritis entirely disappeared.
2. 17 year-old female was completely disabled by pain, weakness and numbness of the extremities following an 11 wk. siege of vomiting. She had the pigmentation of pellagra, absent tendon reflexes, absent pallesthesia and position sense in legs and arms, tender skin and muscles and generalized weakness. Anemia and leukopenia were found. She failed to respond to the control diet and placebo injection, but had relief of pain within 45 minutes after the vitamin B_{12} injection and gradually improved with proper diet and supplementation.
3. 58 year-old male alcoholic diabetic had 5 yr. history of gradually increasing neuritis of legs and feet. He had mild cirrhosis or fatty liver. IM vitamin B_{12} stopped the pain within 1 hour.
(*Bean BB et al. An effect of vitamin B_{12} on pain in nutritional neuropathy. Am. J. Med. Sci. 220:431-4, 1950*).

Supplementation may be beneficial even without evidence of deficiency.

Case Reports: 2 cases of <u>Bell's palsy</u>, one of about 1.5 yrs. duration and the other of about 4 yrs. duration were treated with "massive" doses of cyanocobalamin (500-1000 mcg daily to every other day for a total of 2000-20,000 mcg) with complete recovery (*Mitra M, Nandi AK. Cyanocobalamin in chronic Bell's palsy. <u>J. Indian Med. Assoc.</u> 33:129-31, 1959*).

Experimental Study: 18 pts. with <u>trigeminal neuralgia</u> and 1 case of <u>glossopharyngeal neuralgia</u> were treated with "massive" doses of cyanocobalamin with the latter cases receiving 1000 mcg IM daily for 10 days. 15/18 showed considerable improvement or complete relief of pain (including the pt. with glossopharyngeal neuralgia), 1 showed moderate improvement and 3 showed little or no immediate improvement (*Surtees SJ, Hughes RR. Treatment of trigeminal neuralgia with vitamin B_{12}. 1:439, 1954*).

Experimental Study: 17 pts. with <u>trigeminal neuralgia</u> received vitamin B_{12} IM daily for 10 days. 6 obtained complete relief lasting 2-8 mo., and 2 obtained satisfactory relief (*Alexander E, Davis CH Jr. Trigeminal neuralgia: Conservative management with massive vitamin B_{12} therapy. <u>N. Carolina Med. J.</u> 14:206-07, 1953*).

Experimental Study: 13 pts. with <u>trigeminal neuralgia</u> received cyancobalamin with the later cases receiving 100 mcg IM daily for 10 days. All achieved "remarkable relief." While 9/13 experienced a prompt and complete remission, 4 pts. who had previously been treated with surgery or alcohol nerve blocks took longer to achieve pain relief (*Fields WS, Hoff HE. Relief of pain in trigeminal neuralgia by crystalline vitamin B_{12}. <u>Neurology</u> 2:131-39, 1952*).

See Also:

Alexander E, Davis CH. *Trigeminal neuralgia: Conservative management with massive B_{12} therapy. <u>North Carolina Med. J.</u> 14:206, 1953.*

- -

<u>Essential Fatty Acids:</u>

Supplementation may be beneficial in <u>Guillain-Barre Syndrome</u>.

Case Reports: Two children who had been severely disabled for 6 and 12 mo. respectively with idiopathic polyneuritis (Guillain-Barre Syndrome) began to recover within a week of starting on a polyunsatuated fatty-acid diet consisting of avoidance of fatty foods and supplementation with sunflower-seed oil 10 ml 3 times daily. They subsequently recovered virtually completely (*Bower BD, Newsholme EA. Treatment of idiopathic polyneuritis by polyunsaturated fatty acid diet. <u>Lancet</u> March 18, 1978, pp. 583-5*).

NEUROMUSCULAR DEGENERATION

See Also: AUTO-IMMUNE DISORDERS (GENERAL)
MULTIPLE SCLEROSIS

NUTRIENTS:

<u>Folic Acid:</u>

Deficiency may cause subacute combined systems degeneration which responds to supplementation in its earlier stages.

Review Article: The clinical signs of subacute system degeneration of the spinal cord can exist in the absence of vitamin B_{12} deficiency in pts. that are severely deficient in folate, and these neurological signs remit during therapy with folate. Although neuropathological and experimental verifications of the relationship between folate deficiency and myelopathy are lacking, a causal relationship appears to be highly probable (*Pincus JH. Folic acid deficiency: A cause of subacute combined system degeneration, in Botez MI, Reynolds EH, Eds. <u>Folic Acid in Neurology, Psychiatry, and Internal Medicine.</u> New York, Raven Press, 1979*).

Case Reports: 2 pts. with subacute combined degeneration of the spinal cord and polyneuropathy had low serum folate levels compared to controls, long-standing GI disease, and deficient folate intake. The D-xylose absorption test gave low values in all pts., while none displayed the classical malabsorption syndrome. They had substantial improvement or recovered after periods ranging from 9-39 mo. of supplementation with oral folic acid 5-15 mg daily (*Botez MI et al. Polyneuropathy and folate deficiency. <u>Arch. Neurol.</u> 35:581-84, 1978*).

<u>Vitamin B_{12}:</u>

Deficiency is well-known to result in subacute combined degeneration of the spinal cord along with dementia, peripheral neuropathy, and optic neuritis which responds to supplementation in its earlier stages.

<u>Vitamin E:</u>

Deficiency (which may be caused by defective absorption of fat-soluble vitamins) is associated with progressive neurologic deterioration, probably due to disordered intracellular peroxidation.

Observational Study: Of 93 children (ages 1 mo.-17 yrs.) with prolonged neonatal cholestatic disorders due to either intrahepatic neonatal cholestasis or to extrahepatic biliary atresia, 64% of the intrahepatic and 77% of the extrahepatic cholestasis gps. were vitamin E deficient based on serum concentrations and the ratios of serum vitamin E concentration to total serum lipid concentration. While neurologic function was normal in vitamin E-sufficient children, between the ages of 1-3 yrs., neurologic abnormalities were present in approx. 50% of the vitamin E-deficient children. By the ages of 8-10 yrs., neurologic dysfunction in the majority of vitamin E-deficient children had progressed to a disabling combination of findings (*Sokol RJ et al. Frequency and clinical progression of the vitamin E deficiency neurologic disorder in children with prolonged neonatal cholestasis. <u>Am. J. Dis. Child.</u> 139(12):1211-15, 1985*).

Animal Experimental Studies (rats): vitamin E deficiency was associated with the development of muscular weakness (*Evans & Emerson. Minutes and Proceed. of Society for Exp. Biol. & Med., 1940; Einarson L, Ringsted A. Effect of chronic vitamin E deficiency on the nervous system and the skeletal musculature in adult rats. Copenhagen & London, Levin and Munksgaard, 1938*).

Supplementation may be beneficial, especially if deficient.

Experimental Study: Vitamin E deficiency in 14 children with chronic cholestasis was corrected with either oral supplementation of up to 120 IU/kg daily or IM supplementation of 0.8-2.0 IU/kg daily. Neurologic function remained normal in 2 asymptomatic children below age 3 after 15 and 18 mo. of supplementation, while neurologic function became normal in 3 symptomatic chldren below age 3 after 18-32 mo. of supplementation. Restitution of neurologic function was more limited in 9 symptomatic children 5-17 yrs. old (*Sokol RJ et al. Improved neurologic function after long-term correction of vitamin E deficiency in children with chronic cholestasis. N. Engl. J. Med. 313(25):1580-86, 1985*).

Case Report: 23 year-old female with specific vitamin E malabsorption who, starting at age 13, suffered from increasing ataxia and a disturbance of proprioception. There was neither fat malabsorption nor deficiencies of fat-soluble vitamins A,D or K. Serum vitamin E was undetectable, and fasting lipid and lipoprotein concentrations were abnormal. After an initial treatment of alpha-tocopheryl acetate daily for 2 wks., serum vitamin E rose to the normal range. A maintenance dose was continued and, after 15 mo., proprioception (with appreciation of vibration) had marginally improved (*Harding AE et al. Spinocerebellar degeneration associated with a selective defect of vitamin E absorption. New Engl. J. Med. 313(1):32-35, 1985*).

Experimental Study: 4 children (ages 6-17) with chronic cholestasis who developed a slowly progressive neuromuscular disease characterized by ataxia, dysmetria, areflexia, loss of vibratory sensation, and a variable ophthalmoplegia were found to have low serum vitamin E concentrations. Muscle histochemical findings were similar to those described in vitamin E-deficient animals. Alpha tocopherol 0.55-1.42 mg/kg daily IM was required to achieve normal serum vitamin E levels in 3 pts., while 1 pt. achieved normal levels with an oral dosage of 32 mg/kg daily. After normalization of serum concentrations for 12-20 mo., the neurologic disease improved in all 4 pts. (*Guggenheim MA et al. Progressive neuromuscular disease in children with chronic cholestasis and vitamin E deficiency: Diagnosis and treatment with alpha tocopherol. J. Pediatr. 100(1):51-58, 1982*).

Case Report: Pt. with a 25 yr. history of Crohn's disease with multiple small bowel resections presented with bilateral visual field scotomata, generalized motor weakness, a broad-based gait with marked ataxia, brisk reflexes, and a bilateral Babinski response. Serum vitamin E concentration was 0.03 mg/dl (normal 0.8-1.2). Supplementation with 270 IU daily brought complete recovery over a period of 2 years (*Howard L et al. Reversible neurological symptoms caused by vitamin E deficiency in a patient with short bowel syndrome. Am. J. Clin. Nutr. 36:1243-49, 1982*).

Experimental Study: 8/9 cases of amyotrophic lateral sclerosis improved on up to 375 I.U. of alpha tocopheryl acetate "enhanced" with thiamine (*Rosenberger AI. Observations on the treatment of amyotrophic lateral sclerosis with vitamin E. Med. Rec. 154:97-100, 1941*).

Experimental Study: 11/20 cases of amyotrophic lateral sclerosis improved on 60-75 I.U. daily of alpha tocopheryl acetate. The author suggests 300 I.U. for maximal effectiveness (*Wechsler IS. The treatment of amyotrophic lateral sclerosis with vitamin E (tocopherols). Am. J. Med. Sci. 200:765-778, 1940*).

– –

Carnitine:

In patients with neuromuscular diseases, there is a positive correlation between creatinine excretion and carnitine excretion (*Carroll JE et al. Carnitine intake and excretion in neuromuscular diseases. Am. J. Clin. Nutr. 34:2693-8, 1981*).

OBESITY

BASIC DIET:

Low <u>calorie</u> diet.

High <u>fiber</u> diet.

Increases non-caloric bulk to cause satiety with less intake (<u>*Cereal Foods World*</u> *29-11:635*).

- <u>Glucomannan</u>: 3 grams daily

Unabsorbable carbohydrate derived from Konjak root. Absorbs 50 - 200 times its weight of water.

Supplementation may be beneficial.

Experimental Double-blind Study: 20 obese subjects received either glucomannan 1 gm or placebo with 8 oz water 1 hr. prior to each meal. Eating and exercise patterns were unchanged. After 8 wks., there was a significant mean weight loss in subjects using glucomannan and no side-effects were reported (*Walsh DE et al. Effect of glucomannan on obese patients: A clinical study.* <u>*Int. J. Obes.*</u> *8(4):289-93, 1984*).

- <u>Guar Gum</u>:

Supplementation may be beneficial.

Experimental Study: Guar gum reduced hunger in obese subjects and seemed to influence carbohydrate and lipid metabolism in a beneficial way (*Krotkiewski M. Effect of guar gum on body-weight, hunger ratings and metabolism in obese subjects.* <u>*Br. J. Nutr.*</u> *52(1):97-105, 1984*).

Increase intake of <u>raw foods</u>.

Benefits may be due to increased fiber intake.

Experimental Study: 32 hypertensive pts., 28 of whom were obese, received an ave. of 62% of ingested calories as raw foods for a mean duration of 6.7 months. There was a significant mean weight loss of 3.8 kg (*Douglass J et al. Effects of a raw food diet on hypertension and obesity.* <u>*South. Med. J.*</u> *78(7):841, 1985*).

Avoid <u>sugar</u>.

Review Article: The results of several studies suggest that sucrose ingestion can lead to calorie overconsumption and obesity. There is insufficient evidence, however, to conclude that obese people consume a higher proportion of carbohydrates compared to lean people (*Vasselli JR. Carbohydrate ingestion, hypoglycemia and obesity.* <u>*Appetite*</u> *6:53-59, 1985*).

See Also:

Geiseleman PT, Novin D. The role of carbohydrates in appetite, hunger and obesity. <u>*Appetite*</u> *3:203-223(a), 1982*

- -

NUTRIENTS:

Vitamin C:

Supplementation may be beneficial.

> **Experimental Double-blind Study:** 41 females who were about 50% above ideal body weight and who had failed to lose weight on various reducing programs received either ascorbic acid 1 gm 3 times daily or placebo. There was no calorie restriction. After 6 wks., mean weight loss in the experimental gp. was 2.53 kg compared to only 0.95 kg in the control gp. (p less than 0.012). This difference became significant by the second week (*Naylor GJ et al. A double blind placebo controlled trial of ascorbic acid in obesity.* *Nutr. Health* 1985, p. 425).

- -

Coenzyme Q:

May be deficient.

> **Observational Study:** 14/27 (52%) subjects were found to be low in coenzyme Q_{10} (*van Gaal L et al. Exploratory study of coenzyme Q_{10} in obesity, in Folkers K, Yamamura Y, Eds.,* *Biomed. & Clin. Aspects of Coenzyme Q.* Vol. 4. Amsterdam, Elsevier Science Publishers, 1984, pp. 369-73).

If deficient, supplementation may be beneficial.

> **Experimental Controlled Study:** 9 subjects, 5 of whom were deficient in coenzyme Q_{10}, received 100 mg daily of CoQ_{10} along with a 650 kcal diet. After 8-9 wks., mean weight loss in the deficient gp. was 13.5 kg compared to 5.8 kg in the other group (*van Gaal - ibid*).

Evening Primrose Oil: 2 - 4 grams daily

Believed to increase brown fat and Na^+-K^+-ATPase activity and thus to benefit people who fail to lose weight with appropriate diets (estimated to be 1 out of 3 obese people).

> **Negative Experimental Double-blind Study:** 74 women with substantial obesity received either EPO or placebo. After 12 wks., there was no significant difference in weight loss achieved by those taking EPO compared to placebo (*Haslett C et al. A double-blind evaluation of evening primrose oil as an antiobesity agent.* *Int. J. Obes.* 7(6):549-53, 1983).

> **Experimental Study:** Extremely obese pts. investigated on a metabolic unit lost large amts. of weight with evening primrose oil supplementation. Brown fat activation was measured using thermography, since activated brown fat has a higher temperature than ordinary fat or inactive brown fat. In addition, the amount of brown fat in reserve was evaluated by injecting ephedrine. Very obese people had minimal resting brown fat activity and a poor response to ephedrine. In those who lost weight on primrose oil, both resting brown fat activity and the response to ephedrine were dramatically increased after 3-4 weeks. Primrose oil also activated Na^+-K^+-ATPase activity in those for whom enzyme activity was low (*Lowndes RH, Mansel RE. The effects of evening primrose oil (Efamol) on serum lipid levels of normal and obese subjects, in Horrobin DF, Ed.* *Clinical Uses of Essential Fatty Acids.* Montreal, Eden Press, 1982, pp. 37-52).

> **Experimental Study:** 32 normals supplemented their normal diets with 2 gm primrose oil daily and 6 took 4 gms daily. In addition, 6 schizophrenics took 4 gms daily. After 6-8 weeks, about half of those who were more than 10% above ideal weight noted a reduction in appetite and had lost weight without dieting   The higher the starting weight, the greater the weight loss.   There was a

dose/response effect in that those taking 8 gms daily lost more weight than those taking 4 gms daily. People within 10% of ideal body weight showed no weight change (*Vaddadi KS, Horrobin DF. Weight loss produced by evening primrose oil administration in normal and schizophrenic individuals. IRCS J.Med.Sci. 7:52, 1979*).

L-Glutamine:

Said to blunt carbohydrate craving (*Goodwin, Frederick, director of intramural research, Nat. Instit. of Mental Health (U.S.A.) - quoted in APA Psychiatric News December 5, 1986*).

Note: Glutamic acid, like glucose, is a source of energy for the brain, but poorly penetrates the blood-brain barrier. Glutamine, on the other hand, readily penetrates the blood-brain barrier where it is transformed to glutamic acid (Williams Roger J. Nutrition Against Disease. New York, Pitman Publishing Co., 1971).

L-Tryptophan:

Said to reduce the urge for late-night binges (*Goodwin, Frederick, director of intramural research, Nat. Instit. of Mental Health (U.S.A.) - quoted in APA Psychiatric News December 5, 1986*).

ORGANIC MENTAL DISORDER

See Also: ALCOHOLISM   "HYPOGLYCEMIA"
               BIPOLAR DISORDER   INSOMNIA
               DEMENTIA   LEARNING DISABILITIES
               DEPRESSION   PREMENSTRUAL SYNDROME
               HYPERKINESIS   SCHIZOPHRENIA

OVERVIEW:

1. Deficiencies of folic acid and/or vitamin B_{12} are associated with organic mental disorders; deficiencies of the following minerals have also been implicated: calcium, magnesium, phosphorus, potassium, sodium and zinc.

2. Excesses of calcium, copper, potassium or sodium may be associated with organic mental disorders as part of a toxic syndrome.

3. Excessive exposure to toxic metals, such as lead and mercury, may cause organic mental disorders.

4. Food sensitivities have been blamed for causing cognitive and emotional symptoms (especially "spaciness," depression, hyperactivity, memory problems, paranoid trends, and irritability), but there is very little experimental evidence to substantiate these claims.

- -

NUTRIENTS:

Folic Acid: 5 mg. 3 times daily

Folate deficiency, which is found in at least 1/4 of hospitalized psychiatric patients, is associated with a wide variety of psychiatric symptoms including psychosis, depression, confusion, disorientation, and dementia which may be accompanied by neurologic symptoms of weakness, numbness, stiffness and spasticity, both with and without muscular atrophy.

References:

Carney MWP. Psychiatric aspects of folate deficiency, in Botez MI, Reynolds, Eds. Folic Acid in Neurology, Psychiatry, and Internal Medicine. New York, Raven Press, 1979

Botez MI et al. Folate-responsive neurological and mental disorders: Report of 16 cases. Eur. Neurol. 16:230-246, 1977

Howard JS. Folate deficiency in psychiatric practice. Psychosomatics 16:112-15, 1975

Kallstrom B et al. Vitamin B_{12} and folate concentrations in mental patients. Acta Psychiat. Scand. 45:137-52, 1969

Hunter R et al. Serum B_{12} and folate concentration in mental patients. Brit. J. Psychiat. 113:1291-5, 1967

Vitamin B₁₂:

Organic Brain Syndrome (which may include paranoia and violence) is one of the most common psychiatric syndromes associated with B₁₂ deficiency and may occur despite the absence of hematological and neurological evidence of pernicious anemia (*Evans DL et al. Organic psychosis without anemia or spinal cord symptoms in patients with vitamin B₁₂ deficiency. Am. J. Psychiat. 140:218, 1983; Zucker DK et al. B₁₂ deficiency and psychiatric disorders: Case report and literature review. Biol. Psychiat. 16:197-205, 1981*).

If deficient, supplementation may be beneficial.

Case Report: A post-gastrectomy pt. presented with psychosis which responded to vitamn B₁₂ supplementation (*Geagea K, Ananth J. Response of a psychiatric patient to vitamin B₁₂ therapy. Dis. Nerv. Sys. 36(6):343-44, 1975*).

- -

Calcium: 1000 mg. - 1500 mg. daily

Hypoparathyroidism is the most frequent cause of hypocalcemia, and over half the pts. with hypoparathyroidism develop psychiatric symptoms. Cognitive impairment is most frequent, while irritability, agitation, hyperactivity and delusions may also be noted (*Webb WL, Gehi M. Electrolyte and fluid imbalance: Neuropsychiatric manifestations. Psychosomatics 22(3):199-203, 1981*).

Affective and organic symptoms are overwhelmingly dominant in hypercalcemic pts., the majority of whom are women 50 yrs. or older who have been vaguely ill for a prolonged time before the actual endocrinopathy appears. The severity of the psychiatric symptoms seems unrelated to the degree of hypercalcemia (*Alarcon RD, Franceschini JA. Hyperparathyroidism and paranoid psychosis: Case report and review of the literature. Brit. J. Psychiat. 145:477, 1984*). Personality changes characterized by irritability and a lack of initiative and spontaneity are most frequently seen. Depression may be prominent, manifested by a loss of interest, social withdrawal, anorexia, anhedonia, and memory impairment (*Webb WL, Gehi M. Electrolyte and fluid imbalance: Neuropsychiatric manifestations. Psychosomatics 22(3):199-203, 1981*).

Observational Study: Of 54 pts. with hyperparathyroidism, 36 had affective disturbance, 12 had impaired memory, and 5 had acute organic psychosis. 37% experienced moderate personality changes, 21% severe personality changes, and 9% were psychotic. In most cases, the personality changes began with affective disturbance characterized without exception by loss of initiative and spontaneity and by depression. While the personality change developed insidiously for years, the acute organic psychosis had a "violent onset." These changes were wholly reversible with adequate treatment of the underlying disorder (*Petersen P. Psychiatric disorders in primary hyperparathyroidism. J. Clin. Endocrinol. Metabl. 28:1491-95, 1968*).

See Also:

> *Gatewood JW et al. Mental changes associated with hyperparathyroidism. Am. J. Psychiat. 132(2):129-32, 1975*

Copper:

Toxicity may cause brain dysfunction.

Observational Study: 30 pts. with unusually elevated hair copper levels were evaluated. Baseline serum and urine copper levels were normal. Mental symptoms included profound mental fatigue, poor memory, lack of concentration, insomnia, severe depression, apprehension, and irritability along with somatic complaints. Chelation therapy with D-penicillamine often elicited a prompt reduction of symptoms, and 24 hr. urine output of copper during chelation therapy was generally proportional to the hair copper level (*Nolan KR. Copper toxicity syndrome. J. Orthomol. Psychiat. 12:270-82, 1983*).

See Also:

Krischner KN. Copper and zinc in childhood behavior. Psychopharm. Bull. 14(3):58-61, 1978

Magnesium:

Organic brain disorders are part of the deficiency syndrome.

Review Article: Psychiatric symptoms of organic brain syndrome may be the first manifestation of magnesium imbalance; these include personality changes, nervousness, irritability, and restlessness. Depression is a later development (*Webb WL, Gehi M. Electrolyte and fluid imblance: Neuro-pychiatric manifestations. Psychosomatics 22(3):199-203, 1981*).

Review Article: Magnesium deficiency is characterized by neuromuscular irritability and convulsions as well as confusional states and mental depression. During the hyperparathyroid state there is a negative magnesium balance, with increased urinary excretion of magnesium and a variable serum magnesium level due, in part, to the mobilization of magnesium along with calcium from bone. If magnesium is cleared through the kidneys more rapidly than calcium, increased levels of urinary magnesium without elevated serum magnesium can result. While both calcium and magnesium in higher concentrations depress the excitability of the myoneural junction, high magnesium concentrations have a central depressive effect that can be reversed by calcium administration (*Gatewood JW et al. Mental changes associated with hyperparathyroidism. Am. J. Psychiat. 132(2):129-32, 1975*).

Phosphorus:

Hypophosphatemia is associated with complaints of apprehension, irritability, numbness, paresthesias and weakness (*Webb WL, Gehi M. Electrolyte and fluid imbalance: Neuropsychiatric manifestations. Psychosomatics 22(3):199-203, 1981*).

Potassium:

Hypokalemia is frequently associated with a dysphoric mood, tearfulness, weakness, and fatigue. Not uncommonly, a frank organic brain syndrome may also be noted. Decreased intracellar potassium has been noted in depressed pts. compared to controls and pts. who have suicided have been found to have decreased cerebral potassium (*Webb WL, Gehi M. Electrolyte and fluid imbalance: Neuropsychiatric manifestations. Psychosomatics 22(3):199-203, 1981*).

Hyperkalemia frequently results in an organic brain syndrome as part of the toxicity syndrome (*Webb WL, Gehi M. Electrolyte and fluid imbalance: Neuropsychiatric manifestations. Psychosomatics 22(3):199-203, 1981*).

Sodium:

Hyponatremia is frequently associated with apathy, impaired concentration, emotional lability, lethargy, memory impairment, social withdrawal, and anorexia as part of the deficiency syndrome. When severe, disorientation, somnolence, illusions and hallucinations may occur (*Webb WL, Gehi M. Electrolyte and fluid imbalance: Neuropsychiatric manifestations. Psychosomatics 22(3):199-203, 1981*).

Case Report: A 72 year-old female under treatment for subacute bacterial endocarditis was placed on a low salt diet during hospitalization due to congestive heart failure. On her 35th hospital day she became disoriented, confused, rambling in her speech, and frequently drowsy. Her husband noted marked personality changes characterized by irritability, suspiciousness, and a lack of emotional response to him over a period of several days, while previously she had been weak but pleasant, oriented, cooperative and responsive to people around her. During the psychiatric exam she was lying in bed quietly, staring at the ceiling, and talking in word salad. At times she would become drowsy, but she could be aroused. She was disoriented and appeared to be having auditory and visual hallucinations. Her serum sodium was found to be 107 meq/l. By the 8th day following sodium replacement therapy she was oriented, cooperative and pleasant, and her affect was appropriate. There was no evidence of delusional thinking or hallucinations (*Burnell GM, Foster TA. Psychosis with low sodium syndrome. <u>Am. J. Psychiat.</u> 128(10):1313-14, 1972*).

<u>Hypernatremia</u> causes neuropsychiatric signs and symptoms in about 1 out of 4 patients. Irritability and hyperactivity appear early, with a frank organic brain syndrome seen in more severe cases (*Webb WL, Gehi M. Electrolyte and fluid imbalance: Neuropsychiatric manifestations. <u>Psychosomatics</u> 22(3):199-203, 1981*).

<u>Zinc</u>:

Deficiency is associated with apathy, lethargy, amnesia, and mental retardation, often with considerable irritability, depression and paranoia (*Prasad AS et al. Experimental zinc deficiency in humans. <u>Ann. Intern. Med.</u> 89:483, 1978*).

— —

OTHER FACTORS:

Rule out <u>food sensitivities</u>.

Provocative testing with foods and food extracts has been reported to induce cognitive and emotional symptoms.

> **Review Article:** Foods may cause mental and behavioral symptoms by a variety of mechanisms including cerebral allergy, food addiction, hypoglycemias, caffeinism, hypersensitivity to chemical food additives, reactions to vasoactive amines in foods, and reactions to neuropeptides formed from foods (*Rippere V. Some varieties of food intolerance in psychiatric patients: An overview. <u>Nutr. Health</u> 3(3):125-36, 1984*).

> **Negative Experimental Double-blind Study:** 19 pts. with neurotic symptoms who believed their symptoms were due to food allergy were investigated with exclusion diets and open food reintroductions followed by double-blind provocation tests for foods reported to cause reactions. Testing failed to produce evidence that any of them was food-sensitive (*Pearson DJ et al. Food allergy: How much in the mind? An objective clinical and psychiatric study of suspected food hypersensitivity. <u>Lancet</u> 1:1259-61, 1983*).

> **Experimental Double-blind Study:** 30 pts. complaining of psychological symptoms who were found to have elevated MMPI scores noted significantly greater cognitive-emotional symptoms when tested with foods and chemicals than when tested with placebo (*King DS. Can allergic exposure provoke psychological symptoms? a double-blind test. <u>Biol. Psychiat.</u> 16(1):3-19, 1981*).

Rule out <u>heavy metal</u> toxicity.

> **Combined toxicities:**

> **Observational Study:** The relationship between cognitive functioning and hair metal concentrations of lead, arsenic, mercury, cadmium, and aluminum were examined in 69 randomly selected elementary age children. Regression data indicated that increases in <u>arsenic</u> and the interaction of <u>arsenic</u> with <u>lead</u> were significantly related to decreased reading and spelling achievement, and increases in <u>aluminum</u> and

the interaction of <u>aluminum</u> with <u>lead</u> were significantly related to decreased visual-motor performance (*Moon C et al. Main and interaction effects of metallic pollutants on cognitive functioning. J. Learning Disabilites 18(4):217-21, 1985*).

Observational Study: 37 emotionally disturbed children were compared to 107 controls. The disturbed children had significantly higher hair <u>lead</u> and <u>mercury</u> levels, and using discriminant function analysis, subjects could be correctly classified as disturbed or non-disturbed by using <u>lead</u>, <u>mercury</u>, <u>arsenic</u> and <u>aluminum</u> with 77.8% accuracy. Stepwise discriminant analysis showed that <u>lead</u> was the most significant metal in separating the 2 gps., followed by <u>mercury</u>, <u>arsenic</u> and <u>aluminum</u>. There was also a significant positive correlation between <u>lead</u>, <u>mercury</u>, and <u>aluminum</u> levels and ratings on the Walker Problem Behavior Identification checklist (WPBIC) (*Marlowe M et al. J. Orthomol. Psychiat. 12:260-67, 1983*).

<u>Lead</u> toxicity:

Observational Study: 17/31 pts. who had excess blood lead reported 1 or more nonspecific symptoms such as depression, fatigue, irritability, decreased libido and headache. The chief complaint of 4 pts. was severe depressed mood, and depressed mood was prominent in 5 others. Neuropsychological testing demonstrated significant multiple deficits in 14/18 pts. tested (*Schottenfeld RS, Cullen MR. Organic affective illness associated with lead intoxication. Am. J. Psychiat. 141(11):1423-26, 1984*).

See Also:

> *Winneke G et al. Neuropsychological studies in children with elevated tooth-lead concentrations. Int. Arch. Occupation. Environ. Health 51:231-52, 1983*

<u>Mercury</u> toxicity.

Review Article: Mental symptoms from exposure to elemental or organic mercury include: fatigue, irritability, nervousness, shyness, memory loss, lack of concentration, apathy, intellectual decline, depression, anxiety, drowsiness and insomnia (*Kupsinel R. Mercury amalgam toxicity: A major common denominator of degenerative disease. J. Orthomol. Psychiat. 13(4):240-57, 1984*).

See Also:

> *Higgins ITT. Epidemiological approaches to the study of subclinical effects of mercury intoxication, in Hartung R, Dinman BD, Eds. Environmental Mercury Contamination. Ann Arbor, Michigan, Ann Arbor Science Publishers, Inc., 1972*

OSTEOARTHRITIS

See Also: PAIN
RHEUMATISM

NUTRIENTS:

<u>Niacinamide:</u>   1 gram three times daily (taper once effective)
(start with 500 mg. twice daily)
(take with 100 mg. vitamin B complex)

Effects of decreased pain and increased mobility may start to be noted in 2 - 6 weeks. Said to be particularly effective for degenerative arthritis of the knee.

WARNING: May cause nausea or affect liver function studies.

> **Experimental Controlled Study:** 663 pts. receiving niacinamide were shown to have superior scores on an index of joint range of movement than 842 untreated age-matched pts. (*Kaufman W. The use of vitamin therapy to reverse certain concomitants of aging.* J. Am. Geriatr. Soc. *3:927, 1955*).

See Also:

> **Case Reports:** *Kaufman W. Niacinamide: A most neglected vitamin.* J. Int. Acad. Prev. Med., *Winter, 1983*

<u>Pantothenic Acid:</u>

Deficiency may be associated with OA.

> **Animal Experimental Study:** Acute deficiency of PA in the rat resulted in pathologic joint changes which closely resembled those of osteoarthrosis (osteoporosis, calcification of cartilage, and the formation of osteophytes and of lipping) (*Nelson MN et al.* Proc. Soc. Exp. Biol. *73:31, 1950*).

Supplementation may be beneficial.

> **Negative Double-blind Experimental Study:** 47/94 pts. with arthritic conditions (63% with osteoarthrosis) who were previously untreated or who had not responded to previous drug treatment were randomly chosen to receive 2 gm daily of oral calcium pantothenate (starting with 500 mg daily and gradually increasing to 500 mg 4 times daily by day 10), while the rest received placebo. Pts. were permitted to take paracetamol to relieve pain but no other medications were permitted. After 2 mo., daily records kept by pts. failed to show significant reductions in the duration of morning stiffness or degree of disability in either the experimental or control groups. Both gps. reported significant pain relief but neither resulted in any significant reduction in requirements for pain medication. There were no significant between-group differences, and overall assessments by the doctors at the end of the trial gave similar results for active and placebo medication. There was, however, evidence that the sub-gp. of pts. with rheumatoid arthritis may have benefited (*Calcium pantothenate in arthritic conditions. A report from the General Practitioner Research Group.* Practitioner *224:208-11, 1980*).

Experimental Study: Pts. treated with pantothenic acid 12.5 mg twice daily demonstrated a limited, variable improvement starting in 1-2 wks. and ending upon discontinuation of the supplement (*Annand JC. Pantothenic acid and osteoarthritis.* <u>Lancet</u> *2:1168, 1963; Annand JC.* <u>J. Coll. Gen. Practrs.</u> *5:136, 1962*).

Vitamin C:

Supplementation may be beneficial.

Review Article: In the treatment of OA, "certainly vitamin C is always indicated and is harmless in adequate doses" (*Bland JH, Cooper SM. Osteoarthritis: A review of the cell biology involved and evidence for reversibility. Management rationally related to known genesis and pathophysiology.* <u>Seminars in Arthritis & Rheum.</u> *14(2):106-33, 1984*).

Animal Experimental Study: Cartilage taken from guinea pigs with experimental OA fed 2-4 mg vitamin C daily showed classic signs of advanced osteoarthritis while cartilage taken from control guinea pigs who consumed a diet containing 150 mg daily showed only minor arthritic changes with much less cartilage erosion and milder histologic and biochemical changes in and around the OA joint (*Schwartz ER. The modulation of osteoarthritic development by vitamins C and E.* <u>Int. J. Vit. & Nutr. Res.</u> *Suppl. 26, 141-6, 1984*).

In vitro Experimental Study: Ascorbic acid had an anabolic effect on rabbit chondrocytes in a monolayer culture, increasing all growth (proliferation and increase in proteoglycan synthesis) not suppressed by higher concentration of the calf's serum (*Prins APA et al. Effect of purified growth factors on rabbit articular chondrocyte in monolayer culture. Sulfated proteoglycan synthesis.* <u>Arthritis Rheum.</u> *25:1228-38, 1982*).

In vitro Experimental Study: An excess of ascorbic acid was found to be necessary in both human and rabbit chondrocyte protein synthesis (*Krystal G et al. Stimulation of DNA synthesis by ascorbate in culture of articular chondrocytes.* <u>Arthritis Rheum.</u> *25:318-25, 1982*).

Vitamin E: 900 I.U. daily (10 day trial)

A prostaglandin inhibitor (as are non-steroidal anti-inflammatory drugs).

Experimental Single-blind Crossover Study: 29 pts. received 600 mg. of tocopherol and placebo for 10 days each in randomized order. 15 (52%) had a "good analgesic effect" while on tocopherol as compared to 1 (4%) during placebo administration (*Machtey I, Ouaknine, L. Tocopherol in osteoarthritis: A controlled pilot study.* <u>J. Am. Geriat. Soc.</u> *26:328, 1978*).

See Also:

Schwartz ER. The modulation of osteoarthritic development by vitamins C and E. <u>Int. J. Vit. & Nutr. Res.</u> *Suppl. 26, 141-6, 1984*

- -

Sulfur:

May be deficient.

Observational Study: While the cystine content of fingernails in normals is 12%, in arthritics it is only 8.9% (*Sullivan MX, Hess WC. Cystine content of finger nails in arthritis.* <u>J. Bone & Joint Surg.</u> *16:185, 1935*).

Supplementation may be beneficial.

Experimental Study: 100 "arthritics" received I.V. colloidal sulfur. Pain and effusions disappeared in many cases with a return of the cystine fingernail test to normal (*Woldenberg SC. The treatment of arthritis with colloidal sulphur. J. Southern Med. Assoc. 28:875-81, 1935*).

Sulfur baths increase blood sulfur levels.

Observational Study: Following sulfur baths, there was an increase in patients' blood sulfur levels (*Osterberg AE et al. Absorption of sulphur compounds during treatment by sulphur baths. Arch. Derm. Syph. 20:156-66, 1929*).

- -

Glycosaminoglycans: 1200 - 3000 mg. three times daily (one month trial)

Supplementation may be beneficial.

Experimental Study: 28 pts. with severe OA received sub-cut. injections of 300-800 cc of a solution of activated acid-pepsin-digested calf tracheal cartilage ("Catrix-S"). After 3-8 wks., 19 had excellent results, 6 good results, 2 fair results and 1 no benefit. Relief lasted from 6 wks. to over 1 year. There was no evidence of toxicity as assessed both clinically and from lab studies (*Prudden JF, Balassa LL. The biological activity of bovine cartilage preparations. Sem. Arthritis & Rheum. 3(4):287-321, 1974*).

In vitro Experimental Study: An extract of calf costal cartilage plus bone marrow ("Rumalon") was found to stimulate sulfate metabolism in human osteoarthritic cartilage (*Bollet AJ. Stimulation of protein-chondroitin sulfate synthesis by normal and osteoarthritic articular cartilage. Arthrit. Rheum. 11:663-73, 1968*).

See Also:

Experimental Double-blind Study: *Wagenhauser FJ et al. The action of Rumalon, an extract of cartilage and bone marrow: Experimental and clinical investigations. Arch. Int. Rheum. 6:463, 1963*

Green-lipped mussel (Perna Canaliculus) is a rich source of glycosaminoglycans, especially chondroitin-4 and chondroitin-6 sulfate; thus its benefits may be due to their effects.

Experimental Study: 35% of 31 pts. who were supplemented for 6 mo. to 4.5 years benefited (*Gibson RG et al. Perna canaliculus in the treatment of arthritis. Practitioner 224:955-60, 1980*).

See Also:

Green-lipped muscle extract in arthritis. Lancet 1:85, 1981

Double-blind Study: *El-Ghobarey A et al. Quart. J. Med. 47:385, 1978*

Superoxide Dismutase:

Note: Ordinary oral SOD has no effect on tissue levels, although it is conceivable (but unproven) that an enteric-coated pill could escape digestion (Zidenberg-Cherr S et al. Dietary superoxide dismutase does not affect tissue levels. Am. J. Clin. Nutr. 37:5, 1983).

Parenteral supplementation may be beneficial.

References:

Huskisson EC, Scott J. Orgotein in osteoarthritis of the knee joint. Eur. J. Rheumatol. Inflammation 4:212, 1981

Lund-Olesen K, Menander KB. Orgotein: A new anti-inflammatory metalloprotein drug: Preliminary evaluation of clinical efficacy and safety in degenerative joint disease. Curr. Ther. Res. 16:706-17, 1974

<u>Yucca Saponin Extract</u> ("Desert Pride Herbal Food Tablets"): 4 daily (range of 2 - 8)

Supplementation may be beneficial.

Experimental Double-blind Study: 149 arthritis pts., 58.9% considered to have osteoarthritis on the basis of a negative RA fixation test, were randomly given either yucca saponin extract or placebo in periods ranging from 1 wk. to 15 months before re-evaluation. 61% noted less swelling, pain and stiffness versus 22% on placebo. Some improved in days, some in weeks, and some in 3 months or longer (*Bingham R et al. Yucca plant saponin in the management of arthritis. J. Applied Nutr. 27:45-50, 1975*).

- -

OTHER FACTORS:

Rule out <u>food sensitivities</u>.

Non-steroidal anti-inflammatory medications (NSAID's) may increase intestinal permeability to food antigens.

Experimental Controlled Study: OA pts. receiving non-steroidal anti-inflammatory medication excreted significantly more radio-actively labeled EDTA, while untreated pts. did not differ from controls. This suggests that NSAID's are associated with increased intestinal permeability to food antigens (*Bjarnason I et al. Intestinal permeability and inflammation in rheumatoid arthritis: Effects of non-steroidal anti-inflammatory drugs. Lancet November 24, 1984*).

Rule out <u>hydrochloric acid deficiency</u>.

Observational Study: In a gp. of 35 female pts. (ave. age 52), 9 (25.7%) were achlorhydric, while 1 (3%) was hypochlorhydric. By comparison, 2 studies of normal females of similar ages reported an incidence of achlorhydria of 12% and 15.5% (*Hartung EF, Steinbrocker O. Gastric acidity in chronic arthritis. Ann. Int. Med. 9:252-7, 1935*).

Note: While gastric anacidity had been reported in the past to be a relatively common condition which was associated with acne rosacea and a number of other illnesses, the presence of achlorhydria is no longer accepted unless a potent parietal-cell stimulant (such as histamine) is employed in gastric analysis. More recent studies suggest that histamine-fast anacidity is uncommon before the fifth decade of life and, although it probably does not occur in a normal stomach, its presence is not necessarily associated with symptoms (Rappaport EM. Achlorhydria: Associated symptoms and response to hydrochloric acid. New Engl. J. Med. 252(19):802-5, 1955).

OSTEOPOROSIS

See Also: KIDNEY STONES
PERIODONTAL DISEASE

OVERVIEW:

An <u>alkaline ash</u> diet, relatively low in protein (especially animal protein) appears to be beneficial. <u>Alcohol</u>, <u>caffeine</u> and <u>sugar</u> should be avoided. If deficient, the intake of <u>folic acid</u>, <u>pyridoxine</u> and <u>vitamin D</u> should be increased; whether such supplementation is useful otherwise is not yet clear. The use of <u>aluminum-containing anacids</u> should be avoided.

<u>Calcium</u> intake should be 1.0-1.5 gm daily in post-menopausal women, and <u>phosphorus</u> intake should be limited, while <u>magnesium</u> intake should be large enough to insure against deficiency. Supplementation with <u>sodium fluoride</u> may be beneficial, but its disadvantages must be considered.

- -

BASIC DIET:

<u>Alkaline ash</u> diet.

> High acid ash diet (meat and other high protein foods, most cereal grains and other starches) increases calcium excretion and bone loss (*Barzel US. Acid loading and osteoporosis.* <u>*J. Am. Geriatrics Soc.*</u> *September 1982, p.613*).

Restrict <u>meat</u>.

> Lacto-ovo-vegetarian and vegetarian females have less bone mineral loss than omnivorous females, perhaps due to the lower calcium intake, the higher protein intake, or to the higher phosphorus intake among omnivores.

> > **Observational Study:** For men on a high meat diet, long-term calcium and phosphorus balances were 4 and 184 mg, respectively, while for men on a control diet, balances were -15 and 12 mg. The difference was not significant for calcium, but was for phosphorus (*Spencer H et al. Further studies of the effect of a high protein diet as meat on calcium metabolism.* <u>*Am. J. Clin. Nutr.*</u> *37:924-9, 1983*).

> > **Observational Study:** Bone mineral mass in lacto-ovo-vegetarian women was compared with that of omnivorous women. While no significant differences were found in the 20's, 30's or 40's, there was a significant difference in the 50's and older, accelerating with age. At each decade past 50, the omnivorous women had more osteoporosis (*Marsh AG. Cortical bone density of adult lacto-ovo-vegetarian and omnivorous women.* <u>*J. Am. Dietetic Assoc.*</u> *Feb. 1980, pp. 148-51*).

> > **Observational Study:** Bone mineral mass in 48 lacto-ovo-vegetarian women was compared with that of 48 omnivorous women. Before age 60 there was no significant difference. Between the ages of 60 and 89, however, lacto-ovo-vegetarian women had lost 18% of their bone mass compared to 35% in the omnivorous women (*Sanchez IV et al. Bone mineral mass in elderly vegetarian females.* <u>*Am. J. Roentgenol.*</u> *131:542-, 1978*).

See Also:

> *Marsh AG et al. Bone mineral mass in adult lacto-ovo-vegetarian and omnivorous males. <u>Am. J. Clin. Nutr.</u> 37:453-6, 1983*

> *Ellis FR et al. Incidence of osteoporosis in vegetarians and omnivores. <u>Am. J. Clin. Nutr.</u> 25:55-8, 1972*

Restrict <u>protein</u>.

High protein diet is associated with increased calcium loss.

Observational Study: Among a gp. of older subjects, an increase in protein intake from 47 to 112 gm while maintaining calcium, magnesium and phosphorus intakes constant caused an increase in urinary calcium and a decrease in calcium retention. The data indicate that protein-induced hypercalciuria is due to an increase in glomerular filtration rate and a decrease in fractional renal tubular resorption of calcium (*Schuette SA et al. Studies on the mechanism of protein-induced hypercalciuria in older men and women. <u>J. Nutr.</u> 110:305-15, 1980*).

Experimental Controlled Study: 6 adult men received formula diets supplying daily about 1400 mg calcium and 12 or 36 gm of nitrogen. The low N diet contained egg albumin, while the high N diet contained egg albumin and soy protein. Mean daily urinary calcium was 191 mg on the low N diet and 277 mg on the high N diet. Calcium balances on the low and high N diets were -37 mg and -137 mg daily, respectively (*Allen GH et al. Protein-induced hypercalciuria: A longer term study. <u>Am. J. Clin. Nutr.</u> 32:741-9, 1979*).

See Also:

> *Heaney RP, Recker RR. Distribution of calcium absorption in middle-aged women. <u>Am. J. Clin. Nutr.</u> 43:299, 1986*

> *Licata A et al. Acute effects of dietary protein on calcium metabolism in patients with osteoporosis. <u>J. Gerontol.</u> 36:14-19, 1981*

Avoid <u>caffeine</u>.

Increases urinary and fecal calcium loss.

Experimental Study: 31 women ingested decaffeinated coffee at different times to which caffeine had been added. 3 hours afterwards, urinary calcium excretion increased significantly, but only in women taking estrogen, suggesting that caffeine ingestion may offset the beneficial effect of estrogen on calcium metabolism (*Hollingbery PW et al. Effect of dietary caffeine and aspirin on urinary calcium and hydroxyproline excretion in pre- and postmenopausal women. <u>Fed. Proc.</u> 44:1149, 1985*).

Experimental Study: 15 males drank decaffeinated coffee to which 0, 150 or 300 mg caffeine had been added. Total urinary 3 hr. excretion of calcium, magnesium, sodium and chloride increased significantly after caffeine intake, while zinc, phosphorus, potassium, creatinine and volume were unchanged (*Massey LK, Berg TA. The effect of dietary caffeine on urinary excretion of calcium, magnesium, phosphorus, sodium, potassium, chloride and zinc in healthy males. <u>Nutr. Res.</u> 5:1281-84, 1985*).

Observational Study: The caffeine intake of 168 women (ages 36-45) was studied over the long term. Subjects averaged about 2 cups of regular coffee daily and suffered from a net calcium loss of 22 mg daily. The addition of only 1 cup of regular coffee resulted in an additional 6 mg of daily calcium loss. In addition, women who consumed a high amount of caffeine also consumed fewer calcium-rich foods. The authors note that a negative calcium balance of only 40 mg daily is quite sufficient to explain the 1-1.5% loss in skeletal mass annually in postmenopausal women (*Heaney RP, Recker RR. Effects of nitrogen, phosphorus, and caffeine on calcium balance in women. J. Lab. & Clin. Med. 99:46-55, 1982*).

Restrict <u>alcohol</u>.

> **Observational Study:** 8 chronic alcoholics aged 49-61 were found to have a mean density of vertebral cancellous bone which was 58% of normal and a mean density of appendicular cortical bone which was 90% of normal. There was marked reduction in active bone resorption and bone formation (*Bikle DD et al. Bone disease in alcohol abuse. <u>Ann. Int. Med.</u> 103:42-48, 1985*).

> **Observational Study:** Standardized bone samples from men and women who had died suddenly showed that bones of young alcoholics were similar in weight to those of postclimacteric normals (*Saville PD. Changes in bone mass with age and alcoholism. <u>J. Bone & Joint Surg.</u> 47A:492-99, 1965*).

- -

NUTRIENTS:

<u>Folic acid</u>:   5 mg daily

Coenzyme for the conversion of homocysteine (toxic) to methionine. Homocysteine, which is increased in post-menopausal women, interferes with collagen crosslinking leading to a defective bone matrix and osteoporosis.

> *Note: See also "<u>Pyridoxine</u>" below.*

> **Experimental Study:** 5 mg daily for 4 wks substantially reduced homocysteine concentrations (p less than 0.01) both before a methionine load and afterwards (despite the fact that subjects had normal levels of serum and RBC folate) in normal men and pre- and post-menopausal women, suggesting that folic acid may have a prophylactic action against postmenopausal osteoporosis if moderate homocysteinemia promotes its development (*Brattstr:om LE et al. Folic acid responsive postmenopausal homocysteinemia. <u>Metabolism</u> 34(11):1073-7, 1985*).

<u>Pyridoxine</u>:

Promotes the conversion of homocysteine (toxic) to cystathionine. Homocysteine, which is increased in post-menopausal women, interferes with collagen crosslinking leading to a defective bone matrix and osteoporosis. (The incidence of heterozygous homocystinuria due to cystathionine synthase deficiency is about 1 in 70.)

> *Note: See also "<u>Folic acid</u>" above.*

<u>Vitamin D</u>:

Known to be necessary for calcium absorption.

Deficiency is a major cause of osteoporosis.

> **Observational Study:** 82 consecutive hip fracture pts. were compared to 185 controls. Low serum 25-hydroxyvitamin D concentrations were common among patients who were elderly, had poor dietary habits, reduced nutritional status and spent insufficient time in sunlight. OP was more common among them than among controls and was associated with low 25-hydroxyvitamin D levels. Hypocalcemia was also more common (*Harju E et al. High incidence of low serum vitamin D concentration in patients with hip fracture. <u>Arch. Orthoped. & Trauma Surg.</u> 103(6):408-16, 1985*).

Observational Study: Ave. 25-OHD level of 98 women age 65 and older hospitalized for hip fracture was 38% (21 IU) lower than that of 76 matched controls without hip fracture (p less than 0.001). The dietary intake of vitamin D was also significantly lower in pts. (p less than 0.05) than in controls as was sunlight exposure (p less than 0.02). Vitamin D intakes of under 100 IU/day were recorded in 58% of pts. and 41% of the controls (p less than 0.05) (*Baker MR et al. Plasma 25-hydroxy vitamin D concentrations in patients with fractures of the femoral neck. Brit. Med. J. March 3, 1979, p. 589*).

Osteoporotic patients may have a deficit in converting vitamin D to its active form (1,25-dihydroxy vitamin D).

Experimental and Observational Study: The level of 25-hydroxy vitamin D was not found to decrease with age but 1,25 dihydroxy vitamin D was lower in elderly women both with and without hip fractures than it was in normal premenopausal women and normal women within 20 yrs. after menopause. Infusion with a tropic agent for the converting enzyme (bovine parathyroid fragment 1-34) resulted in a higher increase in 1,25 dihydroxy vitamin D for the younger women than for the other groups and the least increase for the elderly women with hip fractures, suggesting that an age-related decrease in the kidney's ability to synthesize 1,25 dihydroxy vitamin D is a contributing factor to the development of senile osteoporosis (*Tsai KS et al. Impaired vitamin D metabolism in women: Possible role in pathogenesis of senile osteoporosis. J Clin. Inves. 73:1668-1672, 1984*).

Observational Study: 15/82 elderly people were deficient in vitamin D (25-hydroxy vitamin D) and 28 more had borderline levels. Even elderly farm workers (who thus spent much of their day outdoors) had significantly lower levels than a youthful control group, suggesting that they had an impairment in vitamin D metabolism rather than inadequate supplies (*Weisman Y et al. Inadequate status and impaired metabolism of vitamin D in the elderly. Israeli J. Med. Sci. 17(1):19-21, 1981*).

Experimental and Observational Study: Decreased calcium absorption was correlated with decreased serum levels of 1,25-dihydroxy vitamin D. 20/24 subjects increased calcium absorption when supplemented with this metabolite (*Gallagher JC et al. Intestinal calcium absorption and serum vitamin D metabolites in normal subjects and osteoporotic patients. J. Clin. Inves. 64:729, 1979*).

Deficiency and resultant disease can be caused by hepatic or renal disease as the vitamin is initially metabolized to 25-hydroxyvitamin D (vitamin D2) in the liver and subsequently converted to 1,25-dihydroxyvitamin D (calcitriol), the active form, in the kidney. Hypoparathyroidism can also be a cause, as parathyroid hormone is necessary for renal activation. (Calcitriol is available by prescription.)

Supplementation may be effective in raising serum vitamin D levels.

Experimental Study: 500 IU daily given to older people with low vitamin D levels resulted in a significant increase by 2 months and levels approaching those of healthy young adults by 6 months (*MacLennan WJ, Hamilton JC. Vitamin D supplements and 25-hydroxy vitamin D concentrations in the elderly. Brit. Med. J. 2:859-61, October 1, 1977*).

Supplementation may be effective in normalizing calcium absorption.

Experimental and Observational Study: 56 pts. had significantly lower mean fractional calcium absorption than 20 age-matched controls (p less than 0.001). Long-term treatment with calcitriol 0.5-0.75 mcg daily (6-24 mo.) significantly increased calcium absorption (p less than 0.001). After treatment, only 1 pt. still had subnormal calcium absorption. Results suggest that insufficient endogenous production of calcitriol may be the major cause of decreased calcium absorption in postmenopausal OP (*Riggs BL, Nelson KI. Effect of long term treatment with calcitriol on calcium absorption and mineral metabolism in postmenopausal osteoporosis. J. Clin. Endocrinol. Metab. 61(3):457-61, 1985*).

Supplementation may be effective in treating postmenopausal women with osteoporosis.

Experimental Double-blind Study: 109 randomly selected elderly women (ages 65-74) received orally either vitamin D_2 15,000 IU weekly or placebo. After 2 yrs., vitamin D significantly reduced the rate of cortical bone loss as measured by hand radiographs (p less than 0.01) (*Nordin BE et al. A prospective trial of the effect of vitamin D supplementation on metacarpal bone loss in elderly women. Am. J. Clin. Nutr. 42(3):470-74, 1985*).

Experimental Double-blind Study: After 1 yr., vitamin D_3 was more effective than estradiol, estradiol with vitamin D_3, or placebo in treating 28 women with post-menopausal OP (*Caniggia A et al. Clinical, biochemical and histological results of a double-blind trial with 1,25-dihydroxyvitamin D_3, estradiol and placebo in post-menopausal osteoporosis. Acta Vitaminol. Enzymol. 6:117-30, 1984*).

Experimental Study: Following long-term treatment with 1,25 dihydroxyvitamin D_3, 62 women with symptomatic OP showed relief from pain and improvement of motility (in <u>all</u> patients) with no side effects, dramatic improvement in previously impaired intestinal calcium transport, non-significant increases in serum calcium, significant increases in 24 hr. urinary excretion of calcium and phosphate, non-significant changes in serum phosphate, serum alkaline phosphatase, and urinary hydroxyproline and non-significant increases in bone mineral content (*Canigglia A et al. The hormonal form of vitamin D in the pathophysiology and therapy of postmenopausal osteoporosis. J. Endocrinol. Invest. 7(4):373-78, 1984*).

- -

Calcium: 1.5 gm. daily for postmenopausal women
(1 gm. daily for premenopausal women over 35)

Women over 35 who ingest less than the above amts. are in negative calcium balance (*Heaney RP et al. Menopausal changes in calcium balance performance. J. Lab. & Clin. Med. 92(6):953-63, 1978*), most likely due to impaired calcium absorption.

Observational Study: 171 early postmenopausal women (ave. age 54 yrs.) who were estrogen-deprived and non-osteoporotic were evaluated. Calcium intake averaged 802 +/- 0.419 mg/day, urine calcium output was 144 +/- 62 mg/day and fractional absorption (estimated using a double tracer method) was 0.266 +/- 0.096. Absorption of calcium in 55% was inadequate at an intake of 800 mg/day and, in 75%, an intake of even 1.5 gm of calcium daily could not maintain a positive calcium balance. Results suggest that poor absorptive performance was due to defective absorption rather than to bone breakdown since urine calcium was positively correlated with absorbed calcium (*Heaney RP, Recker RR. Distribution of calcium absorption in middle-aged women. Am. J. Clin. Nutr. 43:299-305, 1966*).

Experimental Controlled Study: OP pts. displayed a marked reduction in calcium gluconate absorption compared to normal controls (*Spencer H et al. Absorption of calcium in osteoporosis. Am. J. Med. 37:223, 1964*).

Calcium supplementation may prevent osteoporosis.

Negative Double-blind Experimental Study: 43 early postmenopausal women received either estrogen and progesterone, calcium 2 gms daily or placebo. At the end of 2 yrs., bone mineral content in the forearm (measured by single-photon absorptiometry) and in the entire body and spine (measured by dual-photon absorptiometry) remained constant in the estrogen-treated gp. but decreased significantly in the gps. receiving calcium and placebo. In the calcium-treated gp., there was a tendency toward a slowed loss of compact bone in the proximal forearm and total skeleton as compared to the placebo gp., while the loss of trabecular bone (the distal forearm and spine) was the same as in the placebo gp., suggesting that it may have had a minor effect on the loss of cortical, but not trabecular, bone when added to the diets of early postmenopausal women (*Biis B et al.*

Does calcium supplementation prevent postmenopausal bone loss? New Engl. J. Med. *316(4):173-77, 1987).*

Experimental Study: The past and present calcium intake of 90 women ages 19-22 was estimated by a questionnaire. 15 were high calcium consumers (at least 900 mg daily), 52 were ave. (300-900 mg daily) and 23 were low (less than 300 mg daily). Using single-photon densiometry, bone mineral content was found to vary as much as 20% from high calcium to low calcium consumers (*Anderson JJB - reported in* Med. World News *3/10/86*).

NIH Consensus Conference: Calcium intake is commonly insufficient and insufficient intake is associated with decreased bone mineral density. "It seems likely that an increase in calcium intake to 1,000 to 1,500 mg/day beginning well before the menopause will reduce the incidence of osteoporosis in postmenopausal women. Increased calcium intake may prevent age-related bone loss in men as well" (*NIH Consensus Conference: Osteoporosis.* JAMA *252(6):799-802, 1984*).

OP is more common in <u>lactose intolerance</u> due, possibly, to decreased calcium intake due to avoidance of milk products.

Experimental Study: 11/33 women with idiopathic OP had a history of milk intolerance compared to 4/33 matched controls. Although their calcium intakes were comparable, the daily intake of calcium from milk was significantly lower in the OP patients, while their fasting glucose concentrations were significantly higher. OP pts. who demonstrated lactose malabsorption also exhibited a significantly flatter glucose concentration curve during the lactose tolerance test than did the normal women with lactose malabsorption, and lactose tolerance curves were generally flatter in the "normal" OP pts. compared to normal controls. These findings suggest that a disturbance of glucose homeostasis may coincide with asymptomatic minor changes in lactose malabsorption that may predispose to OP (*Finkenstedt G et al. Lactose absorption, milk consumption, and fasting blood glucose concentrations in women with idiopathic osteoporosis.* Brit. Med. J. *292:161-62, 1986*).

Experimental Study: Lactase-deficient subjects absorbed ^{45}Ca from milk and yogurt at least as well as did controls (*Smith TM et al. Absorption of calcium from milk and yogurt.* Am. J. Clin. Nutr. *42:1197-1200, 1985*).

Both acute and chronic hypocalcemia stimulate the release of parathyroid hormone which, in turn, stimulates the osteoclasts to resorb calcified bone (*Hahn TJ. Parathyroid hormone, calcitonin, vitamin D, mineral and bone: Metabolism and disorders, in Mazzaferri EL, Ed.* Textbook of Endocrinology. *Third Edition. New York, Elsevier Science Publishing Co., 1986*).

Supplementation may increase bone density.

Experimental Study: 14 postmenopausal female pts. received a standard diet containing 800 mg calcium daily. After a 12-hour fast, samples of blood and urine were collected for control values and supplementation of 1 gm calcium daily was added to their diets. After 8 days, blood and urine samples were repeated following an overnight fast. Supplementation was found to significantly decrease urinary hydroxyproline and phosphate, indicating reduction in bone resorption, while renal tubular reabsorption of phosphate and plasma phosphate concentration increased, suggesting reduced parathyroid hormone activity (*Horowitz M et al. Effect of calcium supplementation on urinary hydroxyproline in osteoporotic postmenopausal women.* Am. J. Clin. Nutr. *39:857-9, 1984*).

Negative Experimental Study: 103 early postmenopausal women were divided into 3 gps. based on calcium intake over a 2 yr. period. Gp. 1 (#29): calcium intake less than 550 mg. Gp. 2 (#55): calcium intake between 550 mg and 1150 mg. Gp. 3 (#19): calcium intake greater than 1150 mg. All 3 gps. demonstrated continuous bone loss, with yearly levels of 1.9%, 1.6%, and 2%, respectively (no significant differences). Likewise, the changes in mean serum concentrations of calcium, phosphate, and parathyroid hormone were insignificant and did not differ among the groups. In all 3 gps., calcium excretion rose within 3 mo. of starting daily supplementation, with the % rise greatest in gp. one. Calcium excretion rates fell after 3-6 mo. in all pts. When the subjects were stratified according to excretion rate, no differences were seen in the rate of bone loss; conversely, when stratified according to the rate of bone loss, no differences were noted in the initial or final calcium excretion values. These results indicate that a calcium intake of 1000 - 2000 mg had no effect on the loss of bone calcium in early menopause (*Nilas L et al. Calcium supplementation and postmenopausal bone loss. Brit. Med. J. 289:1103-6, 1984*).

Experimental Study: 48 pts. (ave. age 67) were followed over an ave. of 3.5 years. Gp. 1 consisted of 24 postmenopausal women and 1 man over 60 with "typical" causes for their OP. Gp. 2 consisted of men and women (ave. age 47) with OP due to uncommon causes. Initially each pt. received calcium lactate or gluconate supplements according to his or her individual needs; then a particular sex hormonal regimen was added; then a second sex hormonal regimen was substituted for the first; then all hormone therapy was stopped. At each stage, calcium balance studies were conducted. Results indicated that both calcium and sex hormone supplementation improved calcium balance, suggesting that the first line of treatment for most osteoporotic pts. is a high calcium intake, while hormone therapy should be reserved for those pts. with continuing vertebral fractures after 1 yr. of calcium supplementation (*Thalassinos NC et al. Calcium balance in osteoporotic patients on long-term oral calcium therapy with and without sex hormones. Clin. Science 62(2):221-26, 1982*).

Experimental Study: The diets of 20 women (mean age: 70) were supplemented with 3 slices of cheese and 3 calcium capsules daily for 6 months. 11 showed increased bone density, 3 were unchanged, and 6 showed decreased density, suggesting that some elderly persons can benefit from supplementary calcium (*Lee CJ et al. Effects of supplementation of the diets with calcium and calcium-rich foods on bone density of elderly females with osteoporosis. Am. J. Clin. Nutr. 34:819-23, 1981*).

Experimental Placebo-controlled Study: 67 women (ages 37-73) were divided into two groups. One received 750 mg. calcium and 375 mg. vitamin D daily in addition to their regular diet while the other received placebo. After 3 years, bone density increased in group one 12.5% and decreased in group two 6% (*Albanese AA et al. Osteoporosis: Effects of calcium. Am. Family Physician 18(4):160-67, 1978*).

Since post-menopausal women often suffer from achlorhydria which inhibits the absorption of calcium salts under fasting conditions, supplementation with an acidified form of calcium, or taking calcium supplements with meals, may enhance absorption.

Experimental Controlled Study: Compared to normal controls, absorption of calcium from a pH-adjusted solution of calcium citrate under fasting conditions resulted in enhanced calcium absorption for pts. with achlorhydria (*Recker RR. Calcium absorption and achlorhydria. New Engl. J. Med. 313(2):70-73, 1985*).

Supplementation with a small amount of sodium bicarbonate may improve calcium retention in protein-induced hypercalciuria.

Experimental Study: 6 normal women received 44 gm protein in their diets for 16 days followed by 102 gm for 24 days. Calcium, phosphorus and magnesium intakes were held constant at 500, 900 and 300 mg. During the last 10 days, 5.85 gm of sodium bicarbonate was ingested concomitantly. The increase in protein intake significantly increased urinary calcium and net renal acid excretion and the mean calcium balance became negative. The ingestion of sodium bicarbonate alkalinized the urine, reversed the increase in urinary calcium, and the mean net calcium balance became positive (*Lutz J. Calcium balance and acid-base status of women as affected by increased protein intake and by sodium bicarbonate ingestion. Am. J. Clin. Nutr. 39:281-88, 1984*).

- with <u>Vitamin D</u>:

Supplementation is more effective than calcium or vitamin D alone in osteoporosis with calcium malabsorption.

Experimental Study: The effects of calcitriol and calcium, combined or separately, were studied in 45 pts. with OP and calcium malabsorption. Results suggest that calcitriol and calcium suppress bone resorption in OP associated with calcium malabsorption and may be more effective than either given alone (*Need AG et al. 1,25-Dihydroxycalciferol and calcium therapy in osteoporosis with calcium malabsorption. Dose response relationship of calcium absorption and indices of bone turnover.* <u>Miner Electrolyte Metab.</u> *11(1):35-40, 1985*).

<u>Calcium</u> and
<u>Phosphorus</u>:

Calcium balance is significantly affected by the dietary calcium/phosphorus ratio. The optimal Ca/P ratio is estimated to be 1:1, while the typical American diet yields a ratio of 1:2 - 1:4. Ratios of greater than 1:2 enhance bone resorption regardless of calcium intake (*Worthington-Roberts B.* <u>Contemporary Developments in Nutrition.</u> *St. Lewis, Mo., C.V. Mosby Co., 1981, pp. 240-53; Draper HH, Scythes CA. Calcium, phosphorus, and osteoporosis.* <u>Fed. Proc.</u> *40(9):2434-38, 1981*).

Experimental and Observational Studies: In a study of 158 females (ages 20-75), their ave. calcium intake was 600 mg/day with age-related increments of Ca:P ratios and marked loss of bone densities. Confirmation of these relationships was obtained from an experimental study: 38 females (ages 43-65) increased their habitual daily calcium intake from 448 mg/day to 1100 mg/day which reduced Ca:P ratios from 1:1.65 to 1:1.20 and reduced bone density increments from 80 to 110 mils of aluminum after 25-38 months. By contrast, in an unsupplemented control gp. of 42 females (ages 43-67) whose calcium intake was 463 mg/day with a Ca:P ratio of 1:1.70 and whose ave. bone density was 80 mils of aluminum, when studied after 26-42 mo., there was a minimal change in Ca:P ratio and the coefficient of bone density fell to 75 mils of aluminum. Results suggest that treatment of osteoporosis may be fruitless so long as dietary Ca:P ratios are greater than 1:1.25 (*Albanese AA et al. Effects of dietary calcium:phosphorus ratios on utilization of dietary calcium for bone synthesis in women 20-75 years of age.* <u>Nutr. Reports Int.</u> *33(6):879-91, 1986*).

Observational Study: In the U.S. Dept. of Agriculture longitudinal surveys (1971-1979), it was found that, beyond the age range of 19-22, the daily calcium intake of 3,438 females fell from 800 to 500 mg/day while phosphorus consumption remained at approx. 1000 mg/day. As a result, Ca:P ratios of 1:1.4 to 1:1.8 prevailed (*Chinn HI. Effects of dietary factors on skeletal integrity in adults: Calcium, phosphorus, vitamin D and protein. Life Sciences Research Office, Federation of American Societies for Experimental Biology, Bethesda, Md., 1981*).

See Also:

Rottka H et al. The influence of the calcium/phosphorus ratio in the diet on human bone disease: The role of nutritive secondary hyperparathyroidism. <u>Int. J. Vit. Nutr. Res.</u> *51:373, 1981*

Spencer H et al. Effect of phosphorus on the absorption of calcium and on the calcium balance in man. <u>J. Nutr.</u> *108:447-57, 1978*

<u>Copper</u>:

Copper level may influence bone resorption.

In vitro Experimental Study: Mice were injected with [45]$CaCl_2$ 4 days prior to sacrifice and pieces of their calvaria were placed in either a standard incubation medium or an experimental culture containing various concentrations of copper sulphate in the range of normal copper concentrations of humans. The lowest concentration had no effect, while the highest eliminated active resorption of mineral and matrix. However, whereas copper levels were adjusted with soluble copper sulphate ions, only 6% of circulating copper is in a soluble and ionic form; thus the unanswered question of whether bone responds only to soluble copper under *in vivo* conditions is crucial in interpreting these results (*The influence of copper status on bone resorption.* Nutr. Rev. *29(9):347-49, 1981; Wilson T et al. Inhibition of active bone resorption by copper.* Calcif. Tissue Int. *33:35-39, 1981*).

Fluoride:

Clinical studies suggest that sodium fluoride is one of the most potent agents for increasing bone volume in OP patients. Skeletal responses to supplementation include increases in the rate of bone formation, increases in the number of osteoblasts, and heightening of the serum activity of skeletal alkaline phosphatase. Some controlled studies, however, suggest that its effectiveness may be more limited than previously thought (*Editorial: Fluoride and the treatment of osteoporosis.* Lancet *1:547, 1984; Fluoride/calcium in osteoporosis. Letter to the Editor.* New Engl. J. Med. *307(7):441-43, 1982*).

Negative Controlled Experimental Study: 15 post-menopausal OP pts. received 80 mg sodium fluoride daily. Fracture rates of treated pts. were 2.9 new fractures in the first yr. compared to 0.3 in matched controls, while in the second and third yr. fracture rates were approximately equal in both groups. 47% of the treated pts. developed osteoarticular side-effects. In 27% scintigraphy of the ankle was positive, alkaline phosphatase was increased, and radiologic signs of healing stress fractures were present. While total bone density after 3 yrs. was not increased in the treated gp. compared to controls, trabecular bone density was 8% higher (*Dambacher MA et al. Long-term fluoride therapy of postmenopausal osteoporosis.* Bone *7(3):199-205, 1986*).

See Also:

> *Power GR, Gay JD. Sodium fluoride in the treatment of osteoporosis.* Clin. Invest. Med. *9(1):41-43, 1986*

> *Riggs BL et al. Effect of fluoride/calcium regimen on vertebral fracture occurrence in postmenopausal osteoporosis. Comparison with conventional therapy.* N. Engl. J. Med. *306(8):446-50, 1982*

> *Riggs BL et al. Treatment of primary osteoporosis with fluoride and calcium: Clinical tolerance and fracture occurrence.* JAMA *243:446, 1980*

Disadvantages of fluoride include:
1. The bone matrix formed when fluoride is incorporated into the crystalline structure of bone as fluoroapitite is poorly formed and weak.
2. Long-term excessive exposure to fluoride produces osteosclerosis.
3. The therapeutic index is quite narrow, and at the recommended daily dose, supplementation causes significant side effects in 1/3 to 1/2 of pts.

Magnesium:

Deficiencies are common in OP patients.

Observational Study: 16/19 OP pts. had lower than normal trabecular bone magnesium content (by infrared spectrophotometry) and clinical magnesium deficiency (based on Thoren's magnesium loading test) (*Cohen L, Kitzes R. Infrared spectroscopy and magnesium content of bone mineral in osteoporotic women.* Israel J. Med. Sci. *17:1123-5, 1981*).

Magnesium promotes and regulates parathormone (PTH) (*Mahaffee D et al. Magnesium promotes both parathyroid hormone secretion and adenosine 3',5'-monophosphate production in rat parathyroid tissues and reverses the inhibitory effects of calcium on adenylate cyclase. Endocrinol. 110:487-95, 1982*) which, in turn, stimulates the osteoclasts to resorb calcified bone (*Hahn TJ. Parathyroid hormone, calcitonin, vitamin D, mineral and bone: Metabolism and disorders, in Mazzaferri EL, Ed. Textbook of Endocrinology. Third Edition. New York, Elsevier Science Publishing Co., 1986, p. 467*). While acute hypomagnesemia stimulates PTH release, chronic hypomagnesemia is associated with an inappropriately low level of PTH secretion (*Anast CS et al. Impaired release of parathyroid hormone in magnesium deficiency. J. Clin. Endocrinol. Metab. 42:707, 1976*).

Phosphorus:

High phosphorus intakes promote calcium loss through the induction of "nutritional hyper-parathyroidism" (*Jowsey J. Osteoporosis. Postgraduate Med. 60:75-9, 1976*).

Phosphorus intake strongly influences vitamin D metabolism.

> **Experimental Study:** Increases and reductions in oral phosphorus intake in healthy men were found to induce rapidly occurring, large, inverse, and persisting changes in serum 1,25-dihydroxyvitamin D levels due to phosphorus-induced changes in the rate of vitamin D production (*Portale A. Oral intake of phosphorus can determine the serum concentration of 1,25-dihydroxyvitamin D by determining its production rate in humans. J. Clin. Invest. 77:7-12, 1986*).

See Also:

> *Massey LK, Strang MM. Soft drink consumption, phosphorus intake, and osteoporosis. J. Am. Dietetic Assoc. 80:581, 1982*

- -

OTHER FACTORS:

Avoid aluminum-containing anacids.

> Even small amounts bind inorganic phosphorus in the intestine resulting in phosphorus depletion which, in turn, increases fecal calcium excretion resulting in a negative calcium balance. Fecal fluoride is also significantly increased, thus decreasing the intestinal absorption of fluoride (*Spencer H, Kramer L. Osteoporosis: Calcium, fluoride, and aluminum interactions; Spencer H et al. Effect of small doses of aluminum-containing antacids on calcium and phosphorus metabolism. Am. J. Clin. Nutr. 36:32-40, 1982*).

Rule out hydrochloric acid deficiency.

> 40% of post-menopausal women have no basal gastric acid secretion (*Grossman M et al. Basal and histalog-stimulated gastric secretion in control subjects and in patients with peptic ulcer or gastric cancer. Gastroenterol. 45:15-26, 1963*).

Deficiency impairs calcium absorption and increases urinary calcium excretion.

> **Experimental Study:** Absorption of calcium carbonate was compared to the absorption of calcium in a pH-adjusted citrate form in 11 fasting achlorhydric pts. and 9 fasting controls. For the achlorhydric pts., mean calcium absorption was 0.452 for the citrate and 0.042 for the carbonate. For the controls, absorption was 0.243 for the citrate and 0.225 for the carbonate, suggesting that pH and/or the form of calcium salt affects calcium absorption in achlorhydric pts. (*Recker RR. Calcium absorption and achlorhydria. New Engl. J. Med. 313(2):70-73, 1985*).

Negative Experimental Study: A large dose of cimetidine was given to increase intragastric pH but calcium absorption was unaffected, suggesting that gastric acid secretion and gastric acidity do not normally play a role in the absorption of dietary calcium (*Bo-Linn G et al. An evaluation of the importance of gastric acid secretion in the absorption of dietary calcium. J. Clin. Invest. 73:640-7, 1983*).

Note: This study has been criticized on the following grounds:
1. Pts., with the exception of one, were not achlorhydric and thus may have had adequate acidity to dissolve the calcium load.
2. The test meal (pH 5.4) used lowered stomach pH, possibly increasing calcium solubilization.
3. The absorption method required lavage of the GI tract with 7.2 liters of a balanced solution that could have dissolved some of the calcium or increased absorption.
(Calcium absorption and the achlorhydric patient. Capsulations Number 2, August, 1985).

Experimental Study: 4 men with achlorhydria absorbed 0-2% of radiolabelled calcium carbonate. After histalog stimulation in 1 subject, gastric pH dropped from 6.5 to 1.0 and calcium absorption increased from 2% to 10% (*Ivanovich P et al. The absorption of calcium carbonate. Ann. Int. Med. 66:917-23, 1967*).

See Also:

Hunt JN, Johnson C. Relation between gastric secretion of acid and urinary secretion of calcium after oral supplements of calcium. Dig. Dis. Sci. 28:417-21, 1983.

PAIN

See Also: HEADACHE

BASIC DIET:

Avoid <u>coffee</u>.

Has powerful opiate receptor binding activity.

> **In vitro Experimental Study:** Instant coffee powders were found to compete with naloxone for binding to opiate receptors in rat brain membrane preparations irregardless of whether or not they contained caffeine. Instant tea, cocoa, soup powders, stock cubes and extracts of yogurt and cream cheese were without activity. The receptor binding activity resembled that seen with opiate antagonists and its concentration suggests that drinking coffee may be followed by effects mediated via opiate receptors (*Boublik JH et al. Coffee contains potent opiate receptor binding activity. <u>Nature</u> 301:246-48, 1983*).

- -

NUTRIENTS:

<u>Copper</u>:

If deficient, may lower enkephalin levels to affect the endogenous control of pain perception.

> **Experimental Study:** 24 men were placed on a copper-deficient diet. As serum copper concentration decreased, enkephalin levels lowered. When copper levels were replenished, enkephalin levels in the pituitary and central nervous system rose (*Bhathena S et al. Decreased plasma enkephalins in copper deficiency in man. <u>Am. J. Clin. Nutr.</u> 43:42-46, 1986*).

- -

<u>D-Phenylalanine</u> or	250 mg.
<u>D,L Phenylalanine</u>:	750 mg. 15-30 minutes before meals 3 times daily (2 - 21 days for results).
	Double the dose if ineffective for up to another 3 wks.

Side effects: "jitters" or anxiety, headache, hypertension

Inhibits carboxypeptidase A which is involved in enkephalin degradation.

Potentiated in 50% of patients by <u>ASA</u> 325 mg. (or other prostaglandin inhibitor).

Supplementation may be effective for chronic pain, even when standard medications have provided limited or no relief.

> **Negative Experimental Double-blind Crossover Study:** 30 pts. with chronic pain unrelieved by various treatments received either D-phenylalanine 250 mg 4 times daily or lactose placebo. After 4 wks., the gps. were crossed over for an additional 4 weeks. Pain was quantified using a visual analog pain scale and a cold pressor test. Results suggest that DPA is no better than placebo in chronic

pain pts. (*Walsh NE et al. Analgesic effectiveness of D-phenylalanine in chronic pain patients. <u>Arch. Phys. Med. Rehabil.</u> 67(7):436-39, 1986).*

Negative Animal Experimental Study: DPA was not found to exhibit opiate receptor-mediated analgesia in monkeys (*Halpern LM, Dong WK. D-phenylalanine: A putative enkephalinase inhibitor studied in a primate acute pain model. <u>Pain</u> 24:223-27, 1986*).

Experimental Study: 43 pts. (mainly <u>osteoarthritis</u>) were supplemented with DPA 250 mg 3-4 times daily for 4-5 weeks. Significant pain relief was achieved in the last 2 weeks, especially in the pts. with osteoarthritis. The effectiveness of DPA increased with decreasing severity of pain (*Balagot R et al. <u>Adv. Pain Res. Ther.</u> 5:289-292, 1983*).

> *Note: A statistical analysis of the data using a binomial probability distribution revealed the effect of DPA to be insignificant (Walsh NE et al. Letter to the Editor. <u>Pain</u> 409-10, 1986).*

Experimental Double-blind Crossover Study: After 2 wks. of DPA 250 mg 3 times daily, 7/21 chronic pain pts. taken off all other medications noted over 50% pain relief which was not seen or maintained while on placebo. 1 pt. improved while on placebo as the second medication, while 13 pts. noted no significant pain relief from either DPA or placebo. Side effects on DPA and placebo were essentially the same (*Budd K. Use of D-phenylalanine, an enkephalinase inhibitor, in the treatment of intractable pain. <u>Adv. Pain Res. & Therapy</u> 5:305-308, 1983*).

> *Note: The Balagot study (see above) suggests that a longer study period may have resulted in greater therapeutic effects.*

> *Note: A statistical analysis of the data using McNamar's test for the significance of changes revealed the effect of DPA to be insignificant (Walsh NE et al. Letter to the Editor. <u>Pain</u> 409-10, 1986).*

Experimental Study: Normo- and hypertensive headache pts. were treated with 1 or 3 inhibitors of endogenous opioid degradation. The results with D-phenylalanine were inconsistent (*Sicuteri F. Enkephalinase inhibition relieves pain syndromes of central dysnociception (migraine and related headache). <u>Cephalalgia</u> 1(4):229-32, 1981*).

Experimental Study: 10 pts. with chronic benign pain achieved good to total relief with DPA supplementation, usually in as little as 2-3 days. Their conditions included post-surgical low back pain, osteoarthritis, whiplash, rheumatoid arthritis, fibrositis and migraine headaches (*Ehrenpreis S et al. Naloxone reversible analgesia in mice produced by D-phenylalanine and hydrocinnamic acid, inhibitors of carboxypepitase A. <u>Adv. Pain Res. & Therapy</u> Vol. 3, 1978*).

See Also:

> **Review Article:** *Ehrenpreis S et al. D-phenylalanine and other enkephalinase inhibitors as pharmacological agents: Implications for some important therapeutic applications. <u>Acupunct. Electrother. Res.</u> 7(2-3):157-72, 1982*

> **Review Article:** *Seltzer S et al. Perspectives in the control of chronic pain by nutritional manipulation. <u>Pain</u> 11(2):141-48, 1981*

Potentiates acupuncture analgesia.

Experimental Single-blind Study: 15 pts. were divided into acupuncture responsive and non-responsive groups and pre-treatment with DPA or placebo was given. In the responsive group, all showed increases in pain threshold and greater analgesic persistence. In the non-responsive group, half showed increases. Placebo preadministration was ineffective (*Hyodo M et al. Adv. Pain Res. Ther. 5:577-82, 1983*).

Animal Experimental Study: After DPA, acupuncture non-responsive animals became responsive with enhanced analgesic persistence (*Takeshirge M. et al. Parallel individual variations in effectiveness of acupuncture, morphine analgesia, and dorsal PAG-SPA and their abolition by D-phenylalanine. Adv. Pain Res. Ther. 5:563-8, 1983*).

See Also:

> *Cheng R, Pomeranz B. Treatment with D-amino acids and electroacupuncture produces a greater analgesia than either treatment alone; Naloxone reverses these effects. Pain 8:231-6, 1980*

Potentiates morphine analgesia and antagonizes morphine tolerance and dependence in rats (*Hachisu M et al. Relationship between enhancement of morphine analgesia and inhibition of enkephalinase by 2S, 3R 3-amino-2-hydroxy-4-phenylbuanoic acid derivatives. Life Sci. 30:1739-46, 1982*), perhaps because chronic morphine administration increases enkephalinase activity which results in reduced endorphin levels (*Malfroy B et al. High-affinity enkephalin-degrading pepidase in brain is increased after morphine. Nature 276:523-26, 1978*).

L-Tryptophan: 2 - 4 grams daily (1 month trial)
Take with sugar.
Avoid protein for 90 min. before and afterwards.

Supplementation may be benefial.

Review Article: Clinical applications for tryptophan may be as (a) a mild analgesic similar to ASA or acetaminophen which can be used in combination with 1 of them; (b) in combination with diazepam or similar compound to avoid narcotic use; (c) treatment of a possible sub-class of chronic pain pts. with a disorder of serotonergic transmission (*Liberman HR et al. Mood, performance and pain sensitivity: Changes induced by food constituents. J. Psychiat. Res. 17:135-45, 1983*).

Specific effects of supplementation:

1. May raise pain tolerance threshold.

Experimental Double-blind Study (chronic maxillofacial pain): 30 chronic pain pts. were placed on a high carbohydrate, low fat, low protein diet and were randomly assigned to a tryptophan (3 gm daily) or placebo group. After 4 wks., there was a a greater increase in pain tolerance threshold in the tryptophan group, while both gps. noted lower anxiety and depression (*Seltzer S et al. The effects of dietary tryptophan on chronic maxillofacial pain and experimental pain tolerance. J. Psychiat. Res. 17:181-6, 1982-3*).

Experimental Double-blind Study (dental pulp stimulation): 30 normal subjects received either L-tryptophan 2 gms daily in divided doses or placebo. On the eighth day, pain induction through dental pulp stimulation showed pain perception threshold levels to be similar in both groups, while pain tolerance thresholds were significantly higher in the experimental group. Side-effects such as nausea, skin itching, weight loss and mood elevation were more common in the experimental than in the control group (*Seltzer S et al. Alteration of human pain thresholds by nutritional manipulation and L-tryptophan supplementation. Pain 13(4):385-93, 1982*).

Experimental Controlled Study: 30 healthy subjects were placed on a high carbohydrate, low protein, low fat diet which was supplemented with tryptophan 2 gms daily or placebo. While pain perception thresholds (as measured by electrical stimulation of dental pulps) were the same in both gps., pain tolerance levels were significantly higher in the experimental group

(Seltzer S et al. Alteration of human pain thresholds by nutritional manipulation and L-tryptophan supplementation. Pain 13:385-93, 1982).

Experimental Study: 75% success with dental, facial and headache pains unresponsive to other treatments *(Seltzer S et al. Perspectives in the control of chronic pain by nutritional manipulation. Pain 11(2):141-48, 1981).*

2. May restore post-op analgesia in pts. with dorsal rhizotomies and/or cordotomies for intractable pain.

Experimental Study: 5 pts. who had previously undergone dorsal rhizotomy and/or cordotomies for intractable pain, with resulting initial but temporary postoperative sensory deficits leading to the return of pain, were supplemented with L-tryptophan 2 gm daily. After 1 month the analgesic and anesthetic areas began to spread or reappear. In 3-4 months, the maximum sensory deficit imposed by surgery was re-established, and the pts. were essentially pain-free. In addition, 6 pts. with recurrent or persistent facial pain following denervation procedures had a similar result,while 8 pts. with pain due to a peripheral nerve injury showed no change in sensory deficit or pain relief *(King RB. Pain and tryptophan. J. Neurosurg. 53(1):44-52, 1980).*

3. May reverse tolerance to opiates.

Experimental Study: 5 pts. with low back and leg pain on chronic opiate medication were determined to have developed opiate tolerance. Following 2-9 wks. of supplementation with L-tryptophan 4 gm daily, they achieved significant pain relief during the opiate tolerance test and were able to lead more active lives by reducing opiate intake *(Hosobuchi Y et al. Tryptophan loading may reverse tolerance to opiate analgesics in humans: A preliminary report. Pain 9:161-169, 1980).*

4. May reduce reports of clinical pain.

Experimental Placebo-controlled Study (acute pain following root-canal therapy): Subjects given tryptophan 3 gm in 6 divided doses over the first 24 hrs. following the procedure (the period of worst pain) recorded a significantly lower level of pain at 24 hrs. after surgery than those taking placebo (p less than 0.01) *(Shpeen SE et al. The effect of tryptophan on postoperative endodontic pain. Oral Surg. Oral Med. Oral Pathol. 58(4):446-449, 1984).*

Experimental Double-blind Study (chronic maxillofacial pain): 30 chronic pain pts. were placed on a high carbohydrate, low fat, low protein diet and were randomly assigned to a tryptophan (3 gm daily) or placebo group. After 4 wks., there was a greater reduction in reported clinical pain in the tryptophan group, while both gps. noted lower anxiety and depression *(Seltzer S et al. The effects of dietary tryptophan on chronic maxillofacial pain and experimental pain tolerance. J. Psychiat. Res. 17:181-6, 1982-3).*

PARKINSONISM

BASIC DIET:

Low protein diet.

May control the crippling movement fluctuations seen in pts. receiving the combination of L-dopa and carbidopa.

Experimental Study: 11 pts. put on a nearly zero-protein daytime diet demonstrated great sensitivity to L-dopa and reduced movement fluctuations. As a result, the total daily L-dopa dosage could be reduced and all adjuvant therapy to control the fluctuations could be discontinued while the pts. maintained a "near normal clinical state" (*Pincus JH, Barry K. Arch. Neurol. March, 1987*).

- -

NUTRIENTS:

Pyridoxine:

The total dopamine content in the brain is formed by B_6-dependent decarboxylation (*Pfeiffer CC. Mental and Elemental Nutrients. New Canaan, Conn., Keats Publishing Co., 1975*).

WARNING: May counteract the effects of L-Dopa and Levodopa (*Long, James W. Prescription Drugs. N.Y., Harper & Row, 1980*). Zinc supplementation, however, may prevent this from occurring (*Pfeiffer CC. Mental and Elemental Nutrients. New Canaan, Conn., Keats Publishing Co., 1975*).

See Also:

Mars H. Levodopa, carbidopa and pyridoxine in Parkinson's disease. *Arch. Neurol. 30:443-7, 1974*

Hsu TH et al. Effect of pyridoxine on levodopa metabolism in normal and Parkinsonian subjects. *Proceed. Soc. Exp. Biol. Med. 143:577-81, 1973*

Pfeiffer R, Ebadi M. On mechanisms of nullification of CNS effects of L-dopa by pyridoxine in Parkinsonian patients. *J. Neurochem. 19:2175-81, 1972*

Supplementation may be beneficial.

Experimental Study: Supplementation of 10-100 mg pyridoxine daily resulted in better bladder control, steadier gait, and decreased cramps, trembling & rigidity (*Baker AB. Treatment of paralysis agitans with vitamin B_6. J. Am. Med. Assoc. 116:2484, 1941*).

See Also:

Negative Experimental Study: Barker WH et al. Failure of pyridoxine (vitamin B_6) to modify the Parkinsonian syndrome. *Bull. Johns Hopkins Hosp. 69:266, 1941*

Spies TD, Bean WB. Parkinson's disease (paralysis agitans). *Science 91:10, 1940*

<u>Pyridoxine</u> and
<u>Thiamine</u>:

Treatment by intraspinal injection may be beneficial.

Experimental Study: 5 pts. with postencephalitic Parkinsonism obtained temporary relaxation of rigidily following 2-3 intraspinal injections of pyridoxine 5-25 mg and thiamine 5-10 mg. The severity of their tremors, however, was unchanged (*Stone S. Pyridoxine and thiamine therapy in disorders of the nervous system. <u>Dis. Nerv. Sys.</u> 11(5):131-8, 1950*).

<u>Vitamin C</u>:   one month trial

Supplementation may counteract the adverse side-effects of L-Dopa.

Experimental Double-blind Case Study: 62 year-old male had stopped L-Dopa because of intolerable nausea and salivation. L-Dopa was re-instituted along with ascorbic acid. After 4 wks, his ability to move his head increased, salivation decreased, and speech and handwriting improved considerably. Hand coordination improved so markedly that he began to play the organ for the first time in several years. Several times placebo was substituted for vitamin C on a double-blind basis. Each time his condition deteriorated on placebo and improved with vitamin C (*Sacks W. <u>Lancet</u> March, 1975*).

- -

<u>Manganese</u>:

Excessive exposure increases the risk of Parkinsonism. When accumulated by inhalation, it is concentrated in the basal ganglia (*Mena I. Manganese, in Bronner F, Coburn JW, Eds. <u>Disorders of Mineral Metabolism. I. Trace Minerals.</u> New York, Academic Press, 1981, pp. 233-70*).

- -

<u>Leucine</u>:   10 gms. daily (ex. "Vegepro" 2 tbsp. twice daily mixed with juice, milk or water)

5% of "parkinsonian" pts. have <u>olivopontocerebellar atrophy</u> which is often due to glutamate dehydrogenase deficiency causing glutamic acid toxicity (can be ruled out by measuring leukocyte glutamic dehydrogenase) (*Duvoisin RC et al. Glutamate dehydrogenase deficiency in patients with olivopontocebellar atrophy. <u>Neurology</u> 33(10:1322-26, 1983*).

Early trials suggest that some pts. with olivopontocerebellar atrophy will improve with leucine supplementation.

Experimental Study: 3/6 pts improved by 6 months after being supplemented with leucine 10 gms daily, while the disease remained stable for 2/6 (*Duvoisin RC, neurology chairman, U. of Medicine and Dentistry of New Jersey - Rutgers Medical School - quoted in <u>Med. World News</u> November 8, 1982*).

<u>L-Methionine</u>:

Supplementation may be beneficial.

Experimental Study: 15 pts. who had had maximal improvement from standard medications received L-methionine starting with 1 gm/day and increasing gradually to 5 gm/day while medications were continued. After 2 mo., 10/15 were improved. Symptoms responding included activity level, ease of movement, rigidity and dyskinesia, mood, sleep, attention span, muscular strength, concentration, and voice. Tremor and drooling failed to improve in all cases. 2 pts. developed nausea and 1 developed diarrhea (*Smythies JR. Halsey JH. Treatment of Parkinson's disease with L-methionine. <u>South. Med. J.</u> 77:1577, 1984*).

<u>Octacosanol</u>:   300 micrograms 3 times daily

Supplementation may be beneficial.

> **Double-blind Crossover Experimental Study:** 10 pts. with mild to moderate symptoms randomly received either octacosanol in a wheat germ oil base 5 mg 3 times daily with meals or placebo for 6 weeks. Based on a standard self-appraisal rating form, 3/10 significantly improved and none worsened on octacosanol. These 3 and 1 other correctly identified the octacosanol period, while 2 rated the placebo as the active substance and 4 were uncertain. The experimental gp. showed a small but significant average improvement in activities of daily living and mood ratings compared to placebo baselines. Side effects were infrequent. It is possible that the dosage exceeded optimal as other non-study pts. reported that they improved without adverse effects with a daily dosage of 1-2 mg. (*Snider SR. Octacosanol in parkinsonism. <u>Ann. Neurology</u> 16:723, 1984*).

<u>Omega-6 Fatty Acids</u>:

Supplementation with <u>evening primrose oil</u> may reduce tremor.

> Ref.: *Critchley EM. Evening primrose oil (Efamol) in parkinsonian and other tremors: A preliminary study, in Horrobin DF, Ed. <u>Clinical Uses of Essential Fatty Acids</u>. Montreal, Eden Press, 1982, pp. 205-8*

<u>D-Phenylalanine</u>:

Supplementation may be beneficial.

> **Experimental Study:** 15 pts. received DPA 1-250 mg twice daily. After 4 wks., repeat neurological exams revealed significant improvements in rigidity, walking disabilities, speech difficulties and psychic depression, but no improvement in tremor (*Heller B et al. Therapeutic action of D-phenylalanine in Parkinson's disease. <u>Arzneim-Forsch</u> 26:577-79, 1976*).

<u>L-Tryptophan</u>:

Supplementation may be beneficial for pts. receiving <u>levodopa</u>, as competition between tryptophan and levodopa may result in tryptophan malabsorption leading to depression and other side-effects of levodopa treatment (*Levodopa and depression in Parkinsonism. <u>Lancet</u> 1:140, 1971*).

> **Experimental Study:** Mental disturbances were observed in pts. with extremely low tryptophan values and, in 2 cases, IV and oral tryptophan supplementation was followed by considerable improvement of mental symptoms, suggesting that a prophylactic tryptophan or protein treatment during levodopa treatment may be beneficial (*Lehmann J. Tryptophan malabsorption in levodopa-treated parkinsonian patients. <u>Acta Med. Scand.</u> 194:181-89, 1973*).

> **Experimental Controlled Study:** 40 pts. received either levodopa and tryptophan or levodopa and placebo. Levodopa produced striking improvement in ratings of tremor, rigidity, akinesia, gait and posture equally in both groups, while tests of functional ability to do certain tasks showed a significant improvement only in the tryptophan group. Also, only pts. in the tryptophan gp. showed a small but significant improvement in mood and drive (*Coppen A et al. Levodopa and L-tryptophan therapy in parkinsonism. <u>Lancet</u> 1:654-57, 1972*).

<u>L-Tyrosine</u>:   100 mg/ kg daily

Increases dopamine turnover to enhance dopaminergic transmission.

Experimental Study: Supplementation with L-tyrosine 100 mg/kg/day increased CSF levels of tyrosine and homovanillic acid (the major dopamine metabolite) in 23 pts. pretreated with probenecid (a renal tubular blocking agent), suggesting that supplementation with L-tyrosine can increase dopamine turnover in pts. who may benefit from enhanced dopaminergic neurotransmission (*Growdon JH et al. Effects of oral L-tyrosine and homovanillic acid levels in patients with Parkinson's disease. Life Sciences 30:827-32, 1982*).

Deficiency may be due to reduced intake (major sources meats, dairy and eggs) or diminished conversion from phenylalanine.

PERIODONTAL DISEASE

(including GINGIVITIS and PERIODONTITIS)

See Also: OSTEOPOROSIS

BASIC DIET:

Avoid <u>sugar</u>.

Increases plaque accumulation while decreasing chemotaxis and phagocytosis of polymorphonuclear leukocytes (*Ringsdorf W et al. Sucrose, neutrophil phagocytosis and resistance to disease. <u>Dent. Surv.</u> 52:46-8, 1976*).

- -

NUTRIENTS:

<u>Folic acid</u>:   1 mg. daily orally or local application of 0.1% solution

Supplementation or local application may reduce gingival exudate from inflamed and infected gums - which suggests improved tissue health.

Oral Supplementation:

Negative Experimental Study: After 4 wks., pregnant pts. receiving oral folate 5 mg daily failed to demonstrate statistically significant improvements in gingival health (*Thomson ME, Pack ARC. Effects of extended systemic and topical folate supplementation on gingivitis of pregnancy. <u>J. Clin. Periodontal.</u> 9:275-80, 1982*).

Experimental Study: Folate supplementation (4 mg for 60 days) of contraceptive users with normal plasma folate levels improved gingival health (*Vogel RI et al. <u>J. Prev. Dent.</u> 6:221, 1980; <u>J. Dental Res.</u> Vol. 57, 1978*).

Negative Experimental Study: Pts. who ingested 2 mg folic acid twice daily for 30 days showed only minor reduction in gingival inflammation. Plasma folate levels, which were normal, were unaffected by supplementation (*Vogel RI et al. The effect of folic acid on gingival health. <u>J. Periodon.</u> 47:667-8, 1976*).

Local Application:

Experimental Double-blind Study: 60 pts with visible gingivitis rinsed for 1 minute twice daily with either 5 ml of 0.1% folate solution (1 mg/ml) or a placebo. After 4 weeks, the folate gp. was significantly improved compared to the placebo group. Dietary folate did not correlate with treatment results, suggesting a local effect (*Pack ARC. Folate mouthwash: Effects on established gingivitis in periodontal patients. <u>J. Clin. Periodontology</u> 11:619-28, 1984*).

Experimental Study: After 2 wks., pregnant pts. using 1% topical folic acid mouthwash showed significant improvement in gingival health (*Pack ARC, Thomson ME. Effects of topical and systemic folic acid supplementation on gingivitis in pregnancy. <u>J. Clin. Periodontol.</u> 7:402-14, 1980*).

Experimental Double-blind Study: 30 pts. with normal fasting blood folate levels rinsed their mouths daily with 5 cc of a 1 mg/cc folate solution or placebo. After 60 days, experimental subjects showed significant improvement in gingival health compared to controls (*Vogel RI et al. The effect of topical application of folic acid on gingival health. J. Oral Med. 33:20-22, 1978*).

Vitamin A:

Deficiency known to predispose to periodontal disease as it is associated with:
1. keratinizing metaplasia of the gingival epithelium
2. early karyolysis of gingival epithelial cells
3. inflammatory infiltration and degeneration
4. periodontal pocket formation
5. gingival calculus formation
6. increased susceptibility to infection
7. abnormal alveolar bone formation
(*Carranza F. Glickman's Clinical Periodontology. Philadelphia, Pa., WB Saunders, 1984*).

See Also:

> *Cerm:a H et al. Vitamin A level in patients with chronic periodontal disease. Preliminary notice. Acta Univ. Palacki Olomuc. Fac. Med. 107:163-65, 1984*

Vitamin C: 1000 mg. daily

Protects the mucosal barrier against the infiltration of antigenic material such as bacterial endotoxins.

In vitro Experimental Study: Prior treatment with ascorbic acid completely protected fibroblasts in a culture medium against endotoxin challenge (*Aleo JJ. Inhibition of endotoxin-induced depression of cellular proliferation by ascorbic acid. Proc. Soc. Exp. Biol. Med. 164(3):248-51, 1980*).

See Also:

> *Alfano MC et al. Effect of ascorbic acid deficiency on the permeability and collagen biosynthesis of oral mucosal epithelium. Ann. N.Y. Acad. Sci. 258:253-63, 1975*

Subclinical deficiency increases susceptibility to periodontal disease.

Experimental Study: 11 healthy non-smoking males (aged 19-28) ate a rotating 7-day diet deficient only in ascorbic acid (5 mg) which was supplemented with 60 mg/day ascorbic acid for 2 wks., 0 mg/day for 4 wks., 600 mg/day for 3 wks., and 0 mg/day for 4 weeks. No mucosal pathoses or changes in plaque accumulation or probing depths were noted during any of the periods of depletion or supplementation; however, measures of gingival inflammation were directly related to the ascorbic acid status, suggesting that ascorbic acid may influence early stages of gingivitis, particularly crevicular bleeding (*Leggott PJ et al. The effect of controlled ascorbic acid depletion and supplementation on periodontal health. J. Periodontol. 57(8):480-85, 1986*).

Negative Observational Study: Only a weak association between periodontal disease and ascorbic acid deficiency has been shown in an analysis of nutritional and periodontal health data, suggesting that plaque control is more important that vitamin C supplementation in prevention and control of periodontal disease (*Ismail AI et al. Relation between ascorbic acid intake and periodontal diseae in the United States. J. Am. Dental Assoc. 107(6):927-31, 1983*).

Review Article: The work of Olav Alvares, DDS, PhD, U. of Texas at San Antonio, offers "the first concrete evidence that subclinical vitamin C deficiency significantly increases susceptibility to periodontal disease" (*Primate studies indicate that subclinical and acute vitamin C deficiency may lead to periodontal disease. JAMA, 246:730, 1981*).

Animal Experimental Study: Localized periodontal disease was induced in 2 gps. of monkeys by tying a silk thread around a single molar tooth at the gum line. In 2 wks., marginally vitamin C-deficient animals showed 36% greater inflammation in the gingival tissues and a 41% greater periodontal pocket depth around the encircled teeth than a gp. of pair-fed control animals. Also, 23 wks. after the experimental diet began, polymorphonuclear leukocytes of the marginally deficient animals showed a significant reduction in chemotaxis and in phagocytosis compared to pair-fed controls (*Alvares O et al. J. Periodont. Res. 16:628, 1981*).

Animal Experimental Study: Monkeys fed diets with no vitamin C experienced an increase in the permeability of the inside lining of the gingiva that could have contributed to the development of spontaneous scorbutic gingivitis (*Alvares O, Siegel I. Permeability of gingival sulcular epithelium in the development of scorbutic gingivitis. J. Oral Path. 10:40-48, 1981*).

See Also:

> Alvares O et al. the effect of subclinical ascorbate deficiency on periodontal disease in nonhuman primates. *J. Periodontal Res. 16:628-36, 1984*

> Woolfe SN et al. Ascorbic acid and periodontal disease: A review of the literature. *Periodont. Abstr. 28(2):44-56, 1980*

Supplementation results in increased gingival ascorbic acid levels.

Experimental Controlled Study: 11/18 pts. (ages 17-24) with "little" or "slight" periodontal disease received either vitamin C 1 gm daily or placebo. At the end of the trial, ascorbic acid levels were up to 15-20 times higher in the gums of the experimental gp. (*Mallek HM. J. Dent. Res. March, 1979*).

Supplementation may reduce gingival inflammation.

Negative Experimental Placebo-controlled Study: 10 matched non-ascorbic acid deficient subjects received either ascorbic acid 250 mg 4 times daily or placebo. After 1 wk., all pts. were scaled and root planed and received oral hygiene instructions. A gingival biopsy was taken at week 6. Correlations between clinical parameters and ascorbic acid levels over the subsequent 6 wks. revealed no significant differences between the vitamin and placebo gps., suggesting that the use of megadoses of vitamin C in normals does not have a predictable or strong effect on the gingival response to initial therapy (*Woolfe SN et al. Relationship of ascorbic acid levels of blood and gingival tissue with response to periodontal therapy. J. Clin. Periodontol. 11(3):159-65, 1984*).

Vitamin D:

Deficiency is known to impair calcium absorption (*Migicovsky BB, Jamieson JWS. J. Biochem. Physio. 33:202, 1955*).

Vitamin E: 800 mg. daily for 3 weeks (capsules bitten and vitamin applied locally before swallowing)

May be deficient.

Negative Observational Study: Vitamin E levels in pts. with and without periodontal disease were measured. There was no significant difference between the 2 groups (*Slade EW Jr et al. Vitamin E and periodontal disease. J. Periodontol. 47(6):352-54, 1976*).

Supplementation and local application may reduce inflammation.

Experimental Controlled Study: 14 pts. received 800 mg vitamin E daily which they were told to bite open and swish in their mouths before swallowing. After 21 days, changes in gingival fluid indicated reduced inflammation while the control gp. was unchanged (*Goodson JM, U. Calif. School of Dentistry - 1979*).

See Also:

> *Cem:a H et al. Contribution to indication of total therapy with vitamin E in chronic periodontal disease (pilot study).* Acta Univ. Palacki Olomuc. Fac. Med. *107:167-70, 1984*

- -

COMBINED VITAMINS:

Vitamin A,
Vitamin E and
Vitamin K:

> Supplementation with oral application may be beneficial.

> Glutathione reductase is activated and the content of glutathione sulfhydryl gps. is increased in the gingival tissue of patients. Application of antioxidants (vitamins A, E and K) locally and per os normalized the parameters under study and improved the status of the periodontium (*Khmelevski:i, IuV et al. [Effect of vitamins A, E and K on the indices of the glutathione antiperioxidase system in gingival tissues in periodontosis.]* Vopr. Pitan. *(4):54-56, July-Aug., 1985*).

- -

Calcium: 1000 - 1500 mg. daily

Dietary deficiency is associated with alveolar bone loss.

Observational Study: Among denture wearers, those with good underlying bone had a daily calcium intake of about 900 mg while those with bone deterioration had a daily intake of about 500 mg (*Wical KE, Swoope CC. Studies of residual ridge resorption. Part II. The relationship of dietary calcium and phosphorus to residual ridge resorption.* J. Prosthet. Dent. *32(1):13-22, 1974*).

Supplementation may reverse the course of periodontal disease.

Experimental and Observational Study: 10 pts. were found to have an ave. daily calcium intake of 325 milligrams. 6 mo. after supplementation with calcium 500 mg. twice daily, 8/10 had reduction in the size of the pockets of inflammation around the roots of their teeth and all 8 with loose or woobly teeth had some improvement. X-rays revealed that the pattern of jawbone loss was reversed in 7/10, with the appearance of new bone (*Krook L et al. Human periodontal disease: Morphology and response to calcium therapy.* Cornell Vet. *62(1):32-53, 1972*).

See Also:

> **Review Article:** *Aleo J et al. Possible role of calcium in periodontal disease.* J. Periodontal. *55:642-7, 1984*

> *Uhrbom E, Jacobson L. Calcium and periodontitis: Clinical effect of calcium medication.* J. Clin. Periodontol. *11:230, 1984*

Lutwak L et al. Calcium deficiency and human periodontal disease. Isr. J. Med. Sci. 7(3):504-5, 1971

- with <u>Vitamin D</u>:

Supplementation may decrease the rate of alveolar bone loss.

Experimental Controlled Study: 46 denture pts. received calcium 750 mg and vitamin D 375 mg daily or a placebo. After 1 year, the experimental gp. had 34% less bone loss in their upper jaws and 39% less in their lower jaws (*Wical KE, Prussee P. Effects of a calcium and vitamin D supplement on alveolar ridge resorption in immediate denture patients. J. Prosthetic Dent. 41(1):4-11, 1979*).

Magnesium:

Influences the utilization of calcium and phosphate in bones (*Colmore JM et al. Science 172:1339, 1971*).

Supplementation may increase bone density.

Experimental Study: A 1% increase in bone magnesium following supplementation was associated with a 100% increase in alveolar bone density (*Barnett, Louis - reported in Huggins HA. The influence of calcium in the periodontal patient. J. Holistic Med. 2(1):32-9, 1980*).

Phosphorus:

Excess dietary phosphorus impairs calcium absorption (high in meat, grains, potatoes and soft drinks).

It has been theorized that periodontal disease results from a decreased Ca/P ratio by causing secondary hyper-parathyroidism in order to maintain normal serum calcium levels (*Wical KE et al. J. Prosthet. Den. January, 1979; Krook L et al. Cornell Vet. 62:371, 1972*).

Zinc:

Deficiency increases the permeability of gingival tissues to foreign substances.

Animal Experimental Study: Compared to controls, a significant increase in local ^{14}C-bovine serum albumin intake was found in the gingiva, sulcular connective tissue and periosteum and a significant increase in ^{14}C-phenytoin uptake was found in the sulcular connective tissue and periosteum of zinc-deficient rabbits, suggesting that zinc deficiency increases molecular uptake by a number of periodontal tissues. Since these 2 tracer molecules are similar in size and molecular weight to substances known to be cytotoxic originating from oral bacteria, zinc deficiency may decrease host resistance to inflammatory periodontal disease by allowing greater penetration of bacterial products from the gingival sulcus into the adjacent periodontal tissues (*Joseph CE et al. Zinc deficiency changes in the permeability of rabbit periodontium to ^{14}C-phenytoin and ^{14}C-albumin. J. Periodontol. 53:251-56, 1982*).

Serum levels are negatively correlated with marginal alveolar bone loss.

Observational Study: Serum zinc levels were assayed for 51 pts. of varying age and varying degrees of alveolar bone loss as recorded on roentgenograms and found to negatively correlate with marginal alveolar bone loss (*Frithiof L et al. The relationship between marginal bone loss and serum zinc levels. Acta Med. Scand. 207(1):67-70, 1980*).

Topical application may be beneficial.

> **Experimental Study:** A zinc mouthwash containing 18-30 mM soluble zinc markedly reduced plaque extension along the gingival margin over 16 hours, while oral supplementation was ineffective (*Harrap GJ et al. J. Periodont. Res. 18:634-42, 1983*).

- -

<u>Coenzyme Q</u>:   50 mg. daily in divided doses

May be deficient in periodontal disease (*Hansen IL et al. Bioenergetics in clinical medicine. IX. Gingival and leucocytic deficiencies of coenzyme Q_{10} in patients with periodontal disease. Res. Comm. Chem. Pathol. Pharmacol. 14:729, 1976*).

Supplementation may be beneficial.

> **Experimental Double-blind Study:** 56 pts. received either CoQ_{10} or placebo. While the supplemented gp. displayed significant improvement, the control gp. had very little change in periodontal pocket depth or tooth mobility (*Folkers K, Yamamura Y. Biomed. & Clin. Aspects of Coenzyme Q. Vol. 3. Amsterdam, Elsevier/North Holland Biomedical Press, 1981, pp. 109-125*).

> **Review Article:** A review of 7 studies found 70% of 332 pts. to respond favorably to supplementation (*Folkers K, Yamamura Y. Biomed. & Clin. Aspects of Coenzyme Q. Vol. 1. Amsterdam, Elsevier/North Holland Biomedical Press, 1977, pp. 294-311*).

> **Experimental Double-blind Study:** 18 pts. received either CoQ_{10} 50 mg daily or placebo and results were evaluated using a score based on gingival pocket depth, swelling, bleeding, redness, pain, exudate, and looseness of teeth. After 3 wks., all 8 supplemented pts. improved compared to only 3/10 pts. on placebo (p less than 0.01). 8 dentists who were unaware of the study noted "very impressive" acceleration of healing (*Wilkinson EG et al. Bioenergetics and clinical medicine. VI. Adjunctive treatment of periodontal disease with Coenzyme Q_{10}. Res. Commun. Chem. Pathol. Pharmacol. 14:715, 1976*).

- -

OTHER FACTORS:

Rule out <u>hydrochloric acid deficiency</u>.

Reduced gastric acidity impairs calcium absorption which may cause alveolar bone resorption.

> **Experimental Study:** 4 men with achlorhydria absorbed 0-2% of radiolabelled calcium carbonate. After histalog stimulation in 1 subject, gastric pH dropped from 6.5 to 1.0 and calcium absorption increased from 2% to 10% (*Ivanovich P et al. The absorption of calcium carbonate. Ann. Int. Med. 66:917-23, 1967*).

> **Experimental Controlled Study:** 42 pts with alveolar bone resorption had a mean free gastric acidity of 12.4 meq/l and total acidity of 23 meq/l compared to 27.4 meq/l and 44 meq/l respectively in 32 controls (*Brechner J, Armstrong WD. Relation of gastric acidity to alveolar bone resorption. Proc. Soc. Exp. Biol. & Med. 48:98-100, 1941*).

PREGNANCY AND ILLNESS

See Also: HYPERTENSION

BASIC DIET:

Nutritious, well-balanced diet including 60-100 gm. protein.

Multi-vitamin, multi-mineral supplement.

   General Review Article: *Hemminki E, Starfield B. Br. J. Obstet. Gyn. 85:404, 1978*

Avoid alcohol.

   Even mild alcohol ingestion during pregnancy may result in hyperactivity, short attention span and emotional lability in children (*Gold S, Sherry L. Hyperactivity, learning disabilities, and alcohol. J. Learning Disabilities 17(1):3-6, 1984*).

- -

NUTRIENTS:

Folic Acid: 0.8 mg. daily before and during early pregnancy

   Folate is the only vitamin whose requirement doubles in pregnancy. Serum and RBC folate levels decline during pregnancy and some degree of megaloblastic change can be found in substantial minorities of women in late pregnancy (*Truswell AS. Nutrition for pregnancy. Brit. Med. J. July, 1985*).

If deficient, may cause low birth weight.

   Observational Study: The ave. birthweight at all gestational ages of 100 infants with erythroblastosis was lower than that of 200 controls, and there was a strong correlation between low maternal serum folate and the incidence of small-for-dates babies as well as a strong correlation between maternal and cord blood serum folate values, suggesting that a shortage of folic acid available for fetal growth may be the cause (*Gandy G, Jacobson W. Influence of folic acid on birthweight and growth of the erythroblastotic infant. I. Birthweight. Arch. Dis. Child. 52(1):1-6, 1977*).

   See Also:

   Goyal U et al. Effects of folic acid supplementation on birth weight of infants. J. Obstet. Gyn. India 30:104, 1980

Supplementation may prevent neural tube defects.

   Experimental Study: While 24/493 unsupplemented women subsequently delivered babies with neural tube defects, only 3/387 women given periconceptional Pregnavite Forte F (containing folic acid 0.36 mg daily along with vitamins A, B_1, B_2, B_3, B_6, C, D and E and calcium phosphate) delivered babies with such defects. Folate deficiency is believed to account for the differences because the folate antagonist amethopterin causes neural tube defects in animals and pregnant women, and prospective studies have shown that women who later bore babies with neural tube defects had lower RBC folate levels in early pregnancy (*Dobbing J, Ed. Prevention of Spina Bifida and Other Neural Tube Defects. London, Academic Press, 1983*).

Experimental and Observational Study: Half of several hundred women who had delivered children with spina bifida or anencephaly were found to have had a poor diet during the pregnancy which ended with a child with a NTD. 103 of these women received dietary counseling prior to their next pregnancy while 71 controls received no counseling. Of those who improved their diet, all delivered normal children, while all 8/186 newborns with NTD were born to women who ate a poor diet during their first 6 mo. of pregnancy (*Laurence KM. Nutr. & Health 2(3/4), 1983*).

Experimental Study: 80 women who had previously delivered a child with unilateral harelip with or without cleft palate took folate 10 mg daily along with a multivitamin for at least 3 mo. prior to conception and at least until the end of the first trimester. Only 1/85 children was born with a cleft palate while 15/212 children of a similar gp. of women who had no supplementation were born with the deformity. This difference was statistically significant (*Tolarova M. Periconceptional supplementation with vitamins and folic acid to prevent recurrence of cleft lip. Lancet 2:217, 1982*).

Experimental Double-blind Study: 60 of 109 women who previously had delivered a NTD infant were randomly given folic acid 4 mg daily prior to conception and during early pregnancy and 44 complied, while 51 received placebo. None of the supplemented mothers delivered an NTD infant compared to 2/16 non-compliers and 6/51 placebo controls. The difference between the supplemented and unsupplemented gps. was significant (p equals 0.04) (*Laurence KM et al. Double-blind randomized controlled trial of folate treatment before conception to prevent recurrence of neural-tube defects Brit. Med. J. 282:1509, 1981*).

Experimental Study: Women who previously had given birth to 1 or more NTD children were divided into 3 groups. Gp. 1 took Pregnavite Forte F (containing folic acid 0.36 mg daily along with vitamins A, B_1, B_2, B_3, B_6, C, D and E and calcium phosphate) for not less than 28 days prior to conception and until after the second missed period. Gp. 2 conceived within 28 days of starting the supplement or started it after conception but before the estimated time of neural tube closure or missed taking the supplement for more than 1 day. Gp. 3 was unsupplemented. 1/200 women in gp. 1 and none/50 in gp. 2 had NTD infants, while 13/300 in gp. 3 (4%) had NTD infants. There was a statistically significant difference between gps. 1 and 3 (*Smithells RW et al. Apparent prevention of neural tube defects by periconceptional vitamin supplementation. Arch. Dis. Childhood 56:911, 1981*).

See Also:

Laurence KM. Causes of neural tube malformation and their prevention by dietary improvement and preconceptional supplementation with folic acid and multivitamins, in Recent Vitamin Research. CRC Press, 1984

Laurence KM et al. The role of improvement in the maternal diet and preconceptional folic acid supplementation in the prevention of neural tube defects, in Dobbing J, Ed. Prevention of Spina Bifida and Other Neural Tube Defects. London, Academic Press, 1983

Smithells RW et al. Neural tube defects: Prevention by vitamin supplements. Pediatrics 69:498, 1982

Pyridoxine: 20 mg. daily

WARNING: Higher doses may shut off breast milk and thus must be reduced before delivery in nursing mothers (*Marcus RG. Suppression of lactation with high doses of pyridoxine. S. African Med. J. December 6, 1975, pp. 2155-56; Foukas MD. An antilactogenic effect of pyridoxine. J. Obstet. & Gyn. of Brit. Commonwealth August, 1973, pp. 718-20*). Also, the baby could have withdrawal seizures if there is inadequate pyridoxine in commercial formula. Therefore, it is suggested that the mother nurse while continuing to take 20 - 30 mg. pyridoxine daily.

Has been shown in a number of studies to be necessary to keep the laboratory measurements of pyridoxine for pregnant women in the normal range, since it is marginally deficient in about 50% of pregnant women (*Heller S et al. Vitamin B$_6$ status in pregnancy. Am. J. Clin. Nutr. 26(12):1339-48, 1973*).

See Also:

> *Schuster K et al. Vitamin B$_6$ status of low-income adolescent and adult pregnant women and the condition of their infants at birth. Am. J. Clin. Nutr. 34:1731,1981*

> *Reinken L, Dapunt O. Vitamin B$_6$ nutriture during pregnancy.   Int. J. Vit. Nutr. Res. 48:341, 1978*

Given during labor, it may prevent many postnatal adaptation problems by increasing the oxygen-carrying capacity of the blood.

> **Experimental Study:** B$_6$ 100 mg given orally or I.M. at term resulted in greater oxygen affinity *in vitro* (p50) in the newborn's cord blood (*Temesvari P et al. Effects of an antenatal load of pyridoxine (vitamin B$_6$) on the blood oxygen affinity and prolactin levels in newborn infants and their mothers. Acta Paediatrica Scand. 72(4):525-9, 1983*).

Local application as a lozenge may reduce maternal <u>caries</u> which are more common during pregnancy.

> **Experimental Study:** 540 pregnant women received a multiple vitamin with or without 20 mg. pyridoxine as a capsule once daily or as a lozenge (available from <u>Alacer</u>) divided into 3 doses. Although women who received pyridoxine developed less cavities, the difference was significant only for those who received the lozenges (*Hillman RW et al. Am. J. Clin. Nutr. 10:512, 1962*).

May be deficient in women with <u>hyperemesis gravidarum</u> (*Gant VH et al. Vitamin B$_6$ depletion in women with hyperemesis gravidarum. Wien Klin Wochenschr 87:510, 1975*).

Supplementation is said to sometimes be effective in <u>nausea and vomiting of pregnancy</u>.

> Protocol: Start with 50 mg. three times daily. If no relief within 48 hours, increase as needed to 200 mg. three times daily or give I.M.

> > **Negative Experimental Study:** When 180 pregnant women were evaluated to ascertain the relationship between B$_6$ status (pyridoxal 5-phosphate, RBC aspartate aminotransferase activity and stimulation of the latter by PLP) and morning sickness, no correlation was found between B$_6$ and the incidence of morning sickness (*Schuster K et al. Morning sickness and vitamin B$_6$ status of pregnant women. Human Nutrition: Clinical Nutrition 39C:75-79, 1985*).

> > **Experimental Study:** Vitamin B$_6$ alone was compared to B$_6$ plus meclozine. In both gps., approx. 75% experienced complete relief (*Baum G et al. Meclozine and pyridoxine in pregnancy. Practitioner 190:251, 1963*).

> > **Negative Experimental   Study:** No better than placebo in 16 pts. with <u>hyperemesis gravidarum</u> (*Hesseltine HC. Pyridoxine failure in nausea and vomiting of pregnancy. Am. J. Obs. Gyn. 51:82, 1946*).

> > See Also:

> > > *Weinstein BB et al.   Oral administration of pyridoxine hydrochloride in the treatment of nausea and vomiting of pregnancy. Am. J. Obs. Gyn. 47:389-94, 1944*

Supplementation may prevent <u>toxemia of pregnancy</u>.

Experimental Study: 4.4% of women on multivitamins without pyridoxine developed toxemia versus 1.1% of women on multivitamins with 10 mg pyridoxine (*Wachstein M, Graffeo LW. Influence of vitamin B6 on the incidence of preeclampsia. <u>Obstet. Gyn.</u> 8:177, 1956*).

See Also:

Klieger JA et al. Abnormal pyridoxine metabolism in toxemia of pregnancy. <u>Ann. N.Y. Acad. Sci.</u> 166:288, 1969

Note: A case has been reported in which an infant with a partially formed leg (phocomelia) was born to a mother who ingested 50 mg "doses" of B6 daily for 7 months of pregnancy before stopping as they "made her sick." She was also ingesting various other supplements including a multivitamin, vitamin B12 tablets and lecithin and there was no evidence that her supplementation had any connection with the fetal malformation (Gardner LI et al. Phocomelia in an infant whose mother took large doses of pyridoxine during pregnancy. <u>Lancet</u> 1:636, 1985).

<u>Vitamin A:</u>

WARNING: Avoid megavitamin dosages (*Editorial. <u>Lancet</u>, February 9, 1985, p. 319*).

Case Report: 28 year-old woman ingested 150,000 IU vitamin A daily for 2 mo. annually for 4 years as well as for 2 wks. prior to conception and 3 wks. afterwards. The pregnancy was terminated at 23 wks. due to <u>fetal malformations</u> which were found to be typical of vitamin A teratogenicity (*Von Lennep E et al. <u>Prenatal Diag.</u> 5:35-40, 1985*).

<u>Vitamin E:</u>   200 I.U. daily

Supplementation may be effective in preventing <u>habitual abortion</u>.

Review Article: There is reasonable evidence of the prophylactic value of vitamin E in habitual abortion. Conclusive proof is lacking because it would require a controlled study comparing vitamin E against a placebo with no other therapy to rule out interactional effects; however it is difficult to ethically justify withholding all other treatments in habitual aborters (*Marks J. Critical appraisal of the therapeutic value of alpha-tocopherol. <u>Vitam. Hormones</u> 20:573-98, 1962*).

Experimental Study: Of 30 pts. given 150 mg until week 28 who had had usually 2 previous miscarriages in the 2nd or 3rd month, 19 had delivered successfully, 2 were due, 3 were 6 months and 3 were 3 months pregnant. 3 had another miscarriage (*Sutton RV. Vitamin E in habitual abortion. <u>Brit. Med. J.</u> October 4, 1958, p. 858*).

See Also:

Silbernagel WM, Burt, OP. Threatened abortion: Results of treatment in one hundred forty cases. <u>Ohio State Med. J.</u> 39:430, 1943

Shute E. Vitamin E and premature labor. <u>Am. J. Obs. Gyn.</u> 44:271, 1942

Shute E. Vitamin E in habitual abortion and habitual miscarriage. <u>J. Obst. Gyn. Brit. Emp.</u> 49:534, 1942

<u>Vitamin K:</u>

Sub-clinical deficiency is common.

Observational Study: 33/99 pregnant women were found to have evidence of deficiency (*Family Pract. News 14(5):27, 1984*).

Supplementation (along with vitamin C) may be effective for <u>nausea and vomiting of pregnancy</u>. Theorized to work by decreasing placental capillary permeability to prevent transport of a toxin into the maternal circulation.

Experimental Study: Vitamin K_1 (menadione) 5 mg daily along with vitamin C 25 mg daily was effective for 64/70 women within 72 hours (*Merkel RL. The use of menadione bisulfite and ascorbic acid in the treatment of nausea and vomiting of pregnancy: A preliminary report. Am. J. Ob. & Gyn. 64(2):416-18, 1952*).

- -

<u>Calcium:</u> 1 - 1.5 gm. daily during pregnancy
2 gm. daily during lactation
(give 1/2 the amount of magnesium)

WARNING: Hypercalcemia is associated with <u>puerperal psychosis</u>.

Observational Study: The serum calcium of 53 recently delivered mothers with severe puerperal psychosis were compared to that of 35 female psychiatric pts. and 49 normal postnatal women. The mean corrected and ionized serum calcium values of the PP pts. with no personal or family history of psychiatric illness were markedly elevated and were significantly higher than those of the PP pts. with personal or family histories and those of the 2 control groups. Follow-up of 16 PP pts. indicated that the fall in ionized serum calcium levels correlated positively and significantly with improvement in rated symptomatology (*Riley DM, Walt DC. Hypercalcemia in the etiology of puerperal psychosis. Biol. Psychiat. 20:479, 1985*).

Calcium is the only mineral whose requirement doubles during pregnancy (*Truswell AS. Nutrition for pregnancy. Brit. Med. J. July, 1985*).

Deficiency may foster development of <u>toxemia of pregnancy</u>.

Observational Study: The eclampsia incidence and calcium intake for 3 countries, Guatemala (low eclampsia, high calcium), Colombia (high eclampsia, low calcium) and the U.S. (low eclampsia, high calcium) were compared. Crude rates for eclampsia incidence were adjusted to control for age, parity, and prenatal care. Results support an association between calcium intake and the development of eclampsia (*Villar J et al. Epidemiologic observations on the relationship between calcium intake and eclampsia. Int. J. Gynaecol. Obstet. 21(4):271-78, 1983*).

Supplementation may reduce BP during pregnancy.

Experimental Controlled Study: 22 pregnant women received calcium L-aspartate 600 mg daily from 20 wks. of gestation to delivery and the values for the effective pressor dose of angiotensin II were compared with those of 72 unsupplemented pregnant controls. Results suggest that calcium supplementation tends to reduce vascular sensitivity in pregnancy and may prevent the onset of pregnancy-induced hypertension (*Kawasaki N et al. Effect of calcium supplementation on the vascular sensitivity to angiotensin II in pregnant women. Am. J. Obstet. Gynecol. 153(5):576-82, 1985*).

Experimental Controlled Study: 23 women who took 1.5 or 2 gm calcium carbonate daily throughout pregnancy had a mean decrease in diastolic BP of 4-7 mm Hg, with the higher dosage associated with a greater drop. The results were consistent for both white and black women. In contrast, 24 pregnant women given placebo had no such drop in BP. Parathyroid hormone levels dropped with calcium supplementation but rose 25% in the placebo gp. (*Repke, John - reported in Med. World News July 14, 1986*).

Experimental Controlled Study: 36 women with normal single pregnancies (ages 20-35) at 15 wks. gestation were randomly assigned to receive calcium 1 gm daily, 2 gm daily, or placebo.   Baseline BP's, demographic and clinical variables and calcium intakes were not significantly different between groups. The supplemented gps. had significantly lower diastolic BP than the controls between the 20th and 24th wks. of gestation. Thereafter, an increase in the control gp. and the gp. receiving 1 gm calcium was observed, while pts. receiving 2 gm calcium had BP's that remained significantly lower throughout the third trimester (*Belzian JM et al. Preliminary evidence of the effect of calcium supplementation on blood pressure on normal pregnant women. Am. J. Obstet. Gynecol. 146(2):175-80, 1983*).

Supplementation (and/or phosphorus restriction) may prevent or relieve leg cramps.

Review Article: Leg cramps in the pregnant woman may reflect alterations in calcium metabolism (*Pitkin RM. Endocrine regulation of calcium homeostasis during pregnancy. Clin. Perinatol. 10(3):575-92, 1983*).

Experimental Study: 42 pregnant women with leg cramps failed to demonstrate any differences in total serum or ionized calcium concentrations compared to pregnant women without leg cramps. 21 pts. were treated with calcium 1 gm orally twice daily for 2 weeks. Leg cramps ceased in 9/21 and improved in 11/21 while only 3/21 matched controls improved. Treatment increased total serum calcium concentration but did not alter ionized serum calcium (*Hammar M et al. Calcium treatment of leg cramps in pregnancy. Effect on clinical symptoms and total serum and ionized serum calcium concentrations. Acta Obstet. Gynecol. Scand. 60(4):345-47, 1981*).

Experimental Study: Calcium, reduction of milk intake or aluminum hydroxide (to decrease phosphorus absorption) was effective in relieving leg cramps in a gp. of pregnant women. Effective treatment was accompanied by a rise in ionizable calcium and a reduction in blood phosphorus (*Page EW & Page EP. Leg cramps in pregnancy: Etiology and treatment. Obstet. Gyn. 1:94:1953*).

Copper:

Pregnant women may be in negative copper balance unless supplemented.

Experimental and Observational Study: 24 women in their second trimester were found to ingest less than the RDA of copper. Copper retention was -0.02 mg/day until they were supplemented with copper which raised copper retention to 0.89 mg/day (*Taper L et al. Am. J. Clin. Nutr. 41:1184-1192, 1985*).

Iron: supplement if serum ferritin is low

WARNING: Iron supplementation may exacerbate subclinical zinc depletion (*Meadows NJ et al. Lancet 2:1135, 1981*).

Dietary need is known to be increased during pregnancy and amenorrhea and increased iron absorption may not be adequate to make up for the extra demands if storage iron is low.

Experimental Study: 21 pregnant women received supplementation while 21 controls did not. Ferritin fell to 70% of its value at week 16 of amenorrhea in those supplemented versus only 30% in controls. Six and twelve week post-partum levels were still low in the controls (*Wallenburg HCS et* *al. Effect of oral iron supplementation during pregnancy on maternal and fetal iron status. J. Perinat. Med. 12(1):7-12, 1984).*

See Also:

Romslo I et al. Iron requirement in normal pregnancy as assessed by serum ferritin, serum transferrin saturation and erythrocyte protoporphyrin determinations. Brit. J. Obstet. Gyn. 90:101, 1983

Hemminki E, Starfield B. Routine administration of iron and vitamins during pregnancy: Review of controlled clinical trials. Brit. J. Obstet. Gyn. 85:404, 1978

Zinc: Consider supplementation, especially if deficient

Pregnant women ingest only about 2/3 of the recommended dietary allowance of zinc (*Hambridge KM et al. Zinc nutritional status during pregnancy: A longitudinal study. Am. J. Clin. Nutr. 37:429-42, 1983*).

Plasma zinc declines about 30% during pregnancy, while WBC and hair zinc also decline (*Truswell AS. Nutrition for pregnancy. Brit. Med. J. July, 1985*).

Deficiency may foster development of CNS abnormalities.

Observational Study: 259 pregnant women who were either over 40 years of age or had family histories of chromosomal abnormalities had their serum zinc measured during their second trimester. 15 pregnancies were abnormal and in 7/15, mean maternal serum zinc concentration was significantly lower than for the rest of the group (*Buamah PK et al. Maternal zinc status: A determinant of central nervous system malformation. Brit. J. Obst. & Gyn. 91:788-90, 1984*).

Observational Study: Hair zinc of 17 mothers of infants with spina bifida was significiantly higher than that of 30 unselected controls and rose during pregnancy while it decreased in the controls. There was a positive correlation between hair zinc in spina bifida mothers and that of their infants but no such correlation in controls. In addition, mean birth weight and length of spina bifida infants was significantly less than that of the control gp. (*Bergmann, KE et al. Abnormalities of hair zinc concentration in mothers of newborn infants with spina bifida. Am. J. Clin. Nutr. 33:2145, 1980*).

Note: elevated hair zinc usually indicates decreased body zinc.

Deficiency may affect size of baby.

Observational Study: Maternal plasma zinc concentrations of 23 pregnant women carrying small fetuses were significantly higher than those of women carrying large infants both pre- and post- 35 wks. of gestation. In a second study of 12 women with normal pregnancies, there were significant negative correlations between zinc concentrations of maternal plasma and albumin and copper plasma concentration in the third trimester, and mid-arm circumference and ponderal index (a method for determining intra-uterine growth retardation). The authors note that the reason for this inverse relationship between maternal circulating zinc levels and infant birth size is unknown but could be due to anorexia and weight loss causing the transfer of zinc from catabolized tissues to the plasma, while depletion of overall nutrient supply would reduce fetal growth. In support of this hypothesis, the mothers in the study with small infants had 16% lower body weight than mothers with large infants despite almost identical heights (*Fehily D et al. Association of fetal growth with elevated maternal plasma zinc concentration in human pregnancy. Hum. Nutr.: Clin. Nutr. 40C:221-27, 1986*).

Observational Study: Leukocyte zinc concentration declined during pregnancy and was lower in 44 mothers with small-for-gestational-age babies than for 150 mothers with normal size babies at delivery (*Hambridge - op cit*).

Deficiency may foster the development of <u>toxemia of pregnancy</u>.

Observational Study: Low plasma zinc levels were found in women with toxemia (*Cherry FF et al. Am. J. Clin. Nutr. 34:2367-75, 1981*).

Supplementation may reduce the rate of fetal and maternal complications.

Experimental Controlled Study: 179 pts. received zinc aspartate 20 mg between the 12th and 34th wk. of pregnancy while 345 randomly selected controls did not. The control gp. was found to have a higher proportion of both large and small-for-date infants.   Complications during labor (vaginal bleeding, fetal acidosis, uterine inertia) were also higher in the control gp. (*Kynast G, Saling E. Effect of oral zinc application during pregnancy. Gynecol. Obstet. Invest. 21(3):117-22, 1986*).

- -

<u>Citrus Bioflavonoids</u>:   200 mg. three times daily

May be effective in preventing <u>spontaneous abortion</u> and <u>premature labor</u>.

Experimental Study: Many chronic aborters stopped aborting after they were placed on citrus bioflavonoids 200 mg 3 times daily as soon as a period was missed. One pt. who developed uterine bleeding when 3 mo. pregnant began supplementation and delivered a normal baby (*Redman, JC. Letter to the Editor. Med. Trib. April 16, 1980*).

See Also:

Jacobs, WM. Citrus bioflavonoid compounds in Rh-immunized gravidas. Results of a 10-year study. Obst. Gyn. 25:648, 1965

<u>Omega-6 Fatty Acids</u>:

(Evening primrose oil is a source of GLA, precursor to prostaglandin E_1.)

Supplementation may be beneficial in pregnancy-induced <u>hypertension</u>.

Experimental Controlled Study: Pregnancy-induced hypertension is associated with diminished tissue production of E series prostaglandins and an enhanced pressor response to angiotension II (AII). 10 pregnant and 10 non-pregnant subjects were supplemented daily with 3 gm linoleic acid, 32 mg GLA and cofactors. After 1 wk., their pressor response to AII was compared to that of 40 pregnant and 24 non-pregnant unsupplemented controls. While supplementation was not associated with BP changes, the diastolic pressor response to AII in the pregnant subjects was significantly less after treatment and the systolic pressor response was significantly blunted at higher infusion doses, suggesting that supplementation may help to prevent or slow the development of pregnancy-induced hypertension (*O'Brien PMS et al. The effect of dietary supplementation with linoleic acid and linolenic acid on the pressor response to angiotension II: A possible role in pregnancy-induced hypertension? Brit. J. Clin. Pharmacol. 19(3):335-42, 1985*).

PREMENSTRUAL SYNDROME

See Also: "HYPERESTROGENISM"

Premenstrual syndrome can be divided into four subgroups:

PMT-A: ('Anxiety')
nervous tension
mood swings
irritability
anxiety
insomnia

PMT-D: ('Depression')
depression
forgetfulness
crying
confusion

PMT-C: ('Craving')
headache
craving for sweets
increased appetite
heart pounding
dizziness or fainting
fatigue

PMT-H: ('Hyperhydration')
weight gain above 1.4 Kg
swelling of extremities
breast tenderness
abdominal bloating

PMT-A:

Characterized by elevated blood <u>estrogen</u> and <u>low progesterone</u>. Pts. consume excessive <u>dairy products</u> and <u>refined sugars</u>. <u>Pyridoxine</u> 2-800 mg daily reduces blood estrogen, increases progesterone and reduces symptoms under double-blind conditions.

PMT-C:

Associated with <u>increased carbohydrate tolerance</u> and <u>low RBC magnesium</u>. <u>Prostaglandin E_1 (PGE$_1$)</u> may be deficient. Adequate magnesium replacement results in improvement in glucose tolerance and symptoms.

PMT-D:

Mean blood <u>progesterone</u> may be higher than normal during the midluteal phase, and elevated <u>adrenal androgens</u> are observed in some hirsute patients. Other pts. with normal progesterone and estrogens have <u>high hair lead levels</u> and <u>chronic lead intoxication</u>. Treatment depends upon the individual findings.

PMT-H:

Associated with symptoms of <u>water and salt retention</u>, and possibly by <u>elevated serum aldosterone</u>. Vitamin B_6 suppresses aldosterone resulting in diuresis, while <u>vitamin E</u> reduces breast symptoms. <u>Methylxanthines</u> and <u>nicotine</u> should be avoided and <u>sodium</u> limited to 3 gm/day.

(*Abraham GE. Nutritional factors in the etiology of the premenstrual tension syndromes.* <u>*J. Reprod. Med.*</u> *28(7):446-64, 1983; Abraham GE. Premenstrual tension.* <u>*Problems in Obstet. & Gynecol.*</u> *3(12):1-39, 1980).*

BASIC DIET:

Reduce caffeine at least 3 days prior to symptom-onset.

Women who consume large amounts of caffeine are more likely to suffer from PMS.

Observational Study: In a survey of 295 students, the prevalence of PMS, especially with moderate to severe symptoms, increased with greater consumption of caffeine-containing beverages. 61% of women who drank 4.5 to 15 caffeine-containing drinks daily experienced moderate to severe symptoms, while only 16% of women consuming no caffeine experienced moderate to severe symptoms (*Rossignol AM. Caffeine-containing beverages and premenstrual syndrome in young women. Am. J. Public Health 75(11):1335-37, 1985*).

Reduce sugar at least 3 days prior to symptom-onset (PMT-A, PMT-C).

Sugar intake is significantly greater in women with PMT than in normals.

Observational Study: Women with PMT have a significantly greater intake of refined carbohydrates than normals (*Goei GS et al. Dietary patterns of patients with premenstrual tension. J. Applied Nutr. 34(1):4-11, 1982*).

Observational Study: PMT-A pts. were found to consume 2 1/2 times the amount of refined sugar than women without or with mild PMT (*Abraham GE. Magnesium deficiency in premenstrual tension. Magnesium Bulletin 1:68-73, 1982*).

Refined sugar increases the urinary excretion of magnesium, a deficiency of which may contribute to PMT (*Seelig M. Human requirements of magnesium: Factors that increase needs, in Durlach J, Ed. First Int. Sympos. on Magnesium Deficiency in Human Pathology. Paris, Springer, Verlag, 1971, p. 11*).

During the luteal phase, cells have an increased capacity to bind insulin which may be further modified by sugar (*Muggeo M et al. Change in affinity of insulin receptors following oral glucose in normal adults. J. Clin. Endocrinol. Metabol. 44:1206-9, 1977; De Pirro R et al. Insulin receptors during the menstrual cycle in normal women. J. Clin. Endocrinol. Metabol. 47(6):1387-89, 1978*).

Reduce salt to 3 gm/day at least 3 days prior to symptom-onset (PMT-C, PMT-H).

Salt may aggravate PMT-C as it enhances glucose-induced insulin production by facilitating glucose absorption (*Ferrannini E et al. Sodium elevates the plasma glucose response to glucose ingestion in man. J. Clin. Endocrinol. Metab. 54:455, 1982*).

PMT-H is associated with a relative deficiency of dopamine at the renal level (*Kuchel D et al. Catecholamine excretion in 'idiopathic' edema: Decreased dopamine excretion, a pathologic factor: J. Endocrinol. Metab. 44:639, 1977*). Dopamine is natiuretic and diuretic (*McDonald RH et al. Effects of dopamine in man: Augmentation of sodium excretion, glomerular filtration rate and renal plasma flow. J. Clin. Invest. 43:1116, 1964*); thus a deficiency leads to sodium and water retention.

Reduce intake of dairy products and calcium (PMT-A).

Impair absorption of magnesium, a deficiency of which may contribute to PMT (*Seelig M. Human requirements of magnesium: Factors that increase needs, in Durlach J, Ed. First Int. Sympos. on Magnesium Deficiency in Human Pathology. Paris, Springer, Verlag, 1971, p. 11*).

Consumed by PMT-A pts. in significantly higher quantities than by normals (*Goei GS et al. Dietary patterns of patients with premenstrual tension. J. Applied Nutr. 34(1):4-11, 1982; Abraham GE. Magnesium deficiency in premenstrual tension. Magnesium Bulletin 1:68-73, 1982*).

Ca/Mg ratio in the diet appears to be significantly higher in pts. with PMT-A than both normals and other PMT patients (*Abraham, 1982 - ibid*).

Hair calcium levels are significantly more likely to be elevated in PMT-A pts. than in normals (*Abraham GE. Nutritional factors in the etiology of the premenstrual syndrome. J. Reproductive Med. 28(7):446-464, 1983*).

- -

NUTRIENTS:

Pyridoxine: 500 mg. daily   (3 month trial)

May be deficient.

> **Negative Observational Study:** There was no correlation between the severity of PMS symptoms in 210 healthy premenopausal women and plasma pyridoxal-5-phosphate levels (*Richie CD, Singkamani R. Plasma pyridoxal-5^1-phosphate in women with the premenstrual syndrome. Human Nutr.: Clin. Nutr. 40C:75-80, 1986*).

Supplementation may be beneficial.

> (Based on unpublished data, Abraham suggests that B_6 500 mg daily in sustained release form will decrease symptoms of PMT-A, PMT-C and PMT-H. It will also benefit PMT-D, but only when combined with PMT-A (*Abraham GE - personal communication reported in Piesse JW. Nutrition factors in the premenstrual syndrome: A review. Int. Clin. Nutr. Rev. 4(2):54-81, 1984*).

> **Experimental Study:** 70-80% of 630 women taking 80-200 mg B_6 daily reported significant improvement in symptomatology. There were no cases of neuropathy and side effects were minimal (*Brush MG, Perry M. Pyridoxine and the premenstrual syndrome. Lancet 1:1339, 1985*).

> **Experimental Double-blind Study:** 434 pts. with 1 or more of the following cyclic symptoms: tension, irritability, depression, lethargy, lack of coordination, violent feelings, breast tenderness, headache, edema, bloating or acne received B_6 25-100 mg twice daily (adjusted by pts. depending upon relief or side-effects) or placebo. While there was no significant difference in relief of any 1 symptom, overall improvement was noted in 82% of the B_6 gp. compared to 70% of the placebo gp. (p less than 0.02). Pts. who took analgesics during the study were significantly less likely to benefit from either B_6 or placebo (*Williams MJ et al. Controlled trial of pyridoxine in the premenstrual syndrome. J. Int. Med. Res. 13:174-79, 1985*).

> **Experimental Double-blind Crossover Study:** 48 women were given 100 mg. B_6 daily or placebo for 2 months and then changed to the other treatment for 2 months. During B_6 administration 30 subjects reported significant improvement and 6 reported no change; during placebo 10 reported improvement and 20 did not. The difference in favor of B_6 was significant (p less than .001) (*Barr W. Pyridoxine supplements in the premenstrual syndrome. Practitioner 228:425-7, 1984*).

> **Experimental Double-blind Crossover Case Report:** In a multiple crossover trial of B_6 50 mg daily before and during menses for 7 cycles, the results from B_6 vs. placebo were highly significant (p less than 0.008) (*Mattes JA, Martin D. Human Nutr.: Applied Nutr. 36A:131-33, 1981*).

> **Experimental Double-blind Crossover Study:**   After 3 cycles, 21/25 women in all 4 PMT subgroups had responded better to B_6 500 mg daily than to placebo. In all 3 PMT-H pts., B_6 decreased weight

gain below 3 lbs. with concomitant symptom relief (*Abraham GE, Hargrove JT. Effect of vitamin B-6 on premenstrual symptomatology in women with premenstrual tension syndrome: A double-blind crossover study. Infertility 3:155-165, 1980*).

Negative Experimental Double-blind Crossover Study: 13 pts. received either placebo or B$_6$ 50 mg during the luteal phase in randomly alternating fashion from month to month. After 8-12 mo., there was no difference between B$_6$ and placebo (*Stokes J, Mendels J. Pyridoxine and premenstrual tension. Letter to the Editor. Lancet 1:1177-78, 1972*).

> *Note: Negative results may have been due to the relatively low B$_6$ dosage and/or a continuing effect of B$_6$ into the following placebo cycle and/or a longer period than 1 mo. for maximal B$_6$ effects.*

Experimental Study: 58 pts. with premenstrual depression, emotional fatigue and irritability who had been on oral contraceptives for an ave. of 14 months were supplemented with pyridoxine 50 mg daily at the first sign of premenstrual symptoms. 75.8% responded, with 18/58 noting complete resolution, 26/58 noting considerable improvement and 14/58 unchanged. Results were noted within hours or, at the latest, by the next day (*Baumblatt MJ, Winston F. Pyridoxine and the pill. Letter to the Editor. Lancet 1:832, 1970*).

See Also:

> **Experimental Single-blind Study:** *Day JB. Clinical trials in premenstrual syndrome. Curr. Med. Res. Opin. 6 (Suppl. 5):40-45, 1979*

> **Experimental Single-blind Study:** *Kerr GD. the management of the premenstrual syndrome. Curr. Med. Res. Opin. 4 (Suppl. 4):29-34, 1977*

Supplementation with pyridoxine may normalize deficient intracellular magnesium levels.

Experimental Study: 9 females with low RBC Mg levels received vitamin B$_6$ 100 mg twice daily. After 4 wks., RBC Mg levels had normalized (*Abraham GE et al. Effect of vitamin B$_6$ on plasma and red blood cell magnesium levels in premenopausal women. Ann. Clin. Lab. Sci. 11(4):333-36, 1981*).

A co-factor in the conversion of gamma-linoleic acid (GLA) to dihommogamma linolenic acid (DGLA) and of DGLA to prostaglandin E$_1$ (*See "Omega-6 Fatty Acids" below*).

<u>Vitamin A</u>:   100,000 - 300,000 IU daily (2nd half of cycle)

WARNING: close medical supervision is necessary due to possible toxic side-effects

Supplementation may be beneficial.

Experimental Single-blind Study: Pts. received 2-300,000 IU daily premenstrually or placebo. All experimental subjects benefited, compared to 25% of those on placebo (*Block E. The use of vitamin A in premenstrual tension. Acta Obst. Gynec. Scand. 39:586-92, 1960*).

Experimental Study: 218 pts. received 2-300,000 IU daily. 48% had complete symptom relief, 41.2% had a partial effect and 10.8% failed to improve. Results were best for premenstrual headache and worst for PMT-A (*Block - ibid*).

Experimental Study: 100 pts. received 50,000 IU twice daily during the second half of their cycles with good results (*Kleine HO. Vitamin A therapie bei pra menstruellen nervosen Beschwerden. Dtsch. med. Wschr. 79:879-80, 1954*).

Experimental Study: 30 pts. received 200,000 IU daily from day 15 of their cycles until symptom-onset. After 2-6 mo. the majority of pts. were considerably improved. PMT-H responded better than PMT-A. Symptoms did not recur in the year following cessation of vitamin A therapy (*Argonz J, Albinzano C. Premenstrual tension treated with vitamin A. J. Clin. Endocrinol. 10:1579-89, 1950*).

Vitamin E: 300 I.U. daily (2 month trial)
      Increase to 600 I.U. daily if ineffective

Supplementation may be beneficial.

Experimental Study: 150-600 IU daily reduced premenstrual symptoms in women in PMS-A, PMS-C and PMS-D groups (*London RS et al. J. Am. Coll. Nutr. 3(4):351-6, 1984*).

Experimental Double-blind Study: 75 pts. with benign breast disease and PMT randomly received either D,L-alpha-tocopherol 75 IU (#18), 150 IU (#19), or 300 IU (#19) twice daily or placebo (#19). After 2 mo., supplementation significantly improved PMT-A at the 150 IU twice daily dosage, and PMT-C and PMT-D at the 300 IU twice daily dosage, but not PMT-H. Post-menstrually there was a small but significant increase in PMT-H symptoms (*London RS et al. The effect of alpha-tocopherol on premenstrual symptomatology: A double-blind trial. J.Am.Coll.Nutr. 2:115-122, 1983*).

- -

Magnesium: 400 mg. daily

May be deficient.

Observational Study: 26 pts. had significantly lower RBC Mg than 9 normals (p less than 0.01) despite no significant differences in serum Mg levels (*Abraham GE, Lubran MD. Serum and red cell magnesium levels in patients with premenstrual tension. Am. J. Clin. Nutr. 34:1264-66, 1981*).

Magnesium deficiency causes depletion of brain dopamine (*Barbeau A et al. Deficience en magnesium et dopamine cerebrale, in Durlach J, Ed. First Int. Sym. on Magnesium Deficit in Human Pathology. Paris, Vittel, 1973, p. 149*). Since PMT-A is believed to be associated with relative dopamine depletion by excess estrogen in the luteal phase (*Redmond DE et al. Menstrual cycle and ovarian hormone effects on plasma and platelet monamine oxidase (MAO) and plasma dopamine-hydroxylase activities in the Rhesus monkey. Psychosom. Med. 37:417, 1975*), Mg deficiency may contribute to the syndrome.

May reduce glucose-induced insulin secretion (*Curry DL et al. Magnesium modulation of glucose-induced insulin secretion by the perfused rat pancreas. Endocrinology 101:203, 1977*); thus a deficiency could favor the development of PMT-C.

Required for the the conversion of cis-linoleic acid to gamma-linolenic acid by delta-6-desaturase (*Cunnane SC, Horrobin DF. Parenteral linoleic and gamma-linolenic acids ameliorate the gross effects of zinc deficiency. Proc. Soc. Exp. Biol. & Med. 164:583, 1980*) (See "Omega-6 Fatty Acids" below).

Deficiency causes hyperplasia of the adrenal cortex, elevated aldosterone levels and increased extracellular fluid volume (*Cantin M. Hyperaldosteronisme secondaire au cours de la carence en magnesium, in Durlach J. First Int. Sympos. on Magnesium Deficit in Human Pathology. Paris, F. Vittel, 1973, p. 461*). Aldosterone also increases urinary magnesium excretion (*Horton R, Biglieri EG. Effect of aldosterone on the metabolism of magnesium. J. Clin. Endocrinol. 22:1187, 1962*).

Supplementation may be beneficial.

Experimental Study: 192 pts. received magnesium nitrate 4.5-6 gm daily for 1 wk. premenstrually and 2 days menstrually. Nervous tension was relieved in 159/179 (89%); mastalgia in 155/162 (96%);

weight gain in 59/62 (95%); and headache in 16/37 (43%) (*Nicholas A. Traitement du syndrome premenstruel et de la dysmenorrhee par l'ion magnesium, in Durlach J, Ed. First Int. Sympos. on Magnesium Deficiency in Human Pathology. Paris, Springer, Verlag, 1973, pp. 261-3*).

See Also:

Abraham GE. Magnesium deficiency in premenstrual tension. Magnesium Bull. 1:68-73, 1982

- -

Omega-6 Fatty Acids:

linoleic acid → GLA → DGLA → prostaglandin E_1

Example: Evening Primrose Oil (a source of GLA) 500 mg. three times daily

A functional deficiency of essential fatty acids, either due to inadequate linoleic acid intake or absorption or to failure of normal conversion of linoleic acid to GLA, has been postulated to cause abnormal sensitivity to prolactin and the features of PMS (*Horrobin DF. The role of essential fatty acids and prostaglandins in the premenstrual syndrome. J. Reprod. Med. 28(7):465-68, 1983*).

PGE_1 inhibits glucose-induced insulin secretion (*Gugliano D, Torella R. Prostaglandin E_1 inhibits glucose-induced insulin secretion in man. Prostaglandins Med. 48:302, 1979*).

Supplementation may be beneficial.

Experimental Double-blind Study: 30 pts. with severe PMS received EPO 1500 mg twice daily or placebo. After 4 menstrual cycles, EPO-treated pts. showed decreased premenstrual symptoms (particularly depression) more frequently than pts. on placebo. EPO decreased TXB_2 formation (a potent vasodilator) but had no effect on 6-keto-PGF_1 alpha (another potent vasodilator) (*Puolakka J et al. Biochemical and clinical effects of treating the premenstrual syndrome with prostaglandin synthesis precursors. J. Reprod. Med. 39(3):149-53, 1985*).

Experimental Double-blind Crossover Study: Pts. received either EPO or placebo for 2 cycles and the other treatent for a further 2 cycles. Overall improvement with EPO was 60% compared to 40% with placebo. The advantages of EPO were greatest in regard to irritability and depression (*Dept. of Obstetrics, Helsinki U. - reported in Horrobin DF. The role of essential fatty acids and prostaglandins in the premenstrual syndrome. J. Reprod. Med. 28(7):465-68, 1983*).

Experimental Study: 68 pts. with severe PMS who had failed to improve with medications or pyridoxine received EPO 1-2 gm twice daily starting 3 days prior to symptom-onset and continuing to the start of menstruation. 61% reported full relief and 23% partial relief. Of the 36 with mastodynia, 72% reported full relief and 14% partial relief. PMT-A, PMT-D, PMT-C and PMT-H pts. all responded, although cases of PMT-H with severe fluid retention responded poorly (*Brush MG. Evening primrose oil in the treatment of the premenstrual syndrome, in Horrobin DF, Ed. Clinical Uses of Essential Fatty Acids. Montreal, Eden Press, 1982, PP. 155-62*).

PSORIASIS

See Also: RHEUMATOID ARTHRITIS

NUTRIENTS:

Folic Acid:

May be deficient.

> **Experimental Study:** 16/58 (27%) pts. had low serum folate levels, 4/58 (7%) had subnormal RBC folate levels and 16 (27%) had hypersegmented polymorphs in peripheral blood films, while folic acid absorption was normal in all 12 pts. tested. It appears that the high incidence of mild folate deficiency is due to increased utilization of folate by the process and by clinically uninvolved psoriatic skin (*Fry L et al. the mechanism of folate deficiency in psoriasis. Brit. J. Dermatol. 84:539-44, 1971*).

Vitamin A:

The polyamines (putrescine, spermidine and spermine) are increased in psoriasis and lowering of cutaneous and urinary levels is associated with clinical improvement (*Proctor M et al. Lowered cutaneous and urinary levels of polyamines with clinical improvement in treated psoriasis. Arch. Dermatol. 115:945-49, 1979*).

Since Vitamin A inhibits ornithine decarboxylase, the rate-limiting step in endogenous polyamine synthesis (*Haddox M et al. Retinol inhibition of ornithine decarboxylase induction and G1 progression in CHD cells. Cancer Res. 39:4930-38, 1979*), supplementation may be beneficial.

Vitamin B$_{12}$:

Supplementation by injection may be beneficial.

> **Experimental Study:** Vitamin B$_{12}$, triamcinolone or normal saline was injected into lesions with a spring-loaded gun giving a concentration in the epidermis and penetration into the superficial and middle dermis. Triamcinolone caused rapid regression, while normal saline had no effect. Of the 8 pts. who received vitamin B$_{12}$, 6 showed regression of the lesion (*Carslaw RW, Neill J. Vitamin B$_{12}$ in psoriasis. Letter to the Editor. Brit. Med. J. 1:611, 1963*).

> **Negative Double-blind Experimental Study:** 33 pts. with psoriasis for over 2 yrs. who had failed to respond to conventional treatments randomly received 21 injections of either vitamin B$_{12}$ or placebo within 4 wks. Results were assessed at completion and 6 wks. later. There was no difference in results between B$_{12}$ and placebo (*Sneddon JB. Vitamin B$_{12}$ in psoriasis. Letter to the Editor. Brit. Med. J. 1:328, 1963*).

> **Experimental Study:** Good results were obtained with a series of 30 injections of vitamin B$_{12}$ 1000 mcg IM but a shorter series was ineffective. Improvement was often delayed up to 6 wks. after treatment was completed (*Cohen EL. Vitamin B$_{12}$ in psoriasis. Letter to the Editor. Brit. Med. J. 1:125, 1963*).

Negative Experimental Study: Treatment with a series of 15 IM injections of vitamin B_{12} 1000 mcg was ineffective (*Baker H, Comaish JS. Brit. Med. J. December 29, 1962, p. 1729*).

See Also:

Ruedemann R. *Treatment of psoriasis with large doses of vitamin B_{12}: 1,000 micrograms per cubic centimeter. Arch. Dermatol. 69:738, 1954*

- -

Copper:

May be elevated.

Observational Study: Compared to healthy controls, plasma copper levels in psoriatic pts. were significantly higher as measured by atomic absorption spectrophotometry (*Donadini A et al. Plasma levels of Zn, Cu and Ni in healthy controls and in psoriatic patients. Acta Vitaminol. Enzymol. 2:9-16, 1980*).

Nickel:

May be deficient.

Observational Study: Compared to healthy controls, plasma nickel levels in psoriatic pts. were significantly lower as measured by atomic absorption spectrophotometry (*Donadini A et al. Plasma levels of Zn, Cu and Ni in healthy controls and in psoriatic patients. Acta Vitaminol. Enzymol. 2:9-16, 1980*).

Selenium:

Required for activation of glutathione peroxidase, an inhibitor of the 5-lipoxygenase pathway which promotes formation of inflammatory leukotrienes (*White A et al. Role of lipoxygenase products in the pathogenesis and therapy of psoriasis and other dermatoses. Arch. Dermatol. 119:541-7, 1983*).

May be deficient.

Observational Study: The glutathione peroxidase levels of 95 pts. was significantly lower than that of controls (p less than 0.001) (*Juhlin L et al. Blood glutathione-peroxidase levels in skin diseases: Effect of selenium and vitamin E treatment. Acta Dermat. Vener Stockholm 62:211-14, 1982*).

Zinc:

May be deficient.

Observational Study: Compared to healthy controls, plasma zinc levels in psoriatic pts. were significantly lower as measured by atomic absorption spectrophotometry (*Donadini A et al. Plasma levels of Zn, Cu and Ni in healthy controls and in psoriatic patients. Acta Vitaminol. Enzymol. 2:9-16, 1980*).

- -

Essential Fatty Acids:

Patients have changes in fatty acid distribution.

Observational Study: The fatty acid composition of plasma lipid esters (cholesterol esters, triglycerides and phospholipids) and adipose tissue of 20 male pts. and 36 matched controls were examined. In comparison to controls, patients' plasma lipid esters contained significantly lower levels of linoleic acid (18:2 omega 6) and alpha-linolenic acid (18:3 omega 3), and higher levels of dihomo-gamma-linolenic acid (20:2 omega 6). In the patients' adipose tissue, the amt. of alpha-linolenic acid was significantly decreased, while that of arachidonic acid (20:4 omega 6) was increased (*Vahlquist C et al. The fatty-acid spectrum in plasma and adipose tissue in patients with psoriasis. Arch. Dermatol. Res. 278(2):114-19, 1985*).

Supplementation with omega-3 fatty acids may be beneficial.

Experimental Study: 13 pts. were placed on a diet that included concentrated fish oil supplements. After 8 wks., 8/13 showed mild to moderate improvement in skin lesions, correlated with high ratios in epidermal tissue samples of 2 fatty acids found in fish oils in large amounts (*Ziboh VA et al. Arch. Dermatol. November, 1986*).

Glycosaminoglycans (mucopolysaccharides):

Supplementation may be beneficial.

Experimental Study: 38 pts. with severe total-body psoriasis received sub-cut. injections of an extract of activated acid-pepsin-digested calf tracheal cartilege ("Catrix-S"). 19/39 had total remissions within 2 mo. with complete disappearance of the lesions for 6 wks. to more than 1 year, with the ave. being 5 months. 3/38 had an excellent response with little residual disease. 15/38 had a good result, and 1/38 a poor result. 11/16 who did not have a complete remission within 2 mo. went into a complete remission after receiving booster injections every 3 wks. and topical therapy with a 5% activated acid-pepsin-digested calf tracheal cartilege cream ("Psoriacin"). Responding pts developed prompt descaling, although the dilated capillary bed beneath the lesions remained dilated and tender to touch. The authors believe that eventually the capillaries will return to normal and the skin will return to normal thickness (*Prudden JF, Balassa LL. The biological activity of bovine cartilege preparations. Sem. Arthritis & Rheum. 3(4):287-321, 1974*).

Lecithin:

Supplementation may be beneficial.

Experimental Study: 118/ 155 pts. responded during a 10-year study with purified granulated soya phosphatides 15-45 gm daily orally which supplied 0.6 gm each of choline and inositol. Crude lecithin 3-6 gm daily was also given along with small amts. of vitamins A, D, B_1, B_2 and B_6 and calcium pantothenate. When appropriate, crude liver extract, thyroid and reducing diets were utilized, and local applications with various preparations were also provided (*Gross P et al. The treatment of psoriasis as a disturbance of lipid metabolism. N.Y.S. J. of Med. 50:2683-86, 1950*).

- -

TOPICAL APPLICATIONS:

Vitamin D_3:

Topical application may be beneficial.

Experimental Controlled Study: 5 pts. received topical administration of 1,25-dihydroxyvitamin D_3 and a control base. After 2-5 wks. of vitamin D application, all 5 pts. showed definite and in some cases remarkable improvement of the lesions. No systemic toxicity was detected (*Morimoto S et al. Therapeutic effect of 1,25-dihydroxyvitamin D_3 for psoriasis: Report of five cases. Calcif. Tissue Inter. 38:119-22, 1986*).

- -

OTHER FACTORS:

Rule out <u>food sensitivities</u>.

> **Experimental Study:** Pts. improved on a fasting and vegetarian regime (*Lithell H et al. A fasting and vegetarian diet treatment trial in chronic inflammatory disorders. <u>Acta Derm. Vener Stockholm</u> 63:397-403, 1983*).

> **Experimental Study:** 6/6 pts. improved on elimination diets. One improved on a diet which avoided fruits (especially citrus), nuts, corn and milk; the others improved on a diet which avoided acidic foods such as coffee, tomato, soda and pineapple (*Douglass, John M. Psoriasis and diet. Letter to the Editor. <u>California Med.</u> 133(5):450, 1980*).

See Also:

> Bazex A et al. Diet without gluten and psoriasis. <u>Ann. Derm. Syph.</u> 103:648, 1976

Rule out <u>hydrochloric acid deficienciy</u>.

> Supplementation may be beneficial.

>> *Note: While gastric anacidity had been reported in the past to be a relatively common condition which was associated with a number of illnesses, the presence of achlorhydria is no longer accepted unless a potent parietal-cell stimulant (such as histamine) is employed in gastric analysis. More recent studies suggest that histamine-fast anacidity is uncommon before the fifth decade of life and, although it probably does not occur in a normal stomach, its presence is not necessarily associated with symptoms (Rappaport EM. Achlorhydria: Associated symptoms and response to hydrochloric acid. <u>New Engl. J. Med.</u> 252(19):802-5, 1955).*

> **Experimental and Observational Study:** Of 9 pts., 5 had no HCl and only 1 had a normal HCl level. The severity of the condition seemed to correlate with the extent of the HCl deficiency and also seemed to be associated with signs of B complex deficiency. Improvement seemed to be associated with supplemental HCl and vitamin B complex (*Allison JR. The relation of hydrochloric acid and vitamin B complex deficiency in certain skin diseases. <u>Southern Med. J.</u> 38:235-241, 1945*).

> **Observational Study:** 19 pts. underwent a fractional gastric analysis following a routine Ewald test meal. Hypoacidity was defined as values for total and free acids of 1/2 normal or less, while hyperacidity was defined as values 10-15 points above normal or values which were relatively high at the start of the test. 10/19 (52%) of the pts. were found to have hypoacidity, while 5/19 (26%) had normal acid and 4/19 (21%) had hyperacidity. For 5/19 (26%) of the pts., the severity of the eruption correlated with both the presence of GI symptoms and abnormal gastric acid levels (*Ayers S. Gastric secretion in psoriasis, eczema and dermatitis herpetiformis. <u>Arch. Dermatol. Syph.</u> 20:854-57, 1929*).

RAYNAUD'S SYNDROME

See Also: AUTO-IMMUNE DISORDERS (GENERAL)

NUTRIENTS:

Vitamin E:

Supplementation may be beneficial.

Case Reports:
1. 45 year-old male with 6 month history of rapidly deteriorating illness causing ulceration and gangrene was placed on 400 I.U. of d, alpha tocopherol acetate twice daily before meals and local application of emulsified vitamin E drops. The fingers were healed in 8 weeks and remained healed one year later.
2. 37 year-old female with one year history of numbness, tingling and discoloration of the left fifth finger was placed on 100 I.U. of d, alpha tocopherol acetate three times daily 15 minutes before meals. Three weeks later, both the symptoms and the discoloration had improved. Three months later, only a trace of discoloration remained and she was symptom-free. Vitamin E was reduced to 100 I.U. daily and stopped after 6 months. Three years later she remained well.
(*Ayres Jr. S et al. Raynaud's phenomenon, scleroderma and calcinosis cutis: Response to vitamin E. Cutis 11:54-62, 1973*).

- -

Evening Primrose Oil: 1-2 gm 3 times daily

Supplementation may be beneficial.

Experimental Double-blind Study: 21 pts. with either Raynaud's Phenomenon (RP) or RP and systemic sclerosis were given placebo for 2 wks. when they were split into 2 gps., with 10 pts. continuing on placebo and 11 on EPO. Several pts. had symptomatic improvements reaching significance after 6-8 weeks. With colder weather, the placebo gp. experienced more frequent and longer attacks, while the EPO gp. experienced decreased severity of attacks and decreased hand coldness. The majority of pts. on EPO also reported decreased depression and increased energy. Objective measurement of blood flow revealed no change on EPO (*Belch JJ et al. Evening primrose oil (Efamol) in the treatment of Raynaud's phenomenon: A double-blind study. Thromb. Haemost. 54(2):490-94, 1985*).

- -

OTHER FACTORS:

Rule out food sensitivities.

Case Report: 30 year-old female with 25 yr. history of severe recurrent headaches, sore throats and kidney infections developed right index finger pain diagnosed as Raynaud's Disease which worsened despite vasodilators and analgesics. She was admitted to an environmental medical unit where, following a 6 day fast, her symptoms completely cleared and normal color returned to her finger. Digital spasm was provoked by challenge with foods and chemicals. Following discharge she remained almost symptom-free unless she was inadvertently exposed to chemicals. The authors report that they have also been able to identify triggering agents in 9 other patients (*Rea WJ, Suits CW. Cardiovascular disease triggered by foods and chemicals, in Gerrard JW, Ed. Food Allergy: New Perspectives. Springfield, Illinois, Charles C. Thomas, 1980*).

RESTLESS LEGS SYNDROME

BASIC DIET:

Avoid <u>caffeine</u> and other xanthine derivatives (coffee, tea, cola, cocoa).

Experimental Study: 62 pts. with restless legs syndrome and associated symptoms improved on a xanthine-free diet with the temporary addition of diazepam (*Lutz EG. Restless legs, anxiety and caffeinism. <u>J. Clin. Psychiat.</u> Sept. 1978, pp.693-8*).

- -

NUTRIENTS:

<u>Folic Acid:</u>   5 mg. three times daily
(WARNING: should be under medical supervision)

Dietary deficiency can result in a defect in the ability of intestinal cells to absorb folate when the diet is corrected (*Elsborg L. Reversible malabsorption of folic acid in the elderly with nutritional folate deficiency. <u>Acta Haematology</u> 55:140-7, 1976*).

Supplementation may be effective.

Review Article: There are at least 2 clinical forms of RLS: (1) the classic mixed sensorimotor form in which pain, numbness, and lightning stabs of pain in the lower or even the upper limbs are relieved by movement or local massage, and (2) the pure motor or myoclonic form which does not involve any sensory component. The folate-responsive form is exclusively of the mixed type (*Boutez MI et al. Neuropsychological correlates of folic acid deficiency: Facts and hypotheses, in Botez MI, Reynolds EH, Eds. <u>Folic Acid in Neurology, Psychiatry, and Internal Medicine</u>. New York, Raven Press, 1979*).

Experimental Study: 3 women with acquired folate deficiency had mild symptoms of restless legs, depression, muscular and mental fatigue, depressed ankle jerks, diminuation of vibratory sensation in the legs, a stocking type hypoesthesia, and chronic constipation. All 3 recovered with folate treatment (*Boutez, MI et al. Neurologic disorders responsive to folic acid therapy. <u>Can. Med. Assoc. J.</u> 15:217, 1976*).

See Also:

Boutez MI et al. Polyneuropathy and folate deficiency. <u>Arch. Neuro.</u> Sept. 1978 pp. 581-4

Boutez MI. Folate deficiency and neurological disorders in adults. <u>Med. Hypothesis</u> 2:135-40, 1976

<u>Vitamin E:</u>

Supplementation may be beneficial.

Case Reports:

1. A 78 year-old female with a 20 year history of "jumpy" legs up to several times nightly was unresponsive to phenytoin and diphenhydramine. Following 2 months of 300 I.U. daily, she was completely cured.

2. A 37 year-old female with a 10 year history of severe nightly "restless legs" was placed on 300 I.U. daily for 6 wks. and 200 I.U. daily for the following 4 weeks with complete relief.

(*Ayres S, Mihan R. Leg cramps and "restless leg" syndrome responsive to vitamin E. Calif. Med. 111:87-91, 1969*).

- -

L-Tryptophan:

Case Reports:

1. 68 year-old male with chronic renal failure due to malignant hypertension had been on maintenance hemodialysis for 4 years. 3 yrs. ago he developed symptoms of crawling, tingling, and burning sensations in his legs which were most prominent during the evening and on attempts to relax during the daytime. These symptoms led to chronic severe insomnia and depression. Neuro exam revealed no motor weakness or peripheral neuropathy. Clonazepam and hypnotics were ineffective; diazepam 20 mg and propoxyphene 2 tabs were mildly effective. L-tryptophan 1 gm twice daily produced amelioration of both the RLS and the insomnia within 3 days of administration without side effects.

2. 64 year-old man with steroid-dependent chronic obstructive lung disease and steroid myopathy had a 2 yr. history restless legs syndrome causing severe insomnia and depression. Numerous medication trials were unsuccessful. L-tryptophan 2 gm at night produced dramatic amelioration of the insomnia and RLS after 4 nights without side effects.

(*Sandyk R. L-tryptophan in the treatment of restless legs syndrome. Letter to the Editor. Am. J. Psychiat. 143(4):554-5,1986*).

RHEUMATISM

(including "ARTHRITIS", ARTHALGIA, JOINT PAIN, MUSCLE PAIN, TENDINITIS AND TENOSYNOVITIS)

See Also: OSTEOARTHRITIS
PAIN
RHEUMATOID ARTHRITIS

NUTRIENTS:

Pyridoxine:

Supplementation may be beneficial.

Experimental Study: Pts. with tenosynovitis producing numbness, tingling, pain, stiffness and weakness in the shoulders, arms and hands commonly improved in 8-12 wks. while on 100-150 mg pyridoxine hydrochloride daily, while erythrocyte glutamic oxaloacetic transaminase (EGOT) levels (a functional measure of B_6 nutriture) and the severity of rheumatic symptoms showed a close negative correlation, both prior to and following administration of pyridoxine (*Ellis JM. Vitamin B_6 deficiency and rheumatism. Anabolism Winter 1985*).

- -

Copper:

Local application of elemental copper may have some therapeutic value.

Experimental Single-blind Crossover Study: 240 "arthritis/rheumatism sufferers" were randomized into 3 groups. Gp. I wore a copper bracelet for 1 month followed by a "placebo" bracelet for 1 month. Gp. II wore the 2 bracelets in reverse order, while Gp. III wore no bracelets. Of those who noted a difference between the 2 bracelets, more perceived the copper to be more effective (p = less than 0.01). Previous users of copper bracelets deterioriated while wearing the placebo. The average loss of copper from the bracelet was 13 mg.(*Walker, WR & Keats, DM. An investigation of the therapeutic value of the "copper bracelet:" Dermal assimilation of copper in arthritic/rheumatoid conditions. Agents & Actions 6:454,1976*).

- -

OTHER FACTORS:

Rule out food sensitivities.

Experimental Study: 14 pts. with chronic arthralgias were re-challenged with foods already found to be offensive through dietary exclusion and challenges. 8/14 reacted to the re-challenges and 2/14 had doubtful reactions. 6/8 of the reactors developed IgE immune complexes after challenges (PEG precipitation method) while the remainder developed high levels of IgG immune complexes. None of the 4 non-reactors developed IgE or IgG immune complexes (*Brostoff J, Scadding GK. Complexes in food induced arthralgia. Paper presented at the XII International Congress of Allergy and Clinical Immunology, Washington, D.C., October, 1985*).

Experimental Study: While inflammatory arthritis (e.g. rheumatoid arthritis) failed to be influenced by food exclusions and challenges, food challenges did provoke transient synovitis in some pts. with atopic allergy as part of their allergic symptomatology (*Denman AM et al. Joint complaints and food allergic disorders. Ann. Allergy 51:260-3, 1983*).

Experimental Double-blind Study: 30 pts. with "arthritis and rheumatism" were each challenged sub-lingually to 25 foods and chemicals in a double-blind manner. Soy was the most commonly provoking substance (22/30 = 73.3% of pts.), while only 2/30 pts. (6.6%) reacted to placebo. Only 1 pt. had no subjective reactions. In 26 pts. (86%), musculo-skeletal symptoms were evoked (*Mandell M, Conte AA. The role of allergy in arthritis, rheumatism and polysymptomatic cerebral, visceral and somatic disorders: A double blind study. J. Int. Acad. Prev. Med. July, 1982, pp.5-16*).

Experimental Study: In a study performed totally through the mail, over 5000 "arthritis" pts. agreed to avoid members of the nightshade family of plants which includes the white potato, the tomato, eggplant, all peppers (except black) and tobacco. Over 70% reported gradually increasing relief from aches and pains and from some disfigurement over a study period of 7 years (*Childers NF. A relationship of arthritis to the solanaceae (nightshades). J. Int. Acad. Prev. Med. November 1982, pp. 31-7*).

RHEUMATOID ARTHRITIS

See Also: AUTO-IMMUNE DISORDERS (GENERAL)
PAIN
RHEUMATISM

OVERVIEW:

Since <u>malnutrition</u> is common among pts., it should be ruled out. A <u>low fat</u> diet may be beneficial, particularly if it is relatively high in polyunsaturates.

<u>Copper salicylate</u> has been found to be an effective anti-inflammatory agent which may be more potent than aspirin.

<u>Pantothenic acid</u> may be deficient, and there is preliminary evidence that supplementation may be beneficial. The use of <u>iron</u> supplementation is controversial, as is <u>zinc</u> supplementation. While <u>sulfur</u> is an old-fashioned remedy, its use is still not validated by double-blind studies. On the other hand, although more studies are needed, there is increasing evidence that <u>essential fatty acids</u> may be beneficial.

There have been an increasing number of studies in the past few years, some double-blind, demonstrating improvement following food eliminations and worsening following provocation with particular foods.

- -

BASIC DIET:

Rule out <u>malnutrition</u>.

> **Observational Study:** Nearly 3/4 of Alabama pts. with RA showed evidence of malnutrition. It is suggested that these results are primarily due to changes in the way vitamins and handled and nutrients absorbed in RA (*McDuffie FC, Arthritis Foundation - reported in <u>Med. World News</u> July 22, 1985*).

> **Observational Study:** Compared to controls with other types of musculoskeletal disorders, 25% of a gp. of 50 RA pts. were malnourished. The adequacy of dietary intake did not correlate with their nutritional status, but the degree of malnourishment did correlate with the severity of the RA (*Helliwell M et al. <u>Annals Rheum. Dis.</u> 43:386-90, 1984*).

<u>Low fat</u> diet.

> **Case Reports:** 2 pts. with obesity and active RA experienced remission of joint symptoms within days of going on a low-calorie, fat-free weight control formula and remained symptom-free for 9 and 14 mo. respectively. 24-48 hrs. after eating foods which contained a high proportion or all of its calories from fat they experienced short-term exacerbations. Subsequently 4 additional active rheumatoid factor-positive pts. who had fats and oils removed from their diets also experienced remissions. When, after 7 wks., either vegetable oil or animal fat was returned to their diets, they experienced exacerbations within 72 hours. When chicken, cheese, safflower oil, beef or coconut oil were added to the diet, they experienced inflammatory changes affecting joint count, joint swelling and morning stiffness (*Lucas C, Power L. Dietary fat aggravates active rheumatoid arthritis. <u>Clin. Res.</u> 29(4):754A, 1981*; See Also: *Lucas C, Power L. <u>JAMA</u> 4/9/82*).

- with <u>omega-3 fatty acids</u>:

Experimental Study: In 31 patients, a typical high-saturated fat diet was compared to a diet high in polyunsaturated fats, low in saturated fats, and supplemented with 1.8 grams daily of eicosapentaenoic acid. By 12 weeks, morning stiffness was significantly more severe in the control group as their symptoms had lengthened while symptoms in the study group were unchanged. In addition, the study group indicated a significantly greater decrease in the number of tender joints. Reintroduction of the typical diet was followed by substantial deterioration (*Kremer JM et al. Effects of manipulation of dietary fatty acids on clinical manifestations of rheumatoid arthritis.* <u>Lancet</u> *1:184-7, 1985*).

<u>Vegan</u> diet.

May be beneficial due to its low cholesterol and low saturated fat content.

Experimental Study: 20 pts. were placed on a vegan diet following a 7-10 day fast. Also excluded or used sparingly were refined sugar, corn flour, salt, strong spices, alcohol, tea and coffee. After 4 mo., 12 pts. reported some improvement, 5 reported no change, and 3 felt worse. Most felt less pain and were better able to function, although there were no changes in objective measures such as grip strength and joint tenderness (*Sk:oldstam L. Fasting and vegan diet in rheumatoid arthritis.* <u>Scand. J. Rheumatol.</u> *15(2):219-21, 1987*).

- -

NUTRIENTS:

<u>Pantothenic Acid</u>:

Found to be deficient compared to normals, with the degree of deficiency directly related to the severity of symptoms.

Observational Study: The mean level of whole blood pantothenic acid for 66 pts. was significantly lower than that for 29 normals. Moreover, the lower the level of pantothenic acid, the greater the symptom severity. Vegetarian normals had a much higher pantothenate level than did normals consuming a usual balanced diet (*Barton-Wright EC, Elliott WA. The pantothenic acid metabolism of rheumatoid arthritis.* <u>Lancet</u> *2:862-63, 1963*).

Supplementation may be beneficial.

Experimental Double-blind Study: 18 pts. with RA who were previously untreated or who had not responded to previous drug treatment were randomly chosen to receive 2 gm daily of oral calcium pantothenate (starting with 500 mg daily and gradually increasing to 500 mg 4 times daily by day 10), while the rest received placebo. Pts. were permitted to take paracetamol to relieve pain but no other medications were permitted. After 2 mo., daily records kept by pts. in the experimental gp. showed a significant subjective reduction in the duration of morning stiffness (p less than 0.01), degree of disability (p less than 0.04) and severity of pain (p less than 0.01) compared to baseline, while controls failed to report significant improvements. Analysis of co-variance between gps. revealed a significant difference in the reduction of disability (p less than 0.04), although the duration of morning stiffness and severity of pain differences were not significant (*Calcium pantothenate in arthritic conditions. A report from the General Practitioner Research Group.* <u>Practitioner</u> *224:208-11, 1980*).

Experimental Study: 20 pts. received calcium-D-pantothenate 50 mg IM daily leading to temporary alleviation of symptoms after 7 days along with an increase in whole blood pantothenate. Another 21 days of injections failed to result in further improvement. After discontinuation, blood levels fell to their initial values by the end of 1 month with concomitant reappearance of symptoms, suggesting that abnormal pantothenate metabolism is due to some other factor. Since royal jelly is rich in pantothenic acid in its free state as well as in other 10-carbon straight chain fatty acids, 20 pts. received a mixture of royal jelly and pantothenic acid 50 mg of each IM daily. By 28 days, 14 pts. (70%) noted an improvement in general condition and joint mobility along with a fall in ESR coincident with rising blood levels which lasted until blood levels returned to previous values 2 mo. following discontinuation of the injections. 10 vegetarians with RA all improved on the same regime by 14 days with a greater rise in whole blood pantothenate levels than in the non-vegetarian arthritics. Preliminary results with oral supplementation has been encouraging (*Barton-Wright EC, Elliott WA. The pantothenic acid metabolism of rheumatoid arthritis. Lancet 2:862-63, 1963*).

Vitamin C:

May be deficient.

> **Review Article:** Leucocyte and plasma concentrations of ascorbate are significantly decreased in RA (*Mullen A, Wilson CWM. The metabolism of ascorbic acid in rheumatoid arthritis. Proc. Nutr. Sci. 35:8A-9A, 1976; Sahud MA, Cohen RJ. Effect of aspirin ingestion on ascorbic-acid levels in rheumatoid arthritis. Lancet 1:937-38, 1971*) possibly because of increased degradation and excretion due to the greatly enhanced rates of oxidation of ascorbate in inflammation in activated neutrophils (*Roberts P et al. Vitamin C and inflammation. Med. Biol. 62:88, 1984*).

Vitamin K (menadione):   5 - 10 mg. three times daily

May stabilize the synovial linings of affected tissue.

> **In vitro Experimental Study:** Hydrogen-accepting molecules, especially menadione, stabilized the lysosomal membranes of synovial lining cells of human rheumatoid tissue and decreased the excessively reductive cytoplasmic pH, while ascorbate, a hydrogen donor, did the opposite (*Chayen J et al. The effect of experimentally induced redox changes on human rheumatoid and non-rheumatoid synovial tissue in vitro. Beitr. Path. Bd. 149:127, 1973*).

— —

Copper: copper salicylate: 1-2 64 mg. tabs daily with meals
          (maximum of 10 days per treatment)

Serum copper concentrations are elevated (*Niedermeier W, Griggs JH. Trace metal composition of synovial fluid and blood serum of patients with rheumatoid arthritis. J. Chron. Dis. 23:527-36, 1971*). Synovial fluid copper concentrations are 3 times that of normals due to elevated ceruloplasmin which may reflect elevated serum copper and increased permeability of the synovial membrane to ceruloplasmin (*Niedermeier W. Concentration and chemical state of copper in synovial fluid and blood serum of patients with rheumatoid arthritis. Ann. Rheum. Dis. 24:544, 1965*).

Serum copper levels are directly related to length and severity of the disease and return to normal with remission but do not reflect copper balance in the body. The rise in serum copper seen in RA is associated with a fall in liver copper stores as well as an increased rate of synthesis of ceruloplasmin and an increase of ceruloplasmin within synovial fluid (*Sorenson J. in The Anti-inflammatory Activities of Copper Complexes, Metal Ions and Biological Systems. Marcel Dekker, 1982 pp. 77-125*).

See Also:

> *Brown DH et al. Serum copper and its relationship to clinical symptoms in rheumatoid arthritis. Ann. Rheum. Dis. 38(2):174-6, 1979*

Supplementation with <u>copper salicylate complex</u> may be beneficial and is more effective in animal models of inflammaton than aspirin or copper alone.

> **Animal Experimental Study:** Shown to have both an anti-inflammatory and an analgesic effect upon arthritic rats (*Jacka T et al. Copper salicylate as an anti-inflammatory and analgaesic agent in arthritic rats. <u>Life Sci.</u> 32:1023, 1983*).

> **Review Article:** Copper's anti-inflammatory effect appears to be related to its ability to form complexes which serve as selective antioxidants, thus reducing the localized tissue inflammation which has resulted from enhanced oxidant damage (*Sorenson J. Copper aspirinate: A more potent anti-inflammatory and anti-ulcer agent. <u>J. Intern. Acad. Prev. Med.</u> pp.7-21, 1980*).

> **Experimental Study:** Oral copper salicylate (60 mg twice daily) was compared with salicylic acid and copper acetate in equal doses in pts. with RA and rheumatism-like degenerative diseases. The copper salicylate was more effective than either salicylic acid or copper acetate and produced reduction in morning stiffness, increased joint mobility and reduced need for other drugs (*Hangarter W. Copper salicylate in rheumatoid arthritis and rheumatism-like degenerative diseases. <u>Med. Welt.</u> 31:1625, 1980*).

> **Experimental Study:** 89% of 1140 pts. treated with short-term I.V. copper salicylate showed remission of fever, increased joint mobility, decreased swelling, and normalization of ESR for an average of 3 years (*Hangarter W. <u>Inflammation</u> 2:217, 1977*).

> **Review Article:** Copper salicylates are believed to be the best copper complex for the treatment of arthritic pain based on rat studies and uncontrolled human trials (*Sorenson JRJ, Hangarter W. Treatment of rheumatoid and degenerative diseases with copper complexes: A review with emphasis on copper-salicylate. <u>Inflammation</u> 2:217, 1977*).

> See Also:

>> *Bland, J. Copper salicylates and complexes in molecular medicine. <u>Int. Clin. Nutr. Rev.</u> 4(3):130-4, 1984*

>> *Sorenson JRJ. Copper chelates as possible active forms of anti-arthritic agents. <u>J. Med. Chem.</u> 19:135, 1976*

>> *Williams DA et al. Synthesis and biological evaluation of tetrakisu(acetylsalicylato)-dicopper (II). <u>J. Pharm. Sci.</u> 65:126, 1976*

Local application of elemental copper may have some therapeutic value.

> **Experimental Single-blind Crossover Study:** 240 "arthritis/rheumatism sufferers" were randomized into 3 groups. Gp. I wore a copper bracelet for 1 month followed by a "placebo" bracelet for 1 month. Gp. II wore the 2 bracelets in reverse order, while Gp. III wore no bracelets. Of those who noted a difference between the 2 bracelets, more perceived the copper to be more effective (p = less than 0.01). Previous users of copper bracelets deteriorioated while wearing the placebo. The average loss of copper from the bracelet was 13 mg.(*Walker, WR & Keats, DM. An investigation of the therapeutic value of the "copper bracelet:" Dermal assimilation of copper in arthritic/rheumatoid conditions. <u>Agents & Actions</u> 6:454,1976*).

<u>Iron</u>:

Significantly elevated in synovial fluid compared to normals, and significantly reduced in serum (*Niedermeier W, Griggs JH. Trace metal composition of synovial fluid and blood serum of patients with rheumatoid arthritis. <u>J. Chron. Dis.</u> 23:527-36, 1971*).

The iron content of synovial membrane is markedly increased (*Muirden KD, Senstar GB. Iron in the synovial membrane in rheumatoid arthritis and other joint diseases. <u>Ann. Rheum. Dis.</u> 27:38, 1968*) and iron deposits in the membrane can regularly be seen histologically (*Senatar GB, Muirden KD. Concentration of iron in synovial membrane, synovial fluid and serum in rheumatoid arthritis and other joint diseases. <u>Ann. Rheum. Dis.</u> 27:49, 1968*).

The advisability of supplementation is controversial.

Review Article: The combination of microcytic anemia and a plasma ferritin concentration of less than 110 micrograms/l predicts that oral iron supplementation will result in increases in HGb concentration, red cell MCV and red cell ferritin contents (*Davidson A et al. Red cell ferritin content: A re-evaluation of indices for iron deficiency in the anaemia of rheumatoid arthritis. <u>Brit. Med. J.</u> 289:648-50, 1984*).

Experimental Study: Iron supplementation had positive results (*Hansen M et al. Serum ferritin and the assessment of iron deficiency in rheumatoid arthritis. <u>Scand. J. Rheumatol.</u> 12:3353-59, 1983*).

Review Article: Iron supplementation may be contraindicated due to the possibility of the formation of highly reactive hydroxy radicals from hydrogen peroxide and iron salts by superoxide and ascorbate-dependent mechanisms (*Rawley DA, Halliwell B. Formation of hydroxyl radicals from hydrogen peroxide and iron salts by superoxide and ascorbate-dependent mechanisms: Relevance to the pathology of rheumatoid disease. <u>Clin. Sci.</u> 64:649-53, 1983*).

Single-blind Case Report: 39 year-old female pt. whose peripheral synovitis worsened both subjectively and objectively within 48 hrs. of ingesting ferrous sulphate 200 mg 3 times daily, while placebo caused no change. Serum ferritin rose from 30-50 mcg/l while her symptoms exacerbated on iron, but returned to 15 mcg/l one month after iron was stopped (*Blake D, Bacon P. <u>Lancet</u> 1:623, 1982*).

Review Article: Since serum ferritin is also an acute phase reactant in clinically active disease, its level may also correlate with disease activity and thus may not accurately reflect the degree of iron deficiency (*Rothwell RS, Davis P. Relationship between serum ferritin, anemia, and disease activity in acute and chronic rheumatoid arthritis. <u>Rheumatol. Int.</u> 1(2):65-7, 1981*).

<u>Manganese:</u>

Total body turnover is low in pts. but is restored to normal with corticosteroid therapy. RBC Mn levels, however, are higher than in normals (*Cotzias GC et al. Slow turnover of manganese in active rheumatoid arthritis and acceleration by prednisone. <u>J. Clin. Invest.</u> 47:992, 1968*).

<u>Selenium:</u>

May be deficient.

Observational Study: 26 girls with juvenile chronic arthritis had a significantly decreased plasma selenium compared to controls. Blood glutathione peroxidase was also slightly lower in pts. and was significantly lower among pts. with high to medium disease compared to those with low disease activity (*Johansson V et al. Nutritional status in girls with juvenile chronic arthritis. <u>Human Nutr.: Clin. Nutr.</u> 40C:57-67, 1986*).

Observational Study: 87 pts. were found to have significantly lower serum selenium levels than controls. Reduction in serum Se was most pronounced in pts. with active, disabling disease of long duration. There was a significant inverse correlation between serum Se and certain parameters of disease severity as well as a significant positive correlation between serum Se and hemoglobin concentration (*Tarp U et al. Low selenium level in severe rheumatoid arthritis. Scand. J. Rheumatol. 14:97, 1985*).

Observational Study: Plasma selenium levels in pts. were significantly lower than those of controls (*Aeseth J et al. Trace elements in serum and urine of patients with rheumatoid arthritis. Scand. J. Rheumatol. 7:237-40, 1978*).

Sulfur:

May be deficient.

Observational Study: While the cystine content of fingernails in normals is 12%, in "arthritics" it is only 8.9% (*Sullivan MX, Hess WC. Cystine content of finger nails in arthritis. J. Bone & Joint Surg. 16:185, 1935*).

Supplementation may be beneficial.

Experimental Study: 100 "arthritics" received I.V. colloidal sulfur. Pain and effusions disappeared in many cases with a return of the cystine fingernail test to normal (*Woldenberg SC. The treatment of arthritis with colloidal sulphur. J.Southern Med. Assoc. 28:875-81, 1935; See Also: Neligan AR, Salt HB. Sulphur in rheumatoid arthritis. Lancet 2:209, 1934*).

May be absorbed through the skin.

Experimental Study: Blood sulphur levels rose following sulphur baths (*Osterberg AE et al. Absorption of sulphur compounds during treatment by sulphur baths. Arch. Derm. Syph. 20:156-66, 1929*).

Zinc: 20 - 50 mg. three times daily

Synovial fluid levels are significantly elevated compared to normals, while serum levels are significantly reduced (*Niedermeier W, Griggs JH. Trace metal composition of synovial fluid and blood serum of patients with rheumatoid arthritis. J. Chron. Dis. 23:527-36, 1971*) and urinary zinc is higher.

Observational Study: Compared to age- and sex-matched controls, mean serum zinc levels in 28 pts. was significantly lower (72.53 vs. 105.12 mcg/ml) and 24 hr. urinary zinc was higher (*Pandey SP et al. Zinc in rheumatoid arthritis. Indian J. Med. Res. 81:618-20, 1985*).

Zinc levels are related to the degree of inflammation, but plasma and cellular zinc levels differ in the nature of this relationship.

Experimental and Observational Study: Markedly reduced cellular zinc values were found in pts. compared to healthy subjects but were unrelated to inflammatory activity or disease duration. Plasma zinc was reduced in the majority of the patients and was negatively correlated to the inflammatory activity as estimated by ESR and serum orosomucoid. Corticosteroid therapy induced a significant elevation of cellular zinc while plasma zinc was unchanged (*Svenson KL et al. Reduced zinc in peripheral blood cells from patients with inflammatory connective tissue diseases. Inflammation 9(2):189-99, 1985*).

Experimental Study: Plasma zinc levels were significantly lower in pts. on NSAID's than in those on levamisole and penicillamine. In addition, plasma zinc levels correlated positively with serum albumin, and negatively with both ESR and serum globulin, suggesting that it is one of the nonspecific features of inflammation (*Balogh Z et al. Plasma zinc and its relationship to clinical symptoms and drug treatment in rheumatoid arthritis. Ann. Rheum. Dis. 39(4):329032, 1980*).

Zinc supplementation may result in lessened disease activity.

Negative Experimental Double-blind Study: 22 pts. with severe long-standing RA received oral zinc sulphate 220 mg 3 times daily 1 hr. before meals or placebo. 6/22 had subjective but not objective improvement for 6 mo. but then deteriorated. In the whole gp., neither the number of affected joints, the ARA grading, the functional classification, ESR, hemoglobin, hematocrit, or platelet count changed significantly. The main side-effect was nausea (*Rasker JJ, Kardaun SH. Lack of beneficial effect of zinc sulphate in rheumatoid arthritis. Scand. J. Rheumatol. 11:168-70, 1982*).

Experimental Double-blind Crossover Study (psoriatic <u>arthritis</u>): 24 pts. with negative tests for rheumatoid factors, LE cells and antinuclear antibodies experienced reduction in signs and symptoms of RA following supplementation with zinc sulphate 220 mg 3 times daily for 6 wks. accompanied by reduction of serum immunoglobulins and an increase in serum albumin. Only joint pains were significantly reduced following the initial study; however, during a subsequent 24 wk. open trial, morning stiffness and improvement in their overall condition reached significance. There was no improvement in psoriatic lesions and severe side-effects were not seen (*Clemmensen OJ et al. Psoriatic arthritis treated with oral zinc sulphate. Brit. J. Dermatol. 103:411-15, 1980*).

Experimental Double-blind Study: 12/24 treatment-resistent pts. received 50 mg. zinc 3 times daily for 12 wks. while the rest received placebo, then all 24 pts. received zinc for 12 more weeks. There were significant improvements in joint swelling, morning stiffness, walking time and subjective symptoms during the first part of the study with continuing, impressive improvement in the second part (*Simkin PA. Oral zinc sulphate in rheumatoid arthritis. Lancet 2:539, 1976*).

See Also:

> *Simkin PA. Treatment of rheumatoid arthritis with oral zinc sulfate. Agents Actions [Suppl] 8:587-96, 1981*

> **Negative Experimental Study:** *Job C et al. Zinc sulphate in the treatment of rheumatoid arthritis. Arthritis Rheum. 23:1408, 1980*

One effect of zinc which may explain its benefits is the lowering of elevated serum copper levels.

Case Report: *Pfeiffer, Carl. Zinc and Other Micro-Nutrients. Keats Publishing, 1978, p.51*

- -

<u>Bromelain</u>: 2250 mg. twice daily

A proteolytic enzyme derived from the pineapple plant with known anti-inflammatory properties.

Experimental Study: 25 pts. with stages II or III RA, along with 1 pt. with both RA and osteoarthritis, 2 pts. with OA alone and 1 pt. with gout had residual joint swelling and impairment in mobility following long-term corticosteroid therapy. Their doses were tapered to small maintenance doses and they received enteric-coated bromelain 20-40 mg 3-4 times daily with each mg equal to 2500 Rorer units of activity. In most pts. residual joint swelling was significantly reduced (p less than 0.01) and joint mobility was increased soon after supplementation was started. After 3 wks.- 13 mo. of observation, 8/29 (28%) had excellent results, 13/29 (45%) good results, 4/29 (14%) fair results and 4/29 (14%) poor results. The pt. with gout had poor results. One of the OA pts. had good results, the other fair results. It seemed that smaller amts. of steroids were needed when bromelain was given concurrently. There were no side-effects (*Cohen A, Goldman J. Bromelains therapy in rheumatoid arthritis. Pennsyl. Med. J. 67:27-30, June 1964*).

Catechin:

A naturally occurring flavonoid.

Able to inhibit the breakdown of collagen caused by either free radicals or enzymes (hyaluronidase, collagenase, and pepsin) as well as to crosslink directly with collagen fibers and inhibit procollagen biosynthesis (*Blumenkrantz N, Asboe-Hansen G.   Effect of (+)-catechin on connective tissue.   Scand. J. Rheumatol. 7:55-60, 1978*).

Glycosaminoglycans (mucopolysaccharides):   1200 - 3000 mg. three times daily

Supplementation may be beneficial.

> **Experimental Study:** 67% of 55 pts. treated for 6 months to 4.5 years with perna canaliculus (green-lipped mussel), a rich source of glycosaminoglycans, benefited (*Gibson RG et al.   Perna canaliculus in the treatment of arthritis.   Practitioner 224:955-60, September, 1980*).

> **Experimental Double-blind Study:** 28 pts. on NSAID's were supplemented with perna canaliculus 350 mg 3 times daily or placebo for 6 months with significant benefit to the experimental gp. as compared to controls (*El-Ghobarey A et al.   Quart. J. Med. 47:385, 1978*).

> **Experimental Study:** 9 pts. received sub-cut. injections of an activated acid-pepsin-digested calf tracheal cartilege extract ("Catrix-S") over a period of 10-35 days followed by booster doses every 3-4 wks depending upon pt. response. 3/9 had an excellent response, while the other 6 had a good response (*Prudden JF, Balassa LL.   The biological activity of bovine cartilage preparations.   Sem. Arthritis & Rheum. 3(4):287-321, 1974*).

> See Also:

> > *Green-lipped mussel extract in arthritis. Editorial. Lancet 1:85, 1981*

> > *Gibson RG, Gibson SL. Green-lipped mussel extract in arthritis. Letter to the Editor. Lancet 1:439, 1981*

> > *Highton TC, McArthur AW.   Pilot study in the effect of New Zealand Green Mussel on rheumatoid arthritis. NZ Med. J. March 12, 1975, p.261*

L-Histidine: 1000 mg. 2-3 times daily between meals (several month trial)

Markedly depressed (while other amino acids are normal) (*Gerber DA et al.   Free serum histidine levels in patients with rheumatoid arthritis and control subjects following an oral load of free L-histidine. J. Clin. Inves. 55:1164, 1975; Gerber DA et al.   Specificity of a low free serum histidine concentration for rheumatoid arthritis. J. Chron. Dis. 30:115, 1977*).

Supplementation may be of benefit.

> **Experimental Double-blind Study:** Pts. were treated with oral L-histidine 4.5 gm daily or placebo. After 30 weeks no clinical measurement showed an advantage of histidine over placebo, although a small decrease in rheumatoid factor titer and a small increase in hematocrit were found only in the histidine group and there was suggestive evidence of a beneficial effect of histidine in pts. with more active and prolonged disease (*Pinals RS et al.   Treatment of rheumatoid arthritis with L-histidine: A randomized, placebo controlled, double-blind trial. J. Rheumatol. 4(4):414-19, 1977*).

See Also:

> *Ambanelli U et al. [Histidine in the treatment of rheumatoid arthritis.] Clin. Ter. 72(2):113-27, 1975*

One effect may be to lower elevated levels of heavy metals such as copper and iron in affected joints.

Experimental Study (elevated copper and iron in joint fluid): *Niedermeier W, Griggs JH. J. Chronic Dis.23:527-536, 1971*

Omega-3 Fatty Acids:

("MaxEPA" is a refined source with 18% eicosapentaenoic acid.)

Supplementation may be beneficial.

Experimental Controlled Study: 17 pts. were placed on a high polyunsaturated fat, low saturated fat diet and supplemented with "MaxEPA" (Scherer) 10 capsules (1.8 gm EPA) daily, while 20 controls received a typical American diet and placebo capsules. After 12 wks., the EPA gp. had significantly less morning stiffness (as stiffness had worsened only in the control gp.). Joints were also less tender and HGb improved, but these measures did not reach significance. A rapid deterioration with increased pain and stiffness was seen in treated pts. compared to controls upon cessation of the experimental diet (*Kremer JM et al. Effect of manipulation of dietary fatty acids on clinical manifestations of rheumatoid arthritis. Lancet 1:184-7, 1985*).

Experimental Controlled Study: 12/17 pts. randomly received 10 fish oil capsules daily for 14 wks., while 7 received placebo. During the first 6 wks., all 19 also received a NSAID. After 6 wks., the fish-oil cohort showed a significant reduction in the number of painful joints compared to controls. This relief disappeared after withdrawal of NSAID therapy, although pts. did not regress from their baseline status as usually happens when NSAIDs are withdrawn, suggesting that fish oil has an anti-inflammatory effect (*Sperling RI - reported in Med. World News July 14, 1986*).

Omega-6 Fatty Acids:

Example: Evening Primrose Oil: 1 gram four times daily (3 month trial)

Early studies suggest:
1. Relatively ineffective in pts. receiving more than trivial doses of steroids or non-steroidal anti-inflammatory drugs, although it may permit their dosage to be reduced after 1-3 months.
2. The effects do not usually become apparent in less than 4-12 weeks.
3. Some of the pts. who show the best long-term response have a transient worsening in the first 1-2 weeks.
4. The course of the disease may actually be stopped in some patients.
(*Horrobin DF. The importance of gamma-linolenic acid and prostaglandin E_1 in human nutrition and medicine. J. Holistic Med. 3:118-139, 1981*).

Supplementation may be comparable to non-steroidal analgesics.

Experimental Study: When combined with the cofactors zinc, ascorbic acid, niacin and pyridoxine, primrose oil was as effective as conventional treatment for 20 pts. switched to it from non-steroidal analgesics (*Hansen TM et al. Treatment of rheumatoid arthritis with prostaglandin E_1 precursors cis-linoleic acid and gamma-linolenic acid. Scand. J. Rheum. 12:85, 1983*).

Experimental Study: Several pts. were given 2.1 gm. primrose oil daily. After 3 months of treatment, results were seen which suggest that it may be effective (*McCormick JN et al. Immunosuppressive effect of linoleic acid. Lancet 2:508, 1977*).

In vitro Experimental Study: *Mucosal mast cells. III. Effect of quercetin and other flavonoids on antigen induced histamine secretion from rat intestinal mast cells. J. Allergy Clin. Immunol. 73:819-23, 1984*

D,L Phenylalanine: 750 mg 15-30 minutes before meals 3 times daily (2-21 days for results).
Double the dose if ineffective for up to another 3 weeks.

Supplementation may be beneficial.

Case Report: A 47 year-old woman with an 18 year history of RA had marked inflammation and swelling of the dorsum of her hands causing the MCP joints to become hidden. Seven days after starting DLPA her pain had faded and the swelling was so greatly reduced that the knuckles were visible. In addition there was dramatic improvement in joint flexibility (*Study reported in Hopkins P. Phenylalanine & relief of chronic pain. Anabolism vol. 4 no. 2, 1985*).

Quercitin:

RA is characterized by substantially increased numbers of mast cells in synovial membranes and fluids. Degranulation of these mast cells are believed to be a major factor in the tissue destruction. Quercetin is a potent inhibitor of mast cell degranulation.

Superoxide Dismutase:

Note: Oral SOD has no effect on tissue levels, although it is conceivable (but unproven) that an enteric-coated pill could escape digestion (Zidenberg-Cherr S et al. Dietary superoxide dismutase does not affect tissue levels. Am. J. Clin. Nutr. 37:5, 1983).

Parenteral supplementation may be beneficial.

Experimental Double-blind Study: 30 pts. with active classical RA affecting the knee received intra-articular injections of orgotein (ZnCu superoxide dismutases) 4 mg/wk or aspirin for 6 weeks. After 12 wks., clinical and biochemical assessments showed that orgotein was superior to aspirin and resulted in significant improvement. Changes in synovial fluid suggest that the anti-inflammatory properties of orgotein may lie in its effect on proliferating synovia (*Goebel KM et al. Intrasynovial orgotein therapy in rheumatoid arthritis. Lancet 1:1015-17, 1981*).

See Also:

Menander-Huber KB. Orgotein in the treatment of rheumatoid arthritis. Eur. J. Rheumatol. Inflammation 4:201, 1981

Walravens M, Dequeker J. Comparison of gold and orgotein treatment in rheumatoid arthritis. Curr. Ther. Res. 20:62, 1976

Tryptophan:

Supplementation may be beneficial.

Animal Experimental Study: Tryptophan had a marked effect in reducing the edema of adjuvant arthritis induced in rat paws compared to controls (*Rand SA, Forst MB. Treatment of adjuvant arthritis with nonsteroidal agents: A comparative study. J. Am. Podiatry Assoc. 70(2):65, 1980*).

Animal Experimental Study (rat): Both L- and DL-tryptophan were orally effective in suppressing both acute inflammatory exudate formation and the proliferative phase of inflammation in an animal model, with their efficacy equivalent to that of pheylbutazone (*Madan BR et al. Anti-inflammatory activity of L-tryptophan and DL-tryptophan. Indian J. Med. Res. 68:708-13, 1978*).

Experimental Study: Patients treated for depression with tryptophan had relief of arthritis (*Broadhurst AD. Tryptophan and rheumatic diseases. Brit. Med. J. August 13, 1977, p.456*).

Yucca Saponin Extract ("Desert Pride Herbal Food Tablets"): 4 daily (range of 2 - 8)

Supplementation may be beneficial.

Experimental Double-blind Study: 149 arthritis pts., 41.1% with a positive RA fixation test, were randomly given either yucca saponin extract or placebo in periods ranging from 1 wk. to 15 months before re-evaluation. 61% noted less swelling, pain and stiffness versus 22% on placebo. Some improved in days, some in weeks, and some in 3 months or longer (*Bingham R et al. Yucca plant saponin in the management of arthritis. J. Applied Nutr. 27:45-50, 1975*).

- -

OTHER FACTORS:

Rule out food sensitivities.

Fasting and some elimination diets may produce temporary improvement; when successful, subsequent food challenges may produce exacerbations.

Experimental Double-blind Case Report: 52 year-old white female with an 11 yr.history of joint pain, tenderness, swelling and stiffness fulfilled the criteria for active RA and achieved only fair results from NSAIDs. She was placed on a baseline diet for 6 days, a 3-day mineral water fast and vanilla-flavored Vivonex for 2 days. She was then challenged with encapsulated lyophilized foods or D-xylose placebo. Within 24 hrs. of starting the water fast, there was noticable symptomatic relief which was sustained on Vivonex. There were no notable responses to 52 placebo challenges, but she responded with symptomatic deterioration and worsening of ESR and other peak responses to cow's milk challenge on 4 separate occasions. While no elevation of IgE antibodies to foods was noted, she did have mildly increased amts. of IgG anti-milk and large amts. of IgG$_4$ anti-milk antibodies and IgG- and milk-containing circulating immune complexes were marginally elevated 48 hrs. following one of the milk challenges (*Panush RS et al. Food-induced (allergic) arthritis. Arthritis Rheum. 29(2):220-26, 1986*).

Experimental Single-blind Study: After 2 wks. in which all previous therapy was withdrawn and a normal diet consumed, 45 pts. were randomly divided into an immediate dietary gp. (Gp. B) and a control gp. which received placebo for 6 wks. prior to dietary therapy (Gp. C). Foods producing symptoms in Gp. B following a hypoallergenic dietary baseline were eliminated. When compared to the scores of Gp. C during their placebo period, Gp. B did better for all 13 subjective and objective variables measured for which the differences were significant, while Gp. C during its subsequent diet did better than during the placebo period for all 12 variables which showed significant differences. 33/45 (73%) of pts. considered their condition to be "better" or "much better" following dietary therapy (*Darlington LG et al. Placebo-controlled, blind study of dietary manipulation therapy in rheumatoid arthritis. Lancet February 1, 1986, pp. 236-38*).

Case Report: A 14 year-old female with Juvenile RA for 6 yrs. had both IgG and IgM antibodies to milk and responded in 3 wks. to the removal of milk products from her diet with return of symptoms on 4 occasions following reintroduction of milk products. She was seronegative and lactase deficient and had a family history of milk allergy (*Ratner D et al. Juvenile rheumatoid arthritis and milk allergy. J. Royal Soc. Med. 78(5):410-13, 1985*).

Experimental Study: 43 pts. with definite or classical RA underwent a water fast lasting about 7 days. Seven objective and subjective parameters of disease activity all significantly improved during the fast (*Kroker GF et al. Fasting and rheumatoid arthritis: A multicenter study. Clin. Ecol. 2:137-144, 1984*).

Experimental Study: 23 pts. with definite or classical RA who were water fasted about 7 days with significant improvement (*see Kroker GF et al - ibid*) underwent subsequent food challenges. Reactive foods (especially corn, wheat and animal protein) provoked frequent and intense reactions with significant deterioration of objective and subjective parameters of disease activity (*Marshall R et al. Food challenge effects on fasted rheumatoid arthritis patients: A multicenter study. Clin. Ecol. 2:181-190, 1984*).

Experimental Double-blind Study: 11/26 pts. were placed on a diet free of additives, preservatives, fruit, red meat, herbs and dairy products, while 15/26 were placed on a "placebo diet" with random food exclusions. After 10 weeks, there were no clinically important differences between groups. Two pts. on the experimental diet improved notably, elected to remain on it, have continued to improve, and noted exacerbations of disease upon challenges of certain of the excluded foods (*Panush RS et al. Diet therapy for rheumatoid arthritis. Arth. Rheum. 26:462-71, 1984*).

Experimental Crossover Study: 13 RA pts. were fasted for 7 days in comparison to a control regimen. During fasting joint inflammation and ESR decreased while during the control regimen the joints were unchanged or worse and ESR was unchanged. Improvement in joint inflammation was associated with enchancement of neutrophil bactericidal capacity (*Uden AM et al. Neutrophil functions and clinical performance after total fasting in patients with rheumatoid arthritis. Ann. Rheum. Dis. 42(1):45-51, 1983*).

Experimental Study: 14 pts. with classical RA and 7 healthy controls followed a diet of diluted fruit and vegetable juices for 10 days. Both pts. and healthy controls developed reduced plasma levels of complement factor 3 (C_3), orosomucoid and haptoglobin, although only the decreases in C_3 and orosomucoid were greater in the pt. group (*Skoldstam L et al. Specific plasma proteins as indices of inflammation during a modified fast in patients with rheumatoid arthritis. Scand. J. Rheumatol. 12(2):161-5, 1983*).

Experimental Study: 5 RA pts. underwent fasting and subsequently were placed on a lactovegetarian diet. During fasting, disease activity (measured by a clinical 6-joint score) decreased and both intestinal and non-intestinal permeability (using low-molecular weight polyethylence glycols as probe molecules) decreased. On the subsequent diet, disease activity and both intestinal and non-intestinal permeability increased again (*Sundquist T et al. Influence of fasting on intestinal permeability and disease activity in patients with rheumatoid arthritis. Scand. J. Rheumatol. 11(1):33-8, 1982*).

Case Report: 38 year-old woman with 11 year history of progressive, erosive seronegative RA who responded poorly to conventional treatment had a passion for cheese and was placed on a dairy-free diet with good results. Challenge with milk and cheese was followed by a pronounced increase in synovitis and changes in immune complexes, IgE antibodies, and heat-damaged red cell clearance rates (*Parke AL, Hughes GRV. Rheumatoid arthritis and food: A case study. Brit. Med. J. 282:2027-9, 1981*).

Experimental Study: 22 pts. (15 sero-positive) followed allergen-exclusion diets. 20 subjectively improved, and 19 reported that certain foods would repeatedly exacerbate arthritic symptoms. Improvement occurred an average of 10 days after the correct exclusions with a maximum of 18 days. Reactions to provocation varied from 2 hours to 2 weeks. Grains were by far the most common allergen (*Hicklin JA et al. The effect of diet in rheumatoid arthritis. Clin. Allergy 10:463, 1980.*)

Experimental Study: 26 pts. with classical RA, all on non-steroidal anti-inflammatory drugs, were involved. 16 were placed on a diet of fruit and vegetable juices and herbal tea for 7-10 days (1 stopped after 2 days), while the other 10 were controls. Most of the 15 experimental pts. felt better by day 5 or 6. At the end of the first diet, 10 reported reduction in pain and stiffness. 5/15 showed objective improvement defined as a greater than 10% decrease in the sedimentation rate with concomitant decrease in joint tenderness, while only 1 of the controls improved. A subsequent 9 week lactovegetarian diet was ineffective for all but 1 pt. (*Skoldstam L et al. Effects of fasting and lactovegetarian diet on rheumatoid arthritis. Scand. J. Rheum. 8:249-55, 1979*).

Symptom provocation during food challenges may be due to the release of serotonin from platelets.

Experimental Study: Exacerbation of arthritis was associated with a fall in serotonin levels and a subsequent increase in 5-hydroxyindoleacetic acid, suggesting that serotonin may be released from platelets during food challenges and that platelet serotonin may contribute to joint inflammation (*Little CH et al. Platelet serotonin release in rheumatoid arthritis: A study in food-intolerant patients Lancet 2:297, 1983*).

Food sensitivities in pts. with RA may be promoted by the use of non-steroidal anti-inflammatory drugs.

Observational Study: Pts. receiving non-steroidal anti-inflammatory medication excreted significantly more radio-actively labeled EDTA, while untreated pts. did not differ from controls. This suggests that NSAID's are associated with increased intestinal permeability to food antigens (*Bjarnason I et al. Intestinal permeability and inflammation in rheumatoid arthritis: Effects of non-steroidal anti-inflammatory drugs. Lancet 2:1171-3, 1984*).

Rule out <u>hydrochloric acid deficiency</u>.

Note: While gastric anacidity had been reported in the past to be a relatively common condition which was associated with acne rosacea and a number of other illnesses, the presence of achlorhydria is no longer accepted unless a potent parietal-cell stimulant (such as histamine) is employed in gastric analysis. More recent studies suggest that histamine-fast anacidity is uncommon before the fifth decade of life and, although it probably does not occur in a normal stomach, its presence is not necessarily associated with symptoms (Rappaport EM. Achlorhydria: Associated symptoms and response to hydrochloric acid. New Engl. J. Med. 252(19):802-5, 1955).

Observational Study: In a gp. of 35 female pts. (ave. age 41) 10 (28.6%) were achlorhydric, while 6 (17%) were hypochlorhydric. By comparison, 2 studies of normal females of similar ages reported an incidence of achlorhydria of 10.8% and 6.5% (*Hartung EF, Steinbrocker O. Gastric acidity in chronic arthritis. Ann. Int. Med. 9:252-7, 1935*).

See Also:

DeWitte TJ et al. Hypochlorhydria and hypergastrinemia in rheumatoid arthritis. Ann. Rheumatic Dis. 38:14-17, 1979

SCHIZOPHRENIA

See Also: ORGANIC MENTAL DISORDER

OVERVIEW:

It is well known that certain specific nutritional deficiency syndromes can produce schizophreniform psychoses or exacerbate schizophrenic symptomatology. Examples are deficiencies of <u>folic acid</u> (the most common vitamin deficiency), <u>ascorbic acid</u>, <u>manganese</u> and <u>zinc</u>. On the other hand, excesses of <u>folic acid</u> or <u>copper</u> can produce a similar picture.

Other than to correct an established abnormality, research on using nutrition to treat schizophrenia is very limited. A number of experimental studies have focused on supplementation with <u>niacin</u>, but the results of double-blind studies have been contradictory.

<u>Food sensitivities</u>, especially to wheat and milk, have been implicated as an etiologic factor. It is not yet known what percentage of schizophrenics, or what schizophrenic sub-group, will respond to food eliminations.

- -

BASIC DIET:

Remove <u>caffeine</u>

> Caffeine is a methyl-xanthine that is absorbed approx. 1 hour after ingestion and has a serum half-life of 3 hours. Animal studies suggest that it can both release norepinephrine and increase norepinephrine synthesis in the CNS. It also appears to increase brain serotonin and has a biphasic effect on dopamine, with an initial increase followed by a prolonged decrease (*Mikkelsen EJ. Caffeine and schizophrenia. <u>Behavioral Med.</u> December, 1980*).

> See Also:

>> **Review Article:** *Mikkelsen EJ. Caffeine and schizophrenia. <u>J. Clin. Psychiat.</u> 39(9),Sept. 1978*

>> *McManamy MC, Schube PG. Caffeine intoxication. <u>New Engl. J. Med.</u> 215:616-20, 1936*

- -

NUTRIENTS:

<u>Folic Acid</u>: 2 mg. daily

> Folate deficiency occurs in approx. 25% of pts. hospitalized in state mental hospitals (*Kallstrom B et al. Vitamin B$_{12}$ and folate concentrations in mental patients. <u>Acta Psychiat. Scand.</u> 45:137-52, 1969; Hunter R et al. Serum B$_{12}$ and folate concentration in mental patients. <u>Brit. J. Psychiat.</u> 113:1291-5, 1967*).

> Folate deficiency is associated with a wide variety of psychiatric symptoms including psychosis, depression, confusion, disorientation, and dementia as well as with neurologic symptoms of weakness, numbness, stiffness and spasticity, both with and without muscular atrophy (*Howard JS. Folate deficiency in psychiatric practice. <u>Psychosomatics</u> 16:112-15, 1975*).

Supplementation may be beneficial.

> **Experimental and Observational Study:** The ave. serum folate in 10 "histapenic" schizophrenics (pts. with low histamine and high copper levels) was 6.0 +/- 3.1 ng/ml compared to 12.3 +/- 6.2 ng/ml in 26 "pyroluric" schizophrenics (normal in copper but deficient in pyridoxine and zinc). Folic acid along with B_{12}, zinc, niacin and vitamin C was effective in the treatment of histapenic schizophrenics resulting in reduction in serum copper and a rise in blood histamine after 5-6 months along with symptomatic improvement. On the other hand, folic acid worsened pts. with high histamine and normal copper levels ("histadelic schizophrenics") who respond to mild antifolate drugs such as phenytoin and agents that decrease histamine such as calcium salts and methionine in doses of 1-2 gm/day (*Pfeiffer CC, Braverman ER. Folic acid and vitamin B_{12} therapy for the low-histamine, high-copper biotype of schizophrenia, in Botez MI, Reynolds EN, Eds.* Folic Acid in Neurology, Psychiatry, and Internal Medicine. *New York, Raven Press, 1979, pp. 483-87*).

See Also:

> *Botez T et al. Neuropsychological disorders responsive to folic acid therapy: A report of 39 cases.* Excerpta Medica Internat. Congress Series *427:202, 1977*

WARNING: Supplementation with folic acid can cause an exacerbation of psychotic behavior if blood levels become elevated.

> **Case Reports:**
> 1. 30 year-old male with schizoaffective illness receiving haloperidol 100 mg daily and lithium carbonate 1800 mg daily had a low RBC folate level and was supplemented with folic acid 3 mg daily. 2 wks. later he began to become more irritable and combative and showed marked verbosity. RBC folate level was found to be elevated. Folic acid was gradually discontinued and his behavior improved.
> 2. 23 year-old male with catatonic schizophrenia and grand mal seizures receiving haloperidol 20 mg daily, diphenylhydantoin 200 mg daily, diazepam 20 mg daily and benztropine 4 mg daily had a low serum folate level and was supplemented with folic acid 1 mg daily. 5 mo. later he gradually became excited and quarrelsome, giggled without reason and showed increased stereotyped behavior. Serum folate level was elevated so folic acid was gradually tapered followed by notable improvement in his behavior.
> (*Prakash R, Petric WM. Psychiatric changes associated with an excess of folic acid.* Am. J. Psychiat. *139(9):1192, 1982*).

Niacin:

Supplementation may be beneficial.

Beneficial effects have been claimed with massive doses which are associated with the potential of serious side-effects (*see below*). The value of this treatment is highly controversial.

Typical regime: 500 mg. three times daily after meals for 3 days; then 1 gm three times daily after meals; then gradually increase dose to 6 - 12 gms daily (alcoholics are said to benefit from still higher doses) (*Ross HM. Megavitamins.* J. Orthomol. Psychiat. *1975*).

Common side effects:
1. Histamine flush: first 3 days; starts in 20 minutes and lasts 1-1 1/2 hours. May be absent once dose is doubled. (ASA 650 mg. 15-30 minutes before may be helpful.)
2. Nausea and vomiting: said to disappear in 2 weeks.

WARNINGS:
1. May increase G.I. irritation
2. May cause abnormal liver function (perform baseline liver function studies and every 6-8 months)
3. May increase blood sugar
4. May increase uric acid
(Reference: *Mosher LR. Nicotinic acid side effects and toxicity: A review. Am. J. Psychiat. 126:9, 1970*)

Alternative to Niacin: Niacinamide (nicotinamide): 1000 mg. 3 times daily after meals

Common side effect: sedation

WARNINGS:
1. May produce depression
2. May cause hepatic toxicity (*Winter SL, Boyer JL. Hepatic toxicity from large doses of vitamin B3 (nicotinamide). New Engl. J. Med. 289 (22):1180-82, 1973*).

Positive Double-blind studies:

Experimental Double-blind Study: The data of a negative experimental double-blind study (*see Wittenborn, 1973 - below*) were analyzed post-hoc to attempt to distinguish a sub-group which benefited from niacin 6 gm daily in additional to standard treatment. Out of the 86 male pts. in the study, a sub-group of 24 pts. did emerge which was distinguished by a history of premorbid close relationships and a stable employment record. At follow-up both at 12 and 24 mo. after supplementation, 10/12 niacin pts. made a good adjustment compared to 5/12 placebo patients. The author cautions that such a post-hoc analysis must be confirmed by prospective experimental studies (*Wittenborn JR. A search for responders to niacin supplementation. Arch. Gen. Psychiat. 31:547-52, 1974*).

Experimental Double-blind Study: 30 pts. were randomly divided into 3 gps. and received either niacin, nicotinamide or placebo, usually in addition to ECT, for 33 days. On follow-up, 10 pts. in the niacin gp. (1 gm 3 times daily) were well an average of 23 out of 26 months and 11 pts. in the nicotinamide gp. (1 gm 3 times daily) were well an average of 26 out of 27 months, while 9 pts. in the placebo gp. were only well an average of 11 out of 23 months (*Osmond H, Hoffer A. Massive niacin treatment in schizophrenia: Review of a nine-year study. Lancet 1:316-20, 1962*).

Note: This study, as well as others by the author, has been criticized on the following grounds:
1. The study population was heterogeneous and included some chronic schizophrenics as well as pts. with toxic and organic psychoses.
2. There was considerable variability in treatments: some only received nicotininc acid, some nicotinic acid plus various other treatments.
3. The control studies were not concurrent.
4. The definition of "well" (return to previous state before illness) is ambiguous.
5. Readmission rates were probably confounded by unreported admissions to other psychiatric facilities.
6. The niacin flush and other side-effects were uncontrolled, suggesting that the double-blind may have been broken by some patients.
(Raft D et al. Nicotinic acid and schizophrenia: A critique. Psychiat. Digest January, 1975, pp. 18-23).

Experimental Double-blind Study: 36 male pts. received either nicotinamide 3 gm daily or placebo in addition to ECT and standard therapy for 5 weeks. When the number of pts. in the hospital each week was calculated, the nicotinamide gp. usually had fewer pts. in the hospital, with the greatest difference occurring wks. 21 and 22 (p less than 0.05). The 17 supplemented pts. spent an ave. of 15 wks. in the hospital compared to 25 wks. for the pts. on placebo (*Denson S. The value of nicotinamide in the treatment of schizophrenia. Dis. Nerv. Sys. 23:167-72, 1962*).

See Also:

Hoffer A. Niacin Therapy in Psychiatry. Springfield, Illinois, Charles C. Thomas, 1962

Negative Double-blind studies:

Note: For a discussion of earlier negative double-blind studies and the negative conclusions reached by the American Psychiatric Association's Task Force on Vitamin Therapy in Psychiatry, see: Megavitamin and Orthomolecular Therapy in Psychiatry. Washington, D.C., American Psychiatric Association, 1973

Review Article: In an attempt to resolve the controversy, the Board of Directors of the Canadian Mental Health Association set up a series of clinical trials utilizing doses of at least 3 gm. daily for as long as 2 years. Six of those studies are summarized which were uniformly negative in their outcome (*Ban TA. Nicotinic acid in the treatment of schizophrenias: Practical and theoretical considerations. Neuropsychobiol. 1:133-45, 1975*).

Negative Experimental Double-blind Study: 86 male schizophrenics initially received niacin 500 mg daily (to assure that the initial niacin flush was experienced equally by both the experimental and placebo gps.) followed by either niacin 3000 mg daily or placebo. After 18 months, analyses of scales rating social adjustment, self-report data, rate of attrition, duration of hospitalization and need for tranquilization failed to reveal an advantage for the niacin group. In addition, 1/3 of the niacin gp. developed a pigmented hyperkeratosis (*Wittenborn JR et al. Niacin in the long-term treatment of schizophrenia. Arch. Gen. Psychiat. 28:308-15, 1973*).

Negative Experimental Double-blind Study: 30 newly-admitted hospitalized pts. received either nicotinic acid 3-8 gm daily according to symptom severity (#9), nicotinamide 3-8 gm daily (#10) or placebo (#11) in addition to standard therapy. Over a 12-wk. period, the nicotinamide gp. showed significant improvement in 12/18 items in the Brief Psychiatric Rating Scale,the nicotinic acid gp. improved on 11 items, and the placebo gp. improved on only 6 items. After 2 years, the nicotinic acid gp. significantly improved on 10 items as did the nicotinamide gp., while the placebo gp. improved in only 6 (p less than 0.05). However, no significant differences in the ave. daily tranquilizer dose or the ave. length of hospitalization was observed between the experimental and control groups (*Ananth JV et al. Nicotinic acid in the treatment of newly admitted schizophrenic patients: A placebo controlled study. Int. J. Clin. Pharmacol. 5:406-10, 1972*).

Note: This study has been criticized because only 6/30 subjects ingested the vitamins or placebo for the full 2 years even though data from all 30 subjects were used; in fact, 1 subject in the nicotinic acid gp. took the vitamin only 14 days and only 7/19 subjects receiving vitamins took them for at least 1 year (Kahan M. Search and Research: Summaries of Megavitamin Studies. Canadian Schizophrenia Foundation, 2229 Broad St., Regina, Saskatchewan, Canada S4P 1Y7).

Pyridoxine: 50 mg. daily - 500 mg. three times daily

Supplementation may be beneficial.

Theoretical Discussion: According to Carl Pfeiffer, Ph.D, M.D., kryptopyrrole, which he claims is found in the urine of 30% of schizophrenics, reacts avidly with all aldehydes. Its reaction with pyridoxal forms a kryptopyrrole-pyridoxal complex which chelates zinc to produce a zinc (as well as a pyridoxine) deficiency ("pyroluria"). Lab findings are eosinophilia, lymphocytosis, elevated bilirubin and depressed immunoglobulin A. These pts. are said to respond "for the most part" to vitamin B_6, Zn and Mn supplementation with progress within 1 wk. and total recovery in 3-4 mo.

(*Pfeiffer CC. The schizophrenias '76. Biol. Psychiat. 2:773-75, 1976; Pfeiffer CC, Bacchi D. Copper, zinc, manganese, niacin and pyridoxine in the schizophrenias. J. Appl. Nutr. 27:9-39, 1975; Pfeiffer CC. Observations on trace and toxic elements in hair and serum. J. Orthomol. Psychiat. 3(4):259-64, 1974*).

Note: In an investigation of Carl Pfeiffer's concept of "pyroluria," urinary pyrrole determinations were performed on 9 schizophrenics taking neuroleptics and 10 healthy controls and the results were compared to the signs and symptoms described by Pfeiffer as characteristic of B$_6$ and zinc deficiency. The results failed to support Pfeiffer's concept. It is suggested that Pfeiffer's observations may have been made on pts. who had acute schizophrenic symptoms secondary to a metabolic disease similar to porphyria which may be associated with psychotic symptoms and pyridoxine deficiency (Cruz R, Vogel WH. Pyroluria: A poor marker in chronic schizophrenia. Am. J. Psychiat. 135(10):1239-1240, 1978).

Case Report: 15 year-old female with schizophrenic symptoms had homocysteinuria due to impaired N^{5,10}-tetrahydrofolate reductase activity. Folate and pyridoxine supplementation resulted in substantial improvement (*Barber GW, Spaeth GL. Successful treatment of homocysteinuria with pyridoxine. J. Pediatr. 75:463-78, 1969*).

See Also:

Brooks SC et al. An unusual schizophrenic illness responsive to pyridoxine HCl (B$_6$) subsequent to phenothiazine and butyrophenone toxicities. Biol. Psychiat. 18(11):1321-28, 1983

- with L-Dopa:

Supplementation may be beneficial.

Experimental Study: 8 pts. with a mean duration of disease of 18.3 yrs. received pyridoxal-5'-phosphate 30 mg and L-Dopa 200 mg daily. By 12 wks., 2/8 showed excellent responses, 3/8 good and 3/8 fair responses. A marked increase in EEG alpha activity occurred starting the 2nd to 4th week in all 8 cases which tended to preceed the clinical improvement. These results contrasted with the results of L-Dopa alone and pyridoxine alone which were each only minimally effective (*Yamauchi M. Effects of L-dopa and vitamin B$_6$ on electroencephalograms of schizophrenic patients: A preliminary report. Folia Psychiatrica et Neurologica Japonica 30(2):121-51, 1976; Kai Y. The effect of L-Dopa and vitamin B$_6$ in schizophrenia. Folia Psychiatrica et Neurologica Japonica 30(1):19-26, 1976*).

Niacin and
Pyridoxine:

Combined supplementation may be more beneficial than either supplement alone.

Experimental Placebo-controlled Study: 30 chronic pts. hospitalized at least 2 yrs. received either (1) nicotinic acid 3 gm daily and pyridoxine placebo, (2) pyridoxine 75 mg daily for 4 wks. per course for 3 courses and nicotinic acid placebo, or (3) nicotinic acid and pyridoxine. After 48 wks., there was significant improvement in both the nicotinic acid gp. and the pyridoxine gp. but not in the combined gp., although the combined gp. was the only one in which the daily ave. phenothiazine dose decreased. There were notable side-effects in all 3 gps. (*Ananth JV et al. Potentiation of therapeutic effects of nicotinic acid by pyridoxine in chronic schizophrenics. Can. Psychiatr. Assoc. J. 18:377-83, 1973*).

Vitamin C:

May be deficient, even with intakes considered to be adequate for normals (*Leitner ZA, Church IE. Nutritional studies in a mental hospital. Lancet 1:565, 1956*).

Observational Study: The vitamin C nutritional status in 20 hospitalized schizophrenics and 15 controls was assessed by loading them with ascorbic acid 1 gm and determining subsequent urinary vitamin C excretion. Prior to loading, the ave. plasma vitamin C level in schizophrenics was significantly lower than that of controls (p less than 0.05). Schizophrenics were found to have a lower vitamin C excretion compared to controls (p less than 0.01). These differences could not be attributed either to differences in ascorbic acid intake (since both gps. received the same diet containing an ave. of 50 mg ascorbic acid daily for at least 2 mo. prior to evaluation) or to differences in ascorbic acid resorption. Regression analyses showed the differences in urinary excretion to be primarily associated with pre-test plasma vitamin C levels (*Suboticanec K et al. Vitamin C and schizophrenia. Acta Med. Iug. 38:299-308, 1984*).

Observational Study: The ave. plasma vitamin C level in 885 psychiatric pts. was 0.51/100 ml compared to 0.87/100 ml in 110 healthy controls. 32% of the pts. had levels below 0.35 mg/100 ml, the threshold which has been associated with detrimental effects on immune responses and behavior (*Schorah CJ et al. Human Nutr.: Clin. Nutr. 37C:447-52, 1983*).

Supplementation may be beneficial.

Animal Experimental Study: Haloperidol was given to rats pretreated with saline or ascorbic acid 1000 mg/kg. to test its ability to block the behavioral response to amphetamine and to elicit catalepsy. Compared to controls, AA-treated rats showed enhanced anti-amphetamine and cataleptogenic effects from haloperidol even though AA at that dosage had no behavioral effect by itself, suggesting that AA helps to modulate the effects of antipsychotic drugs. At higher concentrations, AA blocked the amphetamine response directly, suggesting that it alone could attenuate dopamine-mediated behaviors (*Rebec GV et al. Ascorbic acid and the behavioral response to haloperidol: Implications for the action of antipsychotic drugs. Science 227:438-40, 1985*).

Experimental Double-blind Study: 40 chronic male psychiatric pts. (34 with Schizophrenia) randomly received either ascorbic acid 1 gm daily or placebo. After 3 wks., there was a significant decrease in the MMPI "D" (depression) scale (p less than 0.01) only for the experimental group. The nurse felt that 5 pts. had obviously improved and the doctor agreed in regard to 4 of them; all 5 turned out to be in the experimental group. The Wittenborn Psychiatric Rating Scales showed significant improvement in Paranoid State only for the experimental gp. (p less than 0.05). The 24-hour ascorbic acid urinary excretion in the control gp. was at the very lowest limit of normal. While normal subjects can be saturated with ascorbic acid after 1-2 days of supplementation with 1 gm daily, pts. with borderline or frank scurvy require 7-10 days and the pts. in this study required an ave. of 6 days. These findings suggest that chronic psychiatric pts. may be in a state of "subscurvy" and thus could benefit from ascorbic acid supplementation (*Milner G. Ascorbic acid in chronic psychiatric patients: A controlled trial. Brit. J. Psychiat. 109:294-99, 1963*).

- -

Copper:

May be excessive.

Note: Wilson's Disease, a disease characterized by excessive Cu storage, may present as a schizophrenic syndrome, while "dialysis dementia" is believed to be caused by copper excess.

Negative Observational Study: When CSF copper concentrations were measured using a sensitive flameless atomic absorption spectrophotometric procedure, there were no significant differences between unmedicated and medicated schizophrenics, former heroin addicts, and normal controls. Similarly there were no differences between pt. subgroups with respect to diagnostic subtype, length of hospitalization, race, medication status, platelet monamine oxidase values or CAT scan abnormalities (*Shore D et al. CSF copper concentrations in chronic schizophrenia. Am. J. Psychiatry 140(6):754-57, 1983*).

Review Article:
The hypothesis that excess tissue copper can cause schizophrenia has never been compellingly demonstrated nor convincingly refuted. The following conclusions are suggested by the literature:
1. Copper elevations seem tied to dopamine activity.
2. Elevated copper may be found in schizophrenia.
3. Elevated copper does not produce schizophrenia.
4. Adjusting copper levels affects schizophrenic symptoms but does not cure schizophrenia.
(*Bowman MB, Levis MS. The copper hypothesis of schizophrenia: a review. Neurosci. & Biobehav. Rev. 6:321-8, 1982*).

Negative Observational Study and Review Article: Copper in serum, urine and gastric fluid and serum ceruloplasmin of pts. with acute and chronic schizophrenia, on or off treatment with various major tranquilizers, failed to show significant deviations from normal. Although depletion in body zinc and increases in brain copper have been associated with severe changes in mentation and personality, there are no published, controlled clinical studies which support the hypothesis that administration of of exogenous zinc and/or depletion of body copper is beneficial (*Gillin JC et al. Zinc and copper in patients with schizophrenia. Encephale 8(3):435-44, 1982*).

Theoretical Discussion: According to Carl C. Pfeiffer, Ph.D., M.D., the "histapenic" biotype of schizophenia is frequently due to an environmentally-produced copper overload resulting in a nutrient imbalance characterized by deficiencies in folic acid, vitamin B_{12}, niacin, zinc and manganese. They are usually classified as chronic or process schizophrenics. While paranoia and hallucinations are common in younger pts., depression may predominate in older pts. (*Pfeiffer CC, LaMola S. Zinc and manganese in the schizophrenias. J. Orthomol. Psychiat. 12:215-234, 1983*).

Negative Observational Study: Compared to 6 controls, the CSF copper levels in 8 schizophrenics were significantly lower (*Tyrer SP et al. CSF copper in schizophrenia. Am. J. Psychiatry 136(7):937-39, 1979*).

> *Note: This study has been criticized as follows:*
> *1. The deuterium continuum light source with a limited aspiration flame technique used in this study is hampered by machine noise creating background interference which produces variable, unreliable results.*
> *2. CSF obtained from pts. undergoing evaluation for spinal disc disease (the controls) is usually not considered representative of fluid from normal volunteers (Henkin RI, Agarwal RP. CSF copper concentrations. Letter to the Editor. Am. J. Psychiatry 142(1):143-44, 1985*).

Observational Study: 20% of 240 pts. had elevated serum copper levels (greater than 1.2 mcg/ml) compared to controls (*Pfeiffer CC, Illiev V. A study of zinc deficiency and copper excess in the schizophrenias. Internat. Rev. Biol. Suppl. 1, 1972*).

Experimental Study: Of various supplements tested to increase Cu excretion in pts., the combination of Zn 50 mg, Mn 3 mg and B_6 50 mg was by far the most successful (*Pfeiffer CC - ibid*).

Observational Study: In a study of Cu levels in drinking water across the U.S., every home which had a Cu level greater than what the U.S. Public Health Service considers safe also had at least 1 family member with psychiatric problems (*J. Applied Nutr. Winter, 1975*).

Manganese:

May be deficient.

Observational Study: Hair Mn was low in schizophrenics compared to normal values (*Pfeiffer CC. Observations on trace and toxic elements in hair and serum. J. Orthomolec. Psych. 3(4):259-64, 1974*).

Supplementation may be beneficial.

> WARNING: Supplementation may occasionally elevate blood pressure in people over 40 or cause hypertensive headaches (*Pfeiffer CC, LaMola S. Zinc and manganese in the schizophrenias. J. Orthomol. Psychiat. 12:215-234, 1983*).

> **Experimental Study:** Oral Mn produced a 3-fold increase in Cu excretion in pts. found to have evidence of Cu overload along with low blood histamine ("histapenia") as shown by serum or hair analysis, while the combination of Zn with Mn (10% Zn sulfate and 5% Mn chloride taken as 6 drops twice daily to provide 10 mg Zn and 3 mg Mn) was even more effective in reducing the Cu burden (*Pfeiffer CC, Iliev V. A study of zinc deficiency and copper excess in the schizophrenias, in Pfeiffer CC, Ed. The International Review of Neurobioloby. New York, Academic Press, 1972, p. 141*).

> **Negative Experimental Study:** 30 pts. received suspended Mn dioxide IM. 26 were unchanged, 2 improved and 2 worsened (*Hoskins RG. The manganese treatment of schizophrenic disorders. J. Nerv. Ment. Dis. 79:59, 1934*).

> **Experimental Study:** Of 38 pts. who had been psychotic for 2 wks. to 3 yrs., 22 showed mental and physical improvements with Mn supplementation. Other categories of schizophrenics did not do as well (*English WM. Report of the treatment with manganese chloride of 181 cases of schizophrenia, 33 of manic depression, and 16 other defects of psychoses at the Ontario Hospital, Brockville, Ontario. Am. J. Psychiat. 9:569-80, 1929*).

> **Experimental Controlled Study:** 37% of 30 hospitalized pts. treated with oral and IV Mn were discharged in 1 year compared to 18% of controls (*Reed GE. Use of manganese chloride in dementia praecox. Canad. Med. Assoc. J. 21:96-149, 1929*).

<u>Zinc:</u>   Zinc gluconate 15 mg daily with meals

May be deficient.

> **Negative Observational Study:** Zinc in serum, urine, gastric fluid and hair of pts. with acute and chronic schizrenia, on or off treatment with various major tranquilizers, failed to show significant deviations from normal (*Gillin JC et al. Zinc and copper in patients with schizophrenia. Encephale 8(3):435-44, 1982*).

> **Case Report:** A pt. is described who presented with schizophrenic symptoms and was found to have Zn deficiency and Cu excess (*Stanton MA et al. Zinc deficiency presenting as schizophrenia. Curr. Concepts in Psychiat. 2:1976*).

> **Observational Study:** A 30% reduction in brain Zn content was found in early onset schizophrenics compared to normals (*McLardy T. Hippocampal zinc in chronic alcoholism and schizophrenia. IRCS J. Med. Sci. 2:1010, 1973*).

> **Observational Study:** At autopsy, frontal, occipital and hippocampal portions of brains of schizophrenics were found to have only 50% of the Zn content of control brains (*Kimura I, Kumura J. Preliminary reports on the metabolism of trace elements in neuropsychiatric diseases. I. Zinc in schizophrenia. Proc. Jap. Acad. Sci. 1965, p. 943*).

Deficiency is associated with apathy, lethargy, amnesia, and mental retardation, often with considerable irritability, depression and paranoia (*Prasad AS et al. Experimental zinc deficiency in humans. Ann. Intern. Med. 89:483, 1978*), and elevate brain catecholamine levels (*Wallwork J, Sandstead H. Effect of zinc deficiency on brain catecholamine concentrations in the rat. Fed. Proc. 40:939, 1981*).

Deficiency inhibits omega-6 essential fatty acid metabolism either by blocking linoleic acid desaturation to gamma-linolenic acid or by inhibiting mobilization of dihomogammalinolenic acid from tissue membrane stores (*Cunnane SC, Horrobin DF. Parenteral linolenic and gamma-linolenic acids ameliorate the gross effects of zinc deficiency. Proc. Soc. Exp. Biol. & Med. 164:583, 1980*).

Supplementation (along with pyridoxine) may be beneficial.

WARNINGS: Possible side-effects are occasional nausea, increased sweating, alcohol intolerance and transient worsening of depression or hallucinations. Zinc supplementation may increase grand mal seizures in epileptics, possibly due to it causing a reduction in blood Mn levels, and thus Mn supplementation should be started first (*Pfeiffer CC, LaMola S. Zinc and manganese in the schizophrenias. J. Orthomol. Psychiat. 12:215-234, 1983*).

Review Article: Although depletion in body zinc and increases in brain copper have been associated with severe changes in mentation and personality, there are no published, controlled clinical studies which support the hypothesis that administration of exogenous zinc and/or depletion of body copper is beneficial (*Gillin JC et al. Zinc and copper in patients with schizophrenia. Encephale 8(3):435-44, 1982*).

Animal Experimental Study: Rats given 40 mg/kg B$_6$ absorbed 71% of their dietary Zn while controls receiving 2 mg/kg B$_6$ daily absorbed only 46% (*Evans GW. Normal and abnormal zinc absorption in man and animals: The tryptophan connection. Nutr. Rev. 38:137, 1980*).

Theoretical Discussion: According to Carl Pfeiffer, Ph.D, M.D., kryptopyrrole, which is found in the urine of some schizophrenics, reacts avidly with pyridoxal to form a kryptopyrrole-pyridoxal complex which chelates zinc to produce a zinc (as well as a pyridoxine) deficiency ("pyroluria"). These pts. are said to respond "for the most part" to vitamin B$_6$ and zinc therapy (*Pfeiffer CC. The schizophrenias '76. Biol. Psychiat. 2:773-75, 1976; Pfeiffer CC, Bacchi D. Copper zinc manganese, niacin and pyridoxine in the schizophrenias. J. Appl. Nutr. 27:9-39, 1975*).

Note: In an investigation of Carl Pfeiffer's concept of "pyroluria," urinary pyrrole determinations were performed on 9 schizophrenics on neuroleptics and 10 healthy controls and the results were compared to the signs and symptoms described by Pfeiffer as characteristic of B$_6$ and zinc deficiency. The results failed to support Pfeiffer's concept. It is suggested that Pfeiffer's observations may have been made on pts. who had acute schizophrenic symptoms secondary to a metabolic disease similar to porphyria which may be associated with psychotic symptoms and pyridoxine deficiency (Cruz R, Vogel WH. Pyroluria: A poor marker in chronic schizophrenia. Am. J. Psychiat. 135(10):1239-1240, 1978).

Theoretical Discussion: According to Carl Pfeiffer, Ph.D., M.D., pts. with Cu overload and low blood histamine ("histapenia") will benefit from Zn (along with B$_6$, Mn and Mo) supplementation to decrease the Cu overload (*Pfeiffer CC, Iliev V. A study of zinc deficiency and copper excess in the schizophrenias, in Pfeiffer CC, Ed. The Internat. Rev. of Neurobiol.. New York, Academic Press, 1972, p. 141*). Following supplementation, serum Cu may increase for 1-3 mo. before falling to a normal level. This temporary increase can be avoided by adding d-penicillamine, Mn and B$_6$ (*Pfeiffer CC, LaMola S. Zinc and manganese in the schizophrenias. J. Orthomol. Psychiat. 12:215-234, 1983*).

Observational Study: 11% of 240 schizophrenics had low serum zinc levels (less than 0.8 mcg/ml) compared to normal controls (*Pfeiffer CC, Illiev V. A study of zinc deficiency and copper excess in the schizophrenias. Int. Rev. Neurobiol. Suppl. 1, 1972*).

<u>Omega-6 Fatty Acids</u>:

$$\text{linoleic acid} \rightarrow \text{GLA} \rightarrow \text{DGLA} \rightarrow \text{prostaglandin E}_1$$

Evening primrose oil is a source of GLA, precursor to PGE_1.

Schizophrenics are said to be deficient in linoleic acid, GLA, DGLA, and the 1-series prostaglandins, but have an excess of arachidonic acid and its 2-series prostaglandin derivatives (*Horrobin DF, Huang YS. Schizophrenia: The role of abnormal essential fatty acid metabolism. <u>Med. Hypotheses</u> 10:329-36, 1983*).

In vitro Experimental Study: Red blood cells from pts. contained virtually no DGLA and greatly reduced amts. of linoleic acid from which DGLA can be formed. They contained 3 times the normal amts. of arachidonic acid (*Hitzemann RJ, Garver DL. Abnormalities in membrane lipids associated with deficiencies in lithium counterflow. <u>Soc. of Biol. Psychiat.</u> New Orleans, June, 1981*).

Observational Study: Schizophrenics had higher PGE concentrations in the cerebrospinal fluid than healthy controls, neurotics and pts. admitted for neurological investigation, suggesting that there may be an alteration of PG synthesis or metabolism (*Mathe AA et al. Increased content of immunoreactive prostaglandin E in cerebrospinal fluid of patients with schizophrenia. <u>Lancet</u> 1:16-18, 1980*).

In vitro Experimental Study: Platelets from pts. failed to make PGE_1 normally while those from normals, manics and depressives made substantial amounts (*Abdulla YH, Hamadah K. Effect of ADP on PGE formation in blood platelets from patients with depression, mania and schizophrenia. <u>Brit. J. Psychiat.</u> 127:591-5, 1975*).

Supplementation may be beneficial.

Experimental Study: 3/6 pts. responded to IV PGE_1 (*Kaiya H. Prostaglandin E_1 treatment of schizophrenia. <u>Biol. Psychiat.</u> 19(3):457-63, 1984*).

- with <u>Vitamins B$_3$, B$_6$, C and E</u> and <u>zinc sulfate</u>:

Negative Experimental Study: 10 severely affected chronic pts. whose moods had been stabilized on medications received EPO 4 gm, vitamin C 1 gm, vitamin B$_3$ 200 mg, vitamin B$_6$ 200 mg, vitamin E 40 mg and zinc sulfate 40 mg daily or placebo. Supplementation was stopped after 2 mo. and crossed over for 2 months. Behavior was evaluated every 2 mo. with the MACC Behavioral Adjustment Scale and the Brief Psychiatric Rating Scale. Supplementation was found to have no significant effect (*Holman CP et al. <u>J. Orthomol. Psychiat.</u> 12:302-4, 1983*).

- with <u>Penicillin V</u>:

Experimental Study: 6 chronic pts. inadequately controlled by phenothiazines were treated orally with evening primrose oil 1.2 - 1.8 ml daily and penicillin V (whose actions are compatible with stimulation of the 1-series prostaglandins) 250 mg daily and all other drug therapy was discontinued. 16 wks. later, no pt. had worsened and some showed striking improvement. Two case reports are presented in detail (*Vaddadi KS. Penicillin and essential fatty acid supplementation in schizophrenia. <u>Prostagland. & Med.</u> 2:77-80, 1979*).

<u>Serine</u>:

May be a biologic marker for psychosis.

Observational Study: Plasma serine levels were significantly higher and plasma serine hydroxy-methyltransferase levels significantly lower in 12 psychotic pts. than in 10 nonpsychotics. Two hours after an oral loading dose of serine, however, plasma serine levels were significantly <u>higher</u> in the nonpsychotic subjects. In addition, elimination of serine by psychotics and pts. with a history of psychosis was significantly different from that of nonpsychotics with no history of psychosis. These findings suggest that the absorption of serine is poorer among psychotics (*Wilcox J et al. Biol. Psychiat. 20:41-49, 1985*).

L-Tryptophan:

Tryptophan metabolism may be abnormal.

Observational Study: Dietary intakes of tryptophan and niacin and urinary excretion of metabolites of tryptophan in 7 schizophrenics were compared to 13 controls. Niacin ingestion was lower in schizophrenics than in controls, while all other parameters were not significantly different. Further information was gathered by calculating the correlation coefficients. Results suggest the following interpretations: (1) there is a control mechanism lacking in schizophrenics which determines how much tryptophan is metabolized by the indole and/or kynurenine pathways; (2) tryptophan hydroxylase, the first enzyme in the indole pathway, and pyrrolase, the first enzyme in the kynurenine pathway, may exert this control; (3) dietary manipulation will not affect tryptophan metabolism in schizophrenics; and (4), pyridoxine deficiency does not appear to be involved in the abnormal tryptophan metabolism in schizophrenia (*Payne IR et al. Relationship of dietary tryptophan and niacin to tryptophan metabolism in schizophrenics and nonschizophrenics. Am. J. Clin. Nutr. 27:565-71, 1974*).

Plasma levels may be associated with clinical status.

Observational Study: Plasma tryptophan was low in female schizophrenics and rose during recovery while remaining low in pts. who failed to improve (*Gilmour DG et al. Association of plasma tryptophan levels with clinical change in female schizophrenic patients. Biol. Psychiat. 6:119, 1973*).

Supplementation may be beneficial.

Experimental Double-blind Crossover Study: 12 male pts. alternately received placebo and 1 of 2 dosages of tryptophan. Pts. with high Buss-Durkee Hostility Inventory scores, a high lifetime frequency of aggressive incidents, and normal galvanic skin responses improved (decreased ward incidents, improvement in Brief Psychiatric Rating Scale factors and a lessening of hostility and depressed mood), while pts. with low scores on the BDHI, a low lifetime frequency of aggressive actions, and subnormally reactive galvanic skin responses worsened (worsening of BPRS indicators for depressed mood, conceptual disorganization and anergia) (*Morand C et al. Biol. Psychiat. 18:575-78, 1983*).

Negative Experimental Double-blind Study: After medications were stopped for 1 mo., 8 chronic undifferentiated schizophrenic men who had been relatively unresponsive to psychopharmacologic treatment received placebos for 14 days followed by L-tryptophan, starting at 9-12 gm/day and increasing over 3-4 days to 20 gm/day, administered with or without pyridoxine 100 mg/day, for 11-28 days followed by placebo for about 7 days. Tryptophan did not significantly affect overall mean nurses' ratings of psychosis, depression, anxiety, hallucinations, or delusions. While tryptophan neither improved nor exacerbated the clinical condition of most pts., individual pts.became better or worse, although these effects cannot be definitively attributed to the effects of tryptophan (*Gillin JC et al. Clinical effects of tryptophan in chronic schizophrenic patients. Biol. Psychiatry 11(5):635-39, 1976*).

- -

OTHER FACTORS:

Rule out <u>food sensitivities</u>.

A number of studies suggest that foods, especially <u>wheat</u> and <u>milk</u>, may contribute to schizophrenic symptoms.

Observational Study: The prevalence of overt chronic Schizophrenia was extremely low (only 2 "overtly insane chronic schizophrenics") in adults in remote regions of New Guinea, the Solomon Islands and Micronesia in which little or no grain, beer and milk is consumed, while the prevalence was much higher in the Westernized regions, where the inhabitants were eating Western foods and drinking barley beer (but not consuming milk), suggesting that certain neuroactive peptides from grain glutens may evoke schizophrenia in susceptible persons (*Dohan FC et al. Is schizophrenia rare if grain is rare? Biol.Psychiat. 19:385-99, 1984*).

In vitro Experimental Study: The authors found the amino acid sequence -Pro-Leu-Gly- in a peptide (Pro-Leu-Gly-NH$_2$) generated by enzymatic digestion of alpha-gliadin, a purified gliadin protein from wheat flour, which is similar to that of melanocyte-stimulating-hormone-release-inhibiting factor (MIF). A literature search revealed that the same AA sequence is found in casein, the major protein in cow's milk. They note that animal studies have shown that MIF enhances dopaminergic activity in the CNS and antagonizes both the behavioral and neurochemical effects of neuroleptic drugs. Assuming normal daily intakes of wheat and milk, approx. 150 mg of the tripeptide might be formed daily. 50 mg of MIF has produced EEG changes in normals, and 75 mg has induced mood alterations in clinically depressed subjects (*Mycroft FJ et al. MIF-like sequences in milk and wheat proteins. Letter to the Editor. New Engl. J. Med. 307(14):895, 1982*).

Negative Experimental Double-blind Study: In a randomized manner, 13 pts. were given gluten-free peanut-flour supplementary cookies and 13 were given virtually identical cookies with gluten added. Contrary to expectations, after 10 days the group receiving the gluten-added cookies showed significantly greater improvement on Profile of Mood States measures of tension-anxiety and anger-hostility than controls. Tests and rating scales before and after showed no greater improvement for those receiving the gluten-free cookies than for those receiving the gluten-added cookies (*Storms LH et al. Effects of gluten on schizophrenics. Arch. Gen. Psychiat. 39:323-27, 1982*).

Negative Experimental Double-blind Study: 8 young chronic pts. were maintained on a gluten-, cereal grain- and milk-free diet and challenged with wheat gluten and placebo. While on the diet, each pt. received a daily challenge of 30 gm gluten for 5 wks and a placebo challenge for 8 weeks. Clinical status was not adversely affected by gluten challenge and serum alpha$_1$ glycoprotein measurement demonstrated no evidence of inflammatory response to gluten (*Potkin SG et al. Wheat gluten challenge in schizophrenic patients. Am. J. Psychiat. 138(9):1208-11, 1981*).

Double-blind Case Report: A 14 year-old female with a history of GI intolerance to milk in childhood was challenged with milk and placebo in a double-blind manner. Milk, but not placebo, produced overt psychotic symptoms (*Denman AM. The relevance of immunopathology to research into schizophrenia, in Hemmings J, Ed. Biochemistry of Schizophrenia and Addiction. Lancaster, MTP Press, 1980*).

Observational Study: Psychotic patients (including schizophrenics) could be divided into 2 groups: one whose peripheral blood lymphocytes responded to gluten challenge with production of a leukocyte migration inhibition factor as celiac patients did (despite lack of evidence of malabsorption), and one which responded as normal control subjects did, suggesting that gluten may be involved in biological processes in the brain in certain psychotic individuals (*Ashkenazi A et al. Immunologic reaction of psychotic patients to fractions of gluten. Am. J. Psychiat. 136(10):1306-9, 1979*).

In vitro Experimental Study: Endorphin-like polypeptides ("exorphins") were found to be present in pepsin hydrolysates of wheat gluten and casein, suggesting that peptides derived from some food proteins may be of physiological importance (*Zioudrou C et al. Opioid peptides derived from food proteins. J. Biol. Chem. 254:2446-9, 1979*).

Experimental Study: 14 pts. eliminated milk and cereal grains for 14 weeks. After a 2-wk. drug-free baseline, they received psychotropics and a soy drink for 4 wks., wheat gluten instead of soy for 4 wks. and soy again for 4 wks. The wheat gluten challenge arrested or reversed the improvement in 10 pts. until it was removed. Two of the rating scales were double-blinded. The gluten effect was largely confined to nonparanoid pts. with poor outcomes (*Singh MM, Kay SR. Wheat gluten as a pathogenic factor in schizophrenia. Science 191:401-2, 1976*).

SCLERODERMA

See Also: AUTO-IMMUNE DISORDERS (GENERAL)

NUTRIENTS:

Para-amino benzoic acid:

WARNING: Potential side-effects include skin rash, anorexia, nausea and fever (*Physicians' Desk Reference.* Oradell, N.J., Med. Economics Co., Inc., 1986) as well as vitiligo (*Hughes CG. Oral PABA and vitiligo. J. Am. Acad. Dermatol. 9:770, 1983*) and liver toxicity (*Kantor GR, Ratz JL. Liver toxicity from potassium para-aminobenzoate. Letter to the Editor. J. Am. Acad. Dermatol. 13(4):671-72, 1985*).

Supplementation may be beneficial.

Case Reports:
1. 45 year-old female with 10 yr. history of progressive disease despite a thoracic sympathectomy and most of the accepted therapies. After starting supplementation with potassium para-aminobenzoate 20 gm daily she noted a softening of the skin and a wider range of joint motion. This was the first improvement since the disease began. Dosage was reduced to 10 gm daily and continued indefinitely.
2. 53 year-old female with 6-mo. history of progressive disease. Steroids and physiotherapy were of no benefit, but she improved over 2 years once started on potassium para-aminobenzoate 12 gm daily (*Grace WJ et al. Therapy of scleroderma and dermatomyositis. N. Y. State J. Med. 63:140-44, 1963*).

See Also:

Zarafonetis CJD. Treatment of localized forms of scleroderma. *Am. J. Med. Sci. 243:147, 1962*

Zarafonetis CJD. The treatment of scleroderma: Results of Potassium Para-Aminobenzoate Therapy in 104 cases, in Mills & Moyer, Eds. *Inflammation and Disease of Connective Tissue.* W.B. Saunders Co., 1961, pp. 688-696

Zarafonetis CJD. Treatment of scleroderma. *Ann. Int. Med. 50:343, 1959*

Vitamin E: 800 I.U. of d-alpha tocopheryl acetate daily 15 min. before meals.
Increase to 1600 I.U. if needed; then decrease to minimal maintenance dosage.
Avoid taking iron at the same time.

An experimental progeria-like syndrome in rats with soft tissue calcifications can be prevented by concomitant administration of vitamin E along with the inciting agent.

- with Methyltestosterone:

Animal Experimental Study (rat): A progeria-like syndrome induced by chronic intoxication with dihydrotachysterol was prevented by concurrent D-alpha-tocopherol and methyltestosterone treatment (*Tuchweber B et al. Effect of vitamin E and methyltestosterone upon the progeria-like syndrome produced by dihydrotachysterol. Am. J. Clin. Nutr. 13:238-42, 1963*).

Supplementation may be beneficial.

Experimental Study: 3 patients with systemic sclerosis improved following supplementation with vitamin E as did 3 patients with localized scleroderma (morphea) (*Ayres S et al. Raynaud's phenomenon, scleroderma and calcinosis cutis: Response to vitamin E. Cutis 11:54-62, 1973*).
See Also:

> *Ayres S, Mihan R. Vitamin E (tocopherol): A reappraisal of its value in dermatoses of mesodermal tissues. Cutis 7:35, 1971*

- -

OTHER FACTORS:

Omega-6 Fatty acids:

Supplementation may be beneficial.

Experimental Study: 4 female pts. with systemic sclerosis for 5-13 yrs. duration received EPO (rich in gamma-linolenic acid) 1 gm 3 times daily. After 1 yr. clinical benefits included relief of pain in the extremities, improvement of telangiectasia and skin texture, and healing of ulcers. It is suggested that 6 gms daily may be of greater benefit (*Strong AMM et al. The effect of oral linoleic acid and gamma-linolenic acid (Efamol). Br. J. Clin. Pract. Nov/Dec 1985, p. 444*).

SEBORRHEIC DERMATITIS

NUTRIENTS:

<u>Biotin:</u>

May be deficient in infants. If so, supplementation may be beneficial.

Experimental Study: As biotin was unavailable, infants with extensive seborrheic dermatitis unresponsive to local treatment were fed liver and egg yolk (which have large amts. of biotin) early in the first month or two of life, with good clinical improvement. Those infants with more widespread involvement improved more rapidly when B complex injections (1 cc either once or repeated in 1 wk.) were added (*Nisenson A. Treatment of seborrheic dermatitis with biotin and vitamin B complex. Letter to the Editor. <u>J. Pediat.</u> 81:630-31, 1972*).

See Also:

> *Nisenson A. Seborrheic dermatitis of infants. Treatment with biotin injections for the nursing mother. <u>Pediatrics</u> 44:1014, 1969*

<u>Folic Acid:</u>   2 mg. daily

Supplementation may be beneficial (<u>not</u> for seborrhea sicca).

Experimental Study: Following folic acid supplementation (2.5 mg daily for infants, 5 mg daily for children, and 10 mg daily for adults), 3/5 cases of SD of infancy were much improved, while 17/20 cases of SD in adults responded (9/20 cases much improved, 8/20 improved) (*Callaghan TJ. The effect of folic acid on seborrheic dermatitis. <u>Cutis</u> 3:583-588, 1967*).

<u>Vitamin B$_{12}$:</u> Intramuscular injections

Supplementation may be beneficial.

Experimental Study: 37 pts. were treated with vitamin B$_{12}$ IM 10-30 mcg every wk. to every 3 weeks. Improvement was usually seen after 2 or 3 injections. 16/37 (43.5%) were greatly improved or apparently cured, 16/37 (43.5%) were improved, and 3/37 (8%) were slightly improved (*Andrews GC et al. Seborrheic dermatitis: Supplemental treatment with vitamin B$_{12}$. <u>N. Y. State Med. J.</u> 50:1921-25, 1950*).

<u>Vitamin E:</u>

Supplementation may be beneficial.

Experimental Study: Following 150 mg vitamin E IM 2-3 times weekly in addition to 100-150 mg 3 times daily after meals, 5/8 pts. with dry, scaly skin (ichthyosis or seborrhea sicca) had excellent results and 3 had good results (*Block MT. Vitamin E in the treatment of diseases of the skin. <u>Clin. Med.</u> January 1953, pp. 31-34*).

- -

TOPICAL APPLICATIONS:

Pyridoxine: ointment (50 mg/g) in water-soluble base

(Ex. "Soothing Cream" manufactured by Plus)

Note: initial worsening is considered a positive sign

May be beneficial in seborrhea sicca ("dandruff" - greasy adherent scales on an erythematous base).

Experimental Study: When pyridoxine deficiency was produced by the use of pyridoxine antagonists, a seborrhea-like lesion developed about the eyes, nasolabial fold and mouth, with extension to the eyebrows and skin behind the ears. Many of these cases responded well to the local application of pyridoxine in an ointment base, while little effect was noted when the vitamin was given orally or parenterally (*Schreiner AW et al. Seborrheic dermatitis: A local metabolic defect involving pyridoxine. J. Lab. Clin. Med. 40:121-30, 1952*).

See Also:

Effersoe H. The effect of topical application of pyridoxine ointment on the rate of sebaceous secretion in patients with seborrheic dermatitis. Acta Dermatovener 34:272-77, 1954

Schreiner AW et al. A local defect in the metabolism of pyridoxine in the skin of persons with seborrheic dermatitis of the "sicca" type. J. Invest. Dermatol. 19:95-96, 1952

- -

OTHER FACTORS:

Rule out hydrochloric acid deficiency.

Experimental Study: Of 68 subacute or chronic pts. whose condition had resisted all forms of local treatment, 15 (22%) had no HCl and only 9 (13%) had normal HCl levels. The severity of the condition seemed to correlate with the extent of the HCl deficiency and also seemed to be associated with signs of vitamin B complex deficiency. Improvement of the HCl deficient pts. followed treatment with supplemental HCl and vitamin B complex (*Allison JR. The relation of hydrochloric acid and vitamin B complex deficiency in certain skin diseases. Southern Med. J. 38:235-241, 1945*).

See Also:

Edwards RL. The significance of achlorhydria and hypochlorhydria in dermatosis. Balyeat Hay Fever and Asthma Clinic Proc. 19(1):28-30, 1949

TARDIVE DYSKINESIA

NUTRIENTS:

<u>Niacin:</u> 100 - 500 mg. daily

Supplementation may be beneficial.

    Experimental Study: Supplementation with 1-500 mg daily niacin appeared to be beneficial to 1 pt. with oral and buccal dyskinesias and 1 with oculogyric dyskinesia, as well as 1 pt. with drug-induced parkinsonism. Niacinamide had a similar but less dramatic effect and appeared to be beneficial to 1 out of 2 pts. with oral dyskinesias (*Kunin RA. Manganese and niacin in the treatment of drug-induced tardive dyskinesias. <u>J. Orthomol. Psychiat.</u> 5:4-27, 1976*).

<u>Pyridoxine:</u>

Required for the decarboxylation of dopa to dopamine.

Supplementation may be beneficial.

    Experimental Study: High doses of B_6 reduced the frequency and severity of involuntary movements in pts. (*DeVeaugh-Geiss J, Manion L. High-dose pyridoxine in tardive dyskinesia. <u>J. Clin. Psychiat.</u> 39:573-75, 1978*).

    Experimental Study: Massive doses reversed the movement disorder caused by excessive L-dopa in parkinsonism (*Yahr MD et al. Reversal of L-dopa effects in parkinsonism. <u>Trans. Am. Neurol. Assoc.</u> 95:81-85, 1969*).

- -

<u>Manganese:</u>

Phenothiazines are potent chelators of manganese (*Borg DC, Cotzias GC - quoted in Davies IJT. <u>The Clinical Significance of the Essential Biological Metals</u>. Springfield, Illinois, Charles C. Thomas, 1972, p. 74*) which is found in high concentration in the extrapyramidal system.

Supplementation may be beneficial.

    WARNING: Chronic Mn intoxication may cause potentially irreversible movement and other neurologic disorders (*Weiner WJ et al. Regional brain manganese levels in an animal model of tardive dyskinesia, in Fann WE et al, Eds. <u>Tardive Dyskinesia: Research and Treatment</u>. New York, SP Medical and Scientific Books, 1980, pp. 159-163*).

    Experimental Study: 7 out of 15 cases of withdrawal and tardive dyskinesia were cured following treatment with manganese chelate 5-20 mg 3 times daily, while 3/15 were much improved, 4/15 were improved and only 1/15 was unimproved (*Kunin RA. Manganese and niacin in the treatment of drug-induced tardive dyskinesias. <u>J. Orthomol. Psychiat.</u> 5:4-27, 1976*).

See also:

Hoffer A. Tardive dyskinesia treated with manganese. <u>Can. Med. Assoc. J.</u> 117:859, 1977

- -

<u>Phosphatidyl Choline:</u>   dose equivalent to 2.4 - 6.4 gm. choline

Supplementation may be beneficial.

Negative Experimental Double-blind Crossover Study: 19 pts. were supplemented with either phosphatidyl choline 30 gm daily or placebo for 6 weeks. 13 pts. received the crossover treatment for 6 wks., after which 10/13 were continued on the crossover med. for an additional 6 weeks. Results did not differ between active drug and placebo despite a marked elevation of plasma and RBC choline (*Domino EF et al. Lack of clinically significant improvement of patients with tardive dyskinesia following phosphatidylcholine therapy. <u>Biol. Psychiat.</u> 20(11):1189-96, 1985*).

Experimental Double-blind Crossover Study: TD decreased during lecithin ingestion (25 gm twice daily) in 6 patients and reverted to original levels when stopped. Ratings were blind and independent by 2 psychiatrists who viewed videotapes made for neurological assessment based on the NIMH Abnormal Involuntary Movement Scale shown in random sequence (*Jackson IV, Davis LG, Cohen RK et al. Lecithin administration in tardive dyskinesia: Clinical and medical correlates. <u>Biol. Psychiat.</u> 16:85, 1981*).

Experimental Double-blind Crossover Study: 6 patients with moderate or severe TD significantly improved according to assessments based on the NIMH Abnormal Involuntary Movement Scale following 14 days of treatment with lecithin 50 gm/day while neuroleptic medication was continued. There were no side effects (*Jackson IV, Nuttall EA, Perez-Cruet J. Treatment of tardive dyskinesia with lecithin. <u>Am. J. Psychiat.</u> 136(11):1458-60, 1979*).

Experimental Study: 5 men with mild to severe TD received oral choline chloride (150-200 mg/kg daily) and lecithin (21- 105 gm daily as 20% phosphatidyl-choline) in addition to their regular medications. Both improved abnormal movements in all patients as rated on standardized scales. As pts. on choline all developed GI irritation and a "fishy" odor, lecithin had fewer adverse effects (*Gelenberg AJ et al. Choline and lecithin in the treatment of tardive dyskinesia: Preliminary results from a pilot study. <u>Am. J. Psychiat.</u> 136(6):772-76, 1979*).

See Also:

Growdon JH et al. Lecithin can suppress tardive dyskinesia. Letter to the Editor. <u>New Engl. J. Med.</u> 298:1029-30, 1978

Growdon JH et al. Oral choline administration to patients with tardive dyskinesia. <u>New Engl. J. Med.</u> 297:524-27, 1977

Davis K et al. Choline for tardive dyskinesia. <u>New Engl. J. Med.</u> 193:152, 1975

<u>L-Tryptophan:</u>

Supplementation may be beneficial.

Case Report: 66 year-old female with drug-induced TD, akathisia and insomnia developed severe insomnia and a parkinsonian syndrome 3 mo. after receiving perphenazine and amitriptyline (Triavil 4-50). The parkinsonian syndrome regressed spontaneously, and 3 mo. later the drugs were stopped, but the insomnia was unchanged. One month later she presented with involuntary orofacial dyskinetic movements and akathisia. Reserpine, levodopa, diazepam, propranolol, clonidine, chlorpromazine, amitriptyline, and clonazepam failed to ameliorate symptoms. L-tryptophan, initially 2 gm daily, was increased over 4 wks. to 2 gm 4 times daily combined with nicotinic acid (to reduce metabolism by hepatic tryptophan pyrrolase) and a high carbohydrate, low protein diet. After 4 wks. sleep improved substantially and, as assessed by the AIMS scale, the TD was reduced, and the akathisia was abolished. These effects continued over 3 mo., but 2 attempts to stop L-tryptophan resulted in recurrence of insomnia and exacerbation of TD (*Sandyk R et al. L-tryptophan in drug-induced movement disorders with insomnia. Letter to the Editor. New Engl. J. Med. 314(19):1257, 1986*).

Omega-6 Fatty Acids:

Supplementation may be beneficial.

Negative Double-blind Experimental Study: 16 male pts. with mild-moderate TD of at least 1 year's duration were randomly assigned to receive either evening primrose oil 600 mg or placebo. After 6 wks., there was no significant difference between groups (*Wolkin A et al. Essential fatty acid supplementation in tardive dyskinesia. Am. J. Psychiat. 143(7):912-13, 1986*).

Animal Experimental Study (guinea pigs): Intra-striatal dopamine-induced oral dyskinesias were almost totally abolished after 5 days of pretreatment with intraperitoneal injections of dihomo-gamma-linolenic acid 100 mg/kg. Aspirin, which blocks the conversion of essential fatty acids to prostaglandins, attenuated the anti-dyskinetic effects (*Costall B et al. The antidyskinetic action of dihomo-gamma-linolenic acid in the rodent. Br. J. Pharmacol. 83:733-40, 1984*).

See Also:

Vaddadi KS. Essential fatty acids and neuroleptic drug-associated tardive dyskinesia: Preliminary clinical observations. IRCS J. Med. Sci. 12:678, 1984

- -

COMBINATION TREATMENT:

Ascorbic Acid plus	1.3 - 4 gm. daily
Niacin or Niacinamide plus	1.3 - 4 gm. daily
Pyridoxine HCl plus	250 - 800 mg. daily
D-Alpha Tocopheryl Acetate:	250 - 800 mg. daily

Observational Study: In a survey of the practices of 80 physicians who treated 58,000 pts. with antipsychotic drugs over 10 years plus high dosage vitamins, only 26 pts. were reported to have developed TD, an incidence of less than 0.05% (*Hawkins DR. The prevention of tardive dyskinesia with high dosage vitamins: A study of 58,000 patients. J. Orthomol. Med. 1(1):24-26, 1986*).

Observational Study: Not one case of tardive dyskinesia developed among 10,000 out-patient and 1000 in-patient schizophrenics on phenothiazines receiving the above supplements (*Tkacz C. A preventive measure for tardive dyskinesia. J. Int. Acad. of Preventive Med. 8:5-8, 1984*).

TINNITUS

(including MENIERE'S SYNDROME and SENSORINEURAL HEARING LOSS)

See Also: "HYPOGLYCEMIA" (FUNCTIONAL)

BASIC DIET:

Reduce <u>fat</u> and <u>cholesterol</u>.

May reduce the flow of oxygen and nutrents to the inner ear by increasing erythrocyte aggregation (*Spencer J. Hyperlipoproteinemia and inner ear disease. J. Int. Acad. Metabology 4:38-42, 1975*) and red-cell rigidity (*see "<u>Omega-3 Fatty Acids</u>" below*).

Observational Study: In a study of 49 pts. with idiopathic hearing loss, hearing thresholds were unrelated to low-shear blood viscosity, while hearing impairment at high frequencies was directly related to high-shear blood viscosity and inversely related to plasma viscosity. The derived measure of red-cell rigidity was significantly related at all frequencies to hearing thresholds. The inverse relationship with plasma viscosity was confirmed with a second gp. of 92 patients. Results suggest that increased pure-tone thresholds appear to be related to increased red-cell rigidity (*Browning GG et al. Blood viscosity as a factor in sensorineural hearing impairment. Lancet 1:121-23, 1986*).

Animal Experimental Study: Rats bred to become spontaneously hypertensive and normal controls were subjected to intermittent noise with and without an atherogenic diet. The noise-exposed hypertensive rats fed the atherogenic diet had greater hearing losses than those on the normal diet, with significantly decreased cochlear blood flow. Results suggest that, although hypertension plus an atherogenic diet alone does not produce significant hearing loss, hypertension, a chronic atherogenic diet, and chronic noise are devastating, even when the noise is of a moderate intensity (*Pillsbury HC. Hypertension, hyperlipoproteinemia, chronic noise exposure: Is there synergism in cochlear pathology? Laryngoscope 96(10): 1112-38*).

Observational Study: 33% of 90 pts. with sensorineural hearing loss had hyperlipoproteinemia (*Yanick P, Gosselin EJ. Audiologic and metabolic findings in 90 patients with fluctuant hearing loss. J. Am. Aud. Soc. 2:15-18, 1975*).

Reduction in saturated fats may be beneficial.

Experimental Study: Over 1400 pts. with inner ear symptoms and hyperlipoproteinemia were put on individualized diets and given nutritional counseling. In "most" pts., dizziness cleared promptly, the sensation of pressure in the ears and associated headache was quickly relieved, hearing improved and stabilized (as demonstrated in the pure tone audiogram and in speech discrimination scores) and tinnitus often lessened in severity and sometimes disappeared (*Spencer JT. Hyperlipoproteinemia, hyperinsulinism and Meniere's disease. Southern Med. J. 74:1194-97, 1981*).

Experimental Controlled Crossover Study: Group on low saturated fat diet had superior hearing after 5 years compared to gp. on their usual high saturated fat diet. Four years after gps. crossed over, hearing had improved in the gp. now on the restricted diet and had deteriorated in the gp. on the high saturated fat diet. The incidence of coronary heart disease followed the same pattern. Hearing losses which occurred were usually of the sensorineural type. Audiological findings indicated that the diet may well arrest, if not reverse, hearing loss (*Rosen S et al. Dietary prevention of hearing loss. Acta. Otolaryng. 70:242-47, 1970.*)

Avoid <u>sugar</u>.

Said to cause tinnitus and fluctuant hearing loss by promoting reactive hypoglycemia and consequent adrenalin release which, in turn, causes vasoconstriction in the inner ear.

Observational Study: 58% of of 90 pts. with sensorineural hearing loss had abnormal 5 hour glucose tolerance curves (*Yanick P, Gosselin EJ. Audiologic and metabolic findings in 90 patients with fluctuant hearing loss. J. Am. Audiol. Soc. 2:15-18, 1975*).

Observational Study: 42% of 19 pts. with Meniere's syndrome showed hypoglycemia at some point in a 5 hr. glucose tolerance test compared to 15% of pts. with other diseases (*Weille FR. Hypoglycemia in Meniere's disease. Arch. Otol. 87:129, 1968*).

See Also:

Parkin JL, Tice R. *Hypoglycemia and fluctuant hearing loss. Ann. Otol. 79:992, 1970*

Goldman H. *Treatment of the hypoglycemia of Meniere's syndrome. Trans. Indiana Acad. Ophth. Otolaryngol. 48:7-25, 1965*

Harrill JA. *Headache and vertigo associated with hypoglycemia tendency. Laryngoscope 61:138, 1954*

- -

NUTRIENTS:

<u>Vitamin A</u>:

Deficiency may be associated with inner ear dysfunction.

Review Article: The cochlea has a high concentration of vitamin A and all special sensory receptor cells contain, or are functionally dependent upon, vitamin A (*Chole Q. Vitamin A in the cochlea. Arch. Otorhinolaryngol. 124:379-82, 1978*).

Animal Experimental Study: After feeding young rats a vitamin-A deficient diet, changes in the cuticle of the outer and inner hair cells of the cochlea were seen on electron microscopy (*Lohle E. The influence of chronic vitamin A deficiency on human and animal ears. Arch. Otorhinolaryngol. 234:167-73, 1982*).

Observational Study: Low serum vitamin A levels were associated with decreased auditory function (*Lohle - ibid*).

<u>Vitamin D</u>:

Deficiency may be a cause of otosclerosis and replacement therapy with Vitamin D and calcium may help reverse hearing loss.

Experimental and Observational Study: Abnormally low 25-OH vitamin D levels were found in 10/47 pts. with otosclerosis (mean age = 46 yrs.) and borderline low levels in 2. Raised serum alkaline phosphatase levels were present in 32.6%, calcium in 6.5% and inorganic phosphate in 4.3%. Calcium and vitamin D replacement therapy resulted in significant hearing improvement in 3 out of 16 pts (*Brookes GB. Vitamin D deficiency and otosclerosis. <u>Otolaryngol. Head Neck Surg.</u> 93(3):313-21, 1985*).

Experimental Study: 10 pts with bilateral cochlear deafness and vitamin D deficiency were supplemented with calcium and vitamin D 500-1000 IU daily resulting in unilateral hearing improvement in 2/4 (*Brookes GB. Vitamin D deficiency - A new cause of cochlear deafness. <u>J. Laryngol. Otol.</u> 97(5):405-20, 1983*).

- -

Calcium:

See "<u>Vitamin D</u>" above.

Fluoride:

WARNING: Inhibits the enzyme phosphatase in experimental animals which is critically important for the assimilation of calcium and other minerals (*Yanick, Paul. Solving problematic tinnitus. A clinical scientific approach. <u>Townsend Letter for Doctors</u>. February - March, 1985, p. 31*).

Supplementation (sodium fluoride) may be beneficial in cochlear otosclerosis.

Experimental Study: 94 pts. with cochlear otosclerosis and 98 pts. with stapedial otosclerosis and sensorineural hearing loss received treatment with sodium fluoride. The drug halted or slowed the progression of sensorineural hearing impairment in 63% of the pts. with cochlear otosclerosis and 46% of the pts. with stapedial otosclerosis. Pts. with more rapid rates of progression responded most favorably (*Forquer BD et al. Sodium fluoride: Effectiveness of treatment for cochlear otosclerosis. <u>Am. J. Otol.</u> 7(2):121-25, 1986*).

Magnesium:

Deficiency may cause ototoxicity.

Theoretical Discussion: It is postulated that aminoglycoside drugs cause ototoxicity by depleting magnesium in the hair cells of the cochlea (*Dolev E et al. Is magnesium depletion the reason for ototoxicity caused by aminoglycosides? <u>Med. Hypotheses</u> 10(4):353-58, 1983*).

Potassium and
Sodium:

Electrolyte imbalances may affect the inner ear, since endolymph is higher in potassium and perilymph is higher in sodium (*Yanick P. Holistic applications to ear disorders. <u>J. Int. Acad. Prev. Med.</u> 1983, pp. 24-27*).

Experimental and Observational Study: On the basis of a 24 hr. urinary electrolyte clearance test, pts. with sensorineural hearing loss and hypoglycemia were found to have higher levels of potassium than of sodium and a negative nitrogen balance. Increased salt improved their sodium-potassium balance as well as their nitrogen balance (*Goldman HB. Metabolic causes of fluctuant hearing loss. <u>Otolaryn. Clinics of No. America</u> 8:369, 1975; Tintera JW, Goldman HB. Stress and hypoadrenocorticism: The implications in otolaryngology. <u>Ann. Otol. Rhino. Laryngo.</u> 67:185, 1958*).

Zinc: Zinc Sulfate 600 mg. daily

Supplementation may be beneficial.

Clinical Observation: 20% of elderly pts. with progressive hearing deterioration, most of whom had symptoms of zinc deficiency or a low serum zinc, experienced a slight noticeable improvement, especially in discrimination, with zinc supplementation, while 25% of those with tinnitus noted reduction or sometimes elimination following supplementation. Often it took 3 mo. to 1 yr. to bring low serum zinc levels up to normal. After 3 mo., zinc was omitted for 1 wk. and a serum zinc was drawn. If the level was well above 1.0 (normal range 0.66-1.10 mcg/ml), the supplement was reduced to a maintenance dosage. The most frequent side-effect was nausea and gastric distress, but this is rare if a combination of zinc gluconate and zinc sulfate with vitamin synergists ("Z-Plex" or "Bronson 72"/ Bronson Pharm.) was used (*Shambaugh GE Jr. Zinc: An essential trace element. Clin. Ecology 2(4):203-06, 1984*).

Clinical Observation: 20 pts. with sensorineural hearing loss, tinnitus, or both are described who benefited from supplementation with zinc sulphate 600 mg daily (*Shambaugh GE - interviewed in Geriatrics 38(4):21, 1983*).

- -

Omega-3 Fatty Acids:

Supplementation increases red-cell deformability which may be beneficial (*Browning GG et al. Blood viscosity as a factor in sensorineural hearing impairment. Lancet 1:121-23, 1986*). (*See "Reduce fat and cholesterol" above*).

Experimental Study: Normal subjects received 'MaxEPA,' a fish oil concentrate, 3 gm daily. By 6 wks. there was a significant increase in red-cell deformability and a concomitant reduction in whole blood viscosity but no change in plasma viscosity or hematocrit, suggesting that the effects on blood rheology were mediated by changes in RBC lipid fluidity (*Cartwright IJ et al. The effects of dietary omega-3 polyunsaturated fatty acids on erythrocyte membrane phospholipids, erythrocyte deformability and blood viscosity in healthy volunteers. Atherosclerosis 55(3):267-81, 1985*).

- -

COMBINED TREATMENT:

Clinical Observation: The authors treat pts. with cochlear otosclerosis by prescribing sodium fluoride, calcium and vitamin D (*Balle V, Linthicum FH Jr. Histologically proven cochlear otosclerosis with pure sensorineural hearing loss. Ann. Otol. Rhinol. Laryngol. 93(2 Pt 1):105-11, 1984*).

Experimental Study: Results after individualized diet, nutrition, exercise and stress-reduction program for 130 pts. with hearing loss due to cochlear pathology of unknown etiology:
85% (111/130) had dramatic improvements in hearing levels and in speech understanding ability.
91% (74/82) of those with tinnitus reported dramatic relief.
(*Yanick, P. Holistic applications to ear disorders. J.of the Int. Acad. Prev. Med. 1983, pp. 24-27*)

See Also:

Yanick, P. Nutritional aspects of tinnitus and hearing disorders, in Yanick P Jr, Clark JG, Eds. Tinnitus and its Management. Springfield, Illinois, Charles C. Thomas, 1984

Yanick P. Hearing Instruments 32:12, 1981 & 33:34, 1982

- -

OTHER FACTORS:

Rule out aluminum toxicity.

Said to be common in otosclerosis causing reduced serum phosphate levels and abnormal calcium metabolism (*Yanick, P. Solving problematic tinnitus: A clinical scientific approach. Townsend Letter for Doctors February - March, 1985, p. 31*).

Rule out <u>lead</u> toxicity.

May indirectly affect the ear by causing malfunction in the brain and/or symphathetic nervous system, by inhibiting the enzymatic oxidative processes dependent upon zinc and copper in the mitochondria of the cells of the inner ear, or by depleting the cochlea of phosphorus by forming insoluble salts (*Yanick, P. Nutritional aspects of tinnitus and hearing disorders, in Yanick P Jr, Clark JG, Eds. Tinnitus and its Management. Springfield, Illinois, Charles C. Thomas, 1984*).

TIREDNESS
(including FATIGUE)

See Also: ANEMIA
                DEPRESSION
                "HYPOGLYCEMIA" (FUNCTIONAL)
                ORGANIC BRAIN SYNDROME

NUTRIENTS:

Vitamin B Complex:

Review Article: A restricted intake of some B-complex vitamins - individually and in combination - of approx. less than 35-45% of the RDA may lead to decreased endurance capacity within a few weeks. Supplementation with B-complex vitamins does not improve performance in athletes with a normal biochemical vitamin balance resulting from a well-balanced diet, although it is possible that B-complex supplementation is useful in sports with a high energy expenditure because of the unavoidable consumption of food products with a low nutrient density (*van der Beek EJ. Vitamins and endurance training. Food for running or faddish claims? Sports Med. 2(3):175-97, 1985*).

- Folic Acid:

Deficiency may be associated with easy fatigability.

Experimental Study: 4 pts. with easy fatigability along with other symptoms were found to have deficient levels of folate. As folate levels rose with supplementation, fatigue disappeared (*Clin. Psychiat. News, April, 1976*).

- Pantothenic Acid: 250 mg. daily (calcium pantothenate)

Tiredness is the most prominent deficiency symptom - associated with insomnia, sullenness and depression.

Experimental Controlled Study: One gp. of men received a diet containing pantothenic acid, while another gp. received a diet which excluded it. After 10 weeks, the deprived men were listless and complained of fatigue (*Fox H et al. J. Nutr. Sci. Vitaminol. August, 1976*).

- Pyridoxine:

Supplementation may increase endurance.

Animal Experimental Study (rat): Muscle contractions were maintained longer when pyridoxine was added to normal diet (*Richardson JH, Chenman M. The effect of B6 on muscle fatigue. J. Sports Med. Phys. Fitness 21(2):119-21, 1981*).

418

- Vitamin B$_{12}$:

Supplementation may be reduce tiredness.

Experimental Double-blind Crossover Study: 28 men and women who complained of tiredness but had normal serum B$_{12}$ levels and no physical findings were given injections of hydroxycobalamin 5 mg twice daily for 2 wks. followed by a 2-wk. rest period and then a similar course of placebo injections or the same regimen in reverse order. Those who received placebo first felt significantly better in regard to "general well-being" (p = 0.006) in the second period when they received B$_{12}$. Those who received B$_{12}$ in the first period noted no differences between B$_{12}$ and placebo, which suggests that the effects of B$_{12}$ may persist for a period of at least 4 weeks (*Ellis FR, Nasser S. A pilot study of vitamin B$_{12}$ in the treatment of tiredness. Brit. J. Nutr. 30:277-83, 1973*).

Vitamin C:

Deficiency syndrome may include fatigue.

Review Article: While studies on ascorbic acid depletion have noted no decrease in endurance capacity, a few recent epidemiological surveys have suggested an association between vitamin C deficiency and decreased aerobic power. Supplementation with vitamin C does not improve physical performance in athletes with a biochemical vitamin balance resulting from a well-balanced diet (*van der Beek EJ. Vitamins and endurance training. Food for running or faddish claims? Sports Med. 2(3):175-97, 1985*).

Observational Study: In a survey of vitamin C intake among 411 dentists and their wives, there was a significant inverse relationship between vitamin C intake and fatigue, with the mean number of fatigue symptoms among the low vitamin C users being double that among the relatively high users of vitamin C (*Cheraskin E et al. Daily vitamin C consumption and fatigability. J. Am. Geriat. Soc., 24(3):136-37, 1976*).

- -

Iron:

WARNING: only supplement if deficient - otherwise can be toxic.

Deficiency syndrome is associated with diminished work capacity.

Experimental Controlled Study: The physical work capacity of 75 women was studied. Those with the most severe iron deficiency anemias could stay on a treadmill an average of 8 minutes less than those without anemia, and none of them could perform under the highest work-load conditions, while all of the nonanemic group could. Lactate levels were almost twice as high in the most severely anemic group (*Gardner GW et al. Physical work capacity and metabolic stress in subjects with iron deficiency anemia. Am. J. Clin. Nutr. 30(6):910-17, 1977*).

Magnesium:

Required for ATP synthesis.

Enhances transport of potassium into cells (*see "Potassium" below*).

Experimental Study: Supplementation relieved tiredness in 198/200 people (*In Seelig MS, Cantin M, Eds. Magnesium in Health and Disease: Proceedings of the 2nd International Symposium on Magnesium, Montreal, Quebec, May 30-June 1, 1976. New York, Spectrum Books, 1980*).

Potassium:

Malaise is said to be the most common deficiency symptom when potassium deficits are chronic along with muscular weakness (*Snively WD, Westerman RL. Minnesota Medicine June, 1965*).

> **Observational Study:** Low potassium intake was associated with weaker grip stength (*Judge TG, Cowan NR. Dietary potassium intake and grip strength in older people. Gerontologia Clinica 13:221-6, 1971*).

Zinc: 135 mg. (15 day trial)

Supplementation may improve muscle strength and endurance.

> **Experimental Study:** After 15 days of supplementation with 135 mg zinc daily, isokinetic strength and isometric endurance of leg muscles were significantly improved (*Krotkiewski M et al. Zinc and muscle strength and endurance. Acta Physiol. Scand. 116(3):309-11, 1982*).

- -

Aspartic Acid:

Aspartic acid is converted intracellularly into oxaloacetate, an important substrate in the energy-producing Krebs cycle, and is also a carrier molecule for the transport of potassium and magnesium into the cell.

Supplementation with aspartates may relieve fatigue.

Example: Potassium/Magnesium Aspartate 1 gm twice daily

> **Review Article:** Both uncontrolled and double-blind studies (with a total of nearly 3000 subjects) have found that between 75% and 91% of treated pts. experienced pronounced relief of fatigue during treatment with K^{++} and Mg^{++} aspartates in daily doses of 1 gm of each salt, compared to 5-25% of controls. A beneficial effect was usually noted after 4-5 days, but sometimes 10 days were required. Pts. usually continued treatment for 4-6 wks.; afterwards fatigue frequently did not return. Side effects, which were mild and uncommon, included mild GI distress and dryness of the mouth (*Gaby AR. Aspartic acid salts and fatigue. Curr. Nutr. Therapeut., November, 1982*).

> **Review Article:** The efficacy of aspartates for fatigue is considered unproven as the theoretical basis is questionable and estimation of the relief of fatigue is so subjective that it is extremely difficult to substantiate their effectiveness (*Council on drugs, new, drugs and developments in therapeutics. JAMA 183:362, 1963*).

> **Experimental Double-blind Study:** 87/100 chronically fatigued pts. markedly improved after 5-6 wks. of supplementation (*Formica PE. The housewife syndrome: Treatment with potassium and magnesium salts of aspartic acid. Current Therap. Res. 4:98, March, 1962*).

> **Animal Experimental Study:** Supplementation with aspartates delayed the onset of metabolic exhaustion in rats as measured by the length of time the animals could tread water before sinking to the bottom of the tank (*Rosen H et al. Effects of the potassium and magnesium salts of aspartic acid on metabolic exhaustion. J. Pharmaceut. Sci. 51:592, 1962*).

See Also:

> **Experimental Double-blind Study:** *Hicks J. Treatment of fatigue in general practice: A double-blind study. Clin. Med. January, 1964, p. 85*

Experimental Double-blind Study: *Shaw DL et al.   Management of fatigue: A physiologic approach.   Am. J. Med. Sci. 243:758, 1962*

Carnitine: DL: 1500 mg. twice daily
L: 750 mg. twice daily

Deficiency syndrome may include muscle weakness (*Angelini I et al.   Carnitine deficiency of skeletal muscle.   Neurology 26:633-7, 1976*).

Supplementation may increase endurance.

Experimental Study: 6 long-distance competitive walkers received L-carnitine 4 gm daily. After 2 wks., VO$_2$ max (maximal aerobic power) increased 6% (p less than 0.02) (*Marconi C et al. Effects of L-carnitine loading on the aerobic and anaerobic performance of endurance athletes.   Eur. J. Appl. Physiol. 54(2):131-35, 1985*).

Coenzyme Q: 30 mg. daily in divided doses

Supplementation may improve performance.

Experimental Study: 6 healthy, sedentary males (mean age 21.5 years) performed a bicycle ergometer test before and after receiving CoQ$_{10}$ 60 mg daily for 4-8 weeks. Improvements in work capacity at submaximal heart rate, maximal work load, maximal oxygen consumption, and oxygen transport were noted ranging from 3-12% and starting after about 4 weeks (*Vanfraechem JHP, Folkers KJ.. Coenzyme Q$_{10}$ and physical performance, in Folkers K, Yamamura Y, Eds., Biomed. & Clin. Aspects of Coenzyme Q 3:235-41, 1981*).

N,N Dimethyl Glycine: 1-200 mg. daily

Supplementation may be effective when maximal performance is needed (ex. sports; ischemic heart disease) (*1980 Am. Coll. of Sports Med. annual meeting. Abstracts.   Med. Sci. Sports Exerc. 12:98, 1980*).

L-Glutamine: 500 mg. twice daily for 1 week, then
500 mg. 3 times daily for 1 week, then
1 gm. twice daily for 1 week as a trial

WARNING: Contraindicated in hyperammonemia.

Able to pass through the blood-brain barrier to increase brain levels of glutamate, an excitatory neurotransmitter (*Butterworth et al.   Effect of asparagine, glutamine and insulin on cerebral amino acid neurotransmitters.   J. Can. Sci. Neurol. 7(4):447-50, 1980*).

Inosine:

Supplementation may reduce fatigue by increasing the oxygen-carrying capacity of the blood (*DeVerdier CH, Westman M. Intravenous infusion of inosine in man: Effect on erythrocyte 2,3-diphosphoglycerate concentration and on blood oxygen affinity.   Scand. J. Clin. Lab. Invest. 32(3):205-10, 1973*).

Octacosanol: 375 mg. daily

Supplementation may increase stamina.

Experimental Controlled Study: *Cureton, Thomas.   The Physiologic Effects of Wheat Germ Oil on Humans in Exercise.   Charles C. Thomas, 1972*

<u>Pyridoxine Alpha-ketoglutarate (PAK)</u>:

Supplementation may increase endurance.

> **Experimental Double-blind Study:** 20 runners were supplemented with PAK 30 mg/kg in divided doses or placebo. After 1 month, their endurance rose significantly as evidenced by increased VO_2 Max (p less than 0.005) and reduced lactic acid levels (p less than 0.005). No change was seen in the placebo gp. and neither alpha-ketoglutarate or pyridoxine alone showed positive effects. Results suggest that PAK is complementary to athletic training in improving the capacity for endurance exercise (*Marconi C et al. The effect of an alpha-ketoglutarate-pyridoxine complex on human maximal aerobic and anaerobic performance.* <u>Eur. J. Appl. Physio.</u> *49:307-17, 1982*).

- -

OTHER FACTORS:

Rule out <u>food sensitivities</u>.

Said to sometimes cause an "allergic tension-fatigue syndrome" characterized by sensory and motor hyperactivity and/or sensory and motor fatigue.

> **Clinical Observation:** 75% of a gp. of 50 pts. with tension-fatigue syndrome were found to have a history of nasal, ocular, respiratory, or skin allergy. Over half the pts. treated by an elimination diet had superior to excellent results, while an additional 16/50 had a good response (*Crook WG.* <u>Can Your Child Read? Is He Hyperactive?</u> *Jackson, Professional Books, 1977*).

> **Double-blind Experimental Case Report:** A child presenting with fatigue, irritability, headache and stomach ache had the symptoms reproduced by milk in capsules but not by placebo (*Crook - ibid*).

> **Case Report:** 13 year-old boy hospitalized because of bronchial asthma, musculo-skeletal pains, headache and abdominal pain and findings of pallor and dark circles under his eyes had chocolate and milk removed from his diet. There was marked improvement within 48 hours and reappearance of signs and symptoms with milk reintroduction (*Weinberg EG, Tuchinda M.* <u>Ann. Allergy</u> *31:209, 1973*).

> See Also:

>> **Review Article:** *Rapp DJ. Hyperactivity and the tension-fatigue syndrome, in Gerrard JW, Ed.* <u>Food Allergy: New Perspectives</u>. *Springfield, Illinois, Charles C. Thomas, 1980*

>> **Review Article:** *Speer F. The allergic tension-fatigue syndrome, in Speer F, Ed.* <u>Allergy of the Nervous System</u>. *Springfield, Illinois, Charles C. Thomas, 1970*

>> *Rowe AH. Allergic toxemia and fatigue.* <u>Ann. Allergy</u> *8:72, 1950*

>> *Randolph TG. Allergy as a causative factor in fatigue, irritability, and behavior problems in children.* <u>J. Pediat.</u> *31:560, 1947*

>> *Randolph TG. Fatigue and weakness of allergic origin to be differentiated from "nervous fatigue" or neurasthenia.* <u>Ann. Allergy</u> *3:418, 1945*

Rule out "<u>hypoglycemic fatigue</u>" (episodic tiredness, weakness and apathy relieved by eating).

Case Reports:

Karlan SC, Cohn C. JAMA 130:553, 1946

Alexander F, Portis SA. Psychosomatic Med. 6:191-205, 1944

ULCERATIVE COLITIS

See also: CROHN'S DISEASE

BASIC DIET:

Avoid <u>sugar</u>.

Review Article: A diet high in refined carbohydrate is implicated in the etiology of ulcerative colitis and certain other diseases of the colon. It is suggested that spasm of the smooth muscle is the common pathogenetic mechanism, and the strength of the spasm producing increased pressure in the colonic lumen or wall and the length of time for which the colon has been affected are believed to determine the type of disease resulting. A diet high in refined carbohydrate allows the intense muscle spasm to occur because the physical buffering effect of fecal bulk is considerably reduced (*Grimes DS. Refined carbohydrate, smooth-muscle spasm and disease of the colon.* <u>*Lancet*</u> *1:395-97, 1976*).

See Also:

Thornton JR et al. Diet and ulcerative colitis. <u>Brit. Med. J.</u> February 2, 1980, p. 293

- -

NUTRIENTS:

<u>Folic Acid</u>:

May be deficient due to inadequate diet, malabsorption, or chronic sulfasalazine-induced low-grade hemolysis.

In vitro Experimental Study: Studies on rat lymphocytes demonstrated that sulfasalazine acts as a folate antagonist (*Baum CL et al. Antifolate actions of sulfasalazine on intact lymphocytes.* <u>*J. Lab. Clin. Med.*</u> *97(6):779-84, 1981*).

Observational Study: Of 216 pts. with chronic inflammatory bowel disease, low serum folate levels were found in 59% and low RBC levels in 26%. It is suggested that folate deficiency is of multiple origin: inadequate diet, malabsorption and chronic drug-induced low-grade hemolysis (*Elsborg L, Larsen L. Folate deficiency in chronic inflammatory bowel disease.* <u>*Scand. J. Gastroenterol.*</u> *14:1019-24, 1979*).

See Also:

Halsted CH et al. Sulfasalazine inhibits the absorption of folates in ulcerative colitis. <u>N. Engl. J. Med.</u> 305(25):1513-17, 1981

Supplementation may reduce diarrhea (*Carruthers LB. Chronic diarrhea treated with folic acid.* <u>*Lancet*</u> *1:849, 1946*).

<u>Pantothenic Acid:</u>

May fail to be converted into Coenzyme A in the colonic mucosa.

Observational Study: Colonic tissues of 29 pts. with chronic ulcerative and granulomatous colitis were assayed for pantothenic acid and coenzyme A activity and compared to normal colonic tissues from 31 controls. Compared to normal gut mucosa, CoA activity was markedly low in mucosa from pts. despite the presence of normal amts. of free and bound pantothenic acid, suggesting that there is a block in the conversion of bound pantothenic acid to CoA in diseased mucosa (*Ellestad-Sayed JJ et al. Pantothenic acid, coenzyme A, and human chronic ulcerative and granulomatous colitis. Am. J. Clin. Nutr. 29:1333-38, 1976*).

<u>Vitamin A:</u>   50,000 - 75,000 IU

Absorption may be impaired.

Experimental Controlled Study: 25 UC pts. and 8 healthy controls were orally administrered vitamin A 100,000 USP units. The plasma vitamin A did not rise as high in the pts. with ulcerative colitis as in the control subjects, suggesting that there may be a reflex mechanism operating from the damaged colon that inhibits absorption from the small intestine with an additional factor of diarrhea often present (*Page, RC, Bercovitz Z. The absorption of vitamin A in chronic ulcerative colitis. Am. J. Dig. Dis. 10:174-77, 1943*).

<u>Vitamin D:</u>

May be deficient.

Observational Study: In examining pts. with GI and liver disorders, mild deficiency of vitamin D was common, and severe deficiency (25-OHD levels less than 8 nmol/l) was encountered. Deficiency was more common in pts. with active vs. inactive disease. Plasma 25-OHD levels were significantly correlated with hemoglobin and ESR. Evidence of secondary hyperparathyroidism and osteomalacia was noted (*Dibble JB et al. A survey of vitamin D deficiency in gastrointestinal and liver disorders. Quart. J. Med. 53:119-34, 1984*).

<u>Vitamin K:</u>

May be deficient.

Observational Study: 18/58 (31%) pts. with chronic G.I. disorders were found to have evidence of vitamin K deficiency; all pts. with deficiency had either Crohn's of the terminal ileum or ulcerative colitis treated with sulfasalazine or antibiotics. The mean vitamin E level was lower in pts. with vitamin K deficiency than in those without it (*Krasinski SD et al. The prevalence of vitamin K deficiency in chronic gastrointestinal disorders. Am. J. Clin. Nutr. 41(3):639-43, 1985*).

If deficient, supplementation may normalize prothrombin levels.

Experimental Study: Abnormal prothrombin levels returned toward normal in vitamin K-deficient pts. treated with vitamin K (*Krasinski - ibid*).

- -

<u>Calcium:</u>

May be deficient due to loss of absorptive surfaces, steatorrhea, corticosteroid treatment, and vitamin D deficiency (*Rosenberg IH et al. Nutritional aspects of inflammatory bowel disease. Ann. Rev. Nutr. 5:463-84, 1985*).

Iron:

May be deficient due to chronic blood loss through the gut (*Rosenberg IH et al. Nutritional aspects of inflammatory bowel disease. Ann. Rev. Nutr. 5:463-84, 1985*).

Magnesium:

May be deficient.

Observational Study: Mg depletion as judged by serum and 24 hr. urine concentrations was present in 21/25 pts. with severe disease, 15 of whom required IV nutrition. Mg deficiency was statistically more likely to occur in pts. on IV nutrition taking less than 5 mmol IV Mg/ 24 hr. After discharge, 5 pts. who had received IV nutrition frequently complained of muscle cramps, tetany and bone pain and were found to have recurrent low serum Mg levels over some months (*Russell RI. Magnesium requirements in patients with chronic inflammatory disease receiving intravenous nutrition. J. Am. Coll. Nutr. 4(5):553-58, 1985*).

While serum levels are rarely decreased, intracellular Mg levels are frequently low and may be associated with weakness, anorexia, hypotension, confusion, hyperirritability, tetany, convulsions, and EKG or EEG abnormalities (*Rosenberg IH et al. Nutritional aspects of inflammatory bowel disease. Ann. Rev. Nutr. 5:463-84, 1985*).

Zinc:

May be deficient.

Negative Observational Study: There were no significant differences between plasma zinc levels in 46 pts. with idiopathic UC or proctitis and healthy controls (*Dronfield MW et al. Zinc in ulcerative colitis: A therapeutic trial and report on plasma levels. Gut 18:33, 1977*).

Observational Study: Over half of the pts. with inflammatory bowel disease studied had evidence of zinc deficiency (*Solomons NW et al. Zinc nutrition in inflammatory bowel disease, in Fifth World Congress of Gastroenterology Mexican Society of Gastroenterology: Mexico City, 1974, Abstract: p. 263*).

Supplementation may be beneficial.

Negative Experimental Double-blind Study: 51 pts. randomly received either zinc sulphate 220 mg 3 times daily or placebo. After 4 wks., improvement tended to be slightly greater in those receiving zinc than those given placebo; however, the differences were not significant (*Dronfield - op cit*).

– –

Glycosaminoglycans:

Supplementation may be beneficial.

Experimental Study: 6 pts received sub-cut. injections of an activated acid-pepsin-digested calf tracheal cartilege preparation ("Catrix-S"). 5/6 had responded poorly to traditional treatments. 3/6 had an excellent response: 2 went into total remission but later had recurrences, while 1 showed progressive improvement. 2/6 had a good response: 1 who had been sensitive to sulfasalazine and developed massive edema on prednisone, and 1 who was spared a total colectomy but continued to have 6 movements daily. 1/6 had a fair response which was improved with the addition of prednisone. In an earlier series, oral Catrix powder capsules (3 gm 4 times daily) markedly improved sigmoidoscopic appearance but was unsatisfactory because the long-chain glycosaminoglycan molecule produced an osmotic diarrhea (*Prudden JF, Balassa LL. The biological activity of bovine cartilage preparations. Sem. Arthritis & Rhem. 3(4):287-321, 1974*).

OTHER FACTORS:

Rule out food sensitivities.

Experimental and Observational Study: Based on a symptom survey listing atopic allergic symptoms, 42/59 (71%) pts. were judged to be possibly allergic. In addition, over 50 pts. treated with inhalent allergy hyposensitization and dietary changes consisting of rotation and diversification of allergic foods were considerably improved in both their respiratory and abdominal symptoms, suggesting an allergic diathesis (*Siegel J. Inflammatory bowel disease: Another possible facet of the allergic diathesis. Ann. Allergy 47:92-94, 1981*).

Experimental Study: IgG and IgM antibodies to cow's milk proteins were found to be increased in pts. (*Jewell DP, Truelove SC. Circulating antibodies to cow's milk in ulcerative colitis. Gut 13:796, 1972*).

Experimental Controlled Study: After 1 year, 10/13 pts. on a dairy-free diet had remained symptom-free compared to 5/13 pts. on a "dummy" control diet (*Wright R, Truelove SC. A controlled therapeutic trial of various diets in ulcerative colitis. Brit. Med. J. 2:138, 1965*).

See Also:

Mee AS, Jewell DP. Reaginic hypersensitivity in inflammatory bowel disease, in Pepys J, Edwards AM, Eds. The Mast Cell. London, Pitman, 1979, p.638

Wright R, Truelove SC. A controlled therapeutic trial of various diets in ulcerative colitis. Am. J. Dig. Dis. 11:858, 1966

Rider JA, Moeller HC. Food hypersensitivity in ulcerative colitis: Further experience with an intramucosal test. Am. J. Gastroentero. 37:497, 1962

Rowe AH, Rowe A Jr. Chronic ulcerative colitis: Atopic allergy in its etiology. Am. J. Gastroentero. 34:49, 1960

ULCERS (DUODENAL AND GASTRIC)

BASIC DIET:

High <u>fiber</u> diet.

> **Experimental Controlled Study (<u>duodenal ulcer</u>):** 80 pts. were treated with 1 low-dose anacid tablet 4 times daily. In addition, they were randomly divided to receive either a fiber-rich or a fiber-poor diet. After 4 wks., the ulcer had healed in 67.5% of the fiber-rich and 60% of the fiber-poor gp. (p less than 0.5). Ulcer symptoms did not differ signifiantly between gps. during the treatment period. Constipation was seen in 27.5% of the low-fiber gp. and 10% of the high-fiber gp.(p less than 0.05) (*Rydning A, Berstad A. Fiber diet and antacids in the short-term treatment of duodenal ulcer. <u>Scand. J. Gastroenterol.</u> 20(9):1078-82, 1985*).

> **Experimental Controlled Study (<u>duodenal ulcer</u>):** 73 people with recently healed duodenal ulcers were asked to change diets. On a random basis, 38 were told to eat lots of whole grain bread, porridge made from wheat, barley or oats, and lots of vegetables, while 35 were told to avoid these foods. After 6 months, 28/35 (80%) in the low fiber gp. had suffered a relapse documented by endoscopy compared to 17/38 (45%) in the high fiber gp. (significant at the 0.01 level). 14/15 who ate the least amount of fiber developed new ulcers (*Rydning A et al. Prophylactic effect of dietary fiber in duodenal ulcer disease. <u>Lancet</u> 2:736-39, 1982*).

> **Experimental Controlled Study (normals):** The liquid portion of a meal of water and lightly buttered bread made of white flour and white sugar moved faster from the stomach to the duodenum, was less buffered and was more acidic than that of a meal which differed only in the substitution of whole grain flour and dark brown sugar, suggesting that whole meal bread might benefit those with both duodenal ulcers and non-ulcer dyspepsia (*Grimes DS, Goddard J. Gastric emptying of wholemeal and white bread. <u>Gut</u> 18:725, 1977*).

See Also:

> *Malhotra SL. A comparison of unrefined wheat and rice diets in the management of duodenal ulcer. <u>Postgrad. Med. J.</u> 54:6, 1978*

Avoid snacking and foods found to be irritating.

> Bland diets and strict dietary programs have not been proven effective in controlled studies (*Welsh JD. Diet therapy of peptic ulcer disease. <u>Gastroenterology</u> 72:740-45, 1977*).

Avoid frequent <u>milk</u> ingestion.

> Milk has only a transient neutralizing effect on gastric acidity followed by a rise in acid secretion (*Ippoliti AF et al. The effect of various forms of milk on gastric-acid secretion. <u>Ann. Intern. Med.</u> 84:286-89, 1976*).

> **Experimental Controlled Study:** 65 pts. with duodenal ulcers under treatment with cimetidine were randomly assigned to either a normal hospital diet or one consisting exclusively of milk. Both gps. were allowed to add sugar and fruit as desired. After 4 wks., endoscopic examination showed that the proportion of healed ulcers was significantly higher in the normal diet gp. (78%) than in those given milk (53%) (*Kumar N et al. Effect of milk on patients with duodenal ulcers. <u>Br. Med. J.</u> 293:666, 1986*).

Avoid <u>hot, spicy foods</u>.

Negative Experimental Study: When half of 50 duodenal ulcer pts. were given red chili powder 1 gm with each meal for 4 wks., the rate of ulcer healing (80%) was identical in both groups (*Kumar N et al. Brit. Med. J. 288:1803-04, 1984*).

Avoid <u>alcohol</u>.

Stimulates gastric acid secretion (*Lenz HJ et al. Wine and five percent ethanol are potent stimulants of gastric acid secretion in humans. Gastroenterology 85(5):1082-87, 1983*).

Avoid <u>coffee</u> and strong <u>tea</u>.

Stimulate gastric acid secretion (*Dubey P et al. Dig. Dis & Sci. 29(3):202-06, 1984*).

Avoid <u>sugar</u>.

Experimental Crossover Study (<u>chronic dyspepsia with or without demonstrable peptic ulcer</u>): 41 pts. followed a low-carbohydrate diet (60-70 gm/day) for 3 months followed by a high-carbohydrate diet (the standard "gastric diet") for 3 months. 28/41 felt better on the low-carbohydrate diet, 11 noted no difference and only 2/41 felt better on the high-carbohydrate diet. In order to ascertain whether the reduction in dietary starch or sugar (sucrose) was the cause of symptomatic improvement from the low-carbohydrate diet, the gastric juice of 7 healthy young volunteers was examined following 2 wks. on a high-sugar diet in which dietary starch was reduced by the same amt. that dietary sugar was increased. A test meal before breakfast revealed a 20% increase in peak gastric activity and a 250% increase in peak pepsin activity (*Yudkin J. Eating and ulcers. Letter to the Editor. Br. Med. J. February 16, 1980, pp. 483-84*).

- -

NUTRIENTS:

<u>Bioflavonoids:</u>

Inhibit histamine release (*Amella M et al. Inhibition of mast cell histamine release by flavonoids and bioflavonoids. Planta Medica 51:16-20, 1985*).

Supplementation may be beneficial.

Experimental Study: Supplementation with catechin 1000 mg 5 times daily resulted in reduced histamine levels in gastric tissue (as determined by biopsy) in both normals and in pts. with gastric and duodenal ulcers and acute gastritis (*Wendt P et al. The use of flavonoids as inhibitors of histidine decarboxylase in gastric diseases: Experimental and clinical studies. Naunyn-Schmiedeberg's Arch. Pharma. (Suppl.) 313:238, 1980*).

Animal Experimental Studies (guinea pigs and rats):

Parmar NS, Ghosh MN. Gastric anti-ulcer activity of (+)-cyanidanol-3, a histidine decarboxylase inhibitor. Eur. J. Pharmacol. 69:25-32, 1981

Wendt P et al. The use of flavonoids as inhibitors of histidine decarboxylase in gastric diseases: Experimental and clinical studies. Naunyn-Schmiedeberg's Arch. Pharma. (Suppl.) 313:238, 1980

<u>Pyridoxine:</u>

May be deficient in patients with peptic ulcers (*Sanderson CR, Davis RE. Serum pyridoxal in patients with active peptic ulceration. Gut 16:177, 1975*).

Supplementation may help to heal stress ulcerations.

Animal Experimental Study (<u>stress ulcer</u> - mice): *Lindenbaum ES, Mueller JJ. Effects of pyridoxine on mice after immobilization stress. <u>Nutr. Metabol.</u> 17:368, 1974*

<u>Vitamin A:</u>   Adults: 100,000 I.U.of water-soluble A twice daily
Children: 50,000 I.U. of water-soluble A twice daily

Supplementation may be beneficial.

Experimental Controlled Study (chronic gastric ulcer): 16 pts. were given anacids only, 18 were given antacids plus vitamin A 3x50,000 I.U. orally, and 22 were given anacids, vitamin A and cyproheptadine 3x4 mg. orally daily. After 4 wks., ulcers had completely healed in 3/16 (18%) in gp. one, 7/18 (38%) in gp. two and 8/22 (36%) in gp. three. Ulcer sizes were significantly smaller in gp. one than in gp. two and gp. three (*Patty I et al. Controlled trial of vitamin A in gastric ulcer. <u>Lancet</u> 2:876, 1982*).

Animal Experimental Study (<u>stress ulcer</u> - rat): Of rats subjected to immobilization stress, those given vitamin A developed significantly fewer and smaller stress ulcers (*Schumpelik VV, Farthmann E. Untersuchung zur protektiven wirkung von vitamin A beim stressulkus der ratte. <u>Arzneim-Forsch</u> 26:386, 1976*).

Experimental Controlled Study (<u>stress ulcer</u>): 52 pts. who had had severe physiologic stresses (burns, organ injuries or post-op. organ disturbances) were randomly divided into treatment and control groups. Treatment consisted of water soluble vitamin A 100,000 IU twice daily for adults and 1/2 the dose for children. Additional vitamin A was given if serum vitamin A did not promptly normalize. 63% of the controls but only 18% of the treatment group showed evidence of stress ulcer, a significant difference. Since, in burn pts., serum vitamin A often falls from initially normal levels and returns to normal after pts. receive a high protein diet, the authors speculate that lack of retinal binding protein is responsible for the drop in vitamin A levels (*Chernow MS et al. Stress ulcer: A preventable disease. <u>J. Trauma</u> 12:831, 1972*).

<u>Vitamin C:</u>   1.5 - 4 gm. sodium ascorbate before meals and at bedtime.
For gastric distress: 1.5 gm. in 2 oz. water.

Deficiency positively correlated with incidence of peptic ulcers and gastrointestinal hemorrhage.

Observational Study: The plasma content of reduced ascorbic acid, the leukocyte ascorbic acid and the urinary excretion of ascorbic acid were significantly subnormal in 25 peptic ulcer pts., while dehydroascorbic acid was significantly higher, than in 10 controls (*Dubey SS et al. Ascorbic acid, dehydroascorbic acid, glutathione and histamine in peptic ulcer. <u>Indian J. Med. Res.</u> 76:859-62, 1982*).

Observational Study: 60 hospitalized patients with G.I. hemorrhage (2 with peptic ulcer) were compared to pts. with uncomplicated peptic ulcer and healthy controls. Ascorbic acid levels were significantly lower in the bleeders than in the pts. with uncomplicated peptic ulcers whose levels were significantly lower than those of the healthy controls. Only 6 of the bleeders had clinical evidence of scurvy (*Russell RL et al. Ascorbic acid levels in leucocytes of patients with gastrointestinal hemorrhage. <u>Lancet</u> 2:603-6, 1968*).

Animal Experimental Study (peptic ulcer - gastric, pyloric and duodenal): Guinea pigs fed a diet deficient in vitamin C developed peptic ulcerations (*Smith DT, McConkey M. Peptic ulcers (gastric, pyloric and duodenal) occurence in guinea-pigs fed on a diet deficient in vitamin C. <u>Arch. Int. Med.</u> 51:413-26, 1933*).

See Also:

Crescenzo VM, Cayer D.   Plasma vitamin C levels in patients with peptic ulcer. Response to oral load of ascorbic acid.   Gastroenterology 8:755-61, 1947

Field H et al.   Vitamins in peptic ulcer.   Ann. Int. Med. 14:588-92, 1940

Chamberlin DT, Perkin HJ.   The level of ascorbic acid in the blood and urine of patients with peptic ulcer.   Am. J. Dig. Dis. 5:493, 1938-9

Ingalls TH, Warren HA.   Asymptomatic scurvy.   Its relation to wound healing and its incidence in patients with peptic ulcer.   New Eng. J. Med. 217:443-6, 1937

Supplementation may improve healing.

Experimental Study: 48 pts. (23 with duodenal ulcer, 22 with gastric ulcer and 3 with multiple ulcers) received vitamin C 2 gms IV over 3-4 minutes 3 times weekly for a series of 20 injections. In 35/48 (72%), the ulcers disappeared rapidly during the course of treatment, suggesting that treatment with vitamin C is at least as effective as the classic intravenous therapies (*Debray C et al. [Treatment of gastro-duodenal ulcers with large doses of ascorbic acid.] Semaine Therapeutique (Paris) 44:393-8, 1968*).

See Also:

Nash EC.   A comparative study of an antacid with and without vitamin C in the treatment of peptic ulcer.   Am. Pract. & Digest of Treatments 3:117-20, 1952

- with <u>atropine</u>:

Experimental Study: 48 pts. with duodenal ulcer, 30 pts. with gastric ulcer and 2 pts. with post-operative ulcer received vitamin C 2 gm along with atropine 0.5 mg IV over 3-4 minutes 3 times weekly for a total of 20 injecions. 34/80 (42.5%) had a good result and 39/80 (48.5%) an incomplete result, suggesting that treatment with vitamin C is at least as effective as the classic intravenous therapies (*Debray C et al. [Treatment of gastro-duodenal ulcers with large doses of ascorbic acid.] Semaine Therapeutique (Paris) 44:393-8, 1968*).

- with <u>ferrous sulfate</u>:

Experimental Controlled Study: While, in <u>gastric ulcer</u> pts., the healing index of the gp. given ascorbic acid and ferrous sulfate was significantly higher than that of controls, in <u>duodenal ulcer</u> pts., no significant difference was observed (*Miwa M et al. The therapeutics of peptic ulcers: Clinical evaluation of C-Fe therapy. Tokai J. Exp. Clin. Med. 5(1):41-44, 1980*).

<u>Vitamin E</u>:

Supplementation may protect against stress ulceration.

Animal Experimental Study (<u>stress ulcer</u> - rats): 24 rats were stressed for 12 days by fasting while viewing food and water out of their reach. 12 received vitamin E during the study. When autopsied, the unsupplemented rats developed 78% more gastric ulcerations (*Kangas JA et al. Am. J. Clin. Nutr., September 1972*).

See Also:

*Harris PL et al.   Dietary production of gastric ulcers in rats and prevention by tocopherol ad-
ministration.* Proc. Soc. Exp. Biol. Med. *4:273-77, 1947*

- -

<u>Zinc</u>:   zinc sulfate 220 mg. three times daily

May inhibit stress-induced release of vasoactive agents from gastric mast cells, thus preventing the subsequent microcirculatory changes known to produce mucosal ulceration.

Animal Experimental Study (<u>stress ulcer - rat</u>): Pretreatment with zinc sulfate prevented gastric
ulcer formation in a dose related manner in rats exposed to immobilization and cold stress. It also
prevented the stress-related decline in stomach wall mast cell counts and the increase in microcirculatory blood volume (*Oner G et al. The role of zinc ion in the development of gastric ulcers in rats.*
Eur. J. Pharmacol. *70:241, 1981*).

Animal Experimental Study (<u>stress ulcer - rat</u>): Methacholine caused histamine release which triggered acid secretion leading to ulceration. Zinc supplementation, however, prevented ulceration by
preventing histamine release (*Cho CH, Ogle CW. A correlative study of the antiulcer effects of zinc sulphate in stressed rats.* Eur. J. Pharmacol. *70:241, 1978*).

Experimental Double-blind Study (<u>gastric ulcer</u>): 15 pts. with gastric ulcers were treated randomly
with either zinc or placebo. After 3 wks., the absolute reduction in size of the ulcer crater was 3
times as great in the treated group (statistically significant). Zinc reduced pain markedly within 4
days in some patients. There were no side effects and pretreatment zinc levels were normal (*From-
mer DJ. The healing of gastric ulcers by zinc sulphate.* Med. J. Aust. *2:793, 1975*).

- -

<u>Glutamine</u>:   400 mg. four times daily 1 hour before meals and before retiring

Supplementation may be beneficial.

Experimental Double-blind Study (<u>peptic ulcer</u>): Pts. were given either glutamine or lactose in addition to standard treatment. After 4 weeks, the ulcers of 7/7 pts. on glutamine had healed according
to x-rays compared to 7/14 pts. on lactose (*Shive W et al. Glutamine in treatment of peptic ulcer.*
Texas State J. of Med. *November, 1957, pp. 840-43*).

- -

OTHER FACTORS:

Rule out <u>food sensitivities</u>.

Theoretical Discussion (<u>peptic ulcer</u>): It is argued that all chronic gastroduodenal peptic ulcers result
from localized increase in mucosal susceptibility to acid attack at the interface between a segment of
gastroduodenitis and gastric fundus or duodenal mucosa. Destructive or stimulatory immune reactions
could affect the gastrin-secreting G cells and other paracrine cells causing tropic and inflammatory reactions predisposing to peptic ulceration (*Kirk RM. Could chronic peptic ulcers be localised areas of acid
susceptibility generated by autoimmunity?* Lancet *April 5, 1986, pp. 772-4*).

Observational Study (<u>peptic ulcer</u>): Biopsies obtained from the edges of gastric and duodenal peptic ulcers demonstrate a marked increase of immunoglobulin E containing cells at the lesion edges, suggesting
that mucosal anaphylaxis may be the cause of the lesions (*Andre C et al. Evidence for anaphylactic reactions in peptic ulcer and varioliform gastritis.* Ann. Allergy *51:325-7, 1983*).

Experimental Study (peptic ulcer): Exclusion diets were beneficial (*Siegel J. Immunologic approach to the treatment and prevention of gastrointestinal ulcers. Ann. Allergy 38:27-41, 1977*).

Observational Study (peptic ulcer): 25 out of 43 (58%) allergic children with symptoms suggestive of duodenal ulceration had x-ray evidence of peptic duodenal ulcers (*Rebhun J. Duodenal ulceration in allergic children. Ann. Allergy 34:145-49, 1975*).

Observational Study (peptic ulcer): 98% of pts. with x-ray evidence of peptic ulcer had coexisting upper and lower respiratory tract allergic disease (*Siegel J. Gastrointestinal ulcer - Arthus reaction! Ann. Allergy 32:127-30, 1974*).

Experimental Study (allergic gastritis): Food reactions diminished peristalsis causing delayed gastric emptying time and caused severe hyperemia and edema of the stomach, mainly in the lower one-third (*Pollard HM, Stuart GJ. Experimental reproduction of gastric allergy in human beings with controlled observations on the mucosa. J. Allergy 13:467-73, 1942*).

ULCERS (SKIN)

See Also: WOUND HEALING

NUTRIENTS:

Folic Acid:

Supplementation may be beneficial.

> **Experimental Study:** 3 men and 7 women (ave. age 61) with ulcers due to moderate to advanced peripheral atherosclerosis received 5 mg folic acid orally 3 times daily and 20 mg IM twice weekly. In 6-8 wks., complete healing was achieved in the pts. with smaller ulcers (1-3 cm in diameter), while larger ulcers healed by 12 weeks except for 1 pt. whose ulcer was reduced to 1/2 its former size. The author suggests that healing was due to the vasodilating property of the vitamin (*Kopjas TL. J. Am. Geriat. Soc. March, 1968*).

Vitamin C:

May be deficient.

> **Observational Study:** 23% of 91 paraplegics had low leucocyte ascorbic levels, with the pts. who had decubitus ulcers having lower levels than the others (*Burr RG, Rajan KT. Leucocyte ascorbic acid and pressure sores in paraplegia. Brit. J. Nutr. 28:275-81, 1972*).

Supplementation may be beneficial.

> **Experimental Double-blind Study:** 10/20 pts. with pressure sores received ascorbic acid 500 mg twice daily while controls received placebo. After 1 month ulcers had decreased in size by an average of 84% in the supplemented gp. compared to 43% in the control group, a significant difference (p less than 0.005) (*Taylor TV et al. Ascorbic acid supplementation in the treatment of pressure sores. Lancet 2:544-6, 1974*).

> **Experimental Study:** 7 pts. with decubitus ulcers were given 500 mg ascorbic acid twice daily. After 3 days, biopsies showed enhanced collagen formation (*Burr RG - op cit*).

Vitamin E:

Supplementation may be beneficial.

- with topical application of vitamin E ointment:

> **Clinical Observation and Case Report:** Bedsores, diabetic ulcers and ulcerated surgical incisions responded. A pt. who had previously been treated in 5 different hospitals and clinics without success for extensive ulceration over his lower body was treated with vitamin E 800 IU twice daily and topical applications of vitamin E ointment. The wounds healed completely within 4 months (*Fisher D. The Summary vol. 26, December, 1974.*)

- -

<u>Zinc:</u>

If deficient, supplementation may be beneficial.

Experimental Controlled Study: 7 pts. with low serum zinc and 7 with normal serum zinc randomly received oral zinc sulphate 200 mg 3 times daily with meals, while 7 pts. pts. with low serum zinc and 9 with normal serum zinc served as controls. Within 1 yr., the ulcers were healed in all but 2 of the pts. with low initial serum zinc levels who were unsupplemented. Slowest healing was in the low serum zinc gp. without supplementation, and fastest healing was in the gp. with normal zinc levels receiving zinc (*Haeger K, Lanner E. Oral zinc sulphate and ischemic leg ulcers. <u>Vasa</u> 3(1):77-81, 1974*).

Experimental Double-blind Study: Zinc supplements significantly accelerated the rate of healing of venous leg ulcers, but only in zinc-deficient pts. (*Hallb:o:ok T, Lanner E. Serum zinc and healing of venous leg ulcers. <u>Lancet</u> 2:780-82, 1972*).

See Also:

Dachowski EJ et al. Venous leg ulceration: Skin and serum zinc concentrations. <u>Acta Dermatovener (Stockholm)</u> 55:497-98, 1975

Norris JR, Reynolds RE. The effect of oral zinc sulphate therapy on decubitus ulcers. <u>J. Am. Geriatrics Soc.</u> September, 1971, pp. 793-97

Greaves MW, Skillen AW. Effects of long-continued ingestion of zinc sulphate in patients with venous leg ulceration. <u>Lancet</u> 2:889-891, 1970

Greaves MW, Ive FA. Double-blind trial of zinc sulphate in the treatment of chronic leg ulceration. <u>Brit. J. Dermatol.</u> 87:632-34

- -

TOPICAL APPLICATION:

<u>Vitamin A:</u>

Application may reverse the inhibitory effect of corticosteroids on healing.

Case Report: 18 year-old female receiving a corticosteroid for a skin disease banged her leg and developed an ulceration in the wound which continued to enlarge despite normal medical treatment until vitamin A ointment was applied to the wound 3 times daily. Within 3 days, the wound began to heal. 28 days later, it had completely healed (*Hunt TK et al. Effect of vitamin A on reversing the inhibitory effect of cortisone on healing of open wounds in animals and man. <u>Ann. Surg.</u> 170(4):633-41, 1969*).

<u>Sugar,</u>
<u>Essential Amino Acids,</u> and
<u>Vitamin C:</u>

Application may be beneficial.

Experimental Study: 30 pts. with treatment-resistant bedsores resulting from diabetes, varicose veins or burns were treated with a solution of simple and complex sugars, essential amino acids and vitamin C daily following wound debridement. Response began in 24-73 hours with full healing of the smaller ulcers and successful skin grafting of the larger ones (*Silvetti AN et al. Accelerated wound healing and infection control through the topical application of nutrients. Fed. Proceed. 40(3) Part II p. 922, abstract no. 3929, March 1, 1981*).

URTICARIA (CHRONIC)

See Also: ALLERGY

NUTRIENTS:

Beta Carotene:

Supplementation may be beneficial in <u>solar</u> urticaria (*Pollitt N. Beta-carotene and the photodermatoses. Brit. J. Dermatol. 93:721, 1975*).

Vitamin B$_{12}$:   Intramuscular injections

Supplementation may be beneficial.

> **Experimental Study:** Over 100 pts. were treated with vitamin B$_{12}$ 1000 mcg weekly with relief obtained in the majority (*Simon SW, Edmonds P. Cyanocobalamin (B$_{12}$): Comparison of aqueous and repository preparations in urticaria: Possible mode of action. J. Am. Ger. Soc. 12:79-85, 1964*).

> **Experimental Study:** 9/10 pts. were greatly improved following vitamin B$_{12}$ 1000 mcg IM weekly for 4 weeks (*Simon SW. Vitamin B$_{12}$ therapy in allergy and chronic dermatoses. J. Allergy 22:183-85, 1951*).

Vitamin C:

May be deficient. If so, supplementation may be beneficial.

> **Case Reports:** 7 cases of chronic urticaria are described which were associated with poor dietary habits and deficient levels of blood vitamin C. All responded when citrus fruits were added to the diet (*Rosenberg W. Vitamin C deficiency as a cause of urticaria. Arch. Dermatol. Syph. 37:1010-14, 1938*).

- -

OTHER FACTORS:

Rule out <u>food and chemical sensitivities</u>.

> **Experimental Double-blind Study:** 86/140 children with recurrent urticaria displayed significant improvement on a salicylate-free diet, and nearly 3/4 reacted to double-blind salicylate challenge. Reactions to many other compounds such as preservatives, azo-dyes and brewer's yeast were also observed (*Swain A et al. Salicylates, oligoantigenic diets, and behavior. Lancet 2:41-2, 1985*).

> **Experimental Study:** 67 patients consumed a tyramine and additive-free diet which excluded preserved, artificially colored and flavored foods and drinks, alcoholic beverages, stone fruits, oranges, nuts, strawberries, tomatoes, peas, beans, shellfish, and tyramine-containing foods such as bananas, pineapple and old or fermented cheese. 55% had complete or partial resolution (*Verschave A et al. Pseudo-allergen-free diet in chronic urticaria. Dermatologica 167:256, 1983*).

Experimental Study: 25/137 pts. (18%) with recurrent urticaria were provoked by aspirin, 4% by benzoic acid and 1% by azo dyes (*Hannuksela M. Food allergy and skin diseases. Ann. Allergy 51:269-72, 1983*).

Observational Study: Records of 27 pts. were reviewed. 14/15 thought to be allergic were relieved by allergic therapy (avoidance and sometimes immunotherapy). 2 and possibly 4 pts. not thought allergic were also relieved by allergy therapy, suggesting that pts. should be carefully investigated for allergic reactions (*Catlett JB. Allergic etiology of chronic urticaria-angioedema and response to allergic therapy. Immunol. & Allergy Practice 5(1):21-34, 1983*).

Experimental Study: Recurrent urticaria in 330 pts. was frequently provoked by foods, food dyes and preservatives in amounts that could be present in their diets. Foods were provocative in 30%, drinks in 18% and chocolate and sweets in 10%. 18% were provoked by azo dyes; 22% by aspirin and 16% by yeast (*Juhlin L. Recurrent urticaria: Clinical investigation of 330 patients. Brit. J. Dermatol. 194:369, 1981*).

Experimental Study: 50/158 patients were relieved by a diet free of salicylates, benzoates and azo dyes. 28 of the responders (56%) recalled that ASA exacerbated their skin changes, and all of the responders were intolerant to ASA during the course of urticaria, while none of the non-responders recalled exacerbations from ASA (*Rudzki E et al. Detection of urticaria with food additives intolerance by means of diet. Dermatologica 161(1):57-62, 1980*).

See Also:

Gibson A, Clancy R. Management of chronic idiopathic urticaria by the identification and exclusion of dietary factors. Clin. Allergy 10:699, 1980

Warin WP, Smith RJ. Challenge test battery in chronic urticaria. Brit. J. Dermatol. 94:401, 1976

Doeglas HMG. Reactions to aspirin and food additives in patients with chronic urticaria including the physical urticarias. Br. J. Dermatol. 93:135-44, 1975

Noid HE et al. Diet plan for patients with salicylate-induced urticaria. Arch Dermatol. 109:966, 1974

Rapp DJ. Water as a cause of angio-edema and urticaria. JAMA 221:305, 1972

Juhlin L et al. Urticaria and asthma induced by food and drug additives in patients with aspirin sensitivity. J. Allergy Clin. Immunol. 50:92, 1972

Rule out <u>hydrochloric acid deficiency</u>.

Experimental Study: Of 77 pts., 24 (31%) had no HCl and only 12 (16%) had normal HCl levels. Pts. with urticaria due to food poisoning, drug reactions or infections were excluded. Signs of vitamin B complex deficiency seemed to be correlated with the extent of the HCl deficiency. Treatment of the 84% of patients who presented with diminished HCl levels with vitamin B complex and HCl gave "remarkable" results (*Allison JR. The relation of hydrochloric acid and vitamin B complex deficiency in certain skin diseases. Southern Med. J. 38:235-241, 1945*).

See Also:

Rawls WB, Ancona VC. Chronic urticaria associated with hypochlorhydria or achlorhydria. Rev. Gastroenterol. 18:267, 1951

VASCULAR FRAGILITY
(including SPORTS INJURIES)

NUTRIENTS:

<u>Vitamin C:</u>

Supplementation may be beneficial, especially if deficient.

> **Experimental Study:** 10 pts. with hiatal hernia and esophageal reflux who developed vitamin C deficiency due to intolerance of "acid" foods were supplemented with vitamin C. Subsequently, scattered deficiency symptoms disappeared and both capillary fragility tests and serum ascorbic acid levels returned toward normal (*Hiebert CA. Gastroesophageal reflux and ascorbic acid deficiency. Ann. Thorac. Surg. 24(2):108-12, 1977*).

See Also:

> *Cox BD, Butterfield WJ. Vitamin C supplements and diabetic cutaneous capillary fragility. Br. Med. J. 3:205, 1975*

<u>Vitamin E:</u>

Supplementation may be beneficial.

> **Experimental Study:** 7 cases of purpura due to vascular changes caused by infection, drugs or unknown causes were treated with oral doses of alpha-tocopherol nicotinate 400-600 mg daily. 6/7 showed remarkable improvement of petechiae with their complete disappearance after 5-21 days along with improvements in other clinical symptoms (*Fujii T. The clinical effects of vitamin E on purpuras due to vascular defects. J. Vitaminology 18:125-30, 1972*).

> **Experimental Study:** Capillary permeability was increased in human skin by using chemicals such as histamine, acetylcholine and alpha-chymotrypsin which was then reduced by the administration of alpha tocopherol acetate 450 I.U. for 5-7 days (*Kamimura M. et al. Vitamins 28:129, 1961*).

- -

<u>Zinc:</u>

Deficiency may be associated with senile purpura.

> **Observational Study:** 20 pts. with senile purpura had lower serum zinc levels than 20 controls despite no significant differences in the mean serum concentration of albumin, the main binder of zinc (*Haboubi NY et al. Zinc deficiency in senile purpura. J. Clin. Pathol. 38(1):1189-91, 1985*).

‒ ‒

Bioflavonoids :

Supplementation may be beneficial.

Animal Experimental Study: Various flavonoids were found to reduce capillary permeability in rabbits (*Paris R, Moury J. [Effects of diverse flavonoids upon capillary permeability.] Ann. Pharm. Franc. 22:489-93, 1964*).

Experimental Placebo-controlled Study: The effects of citrus bioflavonoids, ascorbic acid, citrus bioflavonoids and ascorbic acid together, and placebo were compared regarding recovery from athletic injuries. The injury recovery rate in the bioflavonoid gps. was twice as rapid as the ascorbic acid and placebo controls (*Cragin RB. The use of bioflavonoids in the prevention and treatment of athletic injuries. Med. Times 90:529-30, 1962*).

Experimental Double-blind Study: Starting 10 days prior to their initial practice, football players received either placebo or citrus bioflavonoids 600 mg 3 times daily for for the first wk., then 200 mg 3 times daily. While the incidence of injury was similar for both gps., loss of playing time averaged 0.67 days for the treated gp. compared to 2.2 days for the controls (*Miller MJ. Injuries to athletes. Med. Times 88:313-14, 1960*).

Experimental Study: Bioflavonoids minimized capillary bleeding during tonsillectomy and adenoid surgery as well as post-operative bleeding (*Ryan RE. A new aid to tonsil and adenoid surgery. Clin. Med. 5:327, 1958*).

See Also:

Review of Animal Studies: *Gabor M. Pharmacologic effect of flavonoids on blood vessels. Angiologica 9:355-74, 1972*

Gloor M, Fischer H. [Principles of flavonoid therapy.] Fortschr. Med. 89:1025-27, 1971

Lecomte J, Van Cauwenberge H. [Pharmacologic properties of bioflavonoids.] Rev. Med. Liege 26(20):673-81, 1971

‒ ‒

COMBINED SUPPLEMENTATION:

Vitamin C and
Bioflavonoids:

Supplementation may be beneficial.

Experimental Study: The combination of vitamin C 1.5 gm and bioflavonoids (hesperidine methylchalcone 150 mg and esculine 15 mg) given IV reduced the tendency towards capillary bleeding (microscopic hematuria) caused by anti-coagulants in 21 pts. without interfering with normal blood clotting. In 1 pt., a trial of vitamin C alone was unsuccessful (*Shapiro S, Spitzer JM. The use of Cepevit (ascorbic acid plus "p" factors) in drug-induced hypoprothrombinemia. Angiology 5:64-71, 1954*).

See Also:

Kucher AG.   [On the use of vitamins P and C for the prevention of increased capillary fragility in children.]   Vopr. Pitan. 25(2):39-42, 1966

Beiler JM.   Biochemistry of the synergists.   Ascorbic acid and hesperidin.   Exp. Med. Surg. 12:563-69, 1955

Selsman GJV, Horoschak S.   The treatment of capillary fragility with a combination of hesperidin and vitamin C. Am. J. Dig. Dis. 17:92, 1950

VASCULITIS

(including ECCHYMOSES and PURPURA)

See Also: AUTO-IMMUNE DISORDERS (GENERAL)

NUTRIENTS:

<u>Selenium:</u>

Supplementation may be beneficial.

- with <u>Vitamin E:</u>

> **Experimental Study:** 16 pts. with vasculitis were found to have depressed values of glutathione peroxidase compared to normal controls (p less than 0.01) and 2/16 were treated with tablets containing 10 mg tocopheryl succinate and 0.2 mg selenium as Na_2SeO_3. The glutathione peroxidase levels increased slowly within 6-8 wks. and the clinical effect was encouraging (*Juhlin L et al. Blood glutathione-peroxidase levels in skin diseases: Effect of selenium and vitamin E treatment. <u>Acta Derm. Venereal. (Stockh.)</u> 62(3):211-14, 1982*).

OTHER FACTORS:

Rule out <u>food and chemical sensitivities</u> (hypersensitivity vasculitis):

Experimental Study: 10 consecutive pts. with non-specific small vessel vasculitis (petechiae, spontaneous bruising, vascular spasm and recurrent edema) were hospitalized in a unit designed to minimize environmental triggering agents. All medications were stopped. After pts. had reached a basal state free of signs and symptoms of vasculitis, they were challenged with up to 4 less chemically contaminated source foods every 24 hours. All pts. were cleared of evidence of vasculitis in 3-7 days and had their vasculitis reproduced on at least 3 separate occasions, usually within 5 minutes after ingestion (*Rea WJ. Environmentally triggered small vessel vasculitis. <u>Ann. Allergy</u> 38:245-51, 1977*).

Experimental Study: Pts. are described for whom exposure to tree pollen, foods and chemicals triggered small vessel vasculitis (*Theorell H et al. Demonstration of reactivity to airborn and food antigens in cutaneous vasculitis by variation in fibrino peptide and others, blood coagulation, fibrinolysis, and complement parameters. <u>Thromb. Haemost.</u> 36:593, 1976*).

Case Report: 58 year-old while female presented with a 9-year history of recurrent dragging of her right foot. Physical exam revealed extensive noninflammatory purpura, eczema, petechiae, and spontaneous bruising. Her symptoms subsided following a 5-day fast in an environmentally-controlled hospital unit. Challenge testing with several foods was followed by headache within 5 minutes following by severe right-sided pain and spontaneous bruising, culminating in wide-spread noninflammatory purpura. Angiography revealed spasm of the peripheral arteries (*Rea WJ et al. Environmentally triggered large vessel vasculitis, in Johnson H, Spencer JT, Eds. <u>Allergy: Immunology and Medical Treatment</u>. Chicago, Symposia Specialists, 1975, pp. 185-98*).

See Also:

Robinson BWS. Henoch-Schonlein purpura due to food sensitivity. <u>Brit. Med. J.</u> February 19, 1977 p. 510

Siroty RR. Purpura on the rocks - with a twist. <u>JAMA</u> 235:2521, 1976

Michaelsson G et al. Purpura caused by food and drug additives. <u>Arch. Dermatol.</u> 109:49, 1974

Snyder RD. Allergic purpura. <u>Ann. Allergy</u> 26:328, 1968

VITILIGO

NUTRIENTS:

Para Amino Benzoic Acid (PABA):

WARNING: Vitiligo has been reported as being <u>caused</u> by PABA (*Hughes CG. Oral PABA and vitiligo. J. Am. Acad. Dermatol. 9:770, 1983*). Other potential side-effects include skin rash, anorexia, nausea and fever (*Physicians' Desk Reference. Oradell, N.J., Med. Economics Co., Inc., 1986*) as well as liver toxicity (*Kantor GR, Ratz JL. Liver toxicity from potassium para-aminobenzoate. Letter to the Editor. J. Am. Acad. Dermatol. 13(4):671-72, 1985*).

Supplementation may be beneficial.

- with <u>Vitamin B Complex</u>:

Experimental Study: 48 pts. (25 females, 23 males) were studied over 10 months. Most had a history of inadequate diet and symptoms of fatigue, irritability, emotional instability, constipation, headaches and joint pains were common. Pts. received PABA 100 mg 3-4 times daily in addition to vitamin B complex. Later, due to the slowness of the effect, parenteral monoethanolamine PABA 100 mg was added twice daily in order to maintain adequate blood levels. Results were slow, but were striking by 6-7 months of treatment (*Sieve BF. Further investigations in the treatment of vitiligo. Virginia Med. Monthly January 1945, pp. 6-17*).

- -

Copper:

Necessary for the activation of tyrosinase. Decreased tyrosinase activity will impede the conversion of tyrosine to melatonin, resulting in albinism and vitiligo.

References:

Genov D et al. Copper pathochemistry in vitiligo. Clin. Chim. Acta 37:207-11, 1972

Lal S et al. Serum caeruloplasmin in vitiligo. Indian J. Med. Sci. 24(10):678-79, 1970

Sen S. Caeruloplasmin, copper and disease. J. Indian Med. Assoc. 52(4):182-84, 1969

Chorazak T, Rzempoluch E. Etiopathogenesis of vitiligo in the light of our studies. Pol. Med. J. 7(2):494-500, 1968

Supplementation may be beneficial.

Reference:

Bagaeva MI. [Treatment of vitiligo in children with copper sulfate.] Vestn. Dermatol. Vernerol. (3):48-50, March, 1979

- -

Phenylalanine   50 mg/kg

- with UVA light.

> **Experimental Study:** Pts. received phenylalanine 50 mg/kg along with exposure to UVA light 30-45 minutes after ingestion (the time of peak blood concentrations). After 4 mo. (32 treatments), "reasonable" repigmentation occurred. Apart from the repigmentation of hypo-pigmented macules, pts. became able to tolerate more sun than usual, especially at the vitiliginous lesion (*Cormane RH et al. Phenylalanine and UVA light for the treatment of vitiligo. Arch. Dermatol. Res. 277(2):126-30, 1985*).

- -

OTHER FACTORS:

Rule out hydrochloric acid deficiency.

> **Observational Study:** Gastric acid secretion was assessed in 102 consecutive pts. by means of the augmented histamine test. 20/102 (19.6%) were achlorhydric, and 19 of the 20 were female. 8 of the 20 (all females) were found to have pernicious anemia (*Howitz J., Schwartz M. Vitiligo, achlorhydria, and pernicious anemia. Lancet 1:1331-35, 1971*).

> **Experimental and Observational Study:** Of 29 pts., 10 (35%) had no HCl and only 3 (10%) had normal HCl levels. The severity of the condition seemed to correlate with the extent of the HCl deficiency and also seemed to be associated with signs of vitamin B complex deficiency. Good results were obtained following HCl and vitamin B complex supplementation where a definite hypochlorhydria was found (*Allison JR. The relation of HCl and vitamin B complex deficiency in certain skin diseases. Southern Med. J. 38:235-241, 1945*).

> **Experimental Study:** 4 pts. with vitiligo and achlorhydria experienced disappearance of the vitiligo by 2 yrs. after starting hydrochloric acid 15 cc with each meal (*Francis HW. Achlorhydria as an etiological factor in vitiligo, with report of four cases. Nebraska Med. J. 16:25-26, 1931*).

See Also:

> *Allison JR, Curtis AC. Arch. Derm. 72:407, 1955*

> *Ishida K. Jap. J. Derm. Vener. 64:155, 1954*

WOUND HEALING

See Also: ULCERS (ISCHEMIC)

NUTRIENTS:

Pantothenic Acid:

May accelerate the normal healing process.

Animal Experimental Study: In a controlled study, pantothenic acid (20 mg/kg/day) was injected into rabbits and wound healing was observed over a 1 month postoperative period. Chronic pre- and postoperative supplementation significantly increased aponeurosis strength after surgery, slightly, but not significantly, improved skin strength and increased the fibroblast content of the scar (*Aprahamian M et al. Am. J. Clin. Nutr. 578-89, 1985*).

Thiamine:

Deficiency interferes with collagen synthesis.

Animal Experimental Study: Granulation tissue in wounds of thiamine-deficient rats was 1/5 the mass of controls and was greatly deficient in hydroxyproline, confirming that collagen biosynthesis was severely disrupted (*Alvarez OM, Gilbreath RL. Thiamin influence on collagen during the granulation of skin wounds. J. Surg. Res. 32:24-31, 1982*).

See Also:

Alvarez OM, Gilbreath RL. Effect of dietary thiamin on intermolecular collagen crosslinking during wound repair: A mechanical and biochemical assessment. J. Trauma 22:20-24, 1982

Prasad CA, Bose SM. Effect of thiamin deficiency on collagen metabolism. J. Nutr. Sci. Vitaminol. 20:97-102, 1974

Vitamin A:

Ensures that scar tissue is strong and resistent to tearing.

Animal Experimental Study: Rats were fed a vitamin A deficient diet for 2 weeks then divided into 2 groups. One received only a "basal" diet while the other also received additional vitamin A as beta-carotene, retinoic acid or retinyl acetate. After 5 days, the supplemental retinyl acetate and beta-carotene "resulted in increases of 35% and 70%, respectively, over the wound tensile strength of rats fed the basal level of vitamin A" (*Gerber LE, Erdman JW Jr. Wound healing in rats fed small supplements of retinyl acetate, beta-carotene or retinoic acid. Fed. Proc. March 1, 1981, #3453, p. 838*).

Animal Experimental Study: The impairment of wound healing noted in streptozotocin diabetic rats was prevented by supplementation with vitamin A (*Seifter E et al. Impaired wound healing in streptozotocin diabetes. Prevention by supplemental vitamin A. Ann. Surg. 194(1):42-50, 1981*).

Animal Experimental Study: Scars of wounds of rats given vitamin A supplements had greater tensile strength and less risk of breakage than those of controls (*Seitfer E et al. Influence of vitamin A on wound healing in rats with femoral fracture. Ann. Surg. 181(6):836-41, 1975*).

See Also:

> *Hunt TK et al. Effect of vitamin A on reversing the inhibitory effect of cortisone on healing of open wounds in animals and man. Ann. Surg. 170(4):633-41, 1969*

Vitamin C: 500 mg. with meals and at bedtime

Promotes collagen and elastin formation (*Chatterjee IB. Ascorbic acid metabolism. World Rev. Nutr. Diet 30:69-87, 1978*).

Supplementation may be beneficial.

> **Experimental Controlled Study:** A plug of gingival tissue was removed from two subjects and permitted to heal. The procedure was then repeated while the subjects were receiving 250 mg. vitamin C at meals and at bedtime, and again with 500 mg. vitamin C. Compared to the control condition, wound healing was 40% faster at the lower dosage and 50% faster at the higher dosage (*Ringsdorf WM Jr, Cheraskin E. Vitamin C and human wound healing. Oral Surg. 53(3):231-36, 1982*).

> **Experimental Double-blind Study:** 20 patients with bedsores were given either vitamin C 500 mg. twice daily or placebo. After one month, the bedsores of the treated group had decreased an average of 84% in size compared to only a 43% decrease in the placebo group (p less than 0.005) (*Taylor TV et al. Ascorbic acid supplementation in the treatment of pressure-sores. Lancet 2:544-46, 1974*).

Vitamin E:

Supplementation may be beneficial.

> **Animal Experimental Study (rats):** Gingival wounds healed faster in supplemented rats compared to controls (*Kim JE, Shklar G. The effect of vitamin E on the healing of gingival wounds in rats. J. Periodontol. 54:305, 1983*).

> - with topical application of vitamin E ointment:

> > **Clinical Observation and Case Report:** Bedsores, diabetic ulcers and ulcerated surgical incisions responded. A pt. who had previously been treated in 5 different hospitals and clinics without success for extensive ulceration over his lower body was treated with vitamin E 800 IU twice daily and topical applications of vitamin E ointment. The wounds healed completely within 4 months (*Fisher D. The Summary vol. 26, December, 1974.*)

- -

Zinc:

If deficient, supplementation may be beneficial.

> **Review Articles:** A number of studies have found zinc supplementation to have a beneficial effect upon wound healing, while a number of other studies have had negative results. It appears from animal studies that zinc supplementation is only beneficial when deficient; however, zinc nutriture is difficult to evaluate in man as serum zinc concentration may not accurately reflect the total bodily status of zinc metabolism (*Haley JV. Zinc sulfate and wound healing. J. Surg. Res. 27(3):168-74, 1979; Williams KW et al. The effect of topically applied zinc on the healing of open wounds. J. Surg.*

Res. 27:62-67, 1979; Henkin RI. *Zinc in wound healing. Editorial. N. Engl. J. Med. 291(13):675-76, 1974*).

Experimental Study: Supplemental zinc stimulated wound healing, but only in pts. who were zinc-deficient (*Fulghum DD. Ascorbic acid revisited. Arch. Derm. 113(1):91-92, 1977*).

- -

Arginine:

May minimize immediate post-injury weight loss and accelerate wound healing.

Animal Experimental Study (rats): A 1% dietary supplement of arginine HCl accelerated wound healing in injured rats ingesting a commercial diet containing 1.8% arginine (which supports normal growth, reproduction and longevity of healthy rats) (*Seifter E et al. Arginine: An essential amino acid for injured rats. Surgery 84:224-30, 1978*).

See Also:

Barbul A et al. Wound healing and thymotropic effects of arginine: A pituitary mechanism of action. Am. J. Clin. Nutr. 37:786-94, 1983

- -

TOPICAL APPLICATION:

Vitamin A:

Application may reverse the inhibitory effect of corticosteroids on the healing of open wounds.

Case Report: 18 year-old female receiving a corticosteroid for a skin disease banged her leg and developed an ulceration in the wound which continued to enlarge despite normal medical treatment until vitamin A ointment was applied to the wound 3 times daily. Within 3 days, the wound began to heal. 28 days later, it had completely healed (*Hunt TK et al. Effect of vitamin A on reversing the inhibitory effect of cortisone on healing of open wounds in animals and man. Ann. Surg. 170(2):203-6, 1969*).

Animal Experimental Study (rabbits): Wounds of animals receiving cortisone healed normally when they received topical applications of vitamin E (*Hunt TK - ibid*).

PART TWO

APPENDICES

Appendix A

COMMON NUTRIENT DEFICIENCIES

GENERAL:

<u>Hospitalized pts.</u> are frequently nutritionally deficient.

Observational Study: In a 30 mo. study of records of 800 pts. admitted to 2 American hospitals with pneumonia, hip fracture, or inflammatory bowel disease, or in order to have hip, bowel or abdominal surgery, some degreee of malnutrition was found in 55% of all patients (based on: serum albumin below 3.4 g/dl; weight below 90% of ideal body weight; total lymphocyte count below 1400/mm^3; history of recent weight loss). Among the nonsurgical gps., malnourished pts. stayed in the hospital an ave. of 2 days longer than well-nourished pts. while, among the surgical gps., malnourished pts. stayed 5 days longer (*Nutritional therapy saves lives, costs. <u>Med. World News</u> February 24, 1986, p. 99*).

Observational Study: In a study of 3172 hospitalized American pts., 58% were malnourished according to at least 1 of the following indicators: serum albumin, total lymphocyte count, hemoglobin values, and weight-for-height measurement (*Kamath S - reported in <u>Am. Med. News</u> May 24/31, 1985*).

<u>Hospital diets</u> may be nutritionally deficient.

Observational Study: The daily intake of energy, protein, iron and vitamins of pts. on different wards of an English hospital was found to be less than those recommended for healthy adults (*Todd EA et al. What do patients eat in hospital. <u>Human Nutr.: Applied Nutr.</u> 38A:294-97, 1984*).

<u>Parenteral nutrition (TPN)</u> often causes nutritional deficiencies. Within the first week, there are severe deficiencies of phosphorus, potassium, sodium, magnesium and essential fatty acids, while long-term TPN often leads to depletion of Vitamins A and E, folic acid, biotin and pyridoxine as well as zinc, copper, chromium and selenium (*Chipponi J. Total parenteral nutrition (TPN) often causes nutrient deficiencies. <u>Am. J. Clin. Nutr.</u> 35:1112-16, 1982*).

<u>The elderly</u> frequently fail to ingest adequate amounts of certain nutrients.

Observational Study: 403 elderly europeans residing at home were interview in regard to their vitamin and mineral intake. Compared to the Recommended Dietary Allowances, the Joint Nordic Recommendations and the Absolute Minimal Necessary Amounts, folacin intake was low in 100%, cholecalciferol in 62%, pyridoxine in 83%, and zinc in 87% (although the risk of zinc deficiency was only present in 0.5%). Intakes of the other major vitamins and minerals were sufficient. In conclusion, the diet of the elderly, possibly with the exception of folacin, is well above their absolute minimal requirements, but the margin towards malnutrition is small (*Elsborg L et al. The intake of vitamins and minerals by the elderly at home. <u>Int. J. Vitam. Nutr. Res.</u> 53(3):321-29, 1983*).

<u>The elderly</u> are frequently nutritionally deficient.

Observational Study: Status of vitamins B$_1$, B$_2$, B$_6$ and C in 19 hospitalized pts. ages 65-89 were compared to 10 healthy controls. Both thiamine and ascorbic acid deficiencies were common in both gps., while only the pts. were frequently deficient in pyridoxine. Only 1 person in each gp. was deficient in vitamin B2. These deficiencies were not manifested clinically as classic vitamin deficiency syndromes; thus biochemical assays are necessary for their detection (*Keatinge AMB et al. Vitamin B1, B2, B6 and C status in the elderly. Irish Med. J. 76:488-90, 1983*).

Calcium: 1.5 gm. daily for postmenopausal women
              (1 gm. daily for premenopausal women over 35)

Women who ingest less than the above amts. are in negative calcium balance (*Heaney RP et al. Menopausal changes in calcium balance performance. J. Lab. & Clin. Med. 92(6):953-63, 1978*).

NIH Consensus Conference: Calcium intake is commonly insufficient and insufficient intake is associated with decreased bone mineral density. The typical American diet supplies about 450-550 mg daily, well below the RDA. "It seems likely that an increase in calcium intake to 1,000 to 1,500 mg/day beginning well before the menopause will reduce the incidence of osteoporosis in postmenopausal women. Increased calcium intake may prevent age-related bone loss in men as well" (*NIH Consensus Conference: Osteoporosis. JAMA 252(6):799-802, 1984*).

Observational Study: Daily calcium intakes based on 3-day dietary records from the USDA's 1977-8 Nationwide Food Consumption Survey were below the Recommended Dietary Allowance for the majority of the U.S. population, particularly for adult women (*Morgan KJ et al. Magnesium and calcium dietary intakes of the U.S. population. J. Am. Coll. Nutr. 4:195, 1985*).

Calcium is the only mineral whose requirement doubles during pregnancy (*Truswell AS. Nutrition for pregnancy. Brit. Med. J. July, 1985*).

Chromium:

Marginal deficiency is common in Western diets due to the high consumption of refined foods and sugars (*Schroeder HA. The role of chromium in mammalian nutrition. Am. J. Clin. Nutr. 21(3):230-44, 1968; Kumpulainen JT. J. Agricultural & Food Chem. vol. 27, no. 3, 1979*).

Observational Study: In a study of the self-selected diets of 10 males and 22 females (ages 25-65), over 90% of the diets were below the recommended minimum intake of 50 mcg daily (*Anderson RA, Kozlovsky AS. Chromium intake, absorption and excretion of subjects consuming self-selected diets. Am. J. Clin. Nutr. 41:1177-83, 1985*).

Copper:

75% of the daily diets in the United States fail to contain the recommended dietary allowance of copper (*Klevay LM. Biol. Trace Element Res. 5:245-55, 1983*).

Observational Study: Dietary copper levels were determined spectrophotometrically for 22 men and women eating self-selected diets. 81% were found to consume less than 2/3 the RDA for copper, even though the ave. daily protein intake exceeded the RDA (*Holden JM et al. Zinc and copper in self-selected diets. J. Am. Dietet. Assoc. 75:23, 1979*).

Pregnant women may be in negative copper balance unless supplemented.

Experimental and Observational Study: 24 women in their second trimester were found to ingest less than the RDA of copper. Copper retention was -0.02 mg/day until they were supplemented with copper which raised copper retention to 0.89 mg/day (*Taper L et al. Am. J. Clin. Nutr. 41:1184-1192, 1985*).

<u>Folic acid:</u>

Often deficient in <u>the elderly</u> (*Baker H et al. Severe impairment of dietary folate utilization in the elderly. J. Am. Geriat. Soc. 26(5):218-221, 1978*) even despite adequate food intake and daily oral supplementation (*Frank O et al. Superiority of periodic intramuscular vitamins over daily oral vitamins in maintaining normal vitamin titers in a geriatric population. Am. J. Clin. Nutr. 30:630, 1977*).

Observational Study: In a study of 92 elderly Canadians residing in an extended-care facility, 22% were deficient in folic acid. 9.2% were high-risk for a deficiency of RBC folate, while 30.9% were high-risk for serum folate deficiency. The correlation between the 2 levels was significant. The only variable found to correlate with folate deficiency was the length of stay in the facility (*Infante-Rivard C et al. Folate deficiency among institutionalized elderly: Public health impact. J. Am. Geriatr. Soc. 34:211-14, 1986*).

Observational Study: In a study of 403 elderly Danes residing in their own homes, folacin intake (66 mcg mean; range 20-200 mcg) was low in 100% as compared to the Recommended Dietary Allowances (RDA), Joint Nordic Recommendations (NNR) and the Absolute Minimal Necessary Amounts (AMA) (*Elsborg L et al. The intake of vitamins and minerals by the elderly at home. Int. J. Vit. Nutr. Res. 53:321-29, 1983*).

Observational Study: Low serum folate was found in 5-10% of elderly Americans living at home, and 15-20% of those admitted to hospitals or institutions (*Rosenberg IH et al. Folate nutrition in the elderly. Am. J. Clin. Nutr. 36:1060, 1982*).

Review Article: The results of several studies indicate that approx. 30% of the elderly in Great Britain have abnormally low blood folate levels (*Runcie J. Folate deficiency in the elderly, in Botez MI, Reynolds EH. Folic Acid in Neurology, Psychiatry, and Internal Medicine. New York, Raven Press, 1979, pp. 493-99*).

The only vitamin whose requirement doubles in <u>pregnancy</u>. Serum and RBC folate levels decline during pregnancy and some degree of megaloblastic change can be found in substantial minorities of women in late pregnancy (*Truswell AS. Nutrition for pregnancy. Brit. Med. J. July, 1985*).

<u>Iron:</u>

Deficiency is believed to be the most prevalent worldwide nutritional deficiency and the most frequent cause of anemia (*Bernat I. Iron deficiency, in Iron Metabolism. New York, Plenum Press, 1983, pp.215-74*).

The most common nutrient deficiency in American <u>children</u> (*Worthington-Roberts B. Suboptimal nutrition and behavior in children, in Contemporary Developments in Nutrition. St. Louis, Mo., CV Mosby, 1981, pp. 524-62*).

Dietary need is known to be increased during <u>pregnancy</u> and increased iron absorption may not be adequate to make up for the extra demands if storage iron is low.

Experimental Study: 21 pregnant women received supplementation while 21 controls did not. Ferritin fell to 70% of its value at week 16 of amenorrhea in those supplemented versus only 30% in controls. Six and twelve week post-partum levels were still low in the controls (*Wallenburg HCS et al. Effect of oral iron supplementation during pregnancy on maternal and fetal iron status. J. Perinat. Med. 12(1):7-12, 1984*).

See Also:

Romslo I et al. Iron requirement in normal pregnancy as assessed by serum ferritin, serum transferrin saturation and erythrocyte protoporphyrin determinations. Brit. J. Obstet. Gyn. 90:101, 1983

Hemminki E, Starfield B.   Routine administration of iron and vitamins during pregnancy: Review of controlled clinical trials.   Brit. J. Obstet. Gyn. 85:404, 1978

Magnesium:

Dietary intake is often deficient.

Observational Study: Daily magnesium intakes based on 3-day dietary records from the USDA's 1977-8 Nationwide Food Consumption Survey were below the Recommended Dietary Allowance for all age and sex classes, with the exception of children younger than 5 years. Mg consumption was particularly low among adolescent females, adult females, and elderly males; 75-85% of individuals in these gps. ingested less than the RDA (*Morgan KJ et al. Magnesium and calcium dietary intakes of the U.S. population. J. Am. Coll. Nutr. 4:195, 1985*).

Review Article: While the typical American diet provides only 1/2 - 2/3 of the RDA (400 mg), it raises the magnesium requirement to 500-800 mg due to its high content of certain nutritional factors (*Seelig M. Magnesium Deficiency in the Pathogenesis of Disease. New York, Plenum Press, 1980*).

Frequently deficient among pts. admitted to an <u>intensive care unit</u>.

Observational Study: Out of 102 consecutive pts. admitted to a medical ICU, 20% had hypomagnesemia (*Reinhart R et al. Hypomagnesemia in patients entering the ICU. Critical Care Med. 13(6):506, 1985*).

Niacin:

Often deficient in <u>the elderly</u>, even despite adequate dietary intake and oral supplementation (*Frank O et al. Superiority of periodic intramuscular vitamins over daily oral vitamins in maintaining normal vitamin titers in a geriatric population. Am. J. Clin. Nutr. 30:630, 1977*).

Deficient in 30% of <u>institutionalized elderly</u> Americans (*Baker H et al. Vitamin profiles in elderly persons living at home or in nursing homes, versus profiles in healthy subjects. J. Am. Geriatr. Soc. 27:444, 1979*).

Potassium:

Intake frequently deficient in <u>the elderly</u>.

Observational Study: *Abdulla M et al. Dietary intake of potassium in the elderly. Lancet September 20, 1975, p. 562*

Deficient in about 20% of <u>hospitalized patients</u>.

Observational Study: In a study of almost 3000 hospitalized American pts., approx. 20% had plasma potassium concentrations below 3.5 mEq/l (*Surawicz B et al. Clinical manifestations of hypopotassemia. Am. J. Med. Sci. 233:603, 1957*).

Pyridoxine:

Often deficient in <u>the elderly</u>, even despite adequate dietary intake and oral supplementation (*Frank O et al. Superiority of periodic intramuscular vitamins over daily oral vitamins in maintaining normal vitamin titers in a geriatric population. Am. J. Clin. Nutr. 30:630, 1977*).

Observational Study: Deficient in elderly pts. as compared to healthy elderly controls (*Keatinge AMB et al. Vitamin B_1, B_2, B_6 and C status in the elderly. Irish Med. J. 76:488-90, 1983*)

Observational Study: In a study of 403 elderly Danes residing in their own homes, pyridoxine intake was low in 83% as compared to the Recommended Dietary Allowances (RDA) and the Joint Nordic Recommendations (NNR), while only 1% took less than the Absolute Minimal Necessary Amounts (AMA) which is 0.8 mg (*Elsborg L et al. The intake of vitamins and minerals by the elderly at home. Int. J. Vit. Nutr. Res. 53:321-29, 1983*).

Observational Study: 55% of a gp. of elderly Americans were B6-deficient (RDA) (*Bowman BB, Rosenberg IH. Am. J. Clin. Nutr. 35:1142-51, 1982*).

Observational Study: Deficient (RDA) in 30% of institutionalized elderly Americans (*Baker H et al. Vitamin profiles in elderly persons living at home or in nursing homes, versus profiles in healthy subjects. J. Am. Geriatr. Soc. 27:444, 1979*).

Pyridoxine is marginally deficient in about 50% of pregnant women, and studies have shown that supplementation with 20 mg daily may be necessary to keep the laboratory measurements of pyridoxine in the normal range (*Heller S et al. Vitamin B6 status in pregnancy. Am. J. Clin. Nutr. 26(12):1339-48, 1973*).

See Also:

> *Schuster K et al. Vitamin B6 status of low-income adolescent and adult pregnant women and the condition of their infants at birth. Am. J. Clin. Nutr. 34:1731, 1981*

> *Reinken L, Dapunt O. Vitamin B6 nutriture during pregnancy. Int. J. Vit. Nutr. Res. 48:341, 1978*

Riboflavin:

Intake may be deficient in the elderly.

Observational Study: In a study of 403 elderly Danes residing in their own homes, riboflavin intake (2.3 mg mean; range 0.7-5.0 mg) was low in 10% as compared to the Recommended Dietary Allowances (RDA), in 4% as compared to the Joint Nordic Recommendations (NNR), and in 0.5% as compared to the Absolute Minimal Necessary Amounts (AMA) (*Elsborg L et al. The intake of vitamins and minerals by the elderly at home. Int. J. Vit. Nutr. Res. 53:321-29, 1983*).

Frequently marginally deficient in the elderly.

Observational Study: Marginal riboflavin deficiency was found in 30% of Britains over 65 years old (*Powers H, Thornham D. Brit. J. Nutr. 46:257, 1981*).

Frequently marginally deficient in the poor.

Observational Study: In a study of 210 low-socioenomic-status adolescent Americans (ages 13-19), 26.6% of those not on supplements had abnormal RBC glutathione reductase activity (*Lopez R et al. Riboflavin deficiency in an adolescent population in New York City. Am. J. Clin. Nutr. 33:1283-86, 1980*).

Selenium:

Frequently deficient in Western diets.

Deficiency states have been demonstrated for inhabitants of regions where selenium supply is limited, in protein-energy malnutrition, and in pts. on total parenteral nutrition without selenium supplementation (*Neve J et al. Selenium deficiency. Clin. Endocrinol. Metab. 14(3):629-56, 1985*).

It has been estimated that the typical selenium consumption in the U.S. is about 100 mcg, while 250-300 mcg daily can prevent most cancers (*Schrauzer, Gerhard, Ph.D. - 1981*).

<u>Thiamine</u>:

Often deficient in <u>the elderly</u> (*Keatinge AMB et al. Vitamin B₁, B₂, B₆ and C status in the elderly. <u>Irish Med. J.</u> 76:488-90, 1983; Bowman BB, Rosenberg IH. <u>Am. J. Clin. Nutr.</u> 35:1142-51, 1982*), sometimes even when dietary intake appears to be adequate.

<u>Vitamin A</u>:

Intake is occasionally deficient among <u>the elderly</u>.

> **Observational Study:** In a study of 403 elderly Danes residing in their own homes, vitamin A intake (ave. 1500 mcg; range 192-8700 mcg) was low in 14% as compared to the Recommended Dietary Allowances (RDA) and the Joint Nordic Recommendations (NNR), and in 0.5% as compared to the Absolute Minimal Necessary Amounts (AMA) (*Elsborg L et al. The intake of vitamins and minerals by the elderly at home. <u>Int. J. Vit. Nutr. Res.</u> 53:321-29, 1983*).

<u>Vitamin B₁₂</u>:

Often deficient in <u>the elderly</u>, even despite adequate dietary intake and oral supplementation (*Frank O et al. Superiority of periodic intramuscular vitamins over daily oral vitamins in maintaining normal vitamin titers in a geriatric population. <u>Am. J. Clin. Nutr.</u> 30:630, 1977; Elsborg L et al. serum vitamin B₁₂ levels in the aged. <u>Acta Medica Scandinavica</u> 200:309-314, 1976*).

<u>Vitamin C</u>:

20-40% of U.S. <u>women</u> have a vitamin C intake below 70% of the RDA of 60 milligrams daily (*U.S. Dept. of Agriculture*).

Deficiency is common among <u>the chronically sick</u> and and <u>the institutionalized elderly</u>.

> **Observational and Experimental Study:** Chronically sick elderly American women had low intakes and low blood concentrations of vitamin C. Small dietary supplements of vitamin C increased its concentrations in plasma and leukocytes to those found in both the active elderly and the young, confirming that low concentrations among the institutionalized and chronically sick elderly are primarily due to poor intake (*Newton HM et al. The cause and correction of low blood vitamin C concentrations in the elderly. <u>Am. J. Clin. Nutr.</u> 42(4):656-59, 1985*).

Intake may occasionally be deficient in <u>the healthy elderly</u>.

> **Observational Study:** In a study of 403 elderly Danes residing in their own homes, ascorbic acid intake averaged 64 mg with a range of 9-400 mg. This is adequate compared to the recommended daily intakes in England, Canada, the United States and Japan, but low compared to the recommended daily intakes in Holland, West Germany and the USSR. Based on the Joint Nordic Recommendations (NNR) of 60 mg, 24% did not receive enough vitamin C (*Elsborg L et al. The intake of vitamins and minerals by the elderly at home. <u>Int. J. Vit. Nutr. Res.</u> 53:321-29, 1983*).

Other high-risk gps. are men who live alone, individuals who avoid "acid"-containing foods due to dyspepsia or reflux esophagitis, food fadists, pts. undergoing peritoneal dialysis and hemodialysis, and alcoholics (*Reuler JB et al. Adult scurvy. <u>JAMA</u> 253(6):805-7, 1985*).

<u>Vitamin D</u>:

Lack of sunshine (ultraviolet light is necessary for endogenous vitamin D production) can cause vitamin D deficiency.

> **Observational Study:** Vitamin D levels of 23 older people were measured every 3 months for 16 months. In July, their levels were normal. By November, levels had dropped 19%. By February, levels had dropped 65% to a range where 9 had levels consistent with the development of the disease. The May measurement was 62% below the initial measurement, which was equalled again in the next July measurement (*Lawson DE et al. Relative contributions of diet and sunlight to vitamin D state in the elderly.* <u>Brit. Med. J.</u> *2:303-5, August 4, 1979*).

It is recommended that the elderly receive a total supply of 600-800 IU (15-20 mcg) daily of vitamin D (*Parfitt AM et al Vitamin D and bone health in the elderly.* <u>Am. J. Clin. Nutr.</u> *36(5 Suppl.):1014-31, 1982*).

Dietary intake below the RDA (200 IU) is not uncommon.

> **Observational Study:** In a study of 403 elderly Danes residing in their own homes, vitamin D intake (2.4 mcg mean; range 1-26 mcg) was low in 62% as compared to the Recommended Dietary Allowances (RDA) and Joint Nordic Recommendations (NNR) (*Elsborg L et al. The intake of vitamins and minerals by the elderly at home.* <u>Int. J. Vit. Nutr. Res.</u> *53:321-29, 1983*).

> **Observational Study:** In a 5-yr. prospective study, over half of 300 healthy elderly Americans with good incomes had intakes below the RDA and 1/3 were below 100 IU per day. Most of their serum vitamin D levels (25-hydroxy vitamin D) were low compared to a younger control gp. (*Omdahl J et al. Nutritional status in a healthy elderly population: Vitamin D.* <u>Am. J. Clin. Nutr.</u> *36(6):1225-33, 1982*).

May be deficient in <u>the healthy elderly</u>.

> **Observational Study:** In a 5-yr. prospective study, calcidiol was measured in 166 American women and 138 men, all healthy and active and with a mean age of 72. Although 25% took 400 IU daily as a supplement, the majority were consuming less than 100 IU daily. The ave. serum vitamin D level was 15.5 ng/ml compared to 29.1 ng/ml in a younger control gp., and 15% had a serum vitamin D below 8 ng/ml. Vitamin D levels were lower in women than in men. There was an inverse relationship between total serum alkaline phosphatase and serum vitamin D, suggesting chronic bone loss as a result of vitamin D deficiency (*Omdahl J.* <u>Am. J. Clin. Nutr.</u> *36:1225-33, 1982*).

<u>Vitamin K</u>:

Sub-clinical deficiency during <u>pregnancy</u> and in <u>the newborn</u> is common.

> **Observational Study:** 46 normal mother-infant pairs were studied at term. 13 infants (28%) and 7 mothers (15%) were found to be vitamin K-deficient as judged by PIKVA (protein induced by vitamin K absence) status, and maternal PIKVA status correlated with infant status (p less than 0.03) (*Block CA et al. Mother-infant prothrombin precursor status at birth.* <u>J. Pediatr. Gastroenterol. Nutr.</u> *3(1):101-03, 1984*).

<u>Zinc</u>:

Commonly deficient in the Western Diet.

> **Observational Study:** In a study of 403 elderly Danes residing in their own homes, zinc intake (ave. 10 mg; range 4-26 mg) was low in 87% as compared to the Recommended Dietary Allowances

(RDA) and the Joint Nordic Recommendations (NNR) (*Elsborg L et al. The intake of vitamins and minerals by the elderly at home. Int. J. Vit. Nutr. Res. 53:321-29, 1983*).

Observational Study: Dietary zinc levels were determined spectrophotometrically for 22 American men and women eating self-selected diets. 68% were found to consume less than 2/3 the RDA for zinc, even though the ave. daily protein intake exceeded the RDA (*Holden JM et al. Zinc and copper in self-selected diets. J. Am. Dietet. Assoc. 75:23, 1979*).

See Also:

Klevay LM et al. Evidence of dietary copper and zinc deficiencies. JAMA 241(18):1916-18, 1979

Children and teenagers are especially susceptible to zinc deficiency due to their increased requirements for growth and development (*Sanstead HH. Am. J. Clin. Nutr. 26:1251-60, 1973*).

Zinc nutriture is often inadequate during pregnancy.

Observational Study: Pregnant women ingested only about 2/3 of the recommended dietary allowance of zinc (*Hambridge KM et al. Zinc nutritional status during pregnancy: A longitudinal study. Am. J. Clin. Nutr. 37:429-42, 1983*).

Observational Study: Plasma zinc declined about 30% during pregnancy, while WBC and hair zinc also declined (*Truswell AS. Nutrition for pregnancy. Brit. Med. J. July, 1985*).

The elderly are especially susceptible to zinc deficiency due to:
1. lower zinc consumption than younger individuals.
2. poor bioavailability of their dietary zinc.
3. the presence of certain disease states.
4. the use of various medications which affect zinc nutriture.
(*Greger JL. Prevalence and significance of zinc deficiency in the elderly. Geriatr. Med. Today 3(1):24-30, 1984; J. Am. Diet. Assoc. 82:148-53, 1983*).

Severe zinc deficiency can occur with total parenteral nutrition unless supplementation is given (*Goldwasser B et al. Isr. J. Med. Sci. 17:1155-57, 1981*).

Appendix B

DANGERS OF SUPPLEMENTATION

NOTE: Drug interactions should also be considered

<u>Alfalfa</u>:

May produce a <u>lupus-like syndrome</u> or aggravate SLE.

> **Animal Experimental Study (monkey):** Hematologic and serologic abnormalities similar to those observed in human systemic lupus erythematosus developed in monkeys fed alfalfa sprouts. L-canavanine sulfate, a constituent, was incorporated into the diet and reactivated the syndrome (*Malonow MR et al. Systemic lupus erythematosus-like syndrome in monkeys fed alfalfa sprouts: Role of a nonprotein amino acid. <u>Science</u> 216:415-17, 1982*).

See Also:

> **Case Report:** *Roberts JL, Hayashi JA. Exacerbation of SLE associated with alfalfa ingestion. Letter to the Editor. <u>New Engl. J. Med.</u> 308(22):1361, 1983*

<u>Beta-Carotene</u>:

Stored in fatty deposits in the body, especially the liver. Hypercarotenemia is associated with <u>orange discoloration of the skin</u> (esp. palms, soles and naso-labial folds), reversible <u>leukopenia</u>, <u>weakness</u>, <u>enlarged liver</u>, <u>low blood pressure</u> and <u>weight loss</u> (*Vakil DV et al. Hypercarotenaemia: A case report and review of the literature. <u>Nutr. Res.</u> 5:911-17, 1985*).

<u>Calcium</u>:

Usually no adverse effects at customary supplemental doses.

Excessive doses or a calcium:phosphorus ratio above 2:1 due to excess calcium results in <u>reduced bone strength</u> and interferes with vitamin K synthesis and/or absorption, causing internal bleeding (*Calcium: How much is too much? <u>Nutr. Rev.</u> 43(11):345, 1985*).

<u>Carnitine</u>:

Supplementation with DL carnitine 900-1200 mg daily has been associated with a <u>myasthenia-like syndrome</u> in pts. with renal impairment (*McCarty MF. A note on 'orthomolecular' aids for dieting - myasthenic syndrome due to DL-carnitine. <u>Med. Hypotheses</u> December, 1982, pp. 661-62; Bazzato G et al. Myasthenia-like syndrome after DL - but not L - carnitine. <u>Lancet</u> May 30, 1981, p. 1209*).

In clinical studies of L-carnitine, 41% of pts. developed <u>GI side-effects</u> and 11% developed a <u>body odor</u>. In no pt. was it discontinued due to these side-effects, and a decrease in dosage reduced or eliminated them (*<u>FDA Drug Bulletin</u>, June, 1986*).

Copper:

Elevated levels (often due to contaminated drinking water) can be toxic, causing profound mental and physical fatigue, poor memory, severe depression and insomnia (*Nolan KB. Nutr. Rev. 41:318-20, 1983*).

Fluoride:

Inhibits the enzyme phosphatase in experimental animals which is critically important for the assimilation of calcium and other minerals (*Yanick, Paul. Solving problematic tinnitus. A clinical scientific approach. Townsend Letter for Doctors. February - March, 1985, p. 31*).

Folic Acid:

Adverse effects may be seen at higher dosages.

> **Case Reports:** 2 pts. are described who showed exacerbation of psychotic behavior during treatment with folic acid for folate deficiency which was associated with elevated RBC folate levels (*Prakash R, Petrie WM. Psychiatric changes associated with an excess of folic acid. Am. J. Psychiat. 139(9):1192-93, 1982*).

> **Experimental Study:**   14 normal subjects received folic acid 15 mg daily. By 1 mo., 60% had developed GI side-effects (abdominal distension, flatulence, nausea, anorexia), sleep disturbances with vivid dreams, malaise and irritability (*Hunter R et al. Toxicity of folic acid given in pharmacological doses to healthy volunteers. Lancet 1:61-63, 1970*).

Supplementation in the presence of pernicious anemia due to vitamin B_{12} deficiency will cure the anemia but fail to prevent progression of the neuropathology (*Davidson LSP, Girdwood RH. Folic acid as a therapeutic agent. Br. Med. J. 1:587-91, 1947*).

High dose therapy may decrease vitamin B_{12} levels; thus B_{12} supplementation or regular monitoring is indicated (*Hunter R et al. Effect of folic-acid supplement on serum-vitamin-B_{12} levels in patients on anticonvulsants. Lancet 2:50, 1969*).

L-Glutamine:

Megadoses may cause mania.

> **Case Reports:**
> 1. Pt. with no prior psychiatric history was hospitalized with a 1 wk. history of increasing motor and verbal activity culminating in grandiose delusions, hypersexuality, and insomnia. Two wks. earlier, he had begun to ingest up to 4 gm L-glutamine daily.   Symptoms ceased within 1 wk. of stopping the supplement.
> 2. Pt. in psychotherapy with dysthymic disorder began to experience increasing sleep loss, unusually high energy and increased mental acuity and became unusually outgoing and talkative following 1 wk. of ingesting up to 2 gm daily of L-glutamine.
> (*Mebane AH. L-Glutamine and Mania. Letter to the Editor. Am. J. Psychiat. 141(10), October, 1984*).

Iron:

Only supplement if deficient - otherwise can cause subclinical iron excess which may be a contributory cause to hepatic cirrhosis (*Passmore R, Eastwood MA. Davidson and Passmore: Human Nutrition and Dietetics. Edinburgh, Churchill Livingstone, 1986, p. 119*).

GI side-effects (ex. nausea, vomiting, epigastric discomfort) are commonly reported after iron supplementation (*Passmore R, Eastwood MA. Davidson and Passmore: Human Nutrition and Dietetics. Edinburgh, Churchill Livingstone, 1986, p. 463*) which may turn the stools black.

L-Lysine:

May increase cholesterol and triglyceride levels.

> **Animal Experimental Study:** Chicks fed diets with 4% L-lysine developed elevated total cholesterol and triglycerides. No other amino acid had this effect. Addition of arginine failed to reverse these changes; thus they are not mediated by the antagonism between lysine and arginine (*Schmeisser DD et al. Effect of excess dietary lysine on plasma lipids of the chick. J. Nutrition 113(9):1777-83, 1983*).

Manganese:

Supplementation may occasionally elevate blood pressure in people over 40 or cause hypertensive headaches (*Pfeiffer CC, LaMola S. Zinc and manganese in the schizophrenias. J. Orthomol. Psychiat. 12:215-234, 1983*).

Chronic Mn intoxication may cause potentially irreversible movement and other neurologic disorders (*Weiner WJ et al. Regional brain manganese levels in an animal model of tardive dyskinesia, in Fann WE et al, Eds. Tardive Dyskinesia: Research and Treatment. New York, SP Medical and Scientific Books, 1980, pp. 159-163*).

Niacin:

1. Histamine flush: Common side-effect due to histamine release from mast cells. Starts in 20 minutes and can last 1-1 1/2 hours. Usually lessened after 3 days and may disappear at higher doses. Can be minimized by taking niacin with meals and raising the dosage gradually. ASA 300 mg. 15-30 minutes before ingestion may prevent or ameliorate it.
2. Hyperuricemia due to its competition with uric acid for renal excretion is common, although exacerbation of gout or uric acid stone formation is rare (*Buist RA. Editorial: Vitamin toxicities, side effects and contraindications. Int. Clin. Nutr. Rev. 4(4):159-71, 1984; Pfeiffer CC. Mental and Elemental Nutrients. New Canaan, Conn. Keats Publishing, 1975, p. 121*).
3. Hepatic toxicity (perform baseline liver function studies and every 6-8 months) (*Patterson DJ et al. Niacin hepatitis. Southern Med. J. 76(2):239-41, 1983*).

Other side-effects: Pruritis, hyperpigmentation, glucose intolerance.

> References:
>
> *The Medical Letter Vol. 27, No. 695, August 30, 1985*
>
> *Mosher LR. Nicotinic acid side effects and toxicity: A review. Am. J. Psychiat. 126:9, 1970*

Niacinamide (nicotinamide):

Common side effect: sedation

Large doses may cause hepatic toxicity (*Winter SL, Boyer JL. hepatic toxicity from large doses of vitamin B3 (nicotinamide). New Engl. J. Med. :1180, 1973*)

Para-amino Benzoic Acid:

Potential side-effects include skin rash, anorexia, nausea and fever (*Physicians' Desk Reference. Oradell, N.J., Med. Economics Co., Inc., 1986*) as well as vitiligo (*Hughes CG. Oral PABA and vitiligo. J. Am.*

Acad. Dermatol. 9:770, 1983) and <u>liver toxicity</u> (*Kantor GR, Ratz JL. Liver toxicity from potassium para-aminobenzoate. Letter to the Editor. J. Am. Acad. Dermatol. 13(4):671-72, 1985*).

<u>Phenylalanine</u>:

Supplementation may cause <u>anxiety</u>, <u>headache</u> and <u>hypertension</u> and should be avoided by phenylketourics and women who are pregnant or lactating.

<u>Pyridoxine</u>:

Supplementation may cause a <u>sensory neuropathy</u> in doses as low as 200 mg daily over 3 years (usually 2-5 gm daily). The neurotoxicity is believed to be due to exceeding the liver's ability to phosphorylate pyridoxine to the active coenzyme, pyridoxal phosphate. The resulting high pyridoxine blood level could be directly neurotoxic or may compete for binding sites with pyridoxal phosphate resulting in a relative deficiency of the active metabolite (*Parry GJ, Bredesen DE. Sensory neuropathy with low-dose pyridoxine. Neurology 35:1466-68, 1985*). Supplementation in the form of pyridoxal phosphate should thus avoid this danger.

<u>Thiamine</u>:

Toxic side-effects have mostly occurred after IM or parenteral injections and have included <u>generalized urticaria</u>, <u>facial edema</u>, <u>dyspnea</u>, <u>cyanosis</u>, <u>wheezing</u> and <u>anaphylactic shock</u>.

Oral supplementation has very rarely produced side-effects, although <u>nervousness</u>, <u>itching</u>, <u>flushing</u>, <u>shortness of breath</u>, <u>tachycardia</u>, a <u>sensation of</u> <u>heat</u> and <u>perfuse perspiration</u> have been reported. (*Buist RA. Editorial: Vitamin toxicities, side effects and contraindications. Int. Clin. Nutr. Rev. 4(4):159-71, 1984*)

<u>L-Tryptophan</u>:

It has been suggested (*Soukes TL. Toxicology of serotonin precursors. Adv. Biol. Psychiat. 10:160-75, 1983*) that the following gps. not receive large, chronic doses of tryptophan:

1. Pts. with <u>cancer</u> or a history of it
2. Subjects with any source of <u>irritation of the urinary bladder</u>
3. <u>Children</u> and <u>pregnant women</u>
4. <u>Diabetics</u> and pts. with a family history of diabetes
5. Subjects with a history of any <u>scleroderma-like condition</u>
6. Pts. with large flora high in the intestinal tract (e.g. those with <u>achlorhydria</u>)

May aggravate <u>bronchial asthma</u>.

Experimental Double-blind Study: Pts. with <u>bronchial asthma</u> on a low-tryptophan diet improved (*Urge G et al. Effect of dietary tryptophan restrictions on clinical symptoms in patients with endogenous asthma. Allergy 38:211-2, 1983*).

<u>Lupus</u> pts. are said to have decreased serotonin levels, perhaps due to deficient conversion of tryptophan to serotonin. The tryptophan breakdown products may lead to auto-antibody production (*McCormick JP et al. Characterization of a cell-lethal product from the photooxidation of tryptophan: Hydrogen peroxide. Science 191:468-9, 1976*).

Review Article: An abnormal tryptophan metabolism is present with high excretion particularly of kynurenines and xanthurenic acid (*Cardin de'Stefani E, Costa C. [Changes in the metabolism of tryptophan in erythematosus.] Boll. Soc. Ital. Biol. Sper. 60(8):1535-40, 1984*).

Animal Experimental Study: A tryptophan deficient diet increased survival of animals with lupus (*Dubois EL, Ed. Lupus Erythematosus 2nd. Edition. Philadelphia, Lea & Febiger, p. 121*).

Supplementation may be harmful during pregnancy.

Animal Experimental Study: Pregnant hampsters were fed a moderate or high protein diet with varying amts. of tryptophan while, in the control diet, the amt. of tryptophan was equal to 1% of the total protein. When tryptophan was increased 1.8 to 8-fold, there was a decrease in litter size and an increase in mortality of the offspring. As these amts. are well within the range (on a equivalent weight basis) of supplemental doses of tryptophan being used in human studies, results suggest that tryptophan should be used with caution during pregnancy (*Meier AH, Wilson JM. Tryptophan feeding adversely influences pregnancy. Life Sci. 32:1193, 1983*).

Vitamin A:

Hypervitaminosis A is by far the most common cause of vitamin toxicity. The dosage required to produce toxicity is highly variable. While it is possible to receive as much as 1 million IU daily for 5 yrs. without developing toxicity (*Hruban Z et al. Am. J. Pathol. 76:451-61, 1974*), doses as low as 50,000 IU for 2.5 yrs. have been shown to produce toxic effects (*Farris W, Erdman J. JAMA 247:1317-18, 1982*).

Manifestations of chronic toxicity include fatigue, malaise and lethargy, headaches, abdominal discomfort, constipation, insomnia and restlessness. Later, night sweats, alopecia, brittle nails, irregular menses, emotional lability, mouth fissures, dry, scaly, rough, yellowish skin, superficial retinal hemorrhages, exophthalmos, peripheral edema and increased intracranial pressure with headaches, nausea and vomiting may develop (*Buist RA. Editorial: Vitamin toxicities, side effects and contraindications. Int. Clin. Nutr. Rev. 4(4):159-71, 1984*).

May cause abnormal bone growth in young children due to premature epiphyseal closing and thickening of the cortical regions (*Buist RA. Editorial: Vitamin toxicities, side effects and contraindications. Int. Clin. Nutr. Rev. 4(4):159-71, 1984*).

May cause fetal malformations:

Case Report: 28 year-old woman ingested 150,000 IU vitamin A daily for 2 mo. annually for 4 years as well as for 2 wks. prior to conception and 3 wks. afterwards. The pregnancy was terminated at 23 wks. due to fetal malformations which were found to be typical of vitamin A teratogenicity (*Von Lennep E et al. Prenatal Diag. 5:35-40, 1985*).

Hypervitaminosis A is often associated with hypercalcemia and hypercalciuria and calcium deposition in soft tissues may occur (*Buist RA. Editorial: Vitamin toxicities, side effects and contraindications. Int. Clin. Nutr. Rev. 4(4):159-71, 1984*).

Hyperplasia of both liver and spleen may occur with megadosages with elevation of SGOT. Liver biopsies reveal hepatic fibrosis, fat deposition, obstruction of portal blood flow with portal hypertension and sclerosis of vessels (*Buist RA. Editorial: Vitamin toxicities, side effects and contraindications. Int. Clin. Nutr. Rev. 4(4):159-71, 1984*).

Elevated retinol levels may play an important role in the development of some attacks of gouty arthritis (*Marson AR. Letter to the Editor. Lancet 1:1181, 1984*).

Vitamin C:

Diarrhea is the major side-effect of large doses.

Megadoses (over 6 gm daily) may increase <u>urinary oxalate excretion</u> which may be contra-indicated in renal insufficiency and in calcium oxalate stone-formers.

> **Review Article:** Urinary oxalate excretion generally does not increase significantly for both normal subjects and stone-formers with ascorbic acid supplementation unless doses exceed 6 gm daily; however, oxalate excretion even at those high doses is still usually in the range achievable by dietary influences alone. The exceptions derive from anecdotal reports of a small number of cases and from one poorly-controlled trial with unstated methodology and questionable assay techniques (*Piesse JW. Nutritional factors in calcium containing kidney stones with particular emphasis on vitamin C.* <u>*Int. Clin. Nutr. Rev.*</u> *5(3):110-129, 1985*).

> See Also:

> > *McAllister CJ et al. Renal failuure secondary to massive infusion of vitamin C. Letter'to the Editor.* <u>*JAMA*</u> *252(13):1684, 1984*

Contraindicated in cases of <u>iron overload</u> due to its enhancement of iron absorption (*Nienhuis A.* <u>*N. Engl. J. Med.*</u> *304(3):170-71, 1981*).

> Sudden discontinuation of large doses can cause <u>rebound scurvy</u> (*New roles for vitamin C.* <u>*New Scientist*</u> *11:23, 1985; Jakovlieu N.* <u>*Lanachrunestorschune*</u> *3:446, 1958*); thus supplementation should be gradually tapered over several days or weeks.

Vitamin D:

May cause <u>hypercalcemia</u> due to increased intestinal absorption of calcium which can quickly lead to reduction of kidney function (due to nephocalcinosis from deposition of calcium phosphate) and soft tissue calcifications, especially in the joints, blood vessels, stomach, lungs and heart (*Buist RA. Editorial: Vitamin toxicities, side effects and contraindications.* <u>*Int. Clin. Nutr. Rev.*</u> *4(4):159-71, 1984*).

Vitamin E:

Reports of adverse symptoms from large supplemental doses are largely subjective and based on limited observations (*Bieri JG. Medical uses of vitamin E.* <u>*N. Engl. J. Med.*</u> *308(18):1063-71, 1983*).

The most common complaint following large supplemental doses is transient <u>GI disturbances</u> (nausea, flatulence, or diarrhea) (*Bieri JG. Medical uses of vitamin E.* <u>*N. Engl. J. Med.*</u> *308(18):1063-71, 1983*).

Supplementation may exacerbate <u>hypertension</u>. When the oily form is used, this effect is accompanied by an increase in the serum triglycerides:vitamin E ratio; thus the water miscible form is preferred for pts. with <u>cardiovascular disorders</u> and <u>diabetes mellitus</u> (*Buist RA. Editorial: Vitamin toxicities, side effects and contraindications.* <u>*Int. Clin. Nutr. Rev.*</u> *4(4):159-71, 1984*).

As Vitamin E may reduce the insulin requirement, <u>diabetics on insulin</u> should be started on 100 I.U. or less daily and the dosage raised showly with adjustment of the insulin dose (*Vogelsang A. Vitamin E in the treatment of diabetes mellitus.* <u>*Ann. N.Y. Acad. Sci.*</u> *52:406, 1949*).

Zinc:

Excessive zinc intake <u>impairs immune responses</u>, probably due to its adverse effect on copper status (*Copper deficiency induced by megadoses of zinc.* <u>*Nutr. Rev.*</u> *43(5):148-49, 1985*). Similarly, the lowering of copper levels in response to high doses of zinc (above 150 mg daily) may be responsible for causing a marked <u>decrease in HDL cholesterol</u> (*Hooper PL et al. Zinc lowers high-density lipoprotein-cholesterol levels.* <u>*JAMA*</u> *244:1960, 1980; Klevey LM. Interactions of copper and zinc in cardiovascular disease.* <u>*Ann.*</u>

N.Y. Acad. Sci. 355:140-51, 1980; Fischer P et al.   The effect of dietary copper and zinc on cholesterol metabolism. Am. J. Clin. Nutr. 33:1019-25, 1980).

Experimental Study: 11 healthy adult men ingested 150 mg of elemental zinc twice daily. After 6 wks., there was a reduction in lymphocyte stimulation response to phytohemagglutinin as well as chemotaxis and phagocytosis of bacteria by polymorphonuclear leukocytes (*Chandra RK. Excessive intake of zinc impairs immune responses. JAMA 252(11):1443-46, 1984*).

Possible side-effects are occasional <u>nausea</u>, <u>increased sweating</u>, <u>alcohol intolerance</u> and transient worsening of <u>depression</u> or <u>hallucinations</u>. Zinc supplementation may increase <u>grand mal seizures</u> in epileptics, possibly due to it causing a reduction in blood Mn levels, and thus Mn supplementation should be started first (*Pfeiffer CC, LaMola S. Zinc and manganese in the schizophrenias. J. Orthomol. Psychiat. 12:215-234, 1983*).

Appendix C

GUIDELINES FOR NUTRITIONAL SUPPLEMENTATION

NOTE: "Reasonable Dietary Level" refers to the U.S. Recommended Dietary Allowances (1980) adult dietary levels (ages 23-50) suggested for "practically all healthy persons" (except for pregnant or lactating females); "Pharmacologic Dosage Range" refers to the range of intake suggested by the literature for the treatment of specific illnesses

NUTRIENT	REASONABLE DIETARY LEVEL male	female	PHARMACOLOGIC DOSAGE RANGE
Biotin	0-200 mcg		300 - 3000 mcg
Calcium	800 mg		1000 - 1500 mg
Chloride	1700-5100 mg		500 - 2500 mg
Choline	?		500 - 1000 mg
Chromium	50-200 mcg		200 - 300 mcg
Copper	2-3 mg		2 - 4 mg
Fluoride	1.5-4 mg		20-100 mg
Folic Acid	400 mcg		400 - 2000 mcg
Inositol	?		100 - 1000mg
Iodine	150 mcg		100 - 1000 mcg
Iron	10 mg	18 mg	10 - 50 mg
Magnesium	350 mg	300 mg	300 - 800 mg
Manganese	2.5-5 mg		2 - 50 mg
Molybdenum	15-500 mcg		100 - 1000 mcg
Niacin	18 mg	13 mg	100 - 6000 mg
Pantothenic Acid	4-7 mg		50 - 1000 mg
Phosphorus	800 mg		?
Potassium	1875-5625 mg		?
Pyridoxine	2.2 mg	2 mg	10 - 200 mg
Riboflavin	1.6 mg	1.2 mg	10 - 50 mg
Selenium	50-200 mcg		200 - 300 mcg
Sodium	1100-3300 mg		300 - 3000 mg
Sulfur	?		500 - 1000 mg
Thiamine	1.4 mg	1.0 mg	10 - 200 mg
Vitamin A	5000 IU	4000 IU	10,000 - 35,000 IU
Vitamin B_{12}	3 mcg		10 - 1000 mcg
Vitamin C	60 mg		50 - 10,000 mg
Vitamin D	200 IU		400 - 1000 IU
Vitamin E	15 IU	12 IU	100 - 1000 IU
Vitamin K	70-140 mcg		30 - 100 mcg
Zinc	15 mg		20 - 100 mg

Appendix D

LABORATORY METHODS FOR NUTRITIONAL EVALUATION

GENERAL: (Protein Energy Malnutrition)

Laboratory indicators:
1. decreased serum albumin concentration in the absence of liver disease (less than 3.4 g/dL).
2. decreased serum transferrin (seen in starvation earlier than decreased serum albumin).
3. decreased total lymphocyte count (below 1500/ cu mm).
4. decreased 24-hour urine creatinine (roughly proportional to skeletal muscle mass).
(*Wright RA. Commentary: Nutritional assessment. JAMA 244(6):1980*).

Aluminum:

Hair analysis, when properly performed, is a reliable measure of tissue levels (*Yokel RA. Clin. Chem. 28(4):662-665, 1982; Jenkins DW. Toxic Metals in Mammalian Hair and Nails. EPA Report 600/4-79-049 August, 1979 - available through the U.S. National Technical Information Service*). As yet, it cannot be concluded whether aluminum concentrations in hair give a better representation of the body burden than serum aluminum levels do (*De Groot HJ et al. Determination by flameless atomic absorption of aluminum in serum and hair by toxicological monitoring of patients on chronic intermittent haemodialysis. Pharm. Weekbl. [Sci.] 6(1):11-15, 1984*).

Arsenic:

Hair analysis, when properly performed, is a reliable measure of tissue levels (*Jenkins DW. Toxic Metals in Mammalian Hair and Nails. EPA Report 600/4-79-049 August, 1979 - available through the U.S. National Technical Information Service*).

While both hair and urine arsenic levels increase as intake increases, blood arsenic levels do not increase until chronic toxicity is reached (*Valentine JL et al. Environ. Res. 20:24-32, 1979*).

Biotin:

There are no sensitive chemical methods for biotin assay, but the flagellate Ochromonas danica, which has a specific and ultrasensitive biotin requirement, has provided a suitable microbiological assay for measuring biotin in blood, serum, urine, brain and liver (*Baker H. Assessment of biotin status: Clinical implications. Ann. N.Y. Acad. Sci. 447:129-32, 1985*).

The 2 principal criteria of biotin status are blood and urine levels. Blood levels can show extremely wide variation between individuals, so the significance of low plasma levels is uncertain, especially since biotin deficiency seems rare. In children, however, blood and urine levels are more helpful. For example, levels are lower than normal in infants with seborrheic dermatitis and Leiner's Disease who respond to biotin injections (*Whitehead CC. The assessment of biotin status in man and animals. Proc. Nutr. Sci. 40:165-72, 1981*).

Cadmium:

Hair analysis, when properly performed, is a reliable measure of tissue levels (*Jenkins DW. Toxic Metals in Mammalian Hair and Nails. EPA Report 600/4-79-049 August, 1979 - available through the U.S. National Technical Information Service*).

Blood levels are a poor measure of cadmium toxicity as the metal remains in the blood for only a very brief period of time and thus the levels are always extremely low (*Petering HG et al. Trace element content of hair: Cadmium and lead of human hair. Arch. Environ. Health 27:327-30, 1973*).

Calcium:

It is extremely difficult to reliably determine calcium balance in an outpatient setting (*Albanese A. Bone Loss: Causes, Detection and Therapy. New York, Alan R. Liss, Inc., 1977*). Dietary intake is a poor indicator due to such confounding factors as the quantity of fiber and other natural chelators in the diet, the amount of gastric acidity, the ratio of dietary calcium to phosphorus and to magnesium, gut transit time, etcetera, while total serum calcium is subjected to such close homeostatic regulation that it fails to reflect body calcium status.

Ionized calcium, a measure of unbound serum calcium, is perhaps the most useful measure at present when it is low, but values can be normal in the presence of a negative calcium balance.

Hair analysis is of some value, but its results are limited by the fact that a negative calcium balance may by accompanied by elevated hair levels, and by the lack of norms for grey hair which is naturally lower in calcium (*Cranton EM. Update on hair element analysis in clinical medicine. J. Holistic Med. 7(2):120-134, 1985*).

Chromium:

The most dependable criterion for the diagnosis of chromium deficiency may be the correction of impaired glucose tolerance in response to chromium supplementation, but it requires strict control of dietary intake over an extended period.

Although evaluation is hindered by the extremely low levels involved, urinary chromium is a reasonable measure of chromium absorption as the majority of absorbed chromium is excreted in the urine (*Anderson RA, Kozlovsky AS. Chromium intake, absorption and excretion of subjects consuming self-selected diets. Am. J. Clin. Nutr. 41:1177-83, 1985*).

Hair analysis cannot distinguish between contamination by the hexavalent, toxic chromium and the trivalent, nutritional chromium (*Passwater, RA, Cranton EM. Trace Elements, Hair Analysis and Nutrition. New Canaan, Conn., Keats Publishing, Inc., 1983, p. 195*). Moreover, because of the low levels involved, hair chromium content has been considered to be too insensitive to identify any but the most severe deficiencies (*Richman S. Chromium, an overview. Anabolism 1-2:5,12, 1984; Hambridge KM. Chromium nutrition in man. Am. J. Clin. Nutr. 27:505-14, 1974*). A recent study, however, suggests that hair chromium levels may be a useful index of chromium status:

Experimental and Observational Study: Initial hair chromium levels were significantly lower in diabetics than in controls and, after chromium supplementation, mean hair chromium increased by 127 +/- 78 ppb in both diabetic and non-diabetic gps. but only by 17 +/- 90 ppb in the placebo group (*Hunt AE et al. Effect of chromium supplementation on hair chromium concentration and diabetic status. Nutr. Res. 5:131-40, 1985*).

Blood chromium has not been shown to reflect tissue stores (*Mertz W. Physiol. Rev. 49:163-239, 1969*).

Copper:

While no available test is considered to be adequate for subclinical copper deficiency, serum copper may be the best indicator (*Solomons N. Biochemical, metabolic, and clinical role of copper in human nutrition. J. Am. Coll. Nutr. 4:83-105, 1985*).

Hair copper correlates well with copper in levels in other organs, although errors from external contamination of hair (copper-containing fungicides in swimming pools, contaminated water supplies, hair treatments) may occur, and levels are unreliable in the presence of severe liver disease (*Cranton EM. Update on hair element analysis in clinical medicine. J. Holistic Med. 7(2):120-134, 1985*). In addition, hair copper may be normal despite gross copper deficiency (*Bradfield RB et al. Preliminary communication: hair copper in copper deficiency. Lancet 2:343-44, 1980*).

Confirmation of an elevated body copper burden can be provided by a 24 hour urine following a D-penicillamine challenge test. D-penicillamine 250 mg is given orally every 6 hrs. away from meals and the urine test is performed on the third day of treatment (*Walshe JM. The discovery of the therapeutic use of D-penicillamine. J. Rheumatol. (Suppl.) 7:3-8, 1981*).

Folic Acid:

A low serum folate is the earliest sign of folate deficiency; later the urine formiminoglutamic acid (FIGLU) level rises. High FIGLU excretion also occurs, however, in vitamin B_{12} deficiency and in liver disease; thus it is not specific for folate deficiency (*Herbert V. Experimental nutritional folate deficiency in man. Trans. Assoc. Am. Phys. 75:307-20, 1962*). RBC folate concentrations reflect body folate stores, while serum folate tends to reflect recent dietary intake (*Nutrition & the M.D. 12(7), July, 1986*).

Serum folate is highly correlated with CSF folate and better correlated with CSF folate than is RBC folate. However, it is not known in man whether a low CSF folate is necessarily accompanied by a fall in brain folate level, but experimental studies have suggested that the latter falls last, when stores elsewhere are severely depleted (*Reynolds EH. Interrelationships between the neurology of folate and vitamin B_{12} deficiency, in Botez MI, Reynolds EH, Eds. Folic Acid in Neurology, Psychiatry, and Internal Medicine. New York, Raven Press, 1979*).

The determination of hypersegmentation of neutrophils is a useful masure of folate deficiency, although it is unreliable during pregnancy (*Sauberlich HE. Newer laboratory methods for assessing nutriture of selected B-complex vitamins. Ann. Rev. Nutr. 4:377-407, 1984*).

Microbiological assays remain the standard procedure for measuring total folic acid activity, in serum, blood, tissues, and foods. Although a number of commercial radioassay kits are available for measuring folic acid levels in serum and erythrocytes, some uncertanties exist about the validity of the folate values obtained (*Sauberlich HE. Newer laboratory methods for assessing nutriture of selected B-complex vitamins. Ann. Rev. Nutr. 4:377-407, 1984*).

Note: A recent study found that, when chronically ill elderly pts. were compared to healthy young controls, radioimmunoassays showed normal serum and RBC folate concentrations in all elderly pts. and all but 1 of the controls, while microbiological assays showed below normal values of serum folate in 6.8% of the elderly pts. and 12.2% of the controls, and below normal values of RBC folate in 1.8% of pts. and 4.8% of controls, suggesting that radioimmunoassay procedures are superior (Grinblat J et al. Folate and vitamin B_{12} levels in an urban elderly population with chronic diseases. J. Am. Geriatr. Soc. 34:627-32, 1986).

Iron:

Bone marrow aspiration is the procedure of choice, while serum ferritin, an iron storage protein, is a reasonably good indicator of total body iron storage. Serum iron is a poor measure of iron nutriture as iron may be deficient despite the lack of anemia and normal serum iron levels. Like transferrin saturation, it may only become abnormal after iron stores have been completely exhausted (*Finch CA. Editorial: Evaluation of iron status. JAMA 251(15):2004, 1984; Frank P, Wang S. Serum iron and total iron binding capacity compared with serum ferritin in assessment of iron deficiency. Clin. Chem. 27(2):276-79, 1981; Cook JD et al. Serum ferritin as a measure of iron stores in normal subjects. Am. J. Clin. Nutr. 27:681-7, 1974*).

In children, transferrin saturation, hemoglobin and a peripheral blood smear must be done in conjunction with serum ferritin, as ferritin may be normal despite iron deficiency (*Madanat F et al. Serum ferritin in evaluation of iron status in children. Acta Haematol. 71:111, 1984*).

An iron tolerance test may also be useful in determining iron deficiency.

> **Observational Study:** Men with normal iron stores showed little change in plasma iron after ingesting 5, 10 or 20 mg of ferrous sulfate or ferrous fumarate, while plasma iron levels rose significantly when men with a mild iron deficiency took similiar doses of iron (*Crosby WH, O'Neill-Cutting MA. A small dose iron tolerance test as an indicator of mild iron deficiency. JAMA 251(15):1986-87, 1984*).

Hair iron has no known relationship to body levels.

Lead:

Hair analysis, when properly performed, is a reliable measure of tissue levels and the method of choice for diagnosing lead poisoning, although confirmatory studies are necessary (*Passwater, RA, Cranton EM. Trace Elements, Hair Analysis and Nutrition. New Canaan, Conn., Keats Publishing, Inc., 1983; Jenkins DW. Toxic Metals in Mammalian Hair and Nails. EPA Report 600/4-79-049 August, 1979 - available through the U.S. National Technical Information Service*).

Zinc protoporphyrin content is a second choice for diagnosing lead poisoning, while blood lead levels are inadequate as blood rapidly deposits lead into the skeletal tissues and hair (*Passwater, RA, Cranton EM. Trace Elements, Hair Analysis and Nutrition. New Canaan, Conn., Keats Publishing, Inc., 1983, p. 195*).

Magnesium:

A magnesium challenge test is the best method of ascertaining body stores (*Fourth Internat. Sympos. on Magnesium. J. Am. Coll. Nutr. 4:303, 1985*) as serum and RBC magnesium levels remain normal unless magnesium depletion is severe (*Rea WJ et al. Magnesium deficiency in patients with chemical sensitivity. Clin. Ecology 4(1):17-20, 1986*). While on a stable intake of magnesium, a baseline urine is obtained and magnesium chloride or magnesium sulfate 0.2 meq/kg IV is given over a 4 hour period. A second urine is began at challenge and continued over a 24 hour period. Deficiency is defined as less than 80% excretion of the amt. of challenged magnesium (*Jones JE et al. Magnesium requirements in adults. Med. J. Clin. Nutr. 20:632-35, 1967*).

Leucocyte and lymphocyte magnesium levels are better correlated with tissue magnesium levels than are serum levels (*Peter WF et al. Leucocyte magnesium concentration as an indicator of myocardial magnesium. Nutr. Reports Int. 26:105, July 1982; Juan D. Clinical review: The clinical importance of hypomagnesemia. Surgery 5:510-16, 1982*).

RBC magnesium is less reliable as it may vary by a factor of five depending on the age of the red blood cell.

Review Article: While serum levels are rarely decreased, intracellular Mg levels are frequently low in pts. with inflammatory bowel disease and may be associated with weakness, anorexia, hypotension, confusion, hyperirritability, tetany, convulsions, and EKG or EEG abnormalities (*Rosenberg IH et al. Nutritional aspects of inflammatory bowel disease.* <u>*Ann. Rev. Nutr.*</u> *5:463-84, 1985*).

<u>Hair magnesium</u> levels are not always reliable as they tend to be elevated when magnesium is is being lost from bones and are lower in grey hair (*Cranton EM.* *Update on hair element analysis in clinical medicine.* <u>*J. Holistic Med.*</u> *7(2):120-134, 1985*).

Manganese:

<u>Whole blood manganese</u> is considered to be a valid indicator of body manganese and soft tissue levels (*Keen CL et al.* *Whole blood manganese as an indicator of body manganese.* <u>*N. Engl J. Med.*</u> *308:1230, 1983*).

Recent studies suggest that <u>hair manganese</u> may be a reliable indicator of body manganese status (*Cranton EM.* *Update on hair element analysis in clinical medicine.* <u>*J. Holistic Med.*</u> *7(2):120-134, 1985*), although greying hair has a lower concentration than black hair (*Guillard O et al.* *Manganese concentration in the hair of greying ("salt and pepper") men reconsidered.* <u>*Clin. Chem.*</u> *31(7):1251, 1985*).

Mercury:

<u>Hair analysis</u>, when properly performed, is a reliable measure of tissue levels (*Jenkins DW.* <u>*Toxic Metals in Mammalian Hair and Nails.*</u> *EPA Report 600/4-79-049 August, 1979 - available through the U.S. National Technical Information Service*).

<u>Blood mercury</u> is useful for assessing recent methyl mercury exposure (*Berglund F et al.* *[Methyl mercury in fish, a toxologic-epidemiologic evaluation of risks: Report from an expert group.]* <u>*Nord. Hyg. T.*</u> *Suppl. 4, 1971 - published in* <u>*Nord. Hyg. T.*</u> *Suppl. 3, 1970*), but not for assessing exposure to inorganic mercurials (*Friberg L, Nordberg GF.* *Inorganic mercury: Relation between exposure and effects, in Friberg, L, Vostal J, Eds.* <u>*Mercury in the Environment.*</u> *Cleveland, Ohio, Chemical Rubber Co. Press, 1972, pp. 113-139*).

<u>Urinary mercury</u> measurements are unreliable as an indication of mercury poisoning (*Ladd AD et al.* *Absorption and exretion of mercury in man. II. Urinary mercury in relation to duration of exposure.* <u>*Arch. Environ. Health*</u> *6:480-83, 1963*).

Niacin:

Attempts to diagnose deficiency by measuring nicotinic acid in body fluids have proved disappointing. The <u>urinary excretion of 1-N-methylnicotinamide</u>, a nicotinic acid metabolite, is often used as a measure of body reserves (*Passmore R, Eastwood MA.* <u>*Davidson and Passmore: Human Nutrition and Dietetics.*</u> *Eighth Edition.* *London, Churchill Livingstone, 1986, p. 155*), and the excretion ratio of 2-pyridone (another metabolite) to 1-N-methylnicotinamide is the most reliable indicator of niacin nutritional status, especially when high-performance liquid chromatographic techniques are used (*Sauberlich HE et al.* <u>*Laboratory Tests for the Assessment of Nutritional Status.*</u> *Boca Raton, Florida, CRC Press, 1974, pp. 70-74*).

Nickel:

<u>Hair analysis</u>, when properly performed, is a reliable measure of tissue levels when nickel levels are elevated; low hair nickel has no known clinical significance. Due to the possibility of external contamination, blood or urine studies should be performed for confirmation (*Passwater, RA, Cranton EM.* <u>*Trace Elements, Hair Analysis and Nutrition.*</u> *New Canaan, Conn., Keats Publishing, Inc., 1983; Jenkins DW.* <u>*Toxic Metals in Mammalian Hair and Nails.*</u> *EPA Report 600/4-79-049 August, 1979 - available through the U.S. National Technical Information Service*).

Phosphorus:

Plasma phosphate is mainly controlled by renal excretion.

Hair phosphorus has little or no relationship to phosphorous metabolism in the body or to dietary phosphorus intake (*Passwater RA, Cranton EM. Trace Elements, Hair Analysis and Nutrition. New Canaan, Connecticut, Keats Publishing, 1983, p. 61*).

Potassium:

Red blood cell potassium (or whole blood potassium) is superior to serum potassium level as an index of cellular potassium stores (*Bahemuka M, Hodkinson HM. Red-blood-cell potassium as a practical index of potassium status in elderly patients. Age Aging 5:24, 1976*).

> **Experimental and Observational Study:** Serum and red blood cell potassium was measured in 17 pts. with EKG abnormalities. Although some of the abnormalities were typical of potassium deficiency, most were non-specific T wave changes which are commonly attributed (without substantiation) to ischemia. Serum potassium levels were normal but RBC potassium levels were below normal in all cases and returned to normal (as did the EKG abnormalities) after treatment with potassium salts (*Sangiori GB et al. Serum potassium levels, red-blood-cell potassium and alterations of the repolarization phase of electrocardiography in old subjects. Age Aging 13:309, 1984*).

Hair potassium levels do not reflect dietary intake or body stores (*Passwater RA, Cranton EM. Trace Elements, Hair Analysis and Nutrition. New Canaan, Connecticut, Keats Publishing, 1983, p. 85*).

Pyridoxine:

Blood pyridoxine levels may be preferable because of the deficiencies of alternative testing methods: Some B_6-deficient pts., such as those with liver disease, have high pyridoxal-dependent RBC transaminase levels despite low blood pyridoxine. The activity of the RBC aminotransferases increase in thiamin, riboflavin and pantothenate deficiencies and in various disease states. Xanthurenic acid and kyurenine excretion after a tryptophan load most likely represents an aberrant reaction to the load and has no documented clinical significance. In addition, pregnancy and contraceptive pills may render the test abnormal due to inhibition of kynureninase by estrogens (*Sauberlich HE. Newer laboratory methods for assessing nutriture of selected B-complex vitamins. Ann. Rev. Nutr. 4:377-407, 1984; Baker H. Analysis of vitamin status. J. Med. Soc. New Jersey. 80:633-36, 1983*).

Riboflavin:

The procedure most commonly used to evaluate riboflavin nutriture is the measurement of RBC glutathione reductase (EGR) activity and the stimulation of this activity by flavin adenine dinucleotide (FAD) added *in vitro*. The EGR activity is commonly expressed in terms of "activity coefficient" or in terms of percent stimulation, both of which are derived from the stimulating effect of FAD added *in vitro* to the enzyme reaction. Some animal studies suggest that certain deficiencies, such as thiamine, nicotinic acid and pyridoxine, may reduce the apo-enzyme level (*Sharada D, Bamji MS. Erythrocyte glutathione reductase activity and riboflavin concentration in experimental deficiency of some water soluble vitamins. Int. J. Vit. Nutr. Res. 42:43-49, 1972*). Both the age of the subject and the age of the red cell may also influence EGR activity, and the assay may not be valid in subjects with low RBC glucose-6-phosphate dehydrogenase activity (*Sauberlich HE. Newer laboratory methods for assessing nutriture of selected B-complex vitamins. Ann. Rev. Nutr. 4:377-407, 1984*).

Blood riboflavin levels are not necessarily good measures of riboflavin status (*Bamjii MS et al. Relationship between biochemical and clinical indices of B-vitamin deficiency. A study in rural school boys. Br. J. Nutr. 41:431-41, 1979*), although new analytical procedures for measure blood and urinary riboflavin may prove to be useful (*Sauberlich HE. Newer laboratory methods for assessing nutriture of selected B-complex vitamins. Ann. Rev. Nutr. 4:377-407, 1984*).

<u>Selenium</u>:

The only true evidence of selenium deficiency lies in <u>a positive response to selenium therapy</u> (*Neve J et al. Selenium deficiency. Clin. Endocrinol. Metab. 14(3):629-56, 1985*).

<u>Hair selenium</u> correlates well with selenium intake and is clearly superior to whole blood selenium (*Gallagher ML et al. Selenium levels in new growth hair and in whole blood during injection of a selenium supplement for six weeks. Nutr. Res. 4:577-82, 1984; Valentine, JL et al. Selenium levels in human blood, urine and hair in response to exposure via drinking water. Environ. Res. 17:347-55, 1978*).

<u>Blood selenium levels</u> do not correlate (except at the extremes) with selenium intake (*Lane HW et al. Blood selenium and glutathione peroxidase levels and dietary selenium of free living and institutionalized elderly subjects. Proc. Soc. Exp. Biol. Med. 173(1):87-95, 1985*).

<u>Urinary selenium</u> is an inadequate indicator of tissue nutriture (*Neve J et al. Selenium deficiency. Clin. Endocrinol. Metab. 14(3):629-56, 1985*).

<u>Sodium</u>:

<u>Serum sodium levels</u> are commonly used as a measure of sodium nutriture. The principal cation of the extracellular fluid, any change in serum sodium is associated with a fluid shift into or out of the cell. Serum levels, however, do not reflect total body sodium content (*Webb WL, Gehi M. Psychosomatics 22(3):199-203, 1981*).

<u>Hair sodium levels</u> do not reflect dietary intake or body stores (*Passwater RA, Cranton EM. Trace Elements, Hair Analysis and Nutrition. New Canaan, Connecticut, Keats Publishing, 1983, p. 85*).

<u>Thiamine</u>:

The most commonly used procedure for assessing thiamine nutriture has been the measurement of <u>RBC transketolase activity</u> and its stimulation *in vitro* by the addition of thiamine pyrophosphate (<u>TPP effect</u>) Some disease conditions may influence RBC transketolase activity independent of thiamine status. For example, pts. in negative nitrogen balance will have diminished RBC transketolase activity due to insufficient apoenzyme to activate transketolase. In addition, low transketolase in diabetes mellitus and polyneuritis does not reflect a thiamine deficit, while pts. with pernicious anemia may have elevated transketolase levels unrelated to thiamine status (*Sauberlich HE. Newer laboratory methods for assessing nutriture of selected B-complex vitamins. Ann. Rev. Nutr. 4:377-407, 1984*).

Several studies have demonstrated a relationship between RBC transketolase activity and <u>urinary thiamine excretion</u> (*Sauberlich HE. Newer laboratory methods for assessing nutriture of selected B-complex vitamins. Ann. Rev. Nutr. 4:377-407, 1984*).

On a thiamine-deficient diet, a decrease in the <u>blood thiamine level</u> is the earliest sign of a thiamine deficiency (*Baker H. Analysis of vitamin status. J. Med. Soc. New Jersey 80:633-36, 1983*). However, blood thiamine determinations have not been satisfactory primarily because of limitations in methodology, as the decreases in blood thiamine during deficiency are not great (*Sauberlich HE. Newer laboratory methods for assessing nutriture of selected B-complex vitamins. Ann. Rev. Nutr. 4:377-407, 1984*).

<u>Vitamin A</u>:

A <u>liver biopsy</u> is by far the most accurate method of assessing vitamin A status (*Pitt GAJ. The assessment of vitamin A status. Proc. Nutr. Sci. 40:173, 1981*).

Plasma retinol is commonly measured to assess vitamin A status. It should be noted, however, that when insufficient RBP is available, toxicity due to hypervitaminosis A can occur despite a low concentration of plasma retinol; thus, in addition to plasma retinol concentration, it is important that retinol-binding protein also be measured (*Nutr. Rev. 40(10), October, 1982*). Although determination of plasma retinol as the retinol-RBP (retinol-binding protein) complex would appear to be a promising method, the major limitation on its value is that plasma retinol concentration is kept reasonably constant to supply vitamin A to the tissues. While there is some relationship between plasma values and liver content, the plasma content only falls substantially if the liver reserves of retinyl esters are effectively exhausted (*Pitt GAJ. The assessment of vitamin A status. Proc. Nutr. Sci. 40:173, 1981*).

In addition, other factors besides vitamin A nutriture can influence plasma retinol levels. If dietary protein is inadequate, or if various diseases are present, insufficient RBP is synthesized by the liver, and the plasma retinol concentration will fall. Estrogens and oral contraceptives can increase plasma retinol-RBP concentrations. Poor growth depresses, and accelerated growth increases, the plasma retinol concentration, and giving retinoids other than retinol can paradoxically depress plasma retinol concentration as a consequence of diminishing tissue demand for retinol (*Pitt GAJ - ibid*).

Vitamin B_{12}:

While microbiological assays are reliable (*Baker H et al. Vitamin analyses in medicine, in Goodhart RS, Shils, ME, Eds. Modern Nutrition in Health and Disease. Sixth Edition. Philadelphia, Lea & Febiger, 1980, p. 611*), RIA assays are unreliable because they also measure inactive cobalamin analogues (*Cohen KL, Donaldson, Jr RM. Unreliability of radiodilution assays as screening tests for cobalamin (vitamin B_{12}) deficiency. JAMA October 24, 1980, pp. 1942-5; Kolhouse JF et al. Cobalamin analogues are present in human plasma and can mask cobalamin deficiency because current radioisotope dilution assays are not specific for true cobalamin. New Engl. J. Med. 299:787, 1978*).

The Schilling test is a popular test of B_{12} absorption (*Zuckier LS, Chervu LR. J. Nucl. Med. 25:1032, 1984*). Its newer version, the dual-isotope variation, is independent of urine volume and renal function, and is thus the test of choice in the elderly patient (*Lum MC, Mooradian AD. Vitamin B_{12} deficiency: The sepulveda GRECC method. No. 14. Geriatr. Med. Today 5(10):93-97, 1986*).

Serum B_{12} levels are frequently normal despite depressed levels in the cerebrospinal fluid (*van Tiggelen CJM et al. Vitamin B_{12} levels of cerebrospinal fluid in patients with organic mental disorder. J. Orthomol. Psychiat. 12:305-311, 1983*).

Even in the absence of hematological and neurological evidence of pernicious anemia, serum B_{12} levels may be deficient.

Experimental and Observational Study: 4 pts. with presenile dementia for over 4 yrs. failed to show hematologic findings suggesting vitamin B_{12} deficiency, yet their serum B_{12} levels were clearly deficient. B_{12} supplementation did not improve their mental status (*Abalan F, Delile JM. B_{12} deficiency in presenile dementia. Letter to the Editor. Biol. Psychiat. 20(11):1251, 1985*).

Observational Study: Alzheimer pts. had lower serum B_{12} levels at all ages compared to normals and pts. with other forms of dementia, but demonstrated no hematological changes suggestive of B_{12} deficiency (*Cole MG, Prchal JF. Low serum B_{12} in Alzheimer-type dementia. Age Aging 13:101-5, 1984*).

A low serum B_{12}, even without evidence of pernicious anemia, may be associated with organic psychosis (*Evans DL et al. Organic psychosis without anemia or spinal cord symptoms in patients with vitamin B_{12} deficiency. Am. J. Psychiat. 140:218, 1983*).

The determination of hypersegmentation of neutrophils is a useful measure of vitamin B_{12} deficiency, although it is unreliable during pregnancy (*Sauberlich HE. Newer laboratory methods for assessing nutriture of selected B-complex vitamins. Ann. Rev. Nutr. 4:377-407, 1984*).

24-hour urinary methylmalonic acid is not a reliable test as it lacks sensitivity and specificity. MMA excretion is high, for example, in benign methylmalonic aciduria (*Ledley FD et al. Benign methylmalonic aciduria. N. Engl. J. Med. 311:1015-1018, 1984*), and carnitine supplementation may cause MMA levels to decrease (*Roe CR et al. Metabolic response to carnitine in methylmalonic aciduria. Arch. Dis. Child. 58:916-20, 1983*).

Vitamin C:

While serum and plasma ascorbate levels may not always fully reflect vitamin C intakes or the state of tissue ascorbate reserves, within a limited range, serum ascorbate levels show a linear relationship with vitamin C intake and low serum levels indicate low or inadequate intake with probably only partial reserves present (*Sauberlich HE. Vitamin C status: Methods and findings. Ann. N.Y. Acad. Sci. 258:438-49, 1975*).

The leukocyte ascorbic acid concentration tends to respond less readily than does the serum level to recent dietary intake and may be more closely related to tissue stores than are serum levels (*Burr ML et al. Plasma and leukocyte ascorbic acid levels in the elderly. Am. J. Clin. Nutr. 27:144, 1974*), although there is evidence that it may be normal despite other evidence of vitamin C deficiency (*Thomas AJ et al. Is leucocyte ascorbic acid an unreliable estimate of vitamin C deficiency? Age Ageing 13(4):243-47, 1984*).

Erythrocyte and whole-blood ascorbic acid levels appear to be less sensitive indicators of vitamin C deficiency than are serum levels (*Sauberlich HE. Vitamin C status: Methods and findings. Ann. N.Y. Acad. Sci. 258:438-49, 1975*).

Urinary excretion of ascorbic acid declines to undetectable levels in vitamin C depletion and thus could be used to corroborate other findings (*Hodges RE et al. Clinical manifestations of ascorbic acid deficiency in man. Am. J. Clin. Nutr. 24:432, 1971*).

The ascorbic acid saturation test must be carefully conducted and interpreted with caution, but the results can conclusively exclude scurvy as a diagnosis (*Sauberlich HE. Vitamin C status: Methods and findings. Ann. N.Y. Acad. Sci. 258:438-49, 1975; Dutra De Oliveira JE et al. Clinical usefulness of the oral ascorbic acid tolerance test in scurvy. Am. J. Clin. Nutr. 7:630, 1959*).

Results of the lingual ascorbic acid test are not related to changes in ascorbic acid intake and are not consistent with plasma or leukocyte ascorbate concentrations (*Leggott PJ et al. Response of lingual ascorbic acid test and salivary ascorbate levels to changes in ascorbic acid intake. J. Dent. Res. 65(2):131-34, 1986*).

Vitamin D:

Cholecalciferol (vitamin D_3) is the natural vitamin, while ergocalciferol (vitamin D_2) is obtained exclusively from the diet. Each is biologically inert until it undergoes successive enzymatic hydroxylations, at C-25 in the liver and at C-1 in the kidney, to produce 1,25-dihydroxyvitamin D. While intracellular 25-hydroxyvitamin D may serve a specific function, it is unproved and can be regarded as part of the body stores of vitamin D. Measurement of plasma 25-hydroxyvitamin D provides an index of the the bodily reserve of the pro-hormone, and measurement of plasma 1,25-dihydroxyvitamin D an index of prevailing biological action, although the level of 1,25-dihydroxyvitamin D can only be interpreted with reference to the subject's mineral nutrition and the prevailing physiological state (*Stanbury SW. Vitamin D: metamorphosis from nutrient to hormonal system. Proc. Nutr. Soc. 40:179-86, 1981*).

Vitamin E:

Since plasma and serum vitamin E levels are closely correlated with total serum triglycerides (*Farrell PM, Biere JG. Am. J. Clin. Nutr. 28:1381, 1975*), tocopherol to triglyceride serum ratios should be calculated in assessing tocopherol status when plasma or serum vitamin E is being measured. The normal range of this ratio is 35-120 (*Bland J, Prestbo E. Vitamin E: Comparative absorption studies. Int. Clin. Nutr. Rev. 4(2):82-86, 1984*).

The alternative is to measure platelet vitamin E levels, as this measure is unaffected by blood lipids (*Vatasser G et al. Vitamin E concentrations in the human blood plasma and platelets. Am. J. Clin. Nutr. 37:1020-24, 1983*).

Vitamin K:

While prothrombin time and clotting time are commonly used to assess vitamin K, subclinical deficiency is better assessed by methods which quantify the fraction of hepatic prothrombin which fails to become carboxylated in the hepatic reticulum under the influence of vitamin K (*Abnormal plasma prothrombin in the diagnosis of subclinical vitamin K deficiency. Nutr. Rev. 40(10):298-300, 1982*).

Alternative methods are the indirect ratio approach (*Corrigan JJ Jr et al. J. Pediatr. 99:254-57, 1981*) and direct measurement of both native prothrombin and the abnormal species with RIA procedures (*Blanchard RA et al. N. Engl. J. Med. 305:242-48, 1981*).

Zinc:

The most reliable method of diagnosing zinc deficiency is a therapeutic trial (*Editorial: Another look at zinc. Brit. Med. J. 282:1098-99, 1981*).

The zinc tolerance test is perhaps the best available method of determining body zinc nutriture. After a fast, a baseline plasma level is drawn, and an oral loading dose of zinc sulfate 220 mg (50 mg elemental zinc) is given. Two hrs. later, plasma zinc is redrawn. A two or threefold increase in plasma zinc is indicative of zinc adequacy (*Capel ID et al. The assessment of zinc status by the zinc tolerance test in various groups of patients. Clin. Biochem. 15(5):257-60, 1982; Sullivan JF et al. A zinc tolerance test. J. Lab. Clin. Med. 93(3):485-92, 1979*).

WBC zinc is believed to be an useful index of body stores as there is a correlation between leukocyte zinc and muscle zinc levels (*Jones RB et al. The relationship between leukocyte and muscle zinc in health and disease. Clin. Science 60:237-39, 1981*) and, in contrast to RBC zinc, leukocyte zinc is commonly reduced in pts. with liver disease, suggesting tisue zinc deficiency (*Keeling PWN et al. Reduced leucocyte zinc in liver disease. Gut 21:561-64, 1980*).

Sweat zinc, while not yet widely available, may be a useful and sensitive index of zinc status and, in fact, may be more sensitive than either hair or serum (*Davies S. Assessment of zinc status. Int. Clin. Nutr. Rev. 4(3):122-29, 1984*).

Depressed hair zinc levels reliably indicate depletion, but normal or even high values do not rule out low body stores (*Davies S. Assessment of zinc status. Int. Clin. Nutr. Rev. 4(3):122-29, 1984; Pekarek RS et al. Abnormal cellular immune responses during acquired zinc deficiency. Am. J. Clin. Nutr. 32:1466-71, 1979; Hambridge KM et al. Low levels of zinc in hair, anorexia, poor growth and hypogeusia in children. Pediatr. Res. 6:808-74, 1971*). In addition, because standard washing procedures are unable to remove exogenous zinc without reducing endogenous zinc levels, hair levels are unreliable when external zinc contamination is likely to have occurred (*Buckley RA, Dreosti I. Am. J. Clin. Nutr. 40:840-46, 1984*).

Plasma and serum zinc are poor measures of total body zinc stores (*Solomons NW. On the assessment of zinc and copper nutriture in man. Am. J. Clin. Nutr. 32:856-71, 1979*). A moderately low plasma level may simply reflect mobilization of zinc from plasma to the liver and other tissues as part of the normal response to infection or stress (*Wagner PA. Zinc nutriture in the elderly.* Geriatrics. *40:111-13,117-18, 124-25, 1985*). In addition, plasma zinc concentrations depend upon albumin concentration (*Ainley CC et al. Zinc state in anorexia nervosa.* Brit. Med. J. *Vol. 293, October 18, 1986*). Combining measurement of the serum zinc concentration with urinary zinc excretion will provide a more accurate assessment; however, any bodily process that involves the breakdown or rapid turnover of cells (including decreased food intake and starvation) is associated with increased urinary zinc excretion, which may or may not be reflected in serum zinc. Also, stress from any source, including surgery, may cause a redistribution of bodily zinc, and a transient zinc loss may be evident for a few days (*Henkin RI. Zinc in Wound Healing. An Editorial.* N. Engl. J. Med. *291(13):675-76, 1974*).

Red cell zinc, while sometimes low in zinc deficiency, is unreliable as RBC zinc levels are substantially influenced by factors controlling the partitioning of zinc across red cell membranes (*Davies S. Assessment of zinc status.* Int. Clin. Nutr. Rev. *4(3):122-29, 1984*).

A simple zinc taste test which suggests that there will be a favorable response to zinc supplementation uses a test solution made by dissolving zinc sulfate 1 gm in 1 liter of distilled water (0.1% solution). If the subject tasting 5-10 ml notes either no taste or a dry and furry taste developing after a few minutes, zinc supplementation is suggested. Adequate zinc nutriture is suggested by an immediate taste which may be strong and unpleasant (*Bryce-Smith D, Simpson RID. Anorexia, depression, and zinc deficiency.* Lancet *2:1162, 1982*). This test, however, has not been well-validated.

Appendix E

NUTRIENT BIOAVAILABILITY AND INTERACTIONS

NOTE: Drug interactions should also be considered

<u>Calcium:</u>

Best taken at bedtime as more calcium is lost at night and foods may interfere with absorption (*Notelovitz, Morris, professor of ob-gyn, U. of Florida, Gainesville - quoted in <u>Medical Tribune</u> September 26, 1984*).

Should be taken with a meal in the presence of achlorhydria (*Shah BG. Calcium supplementation with anacids. Questions and answers. <u>JAMA</u> 257(4):541, 1987*).

- and <u>Caffeine:</u>

Increases urinary calcium excretion (*Yeh JK et al. <u>J. Nutr.</u> 116(2):273-80, 1986*).

- and <u>Fiber:</u>

Decreases calcium absorption (*Heaney RP et al. <u>Am. J. Clin. Nutr.</u> 36:986-1031, 1982*).

- and <u>Magnesium:</u>

Chronic magnesium deficiency is associated with hypocalcemia (*Mahaffee D et al. Magnesium promotes both parathyroid hormone secretion and adenosine 3',5'-monophosphate production in rat parathyroid tissues and reverses the inhibitory effects of calcium on adenylate cyclase. <u>Endocrinol.</u> 110:487-95, 1982; Anast CS et al. Impaired release of parathyroid hormone in magnesium deficiency. <u>J. Clin. Endocrinol. Metab.</u> 42:707, 1974; Levi J et al. Hypocalcemia in magnesium-depleted dogs: Evidence for reduced responsiveness to parathyroid hormone and relative failure of parathyroid gland function. <u>Metabolism</u> 23:323, 1974*).

Magnesium regulates the neuromuscular activity of the Ca^{++} ion and a deficiency enhances the availability of ionic calcium; thus magnesium is a natural calcium-channel blocker (*Iseri LT, French JH. Magnesium: Nature's calcium blocker. <u>Am. Heart J.</u> July, 1984, p. 188*).

- and <u>Phosphorus:</u>

The ideal Ca/P ratio is 1:1 (*Linkswiler HM, Zemel MB. Calcium to phosphorus ratios. <u>Contemp. Nutr.</u> 4(5), May, 1979*).

High phosphorus intakes (meat, grains, potatoes and soft drinks) promote calcium loss through the induction of "nutritional hyperparathyroidism" in order to maintain normal serum calcium levels in the face of decreased Ca/P ratios (*Jowsey J. Osteoporosis. <u>Postgraduate Med.</u> 60:75-9, 1976*).

- and Phytates:

Decrease calcium absorption (*Goodhart RS, Shils ME. Modern Nutrition in Health and Disease. 6th Edition. Philadelphia, Lee & Febiger, 1980*).

- and Sodium:

Increases urinary calcium excretion (*Heaney RP. Calcium bioavailability. Contemp. Nutr. 11(8), 1986*).

- and Sugar:

Increases urinary calcium concentration.

> **Experimental Study:** In a study of 24 hr. urines of 18 normal subjects, an increase in refined carbohydrates (sugar and sugar products) in a standardized diet caused a significant increase in the number of urines with a calcium concentration above 9 mmol/l (*Thom JA et al. The influence of refined carbohyrate on urinary calcium excretion. Brit. J. Urology 50:459-64, 1978*).

- and Vitamin D:

Promotes calcium absorption and mobilizes calcium from bone (*Passmore R, Eastwood MA. Davidson and Passmore: Human Nutrition and Dietetics. Eighth Edition. London, Churchill Livingstone, 1986, p. 139*).

- and Zinc:

Decreases calcium absorption when a high level of daily supplementation (150 mg) is given along with a low daily dietary calcium intake (*Spencer H et al. Am. J. Clin. Nutr. 35:829, 1982*).

Chromium:

- and Sugar:

Increases urinary chromium loss.

> **Experimental Study:** 27/37 normal subjects had an increase in urinary chromium excretion during a high sucrose diet (35% of calories from sucrose; 15% from complex carbohyrates) compared to a diet with 15% of calories from sucrose and 35% from complex carbohydrates, with the increase ranging from 10-300% (*Kozlovsky AS et al. Effects of diets high in simple sugars on urinary chromium losses. Metabolism 35:515, 1986*).

Copper:

- and Zinc:

Decreases copper absorption when the Zn/Cu ratio is greater than 2.5/1 (*Fischer PWF et al. Am. J. Clin. Nutr. 34:1670, 1981; Van Campen DR. Zinc interference with copper absorption in rats. J. Nutr. 91:473, 1967*).

> **Experimental Study:** Daily ingestion of 150 mg zinc daily (as zinc sulfate 660 mg) produced overt copper depletion with anemia in some pts. (*Prasad AS et al. JAMA 240:2166, 1978*).

Essential Fatty Acids:

- and Vitamin E:

Vitamin E prevents the peroxidation of polyunsaturated fatty acids and thus is recommended whenever they are heavily supplemented (*Chow CK. Nutritional influences on cellular antioxidant defense systems. Am. J. Clin. Nutr. 32:1066-1081, 1979*).

Folic Acid:

- and Pancreatic Enzymes:

Bind with folic acid to form insoluble complexes, thus decreasing folate absorption (*Russell RM et al. Impairment of folic acid absorption by oral pancreatic extracts. Dig. Dis. & Sci. 25(5):369, 1980*).

- and Vitamin B_{12}:

Regulates folic acid metabolism (*Chanarin I et al. Vitamin B_{12} regulates folate metabolism by the supply of formate. Lancet 2:505-7, 1980*).

Iron:

If deficient, oral supplementation is preferred (*Fairbanks VF, Bentler E. Iron deficiency, in Hematology. McGraw Hill, 1983, pp. 466-89*).

Oral supplementation is best absorbed on an empty stomach.

Case Report: Supplemental iron given to a healthy fasting subject increased plasma iron levels by 100% , while the same dose given during or after a meal produced hardly any elevation of plasma iron (*Martinez-Torres C, Layrisse M. Nutritional factors in iron deficiency: Food iron absorption. Clinics in Hematology 2(2):339-52, 1973*).

- and Calcium:

Excessive supplementation may decrease iron absorption in a dose-defined manner leading to iron deficiency anemia. Perhaps 23% of those ingesting more than 2 gm daily are at risk (*Read MH et al. Mineral supplementation practices of adults in seven western states. Nut. Res. 6:375-83, 1986*).

- and Coffee:

Decreases iron absorption.

Experimental Study: In a study of 37 healthy subjects, coffee 1 hr. before eating did not affect iron absorption, while coffee taken with the meal or up to 1 hr. after eating reduced absorbed iron by 39%. This effect was concentration-dependent (*Morck TA et al. Inhibition of food iron absorption by coffee. Am. J. Clin. Nutr., 37(3):416-20, 1983*).

- and Hydrochloric Acid:

If deficient, iron absorption is significantly impaired.

Experimental Study: 25 diabetic pts. with blood counts 4.2 million or less who were under good diabetic control were randomly selected to receive glutamic acid HCl 5 gr 3 times daily before meals which, at the end of 1 month, was replaced by ferrous carbonate 6 3/4 gr 3 times daily. At the end of another month, both supplements were prescribed concomitantly. Following the first month, the RBC increased significantly from 4.06 to 4.56 million, while iron supplementation failed to be followed by a significant change. Following combined supplementation, RBC again increased significantly by 1/4 million. The experiment was replicated with similar results (*Rabinowich IM. Achlorhydria and its clinical significance in diabetes mellitus. Am J. Dig. Dis. 16:322-32, 1949*).

See Also:

> *Conrad ME, Schade SG. Ascorbic acid chelates in iron absorption: A role for hydrochloric acid and bile. Gastroenterol. 55:35, 1968*

> *Jacobs P et al. Role of hydrochloric acid in iron absorption. J. App. Physiol. 19(2):187-8, 1964*

- and Protein:

Beef, lamb, chicken, pork and fish have been shown to enhance iron absorption, while soy decreases it (*Kane AP, Miller DD. In vitro estimation of the effects of selected proteins on iron bioavailability. Am. J. Clin. Nutr. 393-401, 1984*).

- and Tea:

Decreases absorption.

> **Experimental Study:** In a study of 37 healthy subjects, tea taken with a hamburger meal reduced iron absorption by 64% compared to a 39% reduction when coffee was substituted for tea (*Morck TA et al. Inhibition of food iron absorption by coffee. Am. J. Clin. Nutr., 37(3):416-20, 1983*).

- and Vitamin C:

Markedly enhances non-heme iron absorption by keeping ferric iron soluble and available for absorption at the alkaline pH of the duodenum (*Monsen ER. Ascorbic acid: An enhancing factor in iron absorption, in Nutritional Bioavailability of Iron. American Chemical Society, 1982, pp. 85-95; Conrad ME, Schade SG. Ascorbic acid chelates in iron absorption: A role for hydrochloric acid and bile. Gastroenterol. 55:35, 1968*).

Magnesium:

- and Alcohol:

Increases urinary magnesium excretion (*Lindeman RD et al. Magnesium in Health and Disease. Jamaica, N.Y., SP Medical and Scientific Books, 1980, pp.236-45*).

- and Caffeine:

Increases urinary magnesium excretion (*Yeh JK et al. J. Nutr. 116(2):273-80, 1986*).

- and Calcium:

Impairs absorption of magnesium, probably due to competition for a common transport system (*O'Donnell JM, Smith DW. Uptake of calcium and magnesium by rat duodenal mucosa analyzed by means of competing metals. J. Physiol. 229:733, 1973*).

Experimental Study: When dietary Mg was maintained at 250 mg/day, and Ca was increased from 200 mg/day to 1400 mg/day, the Mg balance became negative, but was restored when Mg intake was increased to 500 mg/day (*Spencer H et al. Magnesium in Health and Disease. Jamaica, N.Y., SP Medical and Scientific Books, 1980, pp. 911-19*).

- and <u>Fat</u>:

High levels of fat in the intestinal lumen interfere with magnesium absorption because soaps that are formed from fat and divalent cations like Mg are not absorbed (*Seelig MS. Magnesium Bulletin 31(1a):26-47, 1981*).

- and <u>Phosphorus</u>:

Causes magnesium loss.

Experimental Study: A negative Mg balance was produced when phosphate was increased from the near RDA level of 975 mg daily to 1500 mg daily (*Spencer H et al. Magnesium in Health and Disease. Jamaica, N.Y., SP Medical and Scientific Books, 1980, pp. 911-19*).

- and <u>Pyridoxine</u>:

Supplementation with pyridoxine may normalize deficient intracellular magnesium levels.

Experimental Study: 9 females with low RBC Mg levels received vitamin B_6 100 mg twice daily. After 4 wks., RBC Mg levels had normalized (*Abraham GE et al. Effect of vitamin B6 plasma red blood cell magnesium levels in premenopausal women. Ann. Clin. Lab. Sci. 11(4):333-36, 1981*).

- and <u>Sugar</u>:

High intake of sugar increases the need for magnesium (*Durlack J. Le Diabete 19:99-113, 1971*) and increases urinary Mg excretion (*Lindeman RD et al. Magnesium in Health and Disease. Jamaica, N.Y., SP Medical and Scientific Books, 1980, pp.236-45*).

- and <u>Vitamin D</u>:

Stimulates intestinal magnesium absorption (*Nordin BEC. Plasma calcium and plasma magnesium homeostasis, in Nordin, BEC, Ed. Calcium, Phosphorus and Magnesium Metabolism. New York, Churchill Livingstone, 1976*).

<u>Manganese</u>:

- and <u>Calcium</u>:

Impairs manganese utilization (*Wilgus HS Jr, Dutton AR. Factors affecting manganese utilization in the chicken. J. Nutr. 18:35, 1939*).

- and <u>Iron</u>:

Impairs manganese utilization (*Thomson ABR et al. Interrelation of intestinal transport system for manganese and iron. J. Lab. Clin. Med. 73:6422, 1971*).

- and <u>Phosphorus</u>:

Impairs manganese utilization (*Wilgus HS Jr, Dutton AR. Factors affecting manganese utilization in the chicken. J. Nutr. 18:35, 1939*).

- and <u>Zinc</u>:

May reduce blood manganese levels.

> **Review Article:** Zinc supplementation may increase grand mal seizures in epileptics, possibly by causing a reduction in blood manganese levels, and thus Mn supplementation should be started first (*Pfeiffer CC, LaMola S. Zinc and manganese in the schizophrenias. J. Orthomol. Psychiat. 12:215-34, 1983*).

<u>Phosphorus</u>:

- and <u>Caffeine</u>:

Increases urinary excretion of inorganic phosphate and may cause a negative balance (*Yeh JK et al. J. Nutr.116(2):273-80, 1986*).

- and <u>Calcium</u>:

A calcium to phosphorus ratio above 2:1 due to excess calcium results in reduced bone strength and interferes with vitamin K synthesis and/or absorption, causing internal bleeding (*Calcium: How much is too much? Nutr. Rev. 43(11):345, 1985*).

- and <u>Vitamin D</u>:

Facilitates phosphate absorption (*Passmore R, Eastwood MA. <u>Davidson and Passmore: Human Nutrition and Dietetics</u>. Eighth Edition. London, Churchill Livingstone, 1986, p. 139*).

<u>Potassium</u>:

- and <u>Caffeine</u>:

Increases urinary potassium excretion and may cause a negative balance (*Yeh JK et al. J. Nutr. 116(2):273-80, 1986*).

- and <u>Magnesium</u>:

Potassium deficiency may be refractory in the presence of magnesium depletion (*Whang R et al. Magnesium depletion as a cause of refractory potassium repletion. Arch. Intern. Med. 145(9):1686-89, 1985*) which has been found in 42% of pts. with hypokalemia (*Whang R et al. Predictors of clinical hypomagnesemia. Hypokalemia, hypophosphatemia, hyponatremia, and hypocalcemia. Arch. Intern. Med. 144(9):1794-96, 1984*).

<u>Selenium</u>:

- and <u>Vitamin E</u>:

Deficiency syndromes of both vitamin E and selenium overlap and most can be treated successfully with either nutrient due to their closely-related mechanisms of action (*Combs GF. Assessment of vitamin E status in animals and man. Proc. Nutr. Soc. 40:187-94, 1981*).

Sodium:

- and Caffeine:

Increases urinary sodium excretion and may cause a negative balance (*Yeh JK et al. J. Nutr. 116(2):273-80, 1986*).

Thiamine:

- and Magnesium:

Necessary for the conversion of thiamine into thiamine pyrophosphate, its biologically active form.

> **Case Report:** Pt. with Crohn's disease and chronic diarrhea resulting in thiamine and magnesium deficiency failed to respond to massive IV doses of thiamine until the magnesium deficiency was corrected (*Dyckner T et al. Aggravation of thiamine deficiency by magnesium depletion. A case report. Acta. Med. Scand. 218:129, 1985*).

L-Tryptophan:

- and Niacinamide:

> **Review Article:** The rationale for the addition of niacinamide is that the high rate of catabolism of tryptophan by the liver suggested by animal work can be inhibited with niacinamide (*Young SN, Sourkes TL. The antidepressant effect of tryptophan. Lancet 2:897-98, 1974*). Recent data, however, indicate that niacinamide will not inhibit breakdown of tryptophan in humans at clinical doses following an acute loading (*Green AR et al. Metabolism of an oral tryptophan load: Effect of pretreatment with the putative tryptophan pyrollase inhibitors nicotinamide or allopurinol. Brit. J. Clin. Pharmacol. 10:611-15, 1980*). In addition, in pts. receiving up to 6 gm tryptophan daily along with niacinamide, tryptophan metabolism was still highly variable. Thus it is unlikely that niacinamide is a useful adjunct (*Chouinard G - op cit*).

- and Protein:

Effects protentiated by avoiding protein for 90 minutes before or afterwards (*Fernstrom JD et al. Diurnal variations in plasma concentrations of tryptophan, tyrosine, and other neutral amino acids: Effects of dietary protein intake. Am. J. Clin. Nutr. 32:1912-22, 1979*).

- and Pyridoxine:

May increase brain tryptophan levels by reducing levels of kynurenine which competes with tryptophan for transport.

> **Review Articles:** Kynurenine is derived from tryptophan by the action of tryptophan pyrrolase in the liver and is taken up in the brain and transferred by the same transport carrier as tryptophan where it has a competitively inhibitory effect upon tryptophan equal to that of the competing amino acids (*Moller SE et al. Tryptophan availability in endogenous depression - relation to efficacy of L-tryptophan treatment. Adv. Biol. Psychiat. 10:30-46, 1983*). Supplementation with tryptophan increases the plasma concentration of kynurenine in proportion to the dose given and, after longer-term administration, there is a marked increase in basal kynurenine with a further substantial increase following a further dose of tryptophan. This large increase in kynurenine concentration might reflect a relative saturation of the kynurenine pathway, possibly because of vitamin B_6 depletion since many of the degradative enzymes down the pathway are B_6-dependent. Consistent with this hypothesis are findings that, when tryptophan is given for 7 days with pyridoxine, the basal plasma kynurenine is half that seen in subjects given tryptophan

alone and the peak kynurenine concentration following a single load is the same after long-term pre-treatment with tryptophan plus pyridoxine as after no pre-treatment and only half that seen in subjects who have taken longer-term tryptophan without pyridoxine (*Green AR, Aronson JK. The pharmacokinetics of oral L-tryptophan: Effects of dose and concomitant pyridoxine, allopurinol or nicotinamide administration. Adv. Biol. Psychiat. 10:67-81, 1983*).

- and <u>Sugar</u>:

Effects potentiated by ingesting tryptophan along with carbohydrate to stimulate insulin release which takes up the other amino acids into the tissues, thus improving brain tryptophan intake (*Fernstrom JD. Effects of the diet on brain neurotransmitters. Metabolism 26:207-33, 1977*).

<u>Vitamin A</u>:

- and <u>Vitamin E</u>:

Vitamin A absorption is markedly impaired in vitamin E-deficiency.

Animal Study: Vitamin A levels of vitamin-E-deficient mice remained low after vitamin A injections until they also received vitamin E injections (*Ames SR. Factors affecting absorption, transport and storage of vitamin A. Am. J. Clin. Nutr. 22:934, 1969*).

Vitamin E protects vitamin A from oxidation and by joining with it within the membranous parts of cells in performing its functions (*Tappel AL. Nutrition Today July-August 1973*). It is therefore suggested that vitamin E be added whenever megadoses of vitamin A are desirable.

Case Report: 200,000 units of vitamin A daily produced only slight improvement in a case of Darier' Disease. However, after the addition of 1600 units of vitamin E, 100,000 units of vitamin A produced dramatic improvement (*Ayres S. Darier's Disease: Update on an effective new therapy. Arch. Dermatol. 119:710, 1983*).

<u>Vitamin B$_{12}$</u>:

- and <u>Folic Acid</u>:

High doses of folic acid may decrease B$_{12}$ levels (*Hunter R et al. Effect of folic-acid supplement on serum-vitamin B$_{12}$ levels in patients on anti-convulsants. Lancet 2:50, 1969*).

<u>Vitamin D</u>:

- and <u>Phosphorus</u>:

Phosphorus intake strongly influences vitamin D metabolism.

Experimental Study: Increases and reductions in oral phosphorus intake in healthy men were found to induce rapidly occurring, large, inverse, and persisting changes in serum 1,25-dihydroxyvitamin D levels due to phosphorus-induced changes in the rate of vitamin D production (*Portale A. Oral intake of phosphorus can determine the serum concentration of 1,25-dihydroxyvitamin D by determining its production rate in humans. J. Clin. Invest. 77:7-12, 1986*).

Vitamin E:

- and <u>inorganic Iron</u>:

    (found in mineral supplements, fortified cereals and enriched flour)

    Combines with and inactivates vitamin E in the gut.

- and <u>Selenium</u>:

    Deficiency syndromes of both vitamin E and selenium overlap and most can be treated successfully with either nutrient due to their closely-related mechanisms of action (*Combs GF. Assessment of vitamin E status in animals and man. <u>Proc. Nutr. Soc.</u> 40:187-94, 1981*).

Vitamin K:

- and <u>Calcium</u>:

    Excessive doses of calcium or a calcium to phosphorus ratio above 2:1 due to excess calcium interferes with vitamin K synthesis and/or absorption, causing internal bleeding (*Calcium: How much is too much? <u>Nutr. Rev.</u> 43(11):345, 1985*).

- and <u>Vitamin E</u>:

    A large intake may reduce intestinal absorption of vitamin K and antagonize the effect of vitamin K on coagulation at the level of prothrombin formation (*Bieri JG et al. Medical uses of vitamin E. <u>N. Engl. J. Med.</u> 308(18):1063-71, 1983*).

Zinc:

Supplementation is best taken away from meals, as eggs, milk, and cereal (as well as possibly other foods) will decrease its bioavailability (*Moser PB, Gunderson CJ. Changes in plasma zinc following the ingestion of a zinc multivitamin-mineral supplement with and without breakfast. <u>Nutr. Res.</u> 3:279-84, 1983*).

- and <u>Calcium</u>:

    Decreases zinc absorption in the presence of <u>phytates</u> (*Solomons NW. Mineral interactions in the diet. <u>Contemp. Nutr.</u> 7(7), July, 1982*).

- and <u>Copper</u>:

    Decreases zinc absorption (*Van Campen DR. Copper interference with intestinal absorption of zinc-65 by rats. <u>J. Nutr.</u> 473, 1967*).

- and <u>Folic Acid</u>:

    Decreases zinc absorption.

    Experimental Study: 8 men were fed diets containing 150 mcg folic acid, and 4 of them also received supplementation with an additional 400 mcg of folate daily. Fecal zinc was significantly higher in the supplemented gp. both during the control diet and during a low-zinc diet; no differences were noted in fecal zinc during high zinc intake. During all dietary periods urinary zinc excretion was reduced 50% in the folic acid-supplemented group. These data suggest that folate supplementation may influence zinc homeostasis by forming insoluble chelates which impair absorption (*Milne DB et al. Effect of oral folic acid supplements on zinc, copper, and iron absorption and excretion. Am. J. Clin. Nutr. 39(4):535-39, 1984*).

- and Iron:

Iron supplementation may exacerbate subclinical zinc depletion by competitively inhibiting intestinal absorption when Fe/Zn ratios are greater than 2:1 (*Solomons NW, Jacob RA. Studies on the bioavailability of zinc in humans. Effects of heme and non-heme iron on the absorption of zinc. Am. J. Clin. Nutr. 34:475-82, 1981; Meadows NJ et al. Lancet 2:1135, 1981*).

When deficient, zinc absorption is enhanced (*Pollack S et al. J. Clin. Invest. 44:1470, 1965*).

- and Phytates:

Diets high in vegetable fiber may be associated with poor bioavailability of zinc due to the presence of phytic acid, a zinc-binding compound, in high concentrations (*Navert B et al. A reduction of the phytate content of bran by leavening in bread and its effect on zinc absorption in man. Brit. J. Nutr. 53:47-53, 1985*).

SYNDROMES DUE TO ABNORMAL TISSUE NUTRIENT LEVELS

Aluminum:

    Toxicity associated with:

        Ataxia
        Colic
        GI Irritation

Arsenic:

    Toxicity associated with:

        Alopecia
        Confusion
        Constipation
        Delayed Wound Healing
        Dermatitis
        Diarrhea
        Drowsiness
        Edema
        Fatigue
        GI Complaints
        Headaches
        Limbs Burning or Tingling
        Muscle Pains
        Neuropathy
        Numbness
        Pruritis
        Seizures
        Stomatitis
        Weakness

Biotin:

    Deficiency associated with:

        Alopecia
        Anemia
        Anorexia & Nausea
        Depression
        Fatigue
        Hypercholesterolemia
        Hyperglycemia

        Insomnia
        Muscle Pain
        Muscle Weakness
        Dry, Greyish Skin
        Pale, Smooth Tongue

Cadmium:

    Toxicity associated with:

        Alopecia
        Anorexia
        Anosmia
        Hypertension
        Kidney Damage
        Liver Damage
        Osteoporosis
        Sore Joints
        Dry, Scaly Skin

Calcium:

    Deficiency associated with:

        Agitation
        Brittle Fingernails
        Cognitive Impairment
        Delusions
        Depression
        Eczema
        Hyperactivity
        Hypertension
        Insomnia
        Irritability
        Limb Numbness
        Muscle Cramps
        Nervousness
        Neuromuscular Excitability
        Osteomalacia
        Osteoporosis
        Palpitations
        Paresthesias
        Periodontal Disease

Rickets
Stunted Growth
Tetany
Tooth Decay

Toxicity associated with:

Anorexia
Aphasia (transient)
Ataxia
Depressed Deep Tenson Reflexes
Depression
Irritability
Memory impairment
Muscle weakness
Psychosis

Choline:

Deficiency associated with:

Cardiac Symptoms
Fat Intolerance
Gastric Ulcers
Growth Retardation
Hypertension
Kidney Impairment
Liver Impairment

Chromium:

Deficiency associated with:

Anxiety
Fatigue
Glucose Intolerance
Growth Impairment
Hypercholesterolemia

Toxicity associated with:

Dermatitis
GI Ulcers
Kidney Impairment
Liver Impairment

Copper:

Deficiency associated with:

Alopecia
Anemia (hypochromic, microcytic)
Depression
Dermatoses
Diarrhea

Fatigue
Fragile Bones
Hypercholesterolemia
Respiration Impairment
Weakness

Toxicity associated with:

Depression
Irritability
Joint Pain
Muscle Pain
Nervousness

Essential Fatty Acids:

Deficiency associated with:

Acne
Alopecia
Diarrhea
Eczema
Atrophy of Exocrine Glands
Dry, Brittle Hair
Endocrine Dysfunction
Fatty Degeneration of Liver
Gallstones
Growth Impairment
Immunologic Dysfunction
Impaired Wound Healing
Kidney Dysfunction
Reproductive Failure
Xerosis

Folic Acid:

Deficiency associated with:

Anemia (megaloblastic)
Anorexia
Apathy
Diarrhea
Digestive Disturbances
Dyspnea
Fatigue
Glossitis
Growth Impairment
Headaches
Insomnia
Memory Impairment
Paranoid Ideation
Weakness

Inositol:

Deficiency associated with:

  Alopecia
  Constipation
  Eczema
  Hypercholesterolemia

Iodine:

Deficiency associated with:

  Fatigue
  Cretinism
  Weight Gain

Iron:

Deficiency associated with:

  Anemia (hypochromic, microcytic)
  Angular Stomatitis
  Anorexia
  Brittle Nails
  Confusion
  Constipation
  Depression
  Digestive Disturbances
  Dizziness
  Dysphagia
  Exertional Palpitations
  Fatigue
  Fragile Bones
  Growth Impairment
  Headaches
  Inflammed Tongue
  Irritability

Toxicity associated with:

  Anorexia
  Dizziness
  Fatigue
  Headaches

Lead:

Toxicity associated with:

  Abdominal Pain
  Anorexia
  Anxiety
  Constipation
  Fatigue

  Headaches
  Impaired Coordination
  Indigestion
  Irritability
  Malaise
  Muscle Pains
  Poor Concentration
  Poor Memory
  Restlessness
  Tremors

Magnesium:

Deficiency associated with:

  Anxiety
  Confusion
  Depression
  Hyperactivity
  Hypotension
  Hypothermia
  Insomnia
  Irritability
  Muscle Pains
  Muscle Tremors
  Nervousness
  Neuromuscular Irritability
  Organic Brain Syndrome
  Restlessness
  Seizures
  Sonophobia
  Tachycardia
  Weakness

Manganese:

Deficiency associated with:

  Ataxia
  Atherosclerosis
  Dizziness
  Glucose Intolerance
  Hearing Loss
  Hypercholesterolemia
  Muscle Weakness
  Pancreatic Damage
  Tinnitus

Toxicity associated with:

  Anorexia
  Impaired Judgement
  Parkinsonian-like Neurologic Disorder
  Poor Memory

Mercury:

Toxicity associated with:

Anemia
Anorexia
Ataxia
Colitis
Depression
Dizziness
Drowsiness
Emotional Instability
Erethism
Fatigue
Headaches
Hypertension
Impaired Coordination
Impaired Hearing
Impaired Vision
Insomnia
Irritability
Kidney Damage
Memory Impairment
Metallic Taste
Numbness
Paresthesias
Peripheral Neuritis
Psychosis
Stomatitis
Tremors
Weakness

Niacin:

Deficiency associated with:

Anorexia & Nausea
Canker Sores
Confusion
Depression
Dermatitis
     localized scaly, dark,
       pigmented lesions
Diarrhea
Emotional Lability
Fatigue
Halitosis
Headaches
Indigestion
Insomnia
Irritability
Limb Pains
Memory Impairment
Muscular Weakness
Skin Eruptions

Skin Inflammation

Pantothenic Acid:

Deficiency associated with:

Abdominal Pains
Alopecia
Burning Feet
Coordination Impairment
Depression
Eczema
Faintness
Fatigue
Hypotension
Infections
Insomnia
Irritability
Muscle Spasms
Nausea & Vomiting
Nervousness
Tachycardia
Weakness

Para Aminobenzoic Acid (PABA):

Deficiency associated with:

Constipation
Depression
Digestive Disorders
Fatigue
Greying Hair
Headaches
Irritability

Phosphorus:

Deficiency associated with:

Anorexia
Anxiety
Apprehension
Bone Pain
Fatigue
Irregular Breathing
Irritability
Numbness
Paresthesias
Tremulousness
Weakness
Weight Changes

Potassium:

Deficiency associated with:

Acne
Cognitive Impairment
Constipation
Depression
Edema
Fatigue
Glucose Intolerance
Growth Impairment
Hypercholesterolemia
Hyporeflexia
Hypotension
Insomnia
Muscle Weakness
Nervousness
Polydypsia
Proteinuria
Respiratory Distress
Salt Retention
Slow, Irregular Heartbeat
Xerosis

Toxicity associated with:

Cognitive Impairment
Dysarthria
Dysphasia
Weakness

Pyridoxine:

Deficiency associated with:

Acne
Alopecia
Anemia
Anorexia & Nausea
Arthritis
Cheilosis
Conjunctivitis
Depression
Dizziness
Facial Oiliness
Fatigue
Glossitis
Impaired Wound Healing
Irritability
Nervousness
Neurologic Symptoms
numbness
paresthesias
"electric shock" sensations

Seizures
Sleepiness
Stomatitis
Stunted Growth
Weakness

Riboflavin:

Deficiency associated with:

Alopecia
Blurred Vision
Cataracts
Cheilosis
depression
Dermatitis
dryness with
greasy scaling
Dizziness
Eyes Red, Itching, Burning
Glossitis
Growth Imapirment
Photophobia

Selenium:

Deficiency associated with:

Growth Impairment
Hypercholesterolemia
Pancreatic Insufficiency
Infections
Liver Impairment
Sterility (in males)

Toxicity associated with:

Alopecia
Arthritis
Atrophic, Brittle Nails
Diabetes Mellitus
Garlic Breath Odor
GI Disorders
Irritability
Kidney Impairmnt
Lassitude
Liver Impairment
Metallic Taste
Pallor
Skin Eruptions
Yellowish Skin

Sodium:

Deficiency associated with:

Abdominal Cramps
Anorexia, Nausea & Vomiting
Ataxia
Confusion
Depression
Dermatoses
Dizziness
Emotional Lability
Fatigue
Flatulence
Hallucinations
Headache
Hypotension
Illusions
Infections
Lethargy
Memory Impairment
Muscular Weakness
Seizures
Taste Impairment
Weight Loss

Toxicity associated with:

Anorexia
Cognitive Dysfunction
Congestive Heart Failure
Edema
Hyperactive Deep Tendon Reflexes
Hyperactiviy
Hypertension
Hypertonia
Irritability
Polydypsia
Polyuria
Renal Failure
Seizures
Tremors
Weight Gain

Thiamine:

Deficiency associated with:

Anorexia
Confusion
Constipation
Coordination Impairment
Depression
Digestive Disturbances
Fatigue

Irritability
Memory Loss
Muscle Atrophy
Nervousness
Numbness of Hands and Feet
Pain Sensitivity
Shortness of Breath
Sonophobia
Weakness

Vitamin A:

Deficiency associated with:

Acne
Anosmia
Dry Hair
Fatigue
Growth Impairment
Insomnia
Hyperkeratosis
Infections
Night Blindness
Weight Loss
Xeropthalmia
Xerosis

Toxicity associated with:

Abdominal Pain
Alopecia
Amenorrhea
Cheilosis
GI Disturbances
Hepatomegaly
Hydrocephalus
Irritability
joint Pain
Nausea & Vomiting
Pruritis
Splenomegaly
Weight Loss

Vitamin B$_{12}$:

Deficiency associated with:

Achlorhydria (pathogenetic)
Anemia (macrocytic)
Constipation
Depression
Dizziness
Fatigue
GI Disturbances
Glossitis

Headaches
Irritabiliy
Labored Breathing
Moodiness
Numbness
Palpitations
Psychosis
Spinal Cord Degeneration

Neuromuscular Impairment
   areflexia
   gait disturbance
   ophthalmoplegia
   diminished proprioception
   diminished vibratory sense
Shortened RBC Half-life

Vitamin C:

Deficiency associated with:

Bleeding Gums
Depression
Easy Bruising
Impaired Wound Healing
Irritability
Joint Pains
Loose Teeth
Malaise
Tiredness

Vitamin D:

Deficiency associated with:

Burning in Mouth & Throat
Diarrhea
Insomnia
Myopia
Nervousness
Osteomalacia
Rickets

Vitamin E:

Deficiency associated with:

Vitamin K:

Deficiency associated with:

Hemorrhaging

Zinc:

Deficiency associated with:

Acne
Alopecia
Amnesia
Anorexia
Apathy
Brittle Nails
Delayed Sexual Maturity
Depression
Eczema
Fatigue
Growth Impairment
Hypercholesterolemia
Hypogeusia
Impaired Wound Healing
Impotence
Irritability
Lethargy
Memory Impairment
Paranoia
Sterility
White Spots on Nails

INDEX